Fourth Edition

COMMUNICATION DISORDERS *in* MULTICULTURAL *and* INTERNATIONAL POPULATIONS

Dolores E. Battle, Ph.D.
Professor Emeritus of Speech-Language Pathology
Buffalo State College (State University of New York)
Buffalo, New York

With 16 Contributing Authors

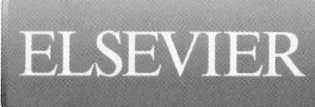

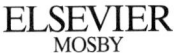

ELSEVIER
MOSBY

3251 Riverport Lane
St. Louis, Missouri 63043

COMMUNICATION DISORDERS IN MULTICULTURAL
AND INTERNATIONAL POPULATIONS

ISBN:978-0-323-06699-0

Copyright © 2012 by Mosby, an imprint of Elsevier Inc.
Copyright © 2002 by Butterworth-Heinemann, an imprint of Elsevier Inc.

Notices

Knowledge and best practice in this field are constantly changing. As new research and experience broaden our understanding, changes in research methods, professional practices, or medical treatment may become necessary.

Practitioners and researchers must always rely on their own experience and knowledge in evaluating and using any information, methods, compounds, or experiments described herein. In using such information or methods they should be mindful of their own safety and the safety of others, including parties for whom they have a professional responsibility.

With respect to any drug or pharmaceutical products identified, readers are advised to check the most current information provided (i) on procedures featured or (ii) by the manufacturer of each product to be administered, to verify the recommended dose or formula, the method and duration of administration, and contraindications. It is the responsibility of practitioners, relying on their own experience and knowledge of their patients, to make diagnoses, to determine dosages and the best treatment for each individual patient, and to take all appropriate safety precautions.

To the fullest extent of the law, neither the Publisher nor the authors, contributors, or editors, assume any liability for any injury and/or damage to persons or property as a matter of products liability, negligence or otherwise, or from any use or operation of any methods, products, instructions, or ideas contained in the material herein.

Library of Congress Cataloging-in-Publication Data or Control Number

Communication disorders in multicultural and international populations / [edited by] Dolores E. Battle ; with 16 contributing authors. — 4th ed.
    p. ; cm.
  Includes bibliographical references and index.
  ISBN 978-0-323-06699-0 (hardcover : alk. paper) 1. Communicative disorders—United States. 2. Transcultural medical care—United States. 3. Multiculturalism—United States. I. Battle, Dolores E.
  [DNLM: 1. Communication Disorders—ethnology. 2. Cultural Diversity. 3. Linguistics. 4. Speech-Language Pathology—methods. WL 340.2]
  RC423.C6425 2012
  616.85′5—dc23

2011021819

Vice President and Publisher: Linda Duncan
Executive Editor: Kathy Falk
Managing Editor: Jolynn Gower
Developmental Editor: Lindsay Westbrook
Publishing Services Manager: Hemamalini Rajendrababu
Project Manager: Anitha Sivaraj
Design Direction: Margaret Reid

Printed in United States of America

Last digit is the print number: 9 8 7 6 5 4 3 2 1

To my family, especially my husband Charles and my children Leslie and Clark, and to the many individuals with communication disabilities and their families, and the families of mankind that connect us all and remind us that effective communication is both a responsibility and a right for all.

Zenobia Bagli, Ph.D.
Audiologist
Gaithersburg, Maryland

Tachelle Banks, Ph.D.
Assistant Professor
Special Education
Cleveland State University
Cleveland, Ohio

Dolores E. Battle, Ph.D.
Professor Emeritus of Speech-Language Pathology
Buffalo State College (State University of New York)
Buffalo, New York

Mara Behlau, Ph.D.
Permanent Professor, Graduate Program in Human
Communicative Disorders
Universidade Federal de São Paulo–UNIFESP
(Federal University of São Paulo) and Centro de Estudos
da Voz-CEV (Center for Voice Studies)
São Paulo, Brazil

Li-Rong Lilly Cheng, Ph.D.
Professor
School of Speech, Language and Hearing Sciences
San Diego State University
San Diego, California

Priscilla Nellum Davis, Ph.D.
Professor
Communicative Disorders
The University of Alabama
Tuscaloosa, Alabama

Helen Grech, Ph.D.
Co-ordinator, Communication Therapy Division
Institute of Health Care
University of Malta, Malta

Ella Inglebret, Ph.D.
Associate Professor
Department of Speech and Hearing
Washington State University
Pullman, Washington

Hortencia Kayser
Director of EBS International
EBS Healthcare
St. Louis, Missouri

Sharynne McLeod, Ph.D.
Professor
Research Institute for Professional Practice, Learning
and Education (RIPPLE)
Charles Stuart University
Bathurst, New South Wales, Australia

Thomas Murry, Ph.D.
Professor of Speech Pathology and Supervisor of Speech
Therapy
Department of Otolaryngology–Neck Surgery
Weill-Cornell Medical College
Cornell University
Adjunct Professor of Biobehavioral Sciences
Teachers College
Columbia University
New York, New York

Constance Dean Qualls, Ph.D.
Chair and Professor of Speech-Language Pathology
State University of New York College at Buffalo
Buffalo, New York

Tommie L. Robinson, Jr., Ph.D.
Scottish Rite Center
Children's Hearing and Speech Center
Children's National Medical Center
Washington, D.C.

Carol Westby, Ph.D.
Bilingual Multicultural Services
Albuquerque, New Mexico

Freda Campbell-Wilson, Ph.D.
Head of Speech Language Pathology
King Faisal Specialty Hospital
Saudi Arabia

Toya Wyatt, Ph.D.
Professor
Department of Human Communication Studies
California State University Fullerton
Fullerton, California

When the first edition of this textbook was published in 1992, the United States and the world were different places than what they are today. We have all become more aware of the world around us. In the past 20 years, we have seen wars in faraway places, such as the Persian Gulf, Iraq, and Afghanistan, being broadcast into our living rooms. We have watched conflict as Bosnia and Herzegovina seceded from Yugoslavia and as Cairo and other nations in the Middle East and Northern Africa underwent political change. We have witnessed genocide in Rwanda and Somalia. The way we travel has been changed by threats of terrorism and the need for security screening at airports. And yet we celebrated global harmony in the Olympic Games in Beijing, Sidney, Calgary, and Vancouver.

The past two decades have also brought changes in health care as we know it. When the first edition of this textbook was published, AIDS and HIV were only whispered about. Dysphagia had only 1457 records on PubMed, as opposed to the 457,000 records today. The laws for ensuring nondiscrimination of children and adults with disabilities have become a part of our everyday lives with the ADA, NCLB, IDEIA, and RIT. Twenty years ago, cochlear implants and genetic mapping of the human genome were in their infancy. Technology, the Internet, online telepractice, and Skype have connected people around the world in ways well beyond our imagination in previous years. And Thomas L. Friedman wrote a book called *The World Is Flat* to bring to our awareness that we cannot think about the world today without thinking about how we are all related and intertwined.

International migration—people moving across national borders—has become one of the challenges and realities of the 21st century. More than 170 million people, about 3% of all humans alive today, live outside their country of birth, up from the estimated 120 million in 1990. If all the world's migrants were in one place, they would create the world's sixth most populous country (after China, India, the United States, Indonesia, and Brazil.) This international migration affects the people living in the major regions of the world, including North and South America, Europe, the Middle East, Asia, and Oceania. Approximately 95,000 people from non-U.S. countries arrive in the United States each day. Although most are nonimmigrant tourists, students, and temporary workers, about 3000 are immigrants or refugees who have been invited to the country to become permanent residents. Another 1000 or more are unauthorized immigrants who enter the country by evading border controls. Regardless of how these people have entered this country or other countries around the world, it is no longer appropriate to consider cultural diversity by historical racial and ethnic groups. More than 11% of residents of the

United States were born in another country. Nearly 96% of residents of the United States speak English well or very well, yet nearly 18% of residents older than 5 years speak a language other than English at home. According to the 2010 Census, although Spanish is by far the most common home language of residents, there are more than 150 languages spoken in the homes of residents.

The U.S. Census Bureau recognized the increasing diversity of the country by the realignment of racial and ethnic groups on the 2000 Census. The realignment recognizes that people are either Hispanic or non-Hispanic by ethnicity and that they may be of one or more racial groups: black or African American, white, Asian, American Indian, Alaskan Native, Native Hawaiian, or Pacific Islander. When one adds to this other dimensions of cultural diversity, such as religion, socioeconomic status, and geographic diversity, the complexity of culture affecting communication and communication disorders is far greater than race and ethnicity.

So, as we began to consider a textbook that would be more consistent with the view of the world that we live in today, it became obvious that the concept of multicultural populations had to be considered more broadly than race and ethnicity in the United States. This edition provides not only a view of communication disorders in the traditional racial and ethnic populations in the United States but also a broader view of populations around the world, including Central and South America, the indigenous peoples of the United States as well as those of Australia, the African diasporas including the peoples of the Caribbean nations, and peoples of Europe and the Middle East. The authors are themselves multicultural and international—they are white, black, Asian, Native American, and Hispanic and come from the United States, Brazil, Australia, Malta, Taiwan, and Saudi Arabia.

Hortencia Kayser looks at bilingual language development in Latino populations in the United States but also at the concepts of disability and development in Central and South America. *Carol Westby* and *Ella Inglebret* expand their presentation of Native Americans in America to include indigenous populations in Canada, Australia, and New Zealand. Recognizing that many of the children of persons who were new immigrants to this country at the time of the first edition of this book have assimilated to varying degrees and are now second- and even third-generation immigrants, *Li-Rong Lilly Cheng* traces the differences in language and concept of disability in first-, second-, and third-generation immigrants from Asian and Pacific Island countries. *Freda Campbell Wilson* discusses the challenges of providing service to persons from the Middle East, which has under gone significant political changes in the past 20 years. Because the immigration of persons from the African diasporas as well as the Caribbean nations has increased, particularly in the cities of the South and Northeast, the discussion of African American or black English is expanded to include consideration of persons from the African diasporas as well.

As in previous editions, the text contains several chapters that focus on specific disorders. *Sharynne McLeod* and *Helen Grech,* well known for their work in language development and international perspectives of phonologic disorders, provide a comprehensive overview of phonology, language, and literacy in English-speaking countries as well as of European languages. *Tom Murry* and *Mara Behlau* provide a comprehensive and innovative overview of cultural and linguistic aspects of voice and voice disorders based on data from countries around the world. *Tommie Robinson* looks at international cultural issues in identification and treatment of fluency disorders, particularly among persons from the African diasporas. *Constance D. Qualls* reviews issues involved in assessment and treatment when persons from culturally and linguistically diverse populations, including new immigrants, have neurologic impairments such as dysphagia.

Hearing impairment and hearing aids and rehabilitation services in developing countries have received worldwide attention through special projects of the World Health Organization and WWHearing. *Zenobia Bagli* provides a comprehensive international review of the advancements made in the identification and treatment of hearing impairments. In this edition, the ICF, IDEIA, NCLB, and RTI present new issues in providing assessment and intervention for children with communication impairments. *Toya Wyatt* approaches the complexities of assessment of communication disorders involving international multicultural clients and families. *Priscilla Davis* and *Tachelle Banks* focus on issues to be considered in providing intervention with culturally and linguistically diverse and international clients and families. The text concludes with a review of the issues to be considered in conducting and reading research on international populations.

This fourth edition of *Communication Disorders in Multicultural and International Populations* provides updated information as well as a new broad perspective of communication impairments in cultural and linguistic diversity around the world. Speech-language pathologists and audiologists providing clinical services will continue to serve growing numbers of clients from a variety of cultural and linguistic backgrounds. Increasing diversity in its many dimensions will shape traditional approaches to assessment and intervention. It is in this spirit that this edition of this textbook is offered.

Dolores E. Battle, Ph. D.
Editor

Contents

Cultural Diversity: Implications for Speech-Language Pathologists and Audiologists

Chapter 1

Communication Disorders in a Multicultural and Global Society

Dolores E. Battle

INTRODUCING A MULTICULTURAL AND GLOBAL SOCIETY

The term *culture* originated from the Latin *colere* meaning to cultivate or improve. Although the term originally referred to agriculture, in the 18th century when the diversity of persons around the world became globally apparent through increased European and world exploration, the term culture evolved to refer to the study of the full range of learned human behavior patterns and experiences. Sir Edward Burnett Tylor (1832-1917), considered the founder of modern anthropology and one of the first scholars to use the term culture in a universal or human sense, defined culture as "that *complex whole* which includes knowledge, belief, art, morals, law, custom, and any other capabilities and habits acquired by man as a member of society" (Tylor, 1871, p. 1). Culture is about the behavior, beliefs, and values of a group of people who are brought together by their commonality. More important, culture is the lens through which one perceives and interprets the world (Vecoli, 1995). It is the filter through which all that one does must pass before entering the collective conscience. Religion, language, customs, traditions, and values are but some of the components of culture. Anthropologists describe culture as a set of interacting systems that perpetuate certain practices and systems through generations. The practices may involve kinship systems, which may encompass mate choice, marriage customs, family relationships and obligations, and household composition, as well as nonkinship relations in various voluntary associations. Religions or belief systems, economic systems, and political systems extend relationships beyond the family and household.

A culture also includes language or communication systems. According to Durant (2010), language systems and speaking behaviors bind communities and shape social life and communication. They help form social identity and group membership and help to organize cultural beliefs and ideologies. All cultures have ways of communicating using a verbal language; classify people according to age and gender (e.g., woman, man, girl, boy) and descent relationships (e.g., wife, mother, uncle, cousin); raise children in some sort of family setting; and have leadership roles for the implementation of community and family decisions. Although all cultures have these and possibly many other universal traits, different cultures have developed their own specific ways of carrying out or expressing them. For instance, people in Deaf cultures frequently use their hands to communicate with sign language instead of verbal language. However, sign languages have grammatical rules just as verbal ones do.

Speech, language, and communication are embedded in culture. Edward T. Hall (1959) said, "Culture is communication. Communication is culture." Culture can be viewed as a system of competencies shared in broad design and deeper principles and varying among individuals. Its specificities are what an individual knows, believes, and thinks about his or her world. Culture is a theory of what one believes his or her fellows know, believe, and mean. It is more than a collection of symbols fit together by the analyst. It is a system of knowledge sharpened and constrained by the way the human brain acquires, organizes, and creates internal models of reality (Keesling, 1974). Culture provides a system of knowledge that allows people of a cultural group to know how to communicate with one another.

The relationship between communication and culture is reciprocal: culture and communication influence each other (Keesling, 1974). Therefore, one cannot understand communication by a group of individuals without a thorough understanding of the ethnographic and cultural factors related to communication in that group. These factors are intricately embedded in the historical, geographic, social, and political histories, which bind a group, give it a sense of *peoplehood,* and give it ethnic identity.

Because the roots of communication are embedded in culture, it is logical to assume that one cannot study communication or communication disorders without reference to the cultural, historical, or societal basis for the communication style or language used by the members of the ethnic or cultural group. The social rules of discourse and narratives (e.g., topic selection, who selects the topic, who initiates the conversation, who ends the conversation, distancing, eye gaze, and sense making) are culturally determined. Who speaks to whom, when, where, and about what must be understood in the context of the culture of both partners in the communicative event if the clinician is to determine the presence or absence of a communication disorder.

Communication behavior and the perception of what constitutes a communication disorder within a particular group are the products of cultural values, perceptions, attitudes, and history. These factors must be considered when determining the communication competence of a particular person within a group. For example, reluctance to speak and failure to initiate a conversation or use a particular narrative style can be appropriate to one culture but inappropriate to another. The impact of a voice disorder can be different for speakers of tonal languages than for speakers of nontonal languages. Expectations of the benefits of rehabilitation for the effects of stroke or traumatic brain injury can also differ across cultural groups.

Terminology

The terms *race* and *ethnicity* are often used interchangeably; however, they have different meanings. Ethnicity refers to a shared culture that forms the basis for a sense of peoplehood based on the consciousness of a common past. For example, Black is considered a race, but Hispanic is considered an ethnicity. Hispanics can be of any race. Race, language, and ancestral customs constitute the major expressions of ethnicity in the United States. Ethnicity is not passed genetically from generation to generation. Rather, ethnicity is constructed and reconstructed in response to particular historical circumstances and changes. In its most intimate form, an ethnic group can be based on face-to-face relationships and political realities that mobilize its members into political self-determination. Joined by the aspirations for political self-determination, ethnicity is used to identify groups or communities that are differentiated by religious, racial, or cultural characteristics and that possess a sense of peoplehood.

An ethnic group is a group of people whose members identify with each other, through a common heritage that is real or assumed, and share cultural characteristics. This shared heritage may be based on putative common ancestry, history, kinship, religion, language, shared territory, nationality, or physical appearance. Members of an ethnic group are conscious of belonging to an ethnic group; moreover, ethnic identity is further marked by the recognition from others of a group's distinctiveness.

Ethnography refers to the fully developed sense of the meaning of a culture and the complex manner in which one comes to understand the intricacies of the culture. The ethnographic understanding of a culture implies a fully developed sense of the complex web of meanings, perceptions, actions, symbols, and adaptations that make a people who they are.

Race refers to the biologic and anatomic attributes and functions, such as skin color, facial features, and hair texture. Two people can be of the same race but differ widely in cultural identity, personal history, and their view of the world. For example, a Korean child reared in a Korean family will have Korean cultural values; however, a transracially adopted Korean child adopted at birth by an African American family has the biologic and genetic characteristics attributed to his or her genetic ancestors but has the cultural values imparted by the adoptive parents.

The 2010 U.S. Census employed categories representing a social-political construct for the race or races that generally reflect a social definition of race recognized in this country. The concept of race took into account social and cultural characteristics as well as ancestry. The race categories included both racial and national-origin groups. The racial groups were identified as white, American Indian/Alaska Native, African American or black, Asian, and Native Hawaiian/other Pacific Islander. Persons were also given the option of identifying as "two or more races." Race and ethnicity were considered separate and distinct identities. Thus, in addition to their race or races, all respondents are categorized by membership in one of two ethnicities, which are "Hispanic or Latino" and "Not Hispanic or Latino." For example, an African American could be identified as "black (Not Hispanic)."

"Hispanic or Latino" was used to refer to "a person of Cuban, Mexican, Puerto Rican, South or Central American or other Spanish culture or origin regardless of race." The term does not refer to those who speak Spanish. For example, many people from the largest country in South America, Brazil, speak Portuguese. Persons in Spain are considered European and are not considered Hispanic. Many Hispanic persons prefer the use of the term *Latino* to refer to their origin in the countries of Central and South America. This distinguished them from persons who are identified only by the language that they speak. Although both terms are used, the term Latino is preferred.

Culture is a term that connotes the implicit and explicit behavior in a variety of areas. Explicit cultural behaviors are visible to the world and include observable features of dress, language, food preferences, customs, and lifestyle. Explicit behaviors are readily visible and are often used to identify the cultural group to observers. These behaviors are the focus of "culture-of-the-month" activities and programs. Implicit cultural variables are those factors that are not easily depicted and observed. They include such factors as age and gender roles within families, child-rearing practices, religious and spiritual beliefs, educational values, fears and attitudes, values and perceptions, and exposure to and adoption of other cultural norms. Implicit cultural values are beneath the surface, relatively invisible; however, they shape the fiber of those who identify as a member of a cultural group.

Multicultural

The term *multiculturalism* emerged in the 1960s in response to recognition of the varieties of racial and ethnic groups that were emerging as educational and political entities in English-speaking countries. It was at first used to refer to cultures by race and ethnicity, particularly blacks in the United States who were gaining political recognition in response to the civil rights movement. Because "culture" has many dimensions, the term *multicultural* is not to be restricted to describe only racial and ethnic minorities. The term has evolved to describe a society characterized by a diversity of cultures with varieties of religions, language, customs, traditions, and values. All individuals have a group identity and an individual identity. The term multicultural is used to describe a society in which people from diverse racial and ethnic backgrounds, socioeconomic groups, age groups, geographic areas, and other variables come together to create a mosaic composed of individuals that form a rich whole. It also includes the cultures defined by socioeconomic class, gender, sexual orientation, ability level versus disability, and other variables that define persons as individuals. The term is used to describe a society in which each individual is respected and valued for his or her contribution to the whole.

In addition to race and ethnicity, one may identify with the culture of deaf persons, persons with a disability, or with gay, lesbian, bisexual, or transgender culture. It is important to realize that the multicultural society is a diverse society of individuals who belong to many different cultural groups or subgroups. In sociology and anthropology, a *subculture* is a group of people with a culture (whether distinct or hidden) that differentiates them from the larger culture to which they belong. For example, Chinese Americans could be considered a subculture of Asian Americans; Cuban Americans could be a subculture of Hispanic or Latino Americans. Because of immigration, emigration, intermarriage, and geographic relocation, many persons identify with one or more cultures or subcultures. Consider a person who was born in Alabama to American parents: a father from Kuwait, Saudi Arabia, whose mother came from Isfahan, Iran; and a mother from Cleveland, Ohio, whose own mother came from a village in the mountains of Slovenia and whose father was a Serb immigrant from Zagreb, Croatia. The mother's family was Baptist, and father's family was Shi'a Muslim. In a sense, all persons are themselves multicultural. Each individual belongs to a unique set of cultures and subcultures that define who they are as individuals and which groups they identify with for a particular activity, practice, or belief.

Multicultural relationships also include the clinician and client and members of the client's family. All persons seeking clinical services are to be considered as individuals with individual cultural values and as belonging to one or more subcultures. All persons providing clinical services are also individuals with individual cultural values. The clinically competent clinician works to bring the persons in the clinical situation into harmony with each other so that the most appropriate clinical services can be provided.

Stereotype

A stereotype is a held popular belief about specific social groups or types of individuals. *Stereotyping* results from the overestimation of association between group membership and individual behavior (Gudykunst & Nishida, 1984). Stereotyping occurs when a person ascribes the collective characteristics associated with a particular group to every member of that group, discounting individual characteristics. Stereotypes can be negative or positive. For example, persons living in Africa may be thought of as living in huts in jungles; Latinos, as poor illegal immigrants; and Asians, as gifted in mathematics and science. Cultural competency requires that clinicians avoid developing stereotypes and keep the individual at the forefront of any clinical encounter.

An *immigrant* is a person who migrates to another country, usually for permanent residence. According to the United Nation's (2005) *World Population Policies Report,* by the end of 2005, the population of the immigrants that were born in a country and currently live in another country reached 191 million. Approximately 75% of international immigrants live in 28 countries, with 20% of the world's immigrants living in the United States. According to the report, in 2005 approximately 39% of immigrants had migrated to less developed or developing countries and 61% had migrated to developed countries of North America and Europe such as Canada, Russia, Germany, Ukraine, France, and Spain. Other countries leading in world immigration include Saudi Arabia, India, United Kingdom, Australia, and China.

BECOMING A MULTICULTURAL SOCIETY: HISTORY OF WORLD IMMIGRATION AND MIGRATION IMMIGRATION

Peoples have been moving about the world since the days of ancient Greeks, Phoenicians, and Romans who "colonized" uninhabited lands for farming, hunting, and gathering in Europe and Northern Africa. Modern colonialism started with the Age of Discovery in the 15th century when sailors from Spain and Portugal discovered new lands across the oceans in the Americas and sought trading routes to Asia. The main European countries that were successful in the Colonial Era were France, Spain, the United Kingdom, the Netherlands, and Portugal. Each of these countries had almost complete power in the world trade from roughly

1500 to 1800. The 17th century saw the creation of the British, French, Dutch, and Swedish colonial empires throughout the world, including the international slave trade in Europe, the Caribbean, and other parts of the world. In the 17th and 18th centuries, English colonists established the framework for the society that would become the United States. They built the colonies in Massachusetts and Virginia and overran the early colonies that had been established by the French and Spanish. The spread of European colonial empires was reduced in the late 18th and early 19th centuries by the American Revolutionary War and the Latin American wars for independence.

The diversity of America was established long before the colonial period. The original American Indians are said to have walked across a land bridge from Siberia thousands of years ago. In 1500, the more than 4.5 million inhabitants of America were divided into hundreds of tribes, each with distinctive cultures, religions, and languages (Vecoli, 1995). The country already was home to American Indians, Spanish, French, Mexican, and other groups who occupied the land that became the United States as the country expanded west. When the first U.S. census was taken in 1790, the United States was already a nation of many cultures. Almost 19% of Americans were of African ancestry; 12% were Scottish and Scotch-Irish; and fewer were German, French, Irish, Welsh, and Sephardic Jews (Vecoli, 1995). The census did not include American Indians or Hispanics.

To preserve the ideals on which the nation was founded, the Naturalization Act of 1790 was passed. It specified that citizenship in the United States was open to "any alien, being a free white person," thus excluding from citizenship of the country those who were not white and those who were enslaved. Those counted as citizens of the United States represented only 48% of the total population of the country. The term immigrant entered into the language to refer to a person who voluntarily moved from his or her own country to another established nation (Population Bulletin, 2003).

First Wave of Immigration: 1820-1880

Population growth in the United States, other than by natural increase, came primarily through three waves of immigration beginning in the 19th century. Between 1820 and 1860, more than 15 million immigrants arrived in the United States, including 4 million immigrants from Germany after the failure of social reform, 3 million each from Ireland and Britain as a result of the potato famine of 1847, and 1 million from Scandinavia who were seeking land available through the Homestead Act. During this period, there was the first major surge in immigration from Asia during the gold rush in the early 1850s and building the railroad. From the 1870s to the early 1880s, the number of persons from China increased from 63,000 to nearly 180,000. (Morrison & Zabusky, 1980; Vecoli, 1995).

By 1882, some Americans became concerned that the newcomers would pose a danger to "American" values and institutions. The slow evolution of a national policy on immigration resulted in a series of laws that progressively restricted immigration or reduced the rights of those who were new to the country (Morrison & Zabusky, 1980). For example, the Chinese Exclusion Act of 1882 denied immigration to Chinese laborers and barred Chinese from acquiring citizenship. As a result of these policies, the Chinese population in the United States had dropped to the 1870 levels.

Second Wave of Immigration: 1880-1920

The second wave of immigration began in 1880 with the beginning of the industrial revolution and ended with the beginning of World War I when 1.2 million immigrants arrived. Advances in transportation technology and the industrial revolutions enabled increasing numbers of people to set off for other parts of the world in search of a better life. This wave brought an additional 18 million immigrants to the United States, including more than 4 million from Italy, 3.6 million from Austria-Hungary, and 3 million from Russia (Vecoli, 1995). Overpopulation in Scandinavia, resulting unemployment, and a desire for freedom led to a significant increase in immigrants from Sweden and Norway, who often relocated to the states of the Midwest, especially Illinois, Minnesota, Michigan, Iowa, and Wisconsin.

In addition to the European immigration during this period, a large number of Asians, primarily from China and Japan, and persons from Greece and the Middle Eastern countries of Lebanon, Turkey, and Syria came. They had language, culture, social institutions, customs, and a collective experience that differed significantly from that of European immigrant groups. The concerns about the differences between Asians and Europeans culminated in the Immigration Acts of 1921 and 1924. These acts denied entry to aliens ineligible for citizenship (i.e., those who were not deemed white) and established national quota systems designed to reduce the number of Southern and Eastern Europeans entering the country and to bar Asians entirely. The laws attempted to freeze the biologic and ethnic identity of the American people by reducing the influence from those not like the early immigrants who had gained political and economic power in the country.

Immigration Pause 1920-1964

The time between 1920 and 1964 marked a hiatus in immigration due to restrictive immigration policies, economic depression, and the effects of two world wars. Immigration after World War II reflected political unrest in Europe and the Middle East. The postwar era brought a renewed interest in immigration to parts of the world. It was followed by a new surge of subsequent changes in laws and immigration policy.

After World War II, the need for migrant farm workers encouraged more than 1 million persons from Mexico to come to the United States. This has continued such that persons from Mexico have been the largest group of immigrants to the United States for the past 60 years. In addition, approximately 20,000 Russians and other displaced individuals immigrated to the United States immediately after World War II (Magocsi, 1995). By 1985, nearly 300,000 Russian Jews had reached the United States and settled in the major cities of the Northeast (Magocsi, 1995). Turkish, Croatian, and Serbian immigration also increased after World War II, including professionals such as engineers and physicians seeking better job opportunities.

Third Wave of Immigration: 1965 to Present

Abhorring the racism of Nazism and stirred by the valor that the Asian Americans and African Americans showed in the fight to protect the freedom of America during World War II and the Korean War, the nation changed the way it thought about race and equality. A combination of international politics and democratic idealism, including the Civil Rights Act of 1964, resulted in the elimination of racial restrictions from American immigration and naturalization policies. The Immigration and Nationality Act of 1965 removed the national origin quotas and opened the United States to immigration from throughout the world by regional quotas. The unexpected consequence of the 1965 Act was the beginning of the third wave of immigration. In 1965, an estimated 75 million people, or less than 3% of the world population, were living outside their country of birth. By 1985, that number had increased to 105 million. There were an estimated 214 million international migrants in the world in 2000, representing an increase of almost 40 million in the first decade of the 21st century and more than double the number of international migrants in 1980 (Hatton & Williamson, 2006; Kent & Mather, 2002).

The third wave of immigration in the United States differs from the previous two waves because the major countries of origin of the immigrants changed. Not only did the total number of immigrants increase steadily to 1 million or more arriving each year, but also the countries of origin changed from being primarily European countries to those of Asia and Latin America (Vecoli, 1995). During the first two waves of immigration, almost 90% of the immigrants originated from Europe. During the 1980s, however, only 12% of the 7.3 million immigrants to the United States originated from European countries.

In the post–Korean War era of the 1970s and the post–Vietnam War era of the early 1980s, there was a significant increase of people immigrating to the United States from the Southeast Asian countries and Pacific Islands, Asia, Central and South America, and the Caribbean. Nearly 85%

of the 7.6 million immigrants since the 1980s have come from Asia, Latin America, and Africa, with Mexico and China having the largest numbers of immigrants, respectively (U.S. Census Bureau, 1996). Between 1980 and 1990, the Hispanic population in the United States grew by 36% with major countries of origin being Mexico, Haiti, the Dominican Republic, and Cuba (U.S. Census Bureau, 1996). More than 2.7 million immigrants came to the United States from the Caribbean, and nearly 2 million came from Mexico alone in 2000 (U.S. Census Bureau, 2000). Between 1990 and 2010, the number of foreign-born residents in the United States increased from 20 million to 40 million while the entire U.S. population grew from 250 million to 310 million. Immigration contributed to a third of the U.S. population growth, and the U.S.-born children and grandchildren of immigrants contributed to nearly half of the entire U.S. population growth (Martin & Midgley, 2010).

The U.S. population increased by 9.7% between 2000 and 2010 (U.S. Census Bureau, 2011). As shown in Table 1-1, the growth in the white population was only 3.4%, whereas the growth in Hispanic population was 37.1% and that in the Asian populations was 36.6%. The growth in the U.S. population was largely due to significant increases in immigration of nonwhite racial and ethnic minority groups.

In addition to the documented legal immigrants to the United States, there are many undocumented or illegal immigrants. Immigration Services estimates that approximately 11.2 million illegal immigrants lived in the United States in 2010 (Passel, 2010). More than 6 million illegal immigrants were from Mexico and more than 1 million from Guatemala, Honduras, and El Salvador. However, many undocumented immigrants also have origins in Canada, Haiti, Poland, and the Philippines.

TABLE 1-1 Population Growth in the United States, 2000-2010

	2000	2010	Change (%)
White	194,552,774	307,006,550	+9.1
Black	34,658,190	39,641,060	+8.7
Hispanic	35,642,379	48,419,324	+37.1
American Indian/Native Alaskan	2,475,956	3,151,284	+32.3
Asian	10,687,312	14,013,954	+36.6
Native Hawaiian/other Pacific Islander	465,614	578,353	+25.0
TOTAL	282,172	307,007	+8.8

Adapted from U.S. Census Bureau (2011). *Statistical abstract of the United States* (122nd ed.). Washington, DC: Author.

The overwhelming majority of legal immigrants settled in California, New York, Texas, Washington, Illinois, Florida, Pennsylvania, Massachusetts, Georgia, and Michigan (U.S. Census Bureau, 2011). In addition to those illegally crossing the borders, a number of undocumented persons enter the country as students, tourists, or temporary workers and remain in the country after their visas have expired. For example, more than 250,000 Chinese intellectuals, scientists, and engineers came to the United States for advanced degrees and stayed after their visas expired or applied for alien resident status. The result of the dramatic increase in immigration is the diversity in the demographic makeup of America.

Global Migration

North America is the world's largest immigration destination. Nearly one-half million persons from Mexico migrate to the United States each year, about one third of whom are undocumented (Passel, 2004). In 2006, more than 11.5 million Mexican immigrants resided in the United States, accounting for 30.7% of all U.S. immigrants and one tenth of the entire population born in Mexico (Batalova, 2008). Canada and the United States include only 5% of the world's population, but they receive more than one half of the world's immigrant population. China, India, Pakistan, and the Philippines account for about 30% of all immigrants to Canada. The 15 independent Caribbean nations have some of the highest immigration rates in the world. Cuba, the Dominican Republic, Haiti, and Jamaica have sent large numbers of immigrants to the United States since 1980. Since 1996, 1.1 million of Colombia's 40 million people have left the country for the United States as well as for Ecuador, Australia, Canada, Spain, and Costa Rica. There are more than 2 million Colombians in Venezuela.

Brazil has been the largest recipient of immigrants in South America for many years. Early immigrants were slaves from Nigeria, Angola, and Benin who were brought to work in the sugar plantations in the northeast region of Salvador. Salvador Bahia remains the largest black city outside of Africa. In the early part of the 20th century, immigrants to Brazil were mostly from countries such as Italy, Germany, Spain, Portugal, and Poland to support farming and mining. After 1920, Brazil attracted more immigrants from Lebanon, Syria, and Japan. As a result, Brazil is a multiethnic country where 99% of the inhabitants speak Portuguese; however, approximately 210 other languages are spoken or signed by the inhabitants.

The movement of between 500,000 and 1 million persons a year in Europe during the 1990s has made migration a major social and political issue in many European countries. The four largest European countries—France, Germany, Italy, and the United Kingdom—include about 66% of European Union (EU) residents but received 88% of EU immigrants in 1995. In 1998, foreign workers made up 6% of the population of the counties in Western Europe (Organization for Economic Cooperation and Development [OECD], 2000). With immigration comes diversity of cultures and languages. In Germany, for example, although most persons learn English as a second language, immigrant languages spoken by sizable communities of first and second generation persons of Eastern European, African, Asian, and Latin American origins include Turkish, Russian, Arabic (by immigrants from Africa and the Middle East), Greek, Dutch, Italian, Polish, Serbo-Croatian (by persons from the former Yugoslavia), and Spanish. In France, as a result of immigration, a number of nonindigenous languages are spoken, including Arabic, Armenian (by recent immigrants arriving from Armenia, Azerbaijan, and Iran), Ababa, Berber, Cambodian, Chinese, Danish, and Dutch. In Asia, most migration is from one Asian country to another; however, many Asians have migrated not only to the United States and Canada but also to the Middle East Gulf nations seeking employment in the oil industry (OECD, 2000).

Although most immigrants leave their country of origin for reunification with their families or to seek a better life through employment of education, some leave their country of origin for fear of being persecuted for reasons of race, religion, nationality, or membership of a particular social group. They become refugees or asylees. The Middle East, which includes Western Asia and Northern Africa, has had major immigration to other parts of the world. Although it makes up only 6% of the world population, it accounts for 45% of the world's refugees, including 1.5 million Afghan refugees to Iran in 2000. The world's largest refugee population lives in Gaza, Jordan, and neighboring countries. In 2000, Africa had nearly one eighth of the world's population and nearly one third of the world's 12 million refugees. The refugees were fleeing domestic turmoil in places such as Rwanda, Somalia, and Darfur. As of December 31, 2005, the countries with the largest source of refugees were Afghanistan, Iraq, Myanmar, Sudan, and the Palestinian territories.

Canada resettles more than 1 in 10 of the world's refugees and is home to persons born in more 100 different countries around the world, with 10 groups having more than 200,000 residents each, including English, French, Scottish, Irish, German, Italian, Chinese, North American Indians, Ukraine, and Dutch (Statistics Canada, 2006). Although Canada is a bilingual country, with English spoken by 59.3% and French spoken by 23.2% of the residents, there are at least 87 other unofficial languages spoken in the country, including North American Indian, aboriginal, and hybrid languages (Lewis, 2009).

Because of colonization and global migration, there are more than 7000 languages spoken in the 196 countries in the world today (Lewis, 2009). The number of ethnic groups is largely unknown. In Asia, there are at least 71 ethnic groups, with 56 ethnic groups in China alone. In Africa, ethnic groups number in the hundreds, with at least

1500 languages and cultures. Australia is also multiethnic country. Although its inhabitants are largely descendants from England, Ireland, Scotland, Italy, Germany, and China, nearly one-half million (2.3%) are of aboriginal descent or from the Torres Strait Islands, and there are at least 40 different languages spoken in the country (Price, 1999).

It is clear that national and worldwide immigration patterns have led to a multiethnic and multicultural world.

ACCULTURATION AND ASSIMILATION

Models of Assimilation

Tens of millions of immigrants with differing cultures have been incorporated into societies around the world by the processes of acculturation and assimilation. *Acculturation* is the process by which newcomers assume the cultural attributes of the receiving country, including its language, cultural norms, behaviors, and values. *Assimilation* is the process of their incorporation into the social and cultural networks of the host society, including work, place of residence, leisure activities, and family. It refers to the process of giving up one's culture and taking on the characteristics of another. Primarily, three models of assimilation and acculturation have been used to explain cultural diversity in the United States. The models can be used to explain cultural diversity in any other country around the world.

Conformity Model

The conformity model of acculturation and assimilation has been favored through much of history. Convinced of their cultural and biologic superiority, early Americans passed laws restricting immigration and citizenship to persons from Western Europe. Nonwhite people were expected to abandon their distinctive cultural, religious, and linguistic values and practices and conform to the American model. Immigrants strove to adopt as much of the American culture as possible so that they could gain the economic and political benefits of being "American." The immigrants believed that the sooner they assimilated into the American culture, the sooner and more easily they could share in the riches of America. In their eagerness to become Americans, they rejected or altered family names and the languages and customs of the "old country" (Morrison & Zabusky, 1980).

Melting Pot Model

A competing model of acculturation and assimilation, the melting pot model is a process whereby, inasmuch as possible, the elements of culture brought by the immigrants are transmuted into a new American culture that embodies cultural variants. The result is an amalgam of the varied cultures and peoples in which no single culture is dominant and all blend into a rich whole. The melting pot ideology provided a rationale for the more liberal immigration policies in the late 1960s. The policy came under attack, however, as the determination of the ethnic groups to retain their individual identity, traditions, and customs increased.

Cultural-Pluralism Model

The cultural-pluralism model offered an alternative to the melting pot model of the 1990s. Cultural pluralism recognizes diversity within the nation. It has been viewed as an internal attitude that predisposes, but does not make compulsory, the display of ethnic identification in interactions. In the cultural-pluralism model, individual cultural identity is valued and accepted; individuals choose to maintain their ethnic identity. Although sharing a common American citizenship and loyalty, ethnic groups maintain and foster their particular languages, customs, and cultural values. They maintain those features of their home culture that identify them with their homeland. For example, although some black persons consider themselves to be black or African American, new immigrants may prefer to retain the identity of their homeland and be recognized for example, as Nigerian or Jamaican.

Levels of Adaptation and Assimilation

The independent variable in the process of acculturation and assimilation is the determination or willingness of the immigrants to assume the culture of America. The degree of adaptation and assimilation varies with each individual and with each group of immigrants. For example, the early immigrants in the first two waves of immigration, influenced by the immigration and naturalization policies of the time, made great efforts to acculturate and assimilate into the fabric of America. The level of assimilation is an important factor to consider in understanding clients and their families. Cheng and Butler (1993) describe six levels of adaptation and assimilation that affect culturally and linguistically diverse immigrants.

At the first level, *reaffirmation,* the people reject the new culture and attempt to maintain or revive native cultural traditions. Chain migrations and preferences in immigration policies allow relatives and friends to group for mutual assistance. They maintain their customary ways by establishing churches, societies, and newspapers and build institutions and communities that reflect and retain their cultural values and language.

At the second level, *synthesization,* people attempt to synthesize a selective combination of cultural aspects of both cultures. For example, they may accept the dress and food of the new culture but retain the native view of health care and education. Through selective assimilation and adaptation, immigrants take from the new culture what they need to survive and keep the traditional cultural beliefs and practices that they value. Although many may gradually adapt the parts of the new culture they chose, many hold dear the culture and language of their ancestors. Rather than shed old country customs, the new immigrants may enroll their children in "cultural schools." Cultural schools ensure that children do not forget the customs of the past.

Such schools allow children to adopt ancestral names and to continue speaking their native language in the home, thus ensuring that a culturally pluralistic country remains.

At the third level, *withdrawal,* people may reject and withdraw from their native culture or the new culture because of cultural conflict. People who reject their native culture become isolated from their cultural peers and do not maintain relationships with individuals other than immediate family members. People who withdraw from the new culture do not learn the language or culture of the new country. Depending on the level of assimilation, these people may experience loneliness and fear when attempts are made to engage in activities and associations to increase adaptation to the new culture.

People at the fourth level, *constructive-marginality,* tentatively accept the two cultures but do not fully integrate into either one. They may believe that they do not belong in either culture and may not be sure of which cultural rule or language to use in a situation.

The fifth level, *biculturalism,* refers to the full involvement of both cultures. Bicultural individuals retain fluency in the native language and obtain fluency in the new language. They are equally comfortable functioning in either culture and can switch between the cultures with relative ease.

At the *compensatory adaptation* level, people become thoroughly integrated into the new culture, rejecting and avoiding identification with the native culture and language. Young adolescents and young adults at this level reject any knowledge of the native country. They are anxious to learn the new language and cultural expectations as quickly and as thoroughly as possible. They may enroll in accent-reduction programs to remove any trace of their native language in their newly adopted language.

Barriers to Assimilation and Acculturation

There are several barriers to assimilation and acculturation, even for those who intend to be fully assimilated into the culture of the new country. Many immigrants experience only limited acculturation and practically no assimilation in their lifetimes. Among the factors that affect the process of acculturation and assimilation are circumstances of immigration, race and ethnicity, class, gender, and the character of community.

Voluntary immigrants, involuntary immigrants, refugees (or asylees) differ in their circumstances of immigration. Voluntary immigrants are usually prepared for the move,

psychologically motivated, and willing to accept the linguistic and cultural changes required to succeed in the new country. Involuntary immigrants, such as those brought to a country in slavery, may be resistant to their new circumstances and may suffer social and political isolation that hamper their attempts at assimilation. Refugees, on the other hand, are forced to leave their country because of adverse domestic, social, or political conditions. Preparation for the move is limited, and many enter the country without knowledge of the language or culture of the receiving country. Like involuntary immigrants, they may have been separated from their families and may have spent days or years in refugee camps before immigrating to the receiving country. As a result, the effects of culture shock are more pervasive on refugees than on voluntary immigrants. Many refugees are eager to assimilate into the receiving country; however, they may live in ethnic enclaves for longer periods of time and have limited access to learning the language and culture of the receiving country.

Vigdor (2008) conducted a major study of the rate of assimilation of immigrants to the United States over the past century. Rate of assimilation is difficult to define. As a measure of assimilation, Vigdor used characteristics that can distinguish immigrants from natives such as economic factors (employment, occupations, education, and home-ownership), cultural factors (ability to speak English, marriage to natives, number of children, and way of dressing), and civic engagement (naturalization, military service). He reported that most immigrants in America are adopting American ways just as quickly as they were in 1990 despite a doubling in their numbers; the rate of assimilation, however, varies with the country of origin. Some of the findings from Vigdor's research are as follows:

- Immigrants of the past quarter-century have assimilated more rapidly than their counterparts of a century ago, even though they are more distinct from the native population on arrival. Immigrants who arrived in the United States after 1995 are culturally assimilating more rapidly than their predecessors.
- Economic and civic assimilation often occurs without significant cultural assimilation.
- Immigrants from developed countries are not necessarily more assimilated than those from less developed countries. Immigrants from Vietnam, Cuba, and the Philippines enjoy some of the highest rates of assimilation. Mexican immigrants experience very low rates of economic and civic assimilation; however, they experience relatively normal rates of cultural assimilation.

Race, especially skin color, has been a dominant factor in barriers to assimilation and acculturation for Asians, Hispanics, African Americans, and Native Americans. Among the important factors limiting acculturation and assimilation is the willingness of the dominant culture to accept those perceived as different. Because it is relatively easy to identify those who differ from the mainstream, by race and skin color, it has been relatively more difficult for Africans and some Asians to assimilate into the American mainstream.

Other factors also affect acculturation and assimilation. Differences in religious practices—particularly those that require dress codes and religious observances that differ from the Christian mainstream and language—have been construed as barriers to assimilation and acculturation. Social class, dictated largely by economic factors, has also limited interactions among different ethnic groups and has limited assimilation and acculturation along class and ethnic lines. Traditional roles for women in various ethnic groups have restricted the acculturation and assimilation experience for some women.

The density of the population and the location of the immigrant communities influence the rate and character of incorporation of some immigrants into the mainstream culture. Most immigrants live in densely populated areas of California, Texas, New York, Florida, New Jersey, and Illinois (Fix & Zimmerman, 1993; U.S. Census Bureau, 2011). Concentration of immigrants in communities in urban cities of the Northeast and in isolated communities of the South and Midwest limits contact between immigrants and the mainstream population and inhibits the processes of acculturation and assimilation. It can be assumed that adults who remain at home or are employed within the community are more likely to hold customs, language, values, and beliefs of the country of origin than children who attend school or adults who are employed outside the community.

The children and grandchildren of immigrants retain fewer of the ancestral cultural values than their ancestors do. This is largely owing to attendance in public schools and the interaction with children from other cultures. The language of the home is often lost or does not keep pace with the growing language skills necessary for academic achievement. Although some second and third generation immigrants choose to abandon their ancestral customs and traditions, many retain a sense of identity and affiliation with their ethnic group through family and community ties.

The models for assimilation and acculturation have come into question in recent years. As the United States enters the 21st century, its future as an ethnically plural society is questioned. There is need for a new paradigm that encompasses the faith of all Americans by embracing them in their many diversities.

CULTURAL DIVERSITY IN A NEW AMERICA

The three waves of immigration, the adoption of the cultural-pluralism model, and the barriers to acculturation and assimilation have resulted in an America that is culturally and linguistically diverse. The 2010 U.S. Census report on ancestry identified more than 207 ancestral groups in response to the question, "What is your ancestry of ethnic origin?" (U.S. Census Bureau, 2011). The largest ancestral groups reported were, in order of magnitude, German, Irish, Italian, and the countries of the United Kingdom, including England, Ireland, Scotland, and Wales. However, there were 2.8 million persons reporting ancestry from sub-Saharan Africa, 1.8 million from other countries in Africa, 2.5 million from the West Indies, and 1.5 million from countries of the Middle East, including Egypt, Iraq, Jordan, and Morocco. The rich complexity of diversity in America is marked by the plethora of groups that reported fewer than 50 thousand members each, including Malta, Carpatho-Rusyns, Cyprus, Kenya, Uganda, Estonia, and New Zealand (U.S. Census Bureau, 2011) (Table 1-1).

Religious Diversity

The importance of religious diversity to the founding of the United States is shown in the guarantee of religious freedom in the First Amendment to the Constitution. Many early settlers from Europe came to the country in search of religious freedom. They were primarily Protestants of many denominations and sects and Roman Catholics. In addition, the Slavic Christian and Jewish immigrants from Central and Eastern Europe established Judaism and orthodoxy as major religious bodies. As a result of Middle East and African immigration, as well as the conversion of many African Americans, the number of persons who identify themselves as Muslim has doubled since 1990 to 1.18 million. Asian immigration has resulted in the number of persons identifying as Hindu and Buddhist doubling to more than 1 million each since 1990. In addition, there are several millions persons who practice as many as 60 other religions in the country (Barrett et al., 2001). Each religion has its own beliefs and practices that affect the identification of communication disorders and the delivery of services to those with communication disorders.

All cultural or ethnic groups have definable implicit characteristics in universal categories of behavior, including views toward education and health care. Many of these beliefs are embedded in religion. Health care in Western or European cultures is based on germ theory (i.e., the theory that a disease or disorder is caused by a germ or a physical malady within the body). To restore health, one must destroy the germ or repair malfunction of the body. For example, by the study of genetics, European medicine hopes to identify the gene related to certain disorders and, by controlling or altering the genetic structure, control the emergence of the disorder. Also, by attempting to identify a specific virus that causes a disease, scientists hope to develop vaccines to control or a medicine to cure the disease. If one can identify the germs or viruses causing or related to the disease, one can control the disease or bring about a cure. Those who hold this view of medicine are more likely to seek health care through medicine or rehabilitation (Stone, 2005).

Non-European and, often, Eastern views of health care see a connection between illness and internal forces.

People who have this point of view believe that health is the result of physical or spiritual harmony with nature and that illness and disease are the result of spiritual or internal disharmony. Eastern medicine and health care is intended to restore harmony. Those with this belief are more likely to seek relief through prayer, incantations, or religious ceremony than through medicine, rehabilitation, or therapy.

Other cultural groups see disease as the result of a specific punishment for an ill deed or religious failing. People with these beliefs are more likely to accept a disorder or illness as a burden that they are obligated to bear. These people do not usually seek assistance from a person who does not share their cultural beliefs (Stone, 2005).

Linguistic Diversity

Racial and ethnic diversity in the United States has also resulted in linguistic diversity. According to data from the 2010 census, more than 55 million persons, or nearly 20% of the population over 5 years of age, speak a language other than English at home. (U.S. Census Bureau, 2011). As shown in Table 1-2, more than 34 million people in the United States speak Spanish or Creole only at home. This represents 61% of all languages other than English spoken at home by persons 5 years of age and older. Other languages spoken by more than 1 million persons at home include Chinese, French (including Patois and Cajun), German, Tagalog, Vietnamese, and Italian. Many other languages are spoken by fewer than 1 million residents, including Arabic, African languages, Greek, Hindi, Persian, Persian, Urdu, and Gujarathi (U.S. Census Bureau, 2011). According to the U.S. Department of Education, National Center for Educational Statistics (2008-09a; 2008-09b), the percentage of students who speak a language other than English is higher among Hispanic and Asian elementary and secondary school students than among elementary and secondary students of other races and ethnicities.

According to the *American Community Survey* (2009), in addition to those who do not speak English at all, more

TABLE 1-2 Languages Spoken at Home by Language, 2008

Language	Number (1000)	Language	Number (1000)
Population 5 yr and older	283,150	Other Indic Languages	653
Speak only English	227,366	Other Indo-European Languages	447
Speak other Language	55,784	Chinese	2466
Spanish or Spanish Creole	34,559	Japanese	440
French (including Patois, Cajun)	1333	Korean	1052
French Creole	646	Mon-Khmer, Cambodian	183
Italian	782	Hmong	190
Portuguese or Portuguese Creole	661	Thai	141
German	1122	Laotian	147
Yiddish	169	Vietnamese	1225
Other West Germanic Languages	277	Other Asian Languages	705
Scandinavian Languages	134	Tagalog	1488
Greek	337	Other Pacific Island Languages	355
Russian	864	Navajo	171
Polish	620	Other Native North American Languages	193
Serbo-Croatian	274	Hungarian	94
Other Slavic Languages	332	Arabic	786
Armenian	231	Hebrew	213
Persian	379	African Languages	742
Gukarathi	333	Other and unspecified languages	126
Hindi	560		
Urdu	353		

From U.S. Census Bureau (2008). *American community survey, b16001: Language spoken at home by ability to speak English for the population 5 years and over.* Washington, DC: Author.

than 5.4% of Americans 5 years of age and older report that they speak English less than very well. In California, 19.9% of residents over the age of 5 years report that they speak English less than very well. This is followed by Texas (14%), New York (13.0%), Hawaii (11.8%), Florida (10.9%), Arizona (10.5%), New Mexico (10.2%), and Illinois (9.2%). Hispanic, Asian, Native Hawaiian/other Pacific Islanders, and American Indian/Native Alaskans had the highest percentages of those who spoke English with difficulty. Black and white students had the lowest percentages of those speaking English with difficulty.

COMMUNICATION DISORDERS IN A MULTICULTURAL SOCIETY

The need for speech-language pathologists and audiologists to understand communication disorders in a multicultural society was recognized soon after the passing of the Civil Rights Act in 1964. There was a growing concern that African American children who spoke African American English were being inappropriately classified as having speech-language disorders. Speech-language pathologists and sociolinguists began the study of communication disorders in multicultural populations in response to the need for understanding the linguistic skills of African American children in schools. In recognition of the growing concern, the American Speech-Language-Hearing Association (ASHA) adopted a position paper on social dialects (ASHA, 1983) that recognized that any dialect of English was a legitimate form of the language and that dialect was not to be considered a pathologic form of English.

Although initially the concern was for African Americans, the need to study cultural diversity in communication disorders grew in direct relationship to the third wave of U.S. immigration and the increase in the number of immigrants from non-European cultural origins. The new immigrants were also more diverse than before, arriving from a broad spectrum of countries encompassing a range of linguistic variables and a diversity of cultural backgrounds. Concerns about cultural and linguistic diversity that once were directed at African American children were directed to immigrants from Spanish-speaking and other non-English-speaking countries. In 1985, ASHA published *Clinical Management of Communicatively Handicapped Minority Language Populations* in recognition of the need to address the needs of those from various cultural and linguistic backgrounds in speech-language and hearing programs (ASHA, 1985).

Communication Disorders in Culturally Diverse Populations

General Demographics

The World Health Organization ([WHO] 2010) estimates that approximately 10% of the world's population or 650 million people around the world are living with disabilities. Of this total, 80% live in low-income countries; most are poor and have limited or no access to basic services, including rehabilitation facilities. The number is increasing owing to the rise of communicable diseases, injuries, falls, violence, and other causes, such as ageing, undernutrition, measles, traumatic brain injury from road crashes, falls, lands mines and blasts, cardiovascular disease, birth defects, mental illness, diabetes, tobacco, malaria, tuberculosis, HIV/AIDS, and maternal and neonatal morbidity (WHO, 2010).

There are no reliable data on the prevalence of speech impairment around the world. However, in 2005, the WHO reported that about 278 million people had moderate to profound hearing impairment; 80% of these individuals live in low and middle-income countries (WHO, 2005). The demography of disability is difficult because disability is not just a status condition, entirely contained within the individual, but is defined differently by various cultures. The WHO recognized the importance of the interaction among the medical condition, body structures and functions, and personal and environmental factors in relation to how a person participates in society. In 1992, the WHO adopted a strategy known as the International Classification of Functioning: Disability and Health (ICF) as a way of coding disability in the context of experiences of people in the environment and their personal resources, body structures, body function, health conditions, and interaction with the environment. Even with the ICF framework, the application of the framework in various countries impedes the compilation of reliable data on the prevalence of disability. Barbotte and associates (2001) reported a review of disability literature that gave disability rates from 3.6% to 66% and low quality of life from disability rates of 1.8% to 26%. Table 1-3 shows the prevalence of disability in selected countries from recent surveys and national surveys.

In the United States, Americans with disabilities constitute the third-largest minority group (after persons of Hispanic origin and African Americans); all three of those minority groups number in the 30-some millions in America. According to the U.S. Census Bureau (2011) disability statistics, 12.1% of noninstitutionalized males and females of all ages, all races, regardless of ethnicity, and with all education levels in the United States reported a disability in 2008.

There are few reliable data on the general incidence or prevalence of communication disorders among culturally and linguistically diverse populations in the United States. Estimates are based on projections from data founded on the general population. Provided that the prevalence of communication disorders among racial and ethnic minorities is consistent with that of the general population, ASHA estimates that 6.2 million, or 10%, of the U.S. population has a disorder of speech, hearing, or language unrelated to the ability to speak English as a native language (ASHA, 2011).

TABLE 1-3 Prevalence of Disability in Selected Countries by Source

Data from Censuses			Data from Surveys		
Country	Year	Percentage of Population with a Disability	Country	Year	Percentage of Population with a Disability
United States	2000	19.4	Australia	2000	20.0
Canada	2001	18.5	Jamaica	2000	15.6
Brazil	2000	14.5	Zambia	2006	13.1
Uganda	2001	3.5	Ecuador	2005	12.1
Mexico	2000	2.3	Nicaragua	2003	10.3
India	2001	2.1	Bangladesh	2000	8.3

Data from United Nations Statistics Division; IBGR (Brazil); INEC (Nicaragua); INEC (Ecuador); INEGI (Mexico); Census of India 2001; Robson, C. (2005). *Educating children with disabilities in developing countries: The role of data sets.* University of Huddersfield, OECD Section. Retrieved from http://siteresources.worldbank.org/DISABILITY/Resources/280658-1172610312075/EducatingChildRobson.pdf; and Barbotte, E., Guillemin, F., Chau, N., & the Lorhandicap Group (2001). Prevalence of impairments, disabilities, handicaps and quality of life in the general population: A review of recent literature. *Bulletin of the World Health Organization, 79* (11), 1047-1055.

Diversity among Children in Special Education

Reliable data on the number of children receiving special education around the world is scant. The difficulty in defining children with a disability in various countries and comparing that information with the number of children receiving regular education increases the problem. Jonsson and Wiman (2001) and Savolainen (2000) provide some information on school enrollment of children with disabilities in several developing countries. They estimate that between 1% and 3% percent of children with disabilities are enrolled in school in developing countries. For example, they report that in the Philippines, only 1.6% of the 3.5 million school-aged children with disabilities were actually enrolled in schools. In Mozambique, only 0.7% of children attending school were children with a disability. Likewise, in Ethiopia, the enrollment rate of children with disabilities was less than 1%. The World Bank (Filmer, 2005) reported the results of 11 national surveys on the education of persons with a disability, including speech, vision, hearing, and physical disabilities. Countries surveyed included Jamaica, Cambodia, Mozambique, Sierra Leone, Pakistan, Spain, and Burundi. The conclusions were that there were gaps of from 15% to 60% between the enrollment of students with a disability and those without a disability in these countries. For example, in Indonesia, 89% of the children aged 6 to 11 years without a disability were enrolled in school; however, only 29% of children with a disability were enrolled in school. Across the 11 surveys, the median gap between the school enrollment for those with a disability and those without was 26% for children aged 6 to 11 years and 31% for those aged 12 to 17 years. In Burundi, however, although there was an enrollment gap among the younger children, there was no gap in school attendance

for the children 12 to 17 years of age; 48% of students both with and without a disability were enrolled in school.

In the United States, since 1975, students with a disability have been guaranteed a free appropriate public education. The Individuals with Disabilities Education Improvement Act (IDEIA also know as IDEA) Amendments of 2004 required that the states report by race and ethnicity the number of preschool- and school-aged children served. Data were collected in five categories: American Indian, Asian/Pacific Islander, black (not Hispanic), Hispanic, and white (not Hispanic). In 2005, 33% of students enrolled in public elementary and secondary schools in the United States were from racial or ethnic minority groups (U.S. Department of Education, National Center for Education Statistics, 2008-09a; 2008-09b). There are disparities, however, in the number of children from racial and ethnic minority groups enrolled in special education under IDEA. The disparities in race and ethnicity distribution of the population of students served by IDEA and the general population of students are shown in Tables 1-4 and 1-5. American Indian/Native Alaskan and black (not Hispanic) children aged 6 to 21 years were nearly 50% (1.5) more likely to be served in IDEA Part B than students of the same age in all other racial and ethnic groups combined (American Indian/Native Alaskan [1.54] and black not Hispanic [1.47], respectively). Conversely, Asian/Pacific Island, white, and Hispanic students were less likely to be served under IDEA Part B than students of the same age in all of the groups combined. In addition, 43.9% of black students were being educated in a regular class, whereas 59.1% of white children were educated in a regular class (Fig. 1-1).

Reasons given for the disproportionate representation of African Americans and Hispanics in special education include (1) poverty, (2) cultural bias in referral and assessment, and (3) unique factors related to race and ethnicity.

TABLE 1-4 Race/Ethnicity of Preschool Children Ages 3 to 5 Years Receiving Special Education and of the General Preschool Population, Fall 2005

	General Population (%)	Special Education Population (%)
White (non-Hispanic)	63.3	64.42
Hispanic	17.2	16.70
Black (non-Hispanic)	15.8	14.55
Asian/Pacific Islander	4.2	3.00
American Indian/ Alaskan Native	0.9	1.34

Adapted from U.S. Office of Special Education Programs (2010). *Twenty-ninth annual report to Congress on the implementation of IDEA.* Washington, DC: U.S. Department of Education.

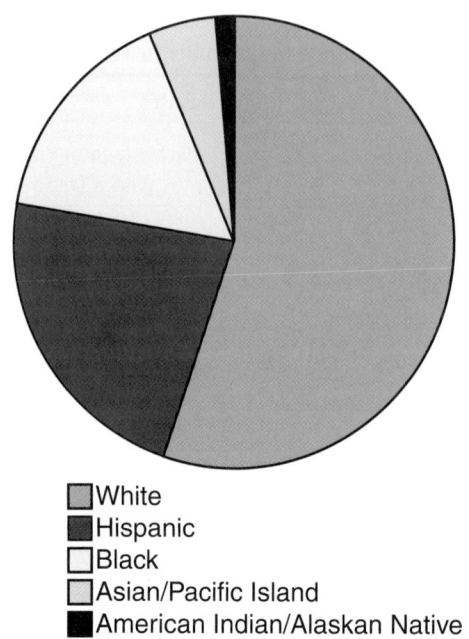

☐ White
■ Hispanic
☐ Black
☐ Asian/Pacific Island
■ American Indian/Alaskan Native

FIGURE 1-1 Public School Enrollment in the United States by race and ethnicity, 2008-2009. *From U.S. Department of Education, National Center for Education Statistics (2008-09b).* Common core of data (CCD): State nonfiscal survey of public elementary/secondary education, version 1a. *Washington, DC: Author.*

Reschly (1996) and Wagner and Blackorg (1996) implicate poverty and the lack of access to health care caused by poverty with resulting low birth weight as factors that affect a population's representation in special education programs. More than 30% of the children with disabilities lived in households in which the annual income (in 1986

TABLE 1-5 Percentage of Students Ages 6 to 21 Years Served by Disability and Race/Ethnicity in the 2005 School Year

Disability	American Indian/ Alaskan Native	Asian/Pacific Islander	Black (Non-Hispanic)	Hispanic	White (Non-Hispanic)
Specific learning disabilities	1.72	1.78	19.89	21.82	54.78
Speech-language impairment	1.32	3.05	15.32	17.78	62.44
Mental retardation	1.23	2.03	32.96	15.00	48.78
Emotional disturbance	1.52	1.15	28.75	10.93	57.65
Multiple disabilities	1.31	2.68	20.84	13.69	61.48
Hearing impairment	1.28	4.97	16.15	22.74	54.87
Orthopedic impairment	0.94	3.49	15.03	20.72	59.83
Other health impairment	1.19	1.50	16.99	10.03	70.29
Visual impairment	1.37	3.99	17.26	18.94	58.44
Autism	0.71	5.27	14.69	11.44	67.89
Deaf-blindness	1.57	5.09	12.56	21.29	59.48
Traumatic brain injury	1.44	2.48	17.01	12.97	66.10
Developmental delay	1.70	2.61	22.22	9.36	62.14
All disabilities	1.5	2.18	20.38	17.82	58.11
Resident population	1.0	3.8	14.8	14.2	66.2

Adapted from Office of Special Education Programs (2010). *Twenty-ninth annual report to Congress on the implementation of IDEA.* Washington, DC: U.S. Department of Education.

dollars) was less than $25,000 (Office of Special Education Programs, 2000). According to the U.S. Department of Health and Human Services (1985), economically disadvantaged children are more predisposed to disorders related to environmental, teratogenic, nutritional, and traumatic factors than other groups. For example, exposure to carbon monoxide and other chemicals and pesticides found in the air, paint, soil, and plumbing of older homes often located in poverty areas has teratogenic effects on the neurologic functions of young children.

The incidence of neurologic impairments, some of which lead to communication disorders, due to the absorption of lead has been found to be higher in nonwhite children than in white children (National Center for Health Statistics, 1994). In addition, although some people from ethnic minority communities have the same types of communication disorders as those in the dominant population, incidences, causes, and effects can be different, indicating different approaches to treatment. For example, stroke is among the three leading causes of death for people of all races and ethnicities, except for American Indian/Alaskan Native males; however, the risk for having a stroke varies. Compared with whites, African Americans have nearly twice the risk for a first stroke. Hispanic Americans' risk falls between the two. Moreover, African Americans and Hispanics are 50% more likely to die after a stroke than are whites (Heron et al., 2009; Lloyd-Jones et al., 2009). Asian Americans tend to have better health, lower mortality, and longer life expectance than other racial ethnic groups, including whites. The racial and ethnic disparities and mortality are largely attributable to group differences in socioeconomic factors such as education, environment, employment, occupation and occupational hazards, and living conditions as well as access to health care.

Access to Health Care

Access to health care and health insurance is a critical issue for the immigrant population in the United States. Few immigrants come to the United States in search of health care. Rather, they are usually in search of employment and improved living conditions. However, there are a number for factors that limit their access to health care. The U.S. health care system is difficult to navigate, particularly when one has limited ability to speak English or to communicate concerns to health care providers. Cultural beliefs and practices may differ for new immigrants. In the home country, for example, health care may be confined to the treatment of disease rather than prevention or early detection through screenings. Because they are more likely to be employed in low-income occupations, they may not have access to employer-sponsored health care. According to a report by the Kaiser Commission (2008), 78% of U.S. citizens had health insurance, but only 22% of immigrants had health insurance. Those who do not speak English are more likely

to be uninsured than those who do. This is particularly true among Hispanics and persons from Korea and Southeast Asia who may not speak English. Immigrants from China, Japan, the Philippines, and southern Asia are more likely to have access to health care through employer-sponsored health care systems (Kaiser, 2008). Undocumented immigrants do not have access to federally sponsored health care programs such as Medicaid or Medicare and are thus not likely to seek the services of health care professionals until health situations are in their later stages. Lack of access to health care affects the physical and mental well-being of families as well as the ability to adapt to the culture of the United States.

For many immigrants, especially children, the immigration process is an event of extraordinary stress. Immigrants are often torn by conflicting social and cultural demands while trying to adapt to an unfamiliar and sometimes hostile and discriminatory environment with limited or no use of the English language. In addition, undocumented immigrants deal with the stress or fear of deportation and separation from family members.

For some immigrants, health worsens in the United States. A study of aggregate data across all immigrant groups found that on virtually every measure of health status, immigrants who had lived in the United States 5 years or less were healthier than those who had lived in the United States more than 10 years (Rumbaut, 1995; Portes & Rumbaut, 2006; New York City Health Department, 2006). The findings were explained by a number of factors, including (1) existing physical conditions that were masked during the early years after immigration, (2) deterioration of health due to limited access to health care, and (3) socioeconomic factors such as exposure to environmental pollutants. The data point to the importance of identifying conditions under which immigrants do well and those that produce negative health outcomes. Among the factors to consider are family networks and social supports, relationships within families, the effect of mobility on children's lives, segmented assimilation into different kinds of contexts, and cultural medical practices from the country of origin.

Rumbaut (1995) and Portes and Rumbaut (2006) found that generation effects and length-of-residence effects have confirmed associations between these variables and health. For example, difficult pregnancies, low birth weight, and infant mortality increased among Hispanic populations with subsequent immigrant generations in the United States. In contrast, Indochinese immigrants in San Diego County who appeared to be at risk for poor infant health due to high levels of unemployment, poverty, welfare dependence, and depression were found to have much lower infant mortality rates than the average resident in San Diego County. This was explained by the nearly universal absence of tobacco, alcohol, and drug abuse among Indochinese women, even though they had less access to prenatal care.

BECOMING A CULTURALLY COMPETENT CLINICIAN

Understanding another culture is a continuous, not discrete, process. Identifying the sources of cultural conflict while providing clinical services to those from cultures different from one's own involves far more than learning about the implicit and explicit variables of a culture. It is important for speech-language pathologists and audiologists to understand the importance of potential sources of cultural conflict in the clinic.

Monocultural assumptions in providing clinical services are not currently relevant. Most literature on communication disorders, intervention, and treatment in multicultural populations assumes that the clinician is a member of the majority culture and that the client is a member of a minority culture. This is a logical conclusion because fewer than 7% of the members of the ASHA identify themselves as nonwhite (ASHA, 2009). It is more accurate to take a broad view of the use of the term *multicultural* or *cross-cultural clinical services*. The clinician and the client may differ by culture, racial and ethnic group, sex, age, socioeconomic class, gender, or religion, to name but a few cultural variables that can affect the clinical interaction. The clinician must look to the various parameters of differences, as well as those of similarity, and construct the clinical management program accordingly. Clinicians realize that they must understand their own culture and cultural assumptions as well as those of the client. Whether there is a cultural conflict must be considered in the interaction. The culturally competent clinician seeks continuous self-assessment regarding cultural differences. The clinician needs knowledge and resources to be competent to provide clinical services in an increasingly culturally diverse world.

As stated in the ASHA Issues in Ethics statement, *Cultural Competence* (2005):

In addition, beliefs and values unique to that individual clinician-client encounter must be understood, protected, and respected. Care must be taken not to make assumptions about individuals based upon their particular culture, ethnicity, language, or life experiences that could lead to misdiagnosis or improper treatment of the client/patient. Providers must enter into the relationship with awareness, knowledge, and skills about their own culture and cultural biases. To best address the unique, individual characteristics and cultural background of clients and their families, providers should be prepared to be open and flexible in the selection, administration, and interpretation of diagnostic and/or treatment regimens. When cultural or linguistic differences may negatively influence outcomes, referral to, or collaboration with, others with the needed knowledge, skill, and/or experience is indicated.

In becoming a culturally competent clinician, it is important to consider culture-bound variables and language-communication-bound variables. Culture-bound conceptualizations have many variables. Among the most important variables in studying communication disorders in the multicultural society is the importance of individuals and groups in the culture, power and distance, time orientation, and several dimensions of verbal and nonverbal communication.

Individualism and Collectivism

Individualism emphasizes independence of the individual. Individuals from cultures of collectivism look after the needs of the entire group as the fundamental unit of concern in their social network. In collectivism, on the other hand, group goals have precedence over individual goals. Individuals from individualistic cultures are supposed to look after themselves and their immediate family. Although individualism and collectivism exist in every culture in varying degrees, cultures in which individualism tends to predominate include but are not limited to the European countries. Cultures in which collectivism tends to predominate include but are not limited to Arab, African, Asian, and Hispanic cultures (Brislin, 1994). Individualism and collectivism play an important role in clinical encounters. These factors affect the client's willingness to establish individual goals and expectations for the individual or the family or group.

The Power-Distance Variable

The power-distance variable focuses on the social relationships between people of different statuses (i.e., superiors and subordinates). This can extend to relationships between men and women. People from high power-distance cultures do not question the orders or suggestions of superiors. On the other hand, people in low power-distance cultures do not necessarily accept superiors' orders. When the clinician and the client are from two different systems, misunderstanding in making and following clinical recommendations is possible.

Time Orientation

Time orientation differs across cultures. When the culture is long-term and future oriented, the establishing of long-term goals and priorities is highly valued. When the focus of the culture is on the past, the establishment of long-term goals is not as relevant as preserving the present and the establishment of short-term, more readily attainable goals. Western cultures are more often oriented toward the future. Many non-Western cultures are focused on the past, as shown by their respect for elders and ancestors.

Nonverbal and Verbal Communication Styles

Language and communication styles are highly correlated with race, culture, and ethnicity. All ethnic groups have communication styles that have major implications for clinical services. These language differences have verbal and nonverbal dimensions.

Nonverbal Communication

In nonverbal communication, information is transmitted by means other than words. This can involve many behaviors, including proxemics, kinesics, eye contact, paralanguage, silence, and directness. Proxemics, or the use of personal space and conversational distance in communication, differs across cultures. Kinesics, or the use of body movements (e.g., facial expressions, smiling, head positioning and nodding, hand shaking, and eye contact), has also been shown to differ across cultures (Battle, 1997). In addition, paralanguage variables such as silence, loudness, inflection, and stress vary across cultures and can affect the clinical relationship.

Verbal Communication

Verbal communication can also vary across cultures. In addition to the barriers created by differences in the linguistic contrasts between the languages of the client and the clinician, differences in word meanings can affect the clinical encounter. The meanings of words such as *bad* or *normal* can vary across cultures. Pragmatics, or the way language is used in greeting, taking compliments, and more ritualized social rules, can affect the clinical encounter. Social distance can also affect the role that the individuals play in the communication process. In Western cultures, conversation tends to be horizontal, with each person in the communication event having equal responsibility and freedom within the conversation. In non-Western cultures, patterns of communication tend to be vertical, with conversation flowing from those of higher prestige to those of lower prestige (Battle, 1997; Sue & Sue, 1990).

CONCLUSION

Culturally competent care requires a commitment to understand and be responsive to the different communication styles, language, and verbal and nonverbal clues, as well as attitudes and values, of all clients and families served. In becoming a culturally competent clinician, it is important that clinicians develop an awareness of their own beliefs as well as the attitudes held by the clients. Multicultural awareness is not an end in itself. It is, rather, a means of increasing a clinician's power, energy, and freedom of choice in a multicultural world (Lynch & Hanson, 2006; Pedersen, 1988). Clinicians need to become culturally aware of their own values and beliefs before they can adjust to the value system of others. Clinicians should understand and value the differences that exist among clients and should develop an awareness of the cultural, verbal, and nonverbal factors that influence the clinical situation. In developing a cultural awareness, the clinician should ask,

"What can I do to serve this client in a culturally appropriate manner?" and "How can I best serve this client according to his or her cultural, as well as clinical, needs?"

Clinicians must develop an understanding of the sociopolitical systems operating in the United States and around the world and of the sociopolitical history experienced by the client. This knowledge helps the clinician appreciate the institutional and historical barriers that affect the client as a member of a particular group. This knowledge can also help the clinician understand the client's response to treatment and interaction in the clinical situation.

Finally, clinicians in a multicultural society must develop skills in interacting with clients from a variety of cultures with myriad cultural and linguistic variables, none of which is the same for different clients (Lynch & Hanson, 2006). Clinicians should be able to send and receive verbal and nonverbal messages appropriately in each culturally different context.

DISCUSSION QUESTIONS

1. Discuss the issues recent immigrants may have in accessing speech language services in the United States. What issues would an American have in accessing services in a sub-Saharan African country? How available are speech-language services in the developed and developing countries? How can effective speech-language and hearing services be provided to people in least developed countries

2. Mrs. A is a 35-year-old woman from Colombia who was admitted to the hospital following a visit to the emergency room with a suspected cerebrovascular accident. She was found to have right hemiparesis, high blood pressure, high cholesterol, oral motor and limb apraxia, and evidence of nonfluent aphasia. She could not communicate verbally or nonverbally and could not walk. The speech-language pathologist was called in for a consult. What factors should the pathologist consider to deliver culturally competent services to the client?

3. Discuss the problems encountered by the plethora of languages spoken in the United States and why this issue is so controversial. Should the United States adopt an English-only policy?

4. Discuss the education that speech-language pathologists should receive in order to provide effective service to clients who speak languages other than English.

REFERENCES

American Community Survey (2009). Washington, DC: U.S. Census Bureau.

American Speech-Language-Hearing Association (1983). Social dialects: A position paper. *ASHA, 25*(1), 23-24.

American Speech-Language-Hearing Association (1985). Clinical management of communicatively handicapped minority language populations. *ASHA, 26*(1), 55-57.

American Speech-Language-Hearing Association (2005). *Cultural competence* [Issues in Ethics]. Retrieved from http://www.asha.org/policy.

American Speech Language Hearing Association (ASHA) (2009). *2000 Membership survey summary report.* Rockville, MD: Author.

American Speech Language Hearing Association (ASHA) (2011). *Communication facts: Focus on culturally and linguistically diverse populations* (2008 ed.). Rockville, MD: Author. Retrieved from http://www.asha.org/research/reports/multicultural.htm.

Barbotte, E., Guillemin, F., Chau, N., & the Lorhandicap Group (2001). Prevalence of impairments, disabilities, handicaps and quality of life in the general population: A review of recent literature. *Bulletin of the World Health Organization, 79*(11), 1047-1055.

Barrett, D., Kurian, G. T., & Johnson, T. M. (2001). *World Christian encyclopedia: A comparative survey of churches and religions* (AD 30-AD 220). London: Oxford University Press.

Batalova, J. (2008). *Mexican immigrants to the U.S.* Migration Information Source. Washington, DC: Migration Policy Institute.

Battle, D. (1997). Multicultural considerations in counseling communicatively disordered persons and their families. In T. Crowe (Ed.), *Applications of counseling in speech-language pathology and audiology* (pp. 118-144). Baltimore: Williams & Wilkins.

Brislin, R. W. (1994). *Intercultural training: An introduction.* Thousand Oaks, CA: Sage.

Cheng, L., & Butler, K. (1993, March). *Difficult discourse: Designing connections to deflect language impairment.* Paper presented at the annual meeting of the California Speech-Language-Hearing Association, Palm Springs, CA.

Durant, A. (2010). Linguistic anthropology. In N. Smelsen & P. B. Baltes (Eds.), *International encyclopedia of social and behavioral science* (pp. 8905-8907), Burlington, MA: Elsevier Ltd.

Filmer, D. (2005). *Disability, poverty & schooling in developing countries: Results from 11 household surveys.* Washington, DC: World Bank.

Fix, M., & Zimmerman, W. (1993). *Educating immigrant children.* Washington, DC: Urban Institute.

Gudykunst, W. B., & Nishida, T. (1984). Individual and cultural influences on understanding reduction. *Communication Monographs, 51,* 23-26.

Hall, E. T. (1959). *The silent language.* New York: Doubleday.

Hatton, T., & Williamson, J. (2006). *Global migration and the world economy: Two centuries of policy and performance.* Cambridge, MA: MIT Press.

Heron, M., Hoyert, D., Murphy, S., Jiaquan, X., Kochanek, K., & Tejada-Vera, B. (2009). Deaths: Final data for 2006. *National Vital Statistics Report, 57*(14).

Jonsson, T., & Wiman, R. (2001). *Education, poverty and disability in developing countries: A technical note prepared for the Poverty Reduction Sourcebook.* Washington, DC: World Bank.

Kaiser Commission (2008). *Health status and health services access and use among U.S. immigrant families.* Washington, DC: Kaiser Commission.

Keesling, R. (1974). Theories of culture. *Annual Review of Anthropology, 3,* 73-97.

Kent, M., & Mather, M. (2002). What drives U.S. population growth? *Population Bulletins,* 1-26.

Lewis, M. P. (Ed.) (2009). *Ethnologue: Languages of the world* (16th ed.). Dallas: SIL International. Retrieved from http://www.ethnologue.com/.

Lloyd-Jones, D., Adams, R., & Carnethon, M. (2009). *Heart disease and stroke statistics: 2009.* Update. A report from the American Heart Association Statistics Committee and Stroke Statistics Subcommittee. *Circulation, 1*(19), e21-e181.

Lynch, E. W., & Hanson, M. J. (Eds.) (2006). *Developing cross-cultural competence: A guide for working with young children and their families* (3rd ed.). Baltimore: Brookes.

Magocsi, P. R. (1995). Russian Americans. In J. Galens, A. Sheets, & R. V. Young (Eds.), *Gale encyclopedia of multicultural America* (pp. 1159-1170). New York: Gale Research.

Martin, P. & Midgley, E. (2003). Immigration: Shaping and Reshaping America. *Population Bulletin 58*(2). Washington, DC: Population Reference Bureau.

Martin, P. & Midgley, E. (2010). Immigration: Shaping and Reshaping America 2010. *Population Bulletin.* Washington. DC: Population Reference Bureau.

Morrison, J., & Zabusky, C. F. (1980). *American mosaic: The immigrant experience in the words of those who lived it.* New York: E. P. Dutton.

National Center for Health Statistics (1994). *Healthy United States, 1993.* Hyattsville, MD: Public Health Service.

New York City Health Department (2006). *Health of immigrants in New York City.* New York: New York City Department of Health & Mental Health.

Office of Special Education Programs (2010). Twenty-Ninth Annual Report to Congress on the Implementation of the Individuals with Disabilities Education Act, Parts B and C. 2007. Washington, DC: Office of Special Education and Rehabilitation Services.

Organization for Economic Cooperation and Development (OECD) (2000). *Database on immigrants in OECD and non OECD countries.* Paris: Author.

Passel, J. S. (2004). *Mexican immigrants in the U.S.: The latest estimates.* Migration Information Source. Washington, DC: Migration Policy Institute.

Passel, J. S. (2010). *Unauthorized immigrant population: National and state trends, 2010.* Washington, DC: Pew Hispanic Center

Pedersen, P. (1988). *A handbook for developing multicultural awareness.* Alexandria, VA: American Association for Counseling and Development.

Portes, A., & Rumbaut, R. (2006). *Immigrant America* (3rd ed.). Berkeley, CA: University of California Press.

Price, C. (1999). Australian population: Ethnic origins. *People and Places, 7*(4), 12-16.

Reschly, D. J. (1996). Identification and assessment of students with disabilities. In *The future of children: Special education for children with disabilities* (vol. 6) (pp. 40-53). Los Angeles: The Center for the Future of Children, The David and Lucille Packard Foundation.

Rumbaut, R. G. (1995). A legacy of war: Refugees from Vietnam, Laos, and Cambodia. In S. Pedraza & R. G. Rumbault (Eds.), *Origins and destinies: Immigration, race, and ethnicity in America* (pp. 583-621). Belmont, CA: Wadsworth.

Savolainen, H., Kokkola, H., & Alasuutari, H. (2001) (Eds.). *Making inclusive education a reality.* Ministry of Foreign Affairs. Helsinki: Niilo Maki Institute.

Statistics Canada (2006). *2006 Community profiles.* Retrieved February 11, 2011 from http://www.statcan.gc.ca.

Stone, J. H. (Ed.) (2005). *Culture and disability: Providing culturally competent services.* Thousand Oaks, CA: Sage.

Sue, D. W., & Sue, D. (1990). *Counseling the culturally different.* New York: Wiley.

Tylor, E. B. (1871). *Primitive culture.* London: J. Murray. Reissues 1958 New York: Harper & Row; 2010: New York: Cambridge University Press.

United Nations Department of Economic and Social Affairs (2005). *World population policies.* New York: Author.

U.S. Census Bureau (1990). *Statistical abstract of the United States* (116th ed.). Washington, DC: U.S. Bureau of the Census.

U.S. Census Bureau (2000). *Statistical abstract of the United States* (120th ed.). Washington, DC: U.S. Bureau of the Census.

U.S. Census Bureau (2008). *American community survey, b16001: Language spoken at home by ability to speak English for the population 5 years and over.* Washington, DC: Author.

U.S. Census Bureau (2011). Statistical Abstract of the United States: 2011 (130th ed.). Washington, DC, 2010. Retrieved from www.census.gov/statab/www/.

U.S. Department of Education, National Center for Education Statistics (2008-09a). *Common core of data (CCD): Public elementary/secondary school universe survey, version 1a; and Local education agency universe survey, version 1a.* Washington, DC: Author.

U.S. Department of Education, National Center for Education Statistics (2008-09b). *Common core of data (CCD): State nonfiscal survey of public elementary/secondary education, version 1a.* Washington, DC: Author.

U.S. Department of Health and Human Services (1985). *Report on the secretary's task force on black and minority health (Vol. 1).* Executive Summary (Pub. No. 491-313/44706) Washington, DC: Department of Health and Human Service.

Vecoli, R. J. (1995). Introduction. In J. Galens, A. Sheets, & R. V. Young (Eds.), *Gale encyclopedia of multicultural America* (pp. xxi-xxvii). New York: Gale Research. Vigdor, J. (2008, May). *Measuring immigrant assimilation in the United States: Civic report 53.* New York: Manhattan Institute.

Wagner, M., & Blackorg, J. (1996). Transition from high school to work or college: How special education students fare. In R. E. Behrman (Ed.), *The future of children: Special education for children with disabilities* (vol. 6) (pp. 103-120). Los Angeles: The Center for the Future of Children, The David and Lucille Packard Foundation.

World Health Organization (2005). *Deafness and hearing impairment fact sheet.* Geneva: Author. Retrieved February 11, 2011, from. www.who.int/mediacentre/factsheets/fs300/en/index.html.

World Health Statistics (2010). World Health Organization Statistical Information System (WHOSIS). Geneva: World Health Organization. Retrieved from www.who.int/whosis/en/.

RESOURCES

American Speech Language Hearing Association. Self assessment for cultural competence. Available at http://www.asha.org/practice/multicultural/self.htm.

ADVANCING EFFECTIVE COMMUNICATION, CULTURAL COMPETENCE, AND PATIENT- AND FAMILY-CENTERED CARE: A ROADMAP FOR HOSPITALS

A resource to help health care professionals learn to communicate with patients regardless of cultural or linguistic differences, sensory impairments, or limitations on ability to communicate with natural speech. Available at http://www.jointcommission.org/Advancing_Effective_Communication/.

GLOBALIZATION 101

Globalization 101 is dedicated to providing information and interdisciplinary learning opportunities on this complex phenomenon. The goal is to challenge you to think about many of the controversies surrounding globalization and to promote an understanding of the trade-offs and dilemmas facing policy-makers. The site covers teaching tools, lesson plans, videos, and in-depth resources on areas such as culture, languages, education, health, religions, and other areas of importance to study of globalization. Available at http://globalization101.org.

WORLD REPORT ON DISABILITY

The World Report on Disability is a major publication from the World Health Organization and World Bank, launched in June 2011. The Report explores current evidence about disability, identifies needs, and highlights what works to improve the lives of people with disabilities in areas including health, rehabilitation, support, environments, education, and employment. The playlist includes the four World Report promotional films on the theme of "What's disability to me?" together with other films that share the human rights emphasis of our disability work. Available at http://www.who.int/disabilities/world_report/en/index.html

Chapter 2

The Cultures of African American and Other Blacks around the World

Dolores E. Battle

A BRIEF HISTORY OF AFRICANS IN THE AMERICAS

The African diaspora includes people of African origin living outside the countries of Africa. The term has been applied to the descendants of the approximately 21 million black Africans who were shipped throughout the world between 1500 and 1900, primarily to the Americas, by way of the transatlantic African slave trade. In the Caribbean, 73% of all residents are descendants of Africa. In South America, 26.6% of the residents are descendants of Africa; in North America, 8.4%; in Europe, 1.2%; and in Asia and Oceania, less than 1%. The largest population of members of the African diaspora is in Brazil, followed by the United States, Colombia, and the Caribbean Islands of Haiti, Dominican Republic, and Jamaica. It also includes blacks in France, Venezuela, the United Kingdom, Cuba, Italy, Peru, Canada, Ecuador, Trinidad and Tobago, and Nicaragua (World FactBook, 2010). Through intermarriage between blacks and nonblacks and their descendants, many persons with African roots have contributed to multiethnic communities throughout the world. In addition, emigration from areas because of warfare and social disruption has further contributed to the worldwide spread of persons from the African countries.

The history of people of African descent in the Americas can be traced to the largest involuntary migration movement in modern times. From the 16th to the 19th centuries, nearly 40 million people from the countries of West Africa were forced to leave their homelands and were sold into slavery. More than 20 million Africans were brought to the Western hemisphere, including the countries of Central and South America, the Caribbean, and North America.

As many as 80% of the inhabitants of the Caribbean countries of Jamaica, Haiti, the Dominican Republic, the Bahamas, and Barbados descended from countries in West Africa. Although they share the common history of slavery, they took on the cultural roots of the British Empire, Spain, France, and the Dutch, which controlled the area during the period of slavery. The British influence remains in the area and can be seen in the customs, models of education, and language and dialects used in the countries once dominated by the British Empire. Many of those in the Caribbean countries speak a dialect of English. Some speak Spanish, such as in Cuba and the Dominican Republic. In Haiti, because of the control of the island by the French, the people speak a Creole of French that is in large part based on French.

The Caribbean descendants of Africa and new African immigrants share a common genealogic root with African Americans, but the history and experiences of the Africans who were brought to the United States in slavery is different (Terrazas, 2009). This distinction is necessary as speech-language pathologists and audiologists come to understand the cultural parameters associated with service delivery to African Americans. It is important to understand that the material that follows cannot be applied uniformly to those in America who appear to have an African heritage. It is important that speech-language pathologists and audiologists identify the ancestral root of the client to determine the specific psychological, cultural, and linguistic variables that affect service delivery to that client.

Persons in the United States who trace their ancestral roots to the North American slave trade are generally considered African Americans. They are culturally and linguistically different from those who trace their roots to the more recent immigrants from the Caribbean islands or the continent of Africa.

Much research about persons of African roots presents them as a homogeneous social group that is different and deficient from mainstream groups. They have diverse social systems, different histories, and different cultures. They differ across many variables, including religion, socioeconomic status, education, use of language, child-rearing practices, and health care beliefs. They share many biologic traits and patterns. The key to understanding members of each group is to recognize the commonalities that they share as well as the differences that are unique to each. Understanding persons from the African diaspora requires understanding the important social constructs that underlie and mask differences and similarities between groups and that affect communication as well as communication disorders. Because of their numbers in the United States, this chapter focuses on African Americans, with the caution that all persons who present as black may not share the cultural or linguistic background of those identified as descendants of the American slaves.

AFRICAN AMERICANS

Hispanics, or Latinos, are the largest ethnic minority group in the United States. African Americans, or blacks, are currently the largest racial minority group in the United States (U.S. Census, 2010). According to the 2011 U.S. Census, 39.9 million persons, or 12.3% of the U.S. population, identify their race as black alone, whereas 42 million identify themselves as black and at least one other race (U.S. Census Bureau, 2011). The census also counted 2.2 million persons who identified themselves as both Hispanic by ethnicity and black by race. The blacks in the United States are largely descendants from West Africa. The history of slavery of Africans in America has involved not only economic conditions but also sociocultural and psychological factors that influence speech and language. Additionally, the vestiges of slavery in the United States have resulted in disparities in the delivery of health care among African Americans, including delivery of speech-language, audiology, and related health care services. This chapter focuses on several of these variables that are important for clinical assessment, intervention, and general access to health care and speech and hearing services.

Black persons of African descent came to the United States by one of three routes: as slaves primarily from West Africa in the 17th and 18th centuries, as immigrants from the Caribbean primarily in the mid to late 20th century, or as immigrants from sub-Saharan Africa in the later part of the 20th century. Nearly 600,000 blacks in America came to the country from the West Indies or Caribbean, including those from Haiti, Barbados, Jamaica, and other areas of the non-Hispanic Caribbean and Central America. More than 1.4 million blacks in the United States were born in Africa. Although the descendants of slaves who have been in this country for many generations prefer to refer to themselves as African Americans, persons from the Caribbean and Africa prefer to refer to themselves by their country of origin, such as Haitian, Cuban, Jamaican, or Nigerian. The groups share some cultural values based on their roots in Africa but also have cultural values that are unique to their individual group or family.

THE AFRICAN AMERICAN FAMILY

Many African Americans came to this country in the 17th an 18th centuries as slaves to support the agriculture programs in the southern part of this country. To understand the structure of the African American family, it is important to understand the importance of the extended families in Africa out of which the black families evolved. In the indigenous societies in Africa, families lived in clusters, villages, or compounds on commonly owned land or living areas. The clusters of cross-residential patterns of the family provided important financial and other support for rearing children and caring for the elderly. The individual family had responsibility for providing financial and nurturing support for the children. The community had a role in socializing and caring for the children of the community.

When the Africans were separated from their families in the transatlantic slave trade, the indigenous family unit was broken; however, the tradition of the family unit continued. The slaves cared for each other and the children without regard for the sanguinity of the family. Although both younger men and women worked in the fields or in the home of the slave owner, the young children were nurtured and socialized by the older women or older children. The child's mother had primary responsibility for child rearing and development; however, all members of the community, particularly the elders, shared the responsibility for social development. Although the slaves were not allowed to marry, the clusters of families formed strong kinship bonds that went beyond blood or legal relationships. The extended family became a sociologic unit consisting of relatives, nonrelatives, and others or fictive kinships who provided support for the members of the family. These bonds continued even though the families were often separated when members of the family were "sold" or were moved to other plantations. Thus, the African American child usually developed a strong sense of social responsibility from his or her earliest years and learned to be respectful, responsible, and supportive member the extended family (Arinze, 1986).

Continuing the historical cross-residential patterns from indigenous Africa, the extended family in African American society includes a kinship web of relatives and nonrelatives who provide social and financial support to the family. The formation of a household often begins with the birth of a child. Children occupy a central place and are raised in a close family group. In the African traditional family, the kin or extended family system includes several generations of elders in addition to stepfamily members, cousins, uncles, aunts, and other relatives living close to one another to form the family. These nonkin or fictive relationships include individuals who consider each other de facto family, including unmarried partners, close family members, foster parents or children, and boyfriends. Young single parents often reside with or near other relatives who provide co-parenting support for the mother and family or in intergenerational families that include the child, the parent and grandparents or great-grand parents (McAdoo, 2007; Simpson, 2008).

HEALTH

According to the National Center for Health Statistics (2011) and Stone (2005), African Americans experience disparities in disease, injury, and disability. According to Ross, (2006), African Americans have the highest rate of severe disability of all racial groups (Ross, 2006). Rates of disability are disproportionate in terms of gender. Women represent more than half of persons with disabilities. African American women (21.7) are second to Hispanic women (21.8) in disability rate. African American women have more multiple disabling conditions. The prevalence of disability among persons reporting as black (24.3%) on the U.S. Census (2000) is higher than those reporting as non-Hispanic whites (18.3%). Also according to the U.S. Census, the higher prevalence was found across all age groups. Among children (ages 5 to 15 years), the rate of disability was 7.0% for African Americans, compared with 5.6% for whites. Among working-aged African Americans (ages 16 to 64 years), 26.4% reported as disabled, compared with 16.8% of whites. Finally, among older adults (ages 65 and older), the rate of disability was 52.8% among African Americans, compared with 40.6% among whites.

Several diseases that are particularly related to speech, language, and hearing disorders have higher prevalence among African Americans than the rest of the population. These diseases include HIV/AIDS, sickle cell disease, stroke, and lead poisoning.

HIV/AIDS

According to the Centers for Disease Controls and prevention (2010), by race and ethnicity, African Americans have a disproportionate rate of HIV/AIDS in the United States. At the end of 2007, blacks accounted for nearly half of all people living with a diagnosis of HIV infection. New HIV infections among blacks have been stable since the early 1990s compared with persons from other races and ethnicities, but blacks continue to account for a higher proportion of cases of all stages of HIV from new infections to deaths.

Sub-Saharan Africa is more heavily affected by HIV/AIDS than any other region of the world. An estimated 22.5 million people are living with HIV in the region—about two thirds of the global total. In 2009, about 1.3 million people died from AIDS in sub-Saharan Africa, and 1.8 million people became infected with HIV. Since the beginning of the epidemic, 14.8 million children have lost one or both parents to HIV/AIDS (United Nations, 2010; World Health Organization, 2004).

HIV/AIDS is related to several types of communication disorders because of opportunistic infections, neurologic complications from the disease, or HIV drugs and drug interactions. The most commonly reported disorders include aphasia, apraxia, dysarthrias, dysphagia, voice disorders,

stuttering, and hearing loss (Zuniga, 2010). The National Institutes of Health (NIH) estimate that as many as 75% of adults with AIDS experience auditory dysfunction as a result of infections or treatment with ototoxic drugs. The more common causes of auditory impairment in the HIV population are otitis media and nasopharyngeal polyps and subcutaneous cysts, which can block the eustachian tubes (American Speech-Language Hearing Association [ASHA], 2011; McNeilly, 2005).

Sickle Cell Anemia

Sickle cell disease, also referred to as *sickle cell anemia*, is a genetic disorder that affects a number of racial groups, but it primarily occurs among persons of African ancestry. According to the Sickle Cell Disease Association of America (2005), the disease originated in at least four places in Africa and in the Indian/Saudi Arabian subcontinent. It exists in all countries of Africa and in areas where Africans have migrated. It is most common in West and Central Africa, where as many as 25% have sickle cell trait and about 1% to 2% of children are born with the disease. In Nigeria, with an estimated population of 90 million, 45,000 to 90,000 babies are born with sickle cell disease each year. In the United States, with a population of more than 270 million, approximately 1000 children are born each year with sickle cell disease. Sickle cell anemia occurs in approximately 1 in 375 live births of African American children. About 1 in 10 African American infants have the sickle cell trait (Davis et al., 2001).

Sickle cell disease results in a misshapen sickle shape to the normally round red blood cells. The clumping of these cells in the veins and capillaries results in blockages in vital organs of the body, producing pain and, in some instances, stroke with resulting aphasia. The clumping can also occur within the stria vascularis, resulting in sensorineural hearing loss that can become progressively permanent with successive sickle cell crises. (See Chapter 12 for a more comprehensive discussion of sickle cell disease and hearing loss.)

In addition to stroke and hearing loss, sickle cell disease may affect speech and language development. Children with sickle cell disease often experience severe pain and anemia. The anemia occurs because the spleen destroys the abnormal, sickled red blood cells faster than the body can produce new cells. Because red blood cells carry oxygen within the body, the activity of the spleen causes a deficiency in the number of these cells, resulting in anemia and accompanying fatigue. Children who are affected by pain and fatigue may not be able to concentrate on their work in school or may have a short attention span.

Stroke

African Americans are 50% more likely to have a stroke, also referred to as *cerebrovascular accident,* than other racial groups. Survivors are at greater risk for long-term complications and disability compared with whites and are less likely to receive rehabilitation for a stroke than whites (Balcazar et al., 2010). More frequent consumption of food that is high in saturated fat and cholesterol may be a factor in increased rates of high blood pressure and heart disease, which may contribute to a high occurrence of stroke with accompanying aphasia among African American populations. There is evidence that there are disparities in the availability and use of rehabilitation services by African Americans compared with whites (Kosoko-Lasaki et al., 2009). Because of decreased access to health care and cultural beliefs of caring for one's own, African Americans do not receive rehabilitation for aphasia and other results of stoke at the same rates as other racial groups. Those that do begin treatment may not continue. The treatment termination rate among African Americans is nearly double that of whites. Higher termination rates of African American clients may result from perceptions of culturally inappropriate intervention, insensitivity to the needs of the client and family, and suspicion of racial discrimination (Balcazar et al., 2010; Sue & Sue, 1990).

Lead Poisoning

Lead poisoning primarily affects children 1 to 11 years of age who live in older homes and neighborhoods in which lead can be ingested. Children who reside in homes with lead pipes and lead-based paint and in neighborhoods that surround lead-smelting factories (that may or may not have been dismantled) are of particular risk for lead poisoning when they ingest food and liquids prepared with water from lead pipes, eat chips of lead paint, play in soil contaminated with lead from factories, and breathe lead-contaminated dust particles. Because these homes and neighborhoods are primarily urban and socioeconomically low income, lead poisoning is an issue potentially affecting anyone who resides in areas in which lead is present and is not strictly an African American issue.

According to the U.S. Department of Health and Human Services (2000), there is no safe level of lead. However, the Health Department considers lead poisoning to have occurred when the blood lead level (BLL) in a person is greater than 10 μg per dL of blood. This is commonly referred to simply as "10." As the BLL rises, the potential for serious developmental problems increases. A BLL above 70 could result in seizure, profound disability, or death. Children who are 1 to 2 years of age are at greatest risk for lead poisoning because of their propensity to put anything into their mouths. These young children, owing to their developing nervous systems, also have an increased susceptibility to the adverse effects of lead (Needleman & Bellinger, 1991).

Lead is a toxic substance that can damage the nervous, circulatory, respiratory, and reproductive systems. In adults, lead poisoning can result in fatigue, memory loss, loss of appetite, headaches, dizziness, and other symptoms. In children, lead poisoning can cause learning disabilities, lowered intelligence quotients or mental retardation, poor attention span, or other neurologic deficits. Speech, language, and reading deficits such as auditory processing difficulties and delayed speech development are also potential effects of lead poisoning among children (Campbell et al., 1995; Pueschels et al., 1996).

AFRICAN AMERICAN ENGLISH

The most prominent linguistic system associated with African Americans is known as *African American English* (AAE) (also known as black English, African American vernacular, or ebonics). AAE is a dialect of *general American English* (GAE). It is a language used by many but not all African Americans. Although it has its roots in the language used by individuals and their descendants brought to the United States through the transatlantic slave trade in the 17th and 18th centuries, AAE cannot be traced to a single ancestral language in Africa or elsewhere (Stockman, 2007). It is not to be confused with the language of blacks who came to the United States more recently from Africa or from other countries, such as the Caribbean, who use the language and dialect of their home language and are not considered to be users of AAE.

The study of AAE has been a focal point of study of cultural and linguistic variables among African Americans since the 1970s in the attempt to understand the social and cultural ramifications of AAE speakers, many of whom were attending integrated schools for the first time as a result of the Civil Rights movement (Smitherman, 1977; Stockman & Vaughn, 1986; Williams & Wolfram, 1976). ASHA adopted a position paper on social dialects (1983) in response to the concern that the use of AAE was a speech disorder that required intervention. The position paper established that AAE is a first language in the homes of many African Americans and is not a disorder. Early study of AAE focused on describing differences between the language systems of mainstream English speakers and the systems used by speakers of African American English, which resulted in AAE being identified as a deficit form of English. More recent approaches have been to describe the differences between GAE and AAE, with a focus on those elements that are contrastive and noncontrastive (Stockman, 2010).

A number of linguistic dialects are spoken among African Americans in the United States. Gullah is spoken by those living on islands off the coasts of South Carolina and Georgia. There are also various dialects spoken by people who immigrated to the United States from the Caribbean and the sub-Saharan African countries. Because African Americans had been generally regarded as homogeneous, there has been little distinction in the use of dialect by Africans according to social class, geographic location, and other factors. In addition, until recently, there has been little research on the development of AAE in oral language or in written language and literacy.

AAE is a systematic, rule-governed, phonological, grammatical, syntactic, semantic, and pragmatic system of language. Although AAE is different from GAE, it maintains enough similarity to GAE to be considered a dialect of American English, not a separate language. It includes not only the verbal spoken word but also nonverbal factors, such as body language, use of personal space, body movement, eye contact, narrative sequence, and modes of discourse. AAE patterns are not exclusive to the dialect because it contains features that are shared by other social and regional dialects, such as Southern English.

Although largely spoken by African Americans, African Americans are not the only people who use AAE. Depending on the level and type of socialization with AAE speakers, some white individuals, Hispanics/Latinos, and Asians use AAE. Within the United States, the density of use of AAE varies from one speaker to the next. Its use is on a continuum that ranges from speakers who do not use the dialect at all to those who use most AAE features in all communicative contexts (Burns et al., 2010; Wyatt, 1991). Age, geographic location, occupation, income, and education are a few factors that have been found to influence the level of use of AAE among speakers (Connor, 2002; Craig & Washington, 2006; Horton-Ikard & Miller, 2004; Labov, 1966; Wyatt, 1991). The use of AAE by children also differs by age, grade in school (with younger children using more features than older children), and gender. Young boys use more AAE features than young girls. Children from lower-income homes use more features than children from middle-income families. In addition, the density of use of features of AAE varies with the communication context, the extent to which the speaker has had experiences with persons who use AAE, and the communication partner. Furthermore, the extent to which a person identifies with the culture of the speech community has been found to influence the use of the dialect (Terrell & Terrell, 1981). Individual speakers can also vary their use of the dialect along the continuum, switching codes depending on the communicative context and communication partner (Washington & Craig, 1998).

Linguistic Features of African American English

AAE is a linguistic system and, as such, contains grammatical, phonosyntactic, semantic, and pragmatic components (Bloom & Lahey, 1978; Lahey, 1988). It is important to consider AAE as more than a list of features but instead as a system that must be viewed in a holistic manner and that is subject to development, particularly in young speakers (Burns & Weddington, 2010; Charity, 2008). Williams and Wolfram (1976) made the first comprehension description of the features of AAE which is the basis of much of the material that follows.

Phonology

The phonology speakers of AAE has been studied less frequently than other areas of AAE even though the use of AAE phonology can identify speakers of AAE, particularly among preschool and school-aged young children (Stockman, 1996a). Despite the numerous representations of the phonology of AAE as different from that of GAE, the inventory of phonemes in AAE is very similar to the inventory in GAE (Pearson et al., 2009). Stockman (1996a, 2006, 2008) observed that typically developing 3-year-old children using AAE accurately produced 15 initial singleton consonants and word-initial clusters of the stop + sonorant type in their conversational speech.

Many of the phonological features of AAE are shared by other dialects of American English, especially Southern American English, including the merger of the vowels /e/ and /i/ before nasals, such that "pen" and "pin" and "ten" and "tin" are pronounced the same. The vowels /iy/ /i/, and /e/ merge before /l/ such that "feel and "fill" and "fail and "fell" are pronounced the same. (Every vowel in GAE is present in AAE except for three phonemic diphthongs: /ar/, /au/, and /ɪ/.)

Every consonant in GAE also occurs in AAE. However, the consonants may be acquired in different orders by children speaking primarily AAE and those speaking primarily GAE. For example, the phoneme /ð/ is often absent in the initial position of words. It is often realized as /d/ such as "dat" for "that," and as /d/ or /v/ in medial and final positions. Recent research has shown that even typically developing children learning AAE have not mastered the use of "th" /ð/ in the initial position by the age of 12 years (Pearson et al., 2009). The researchers have questioned whether voiced "th" /ð/ is actually a phoneme in AAE because the "th" /ð/ is used so infrequently in AAE (Pearson et al., 2009; Stockman, 2006).

The voiceless "th" /θ/ may have a different developmental status in AAE than its voiced counterpart. The voiceless "th" /θ/ is often realized as /t/ or /f/; however, /θ/ is realized as /θ/ in the initial position of words (Green, 2002; Stockman, 1996a, 2006). Velleman, Pearson, and Zurer (2010) found that the phoneme was mastered by age 6 years by typically developing children who use AAE and by age 10 years by AAE-speaking children with speech sound disorders. Also, children whose use AAE as a first language often produce /s/ accurately at an earlier age than do children learning GAE only, whether or not they are typically developing or have a speech sound disorder, even in the final position (Pearson et al., 2009; Velleman & Pearson, 2010)

In addition to similarities in the phonetic inventory, AAE and GAE use the same rules for combining phonemes into words. They have the same consonant clusters in initial word position with few exceptions. The cluster /θ/ is reduced to /r/, /ʃr/ is reduced to /sr/, and /str/ is changed to /skr/. However, because the final position is used infrequently in AAE, children learning AAE generally master use of final consonants and final consonant clusters later than consonants and clusters in the initial and medial position (Burns et al., 2010).

There are three major phonological rules of AAE from which most of the sound features emanate: (1) silencing or substitution of the medial or final consonant in a word, (2) silencing of unstressed initial phonemes and unstressed initial syllables, and (3) silencing of the final consonant in a consonant cluster occurring at the end of a word.

The first phonological rule of AAE is the silencing or substitution of the medial or final consonant in a word. The consonants affected by this rule include voiced and voiceless fricatives. For example, the fricative /ð/ is affected, and AAE speakers may say "dey" for *they*, "nofin" for *nothing*, "toof" for *tooth*, and "brovah" for *brother*. The semivowels /r/ and /l/ are also affected. AAE speakers may say "foe" for *four*, "sto'y" for *story*, and "p'otect" for *protect*.

Voiced stops /b/, /d/, and /g/ are generally affected in the final positions of single-syllable words, usually a consonant-vowel-consonant (CVC) combination. In these words, the final voiced stop is pronounced similarly to the consonant's voiceless cognate /p/, /t/, and /k/. In addition, the vowel in CVC words is lengthened. Examples of these changes occur when speakers say "cap" plus the lengthened vowel for *cab*, "but" plus lengthened vowel for *bud*, and "pik" plus the lengthened vowel for *pig*.

The nasals /m/ and /n/ are also affected by this first phonological rule. Several specific characteristics occur with these nasal consonants. One occurs in CVC-unstressed combinations in a word in which the final consonant in the CVC combination is the /m/ or /n/ (e.g., *mailman*). In these words, the final nasal consonant is silenced, but the quality of nasalization is transferred to the vowel. Some examples of this are "ma" plus the nasalized vowel for *man* and "bu" plus the nasalized vowel for *bun*. This feature is also similar to that which occurs in CVC words such as *pin* and *pen*. In these words, the final nasal consonant /n/ remains intact, but the final consonant nasalizes the adjacent vowels, making these words sound identical.

Other nasalization features in AAE affect the grammatical formulations of the present progressive verb tense *(-ing)* and the articles *a* and *an*. The *-ing* suffix becomes *-in*, as in "singin" and "runnin." The difference between *a* and *an* also becomes neutralized. In this situation, *a* precedes words that begin with a consonant or a vowel, as in "a apple," "a pear," and "a orange," as opposed to *an apple, a pear,* and *an orange*.

According to Stockman (1996a), final consonant silence or absence is most likely to occur under the following conditions:

1. The final consonant is a nasal or a stop (e.g., man, pop).
2. The final consonant or consonant cluster precedes a word that begins with a consonant (e.g., ri*ght* food, be*st* buy) as opposed to a vowel (e.g., ri*ght* on, be*st* of).
3. The final consonant occurs in a monomorphemic cluster (e.g., bent) as opposed to a bimorphophonemic cluster (e.g., can't).
4. The final consonant occurs in a word in which contrastive status can be maintained in its absence (e.g., bad, bean).

The second major phonological rule of AAE is the silencing of unstressed initial phonemes and unstressed initial syllables. Examples of this rule are "bout" for *about,* "cause" for *because*, "matoes" for *tomatoes,* "he uz" for *he was,* and "this un" for *this one*.

The third general rule of AAE is the silencing of the final consonant in a consonant cluster occurring at the end of a word. Examples of this are "des" for *desk,* "min" for *mind,* and "ol" for *old*. This rule also affects the AAE grammatical feature for past tense, as in "miss" for *missed* and "slep" for *slept*. Another feature related to consonant clusters is the use of *skr-* for *str-* in the initial position in words, as in "skring" for *string* and "skreet" for *street*. Additionally, "aks" may be used for *ask*.

Morphosyntactic Features

Although AAE is a variety of GAE, there are systematic contrasts in their linguistic features, with particular emphasis on phonological and morphosyntactic forms. The morphosyntactic forms of AAE have been widely studied because they are often more noticeable and distinct than the phonological features. Like the phonological characteristics, AAE morphosyntactic or grammatical features are systematic and extensive and cannot be simplified into general rules. They affect the use of noun-verb agreement, verb tense, copula and auxiliary forms of the verb to be, modals, negation, pronouns, and demonstratives as well as other morphosyntactic forms voiced "th" /ð/ (Apel & Thomas-Tata, 2009; Connor & Craig, 2006; Craig & Washington, 2004; Ivy & Masterson 2011; Stockman, 1996b).

The variable use of morphosyntactic forms in AAE places obstacles in identifying morphologic impairment, primarily because the linguistic constraints governing the variability of the forms has not yet been fully defined (Seymour et al., 1998). It is particularly difficult to differentiate between speakers of AAE who are typically developing and those who have an impairment. The Diagnostic Evaluation of Language Variation (Seymour, et al, 2000; Seymour et al., 2005) was developed to differentiate those features of AAE that are contrastive and those used by typically developing speakers of GAE.

The morphosyntactic features of the dialect can affect noun-verb agreement, as in "he walk" (for *he walks*). The features also involve the tense of regular past tense verbs (e.g., "cash" for *cashed*) and irregular verbs (e.g., "seen" for *saw* and "done" for *did*). They also affect the future tense of verbs through the use of "gonna" and various reductions of "gonna" (e.g., "I'nga," "I'mon," and "I'ma") and by the silencing of the contraction "ll" for *will*, as in "she miss you" for *she'll miss you*. Other AAE morphosyntactic features include the use of double modals (e.g., "used to couldn't"), the use of "like ta" for *liked to have,* differences in the use of the possessive's morpheme (e.g., "the boy hat" for *the boy's hat*), and differences in the use of the plural morpheme *-s* as in "fifty cent" for *fifty cents.*

Some AAE features attempt to provide regularity to irregular GAE structures. For example, GAE allows for only one comparative or superlative descriptor within a single noun or verb phrase. For example, only *most beautiful* or *prettier* would be allowed in a single phrase. Although GAE does not permit the use of more and most with words ending with an *-er* or *-est* suffix, this combination (e.g., *most prettiest*) is valid in AAE as well as in several other social dialects. The dialectal formulations of comparatives and superlatives can occur in a variety of combinations, serving to carry the comparative or superlative through the entire phrase. Some examples of normal dialectal formulations in this area include "baddest," "mostest," and "worser."

Negative formulations in AAE also regularize GAE rules. The general logic of negatives within a GAE sentence tells us that two negatives cannot be used together because they negate each other and the sentence becomes positive. In AAE, no such philosophical rule exists. Rather, AAE follows the rules for use of negatives that are present in other languages. In Spanish, for example, the negative is carried throughout the sentence. This means that if the sentence is to be negative, every place in the sentence that can be negated is negated. This same rule applies in AAE, resulting in the normal dialectal feature of multiple negation. Some examples of this feature are "He didn't do nothing," "Couldn't nobody do it?" "Nobody didn't do it," and "Ain't no cat can't get in no coop."

Regularization also extends to reflexive pronouns, in which the suffix *-self* can be added to all personal pronouns. The rules used to formulate the first- and second-person reflexive pronouns *myself* and *yourself* can be extended to the third person, as in "hisself" and "theirself."

Some AAE morphosyntactic forms reflect a feature of hypercorrection. This generally means that the speaker has overgeneralized a morpheme to an irregular word that already reflects the function of that morpheme. In all cases of hypercorrection, the speaker does not have sufficient knowledge of the GAE rule for the use of a morpheme. Hypercorrected forms are mostly used by older adult dialectal speakers who have realized that they need a more standard language system but do not have a consistent English model to imitate. Hypercorrected forms occur in the areas of third-person subject-verb agreement (e.g., "I walks," "you walks," and "the children walks"); in pluralization (e.g., "two childrens," "five mens," and "three deers"); and in the use of the possessive morpheme *'s* (e.g., "John's Taylor car")

Other AAE morphosyntactic features occur in the following areas:

- Pronominal apposition
  "*My brother he* bigger than you."
- Demonstratives
  "I want some of *them* candies."
  "I like *these here* pants better than *them there* ones."
- Pronouns
  "*Him* ain't playing." "*Me and her* will go."
  "James got *him* book." "Don't eat that candy 'cause it *mines*."
  "He can dress *hisself*." "I got *me* one of those."
- The use of *have* and *do*
  "I *been* here for hours." "He *have* a bike."
  "He *don't* go." "He always *do* silly things."
- Completed aspects with *done*. This construction is used when an action started and was completed at a certain time in the past.
  "I *done* tried."
- Remote time construction with *been*. This construction is used when an action has taken place in the distant past.
  "I *been* had it there for about three years."
- Indirect questions. Indirect questions follow the same rules as those for formulating direct questions.
  "I wonder was he walking."
  "I wonder where was he going."
- Use of *do* for *if*. This feature is related to the indirect question feature: a clause beginning with *if* is reformulated into a direct question format.
  "I ask' Elon *do he want* to play football."

A major grammatical feature of AAE involves variations in the use of the auxiliary/copula forms of the verb *to be*. The use rules are as follows:

- The silencing of *is, are,* or both in contracted forms.
  "*He* a man," "*He* running home," and "*You* good." Dialectal speakers use *is* and *are* in other sentence contexts, such as in tag questions (e.g., "*He* not home yet, *is* he?"). Also, some dialectal speakers who use a silenced *are* contraction do not use a silenced *is* contraction. Additionally, this feature extends to contractions of *will be* and *would be* ("He *be* here") and ("She *be* happy").
- Neutralization of subject-verb agreement. This construction occurs in past and present forms of *to be*, but neutralization is more frequent in the past tense.
  "*I was* there," "*She was* there," "*You was* there," and "*They was* there." An example of the more infrequently used present tense form is "*They is* here."

- Use of *be* as a main verb for *is*, *are*, or *am*. "I *be* here in the evening" for *I am here in the evening*, "Sometime he *be* busy" for *Sometimes he is busy*, and "They *be* coming" for *They are coming*.
- Use of *be* for habitual tense. In the most prominent feature of AAE, *be* does not specify a tense, but it reflects the African-based habitual tense, which indicates a permanent or consistent quality or condition. "My momma *be* workin' two jobs" means *My mother has been working two jobs for a while*. And the statement, "Don' min' him; he jus' *be* actin' crazy" means *Don't pay any attention to him; acting crazy is his normal tendency.*

Semantic or Lexical Features

Semantics involves the meaning and use of words. Like speakers of other languages or dialects, the lexicon of speakers of AAE is influenced by geographic, economic, regional, sociopolitical, familiar, religious, and racial factors. This means that the person's lexicon is likely to contain words that are unique to the factors that affect the individual's life. For example, Stockman (2010) gives the example of lexical items that are unique to African American culture. The word "finna" or "fitna" is a simplified pronunciation of *fixing to*, which means "imminent action" or "getting ready." The word *hotcomb* refers to a heated metal comb used to straighten African American hair and is common in African American culture but generally unknown in other cultures.

The vocabulary of African Americans can have regional influences. A child living in a predominantly African American neighborhood in an area may have a lexicon that is different from that of a child who lives in a rural area. In some cases, the same lexical item symbolizes different referents. For example, to a rural child, the word *hog* is likely to represent a large pig, but to the urban child, *hog* might symbolize a type of large expensive car or a particular type of motorcycle (Stockman, 2000).

Differences in form and content areas of language can result in communication failures between speakers of different dialects. Some failures can result from differences in pronunciation, grammar, and vocabulary that create intelligibility problems. In the case of different dialects of a language, the actual linguistic differences can be minor but nevertheless implicated in difficulties in communication and in misunderstandings. (See Chapter 13 for a discussion of the performance of African American children on standardized vocabulary tests.)

Pragmatic Functions

Just as there are normal systematic phonological, morphosyntactic, and semantic features of AAE, there are also pragmatic characteristics of the dialect. The rules for communicative interactions used by many African Americans include code switching, eye contact, and narrative style.

Code Switching

Code switching is a major pragmatic feature of the speech of most, if not all, speakers. Code switching involves the speaker's ability to use the linguistic style (formal or informal), dialect, or language that is most appropriate for a particular communication episode. The language used is based on the language, age, race, gender, or level of authority of the person with whom one is speaking; the intended use; and the context of the communicative event. Code switching is used by speakers of AAE when significant changes or decrease in the use of AAE features result in an increased use of GAE (Hester, 1996).

The ability to code-switch or dialect-switch is a skill acquired by school-aged children, including those who use AAE. Craig and Washington (2004) reported the development of code switching of phonological features in students in preschool through grade 5 in oral reading. Of the nine features tracked, only devoicing of the final consonant (e.g., his/hiz) was not produced in the oral reading. Monophthongization of diphthongs, substitution of dental fricatives, and consonant cluster reductions were widely used. Ivy and Masterson (2011) investigated the use of the features of AAE in writing by grade 3 and grade 8 AAE speakers. The results indicated that the grade 3 speakers used the AAE features with relatively equal frequency in their speech and their writing. However, the grade 8 students decreased their use of the six AAE features in their writing. They did, however, use the AAE features when conversing with their peers in informal conversation.

In addition to code switching, speakers may engage simultaneously in style shifting, which refers to changes in the use of features that are predominately oral style or literate. In an examination of the narrative variability of AAE-speaking grade 4 children, Hester (1996) found that the code switching and style shifting among the children varied between narrative tasks (e.g., conversation, story retelling, and story generation). The results of the study imply that clinicians should evaluate an AAE-speaking child's language over a variety of narrative types during the assessment process (Hester, 1996).

Eye Contact

Some African Americans are taught as children that eye contact with an adult during a verbal interchange is disrespectful. Some African American adults may therefore find it difficult to speak to those of authority on an eye-to-eye basis. Judging children and adults for not looking at an examiner or other professional may be a violation of the person's cultural rule for eye contact. This is particularly important in the treatment of dysfluency, as described in

Chapter 9. According to Taylor (1987), African Americans demonstrate attentiveness and respect by using indirect eye contact when they are listeners and direct eye contact when they are speakers. GAE speakers could easily misinterpret the lack of eye contact during listening as inattentive or noncaring behavior.

Narrative Style

Heath (1986) describes four types of narrative styles: (1) patterns used to recount past experiences, (2) patterns used to cast or describe present or future activities or events, (3) patterns used to give accounts of what has been experienced, and (4) fictionalized accounts of storytelling. Despite the variable nature of AAE and the awareness of different narrative styles and genres, investigations of the narratives of AAE have generally been restricted to recounts or narratives of personal experiences (Hester, 1994, 1996). In the 1980s, several investigators studied AAE narratives in terms of oral and literate styles (Collins, 1985; Gee, 1985; Heath, 1982; Michaels & Collins, 1984; Nichols, 1989). In oral language style, meaning is implicit or indirect; that is, it is expressed through the use of idioms, slang, gestures, and changes in voice and pitch in conversations between familiar individuals. In literate language, style meaning is expressed more directly with specific syntactic and morphologic structures as in written language (Olson, 1977; Tannen, 1982; Westby, 1985). Many investigators describe AAE speakers as preferring the oral narrative style because of their relation to the oral tradition of the African ancestry (Baugh, 1983; Erickson, 1984).

Michaels (1981), Nichols (1989), Collins (1985), Gee (1989), Hyter and Westby (1996) and Westby (1985) are among several investigators who studied the oral-literate distinction in the narratives of young children. By analyzing narratives during sharing-time activities for African American and white kindergarten children, Michaels (1981) found that the narrative style used by the AAE-speaking children differed from that used by speakers of GAE. When a particular topic was discussed, speakers of GAE used patterns that involved a fairly strict adherence to a central topic. For example, when a teacher asks a class to talk about things seen and done at a zoo, each child using GAE contributes something appropriate to that main topic. This reflects a topic-centered narrative style. On the other hand, some speakers of AAE engage in a more topic-associated narrative style. With a topic-associated narrative style, a child's statements are not linked by a central topic but by ideas generated from an immediately preceding statement. For example, when a group of children who use this style of discussion is asked to talk about things seen and done at a zoo, the first child may respond that he saw a lion, the second child comments that she saw a lion on the *Circus of the Stars* television special, and the third child adds that she got scared when the performer almost fell off the high wire. The investigators reported that AAE-speaking children's narrative skills are restricted to a topic-associated oral style (Collins, 1985; Michaels, 1981; Nichols, 1989; Westby, 1985).

More recent investigations, however, have found that AAE-speaking children have more flexible narrative styles than was previously thought. Hyon and Sulzby (1994), Hicks (1991), and Hester (1996) studied the use of narrative by kindergarten and grade 1 AAE-speaking children. Hyon and Sulzby (1994) and Champion and associates (1995) reported that African American children used topic-centered and topic-associating features while telling stories to a familiar adult. Hicks (1991) and Hester (1996) found that children who use AAE are able to shift their narrative style according to different task demands. Regardless of the style preferred by the child, African American children can be expected to tell stories and recount events as do other children.

Other Pragmatic Functions

Turn-Taking   Turn-taking rules are somewhat different among African American speakers. In AAE, it is not necessary to wait until the first speaker has completed his or her turn before the next speaker begins. Interruptions are acceptable, and the conversational floor is given to the most assertive and aggressive speaker.

Call and response is an important turn-taking feature of AAE. Call and response is characterized by a choral response to an utterance given by a single person. Largely noticeable within the church and in gospel and rhythm and blues music, call and response is also a feature of conversations among African Americans. There are two specific call-and-response patterns: (1) a statement produced by one person followed by a response by one person and (2) a statement produced by one person followed by responses made by people in a group.

The first type of call and response occurs mostly during a conversational dyad. The response is generally a confirmation or acknowledgment of the speaker's statement. In some instances, the response is confirming (e.g., "I know that's right"). Additionally, the response can denote some element of surprise regarding the content of the statement. In some instances, the call-and-response patterns in a dyad are echoic or hyperechoic. The echoic response duplicates or repeats some portion of the speaker's statement, as in the following conversation:

Speaker: I fixed me some turkey and dressing . . .
Respondent: Um-um! Turkey and dressing!

A pragmatic feature not previously recognized in literature is the hyperechoic response. The hyperechoic response is superimposed on top of the first speaker's utterance. It is a confirmation that the listener not only understands the response but also anticipates, predicts, and verbalizes what the speaker's next words will be while the speaker is talking. If the respondent is wrong, the speaker makes the appropriate adjustments. An example of a hyperechoic response pattern follows:

Speaker: You know I done tried to be fair. But I s'pose you can' teach no ol' . . .

Respondent: Man nothin' new . . . [anticipating "old man, new tricks"]

Speaker: Nothin' new. I know that's right! [echoed and confirmed]

The second type of call-and-response pattern is a statement produced by one person followed by responses made by people in a group. It is typically found in church services, rallies, and other situations with a main speaker and an audience. Audience verbal responses in church include "Yea," "Amen," "Well," "Alright." Nonverbal responses to a speaker's statements include hand clapping, head shaking, and nodding.

Touching During AAE conversations, approval or agreement is demonstrated nonverbally through touching, such as touching the listener's hand or arm. However, the touching of the hair and patting on the head might be considered an insult by speakers of AAE (Roseberry-McKibbin, 1995; Taylor, 1987).

To summarize, it is important to emphasize that social constraints on language are culturally organized and vary from culture to culture and from subculture to subculture. Competent speakers of a language must observe a wide range of sociocultural norms in verbal interaction. For example, competent speakers must know when it is appropriate to address a person using a title and a last name or a first name, they must make vocabulary choices appropriate to their addressee and the social situation, and they must know how to phrase requests without violating rules of etiquette. In many cases, it is the violation of such norms, rather than grammatical or phonological norms, that are the sources of communication failures. The clinical setting, as well as other service-delivery settings, is one in which many people can experience what they believe are violations of their privacy. Compound this with cultural differences in beliefs about what is considered private and pragmatically appropriate, and it becomes easy to envision the barriers of self-defense that clients may erect that block the flow of information necessary for optimal service delivery.

Development of African American English

Morphologic and Syntactic Development

Research on the normal acquisition of AAE morphologic and syntactic patterns is scarce. The few historical data–based studies that have been conducted have largely investigated phonological and morphosyntactic features based on Brown's (1973) set of 14 grammatical morphemes and

suggested that, in addition to sharing linguistic features with other dialects, AAE shares features of normal linguistic development in young children (Blake, 1984; Cole, 1980; Reveron, 1978; Steffensen, 1974; Stockman, 1984, 1986a, 1986b; Stockman & Vaughn-Cooke, 1982). More contemporary studies of the development of language by African American children have aimed at describing the typical language development patterns of AAE preschool children, with particular emphasis on the phonological and morphosyntactic forms.

Blake (1984) and Stockman (1996b, 2006) have both shown that the morphosyntactic development of young children who speak AAE is similar to that of children who use GAE up to the age of 3 years, including the development of the mean length of utterance. Children in homes in which AAE is spoken have a well-developed use of one- and two-word utterances by the age of 18 months, as is observed in homes in which GAE is spoken (Blake, 1984; Steffensen, 1974). Their mean length of utterance increases with age at least to the age of 2.5 years, with increments similar to those of children who speak GAE (Blake, 1984; Stockman, 1984). By the age of 3 years, as with speakers of GAE, elaborated simple sentence with noun/pronoun, verb and verb complements predominate in declarative, imperative, interrogative, and negative forms (Stockman et al., 2009). Also, as with speakers of GAE, at age 4 to 5 years, the frequency of complex sentences and relative clauses including subject and verb phrases increases (Jackson & Roberts, 2001; Oetting & Newkirk, 2008).

Research investigating the development of morphologic features shows that children in homes in which AAE is spoken acquire early morphologic features in the same pattern as children learning GAE, including features to mark the plural, possessive, past tense, and third-person singular (Blake, 1984; Cole, 1980; Oetting & Newkirk, 2008; Reveron, 1978; Ross et al., 2004; Steffensen, 1974; Stockman, 1986a). As with GAE, the morphologic features of AAE involving tense, mood, and aspect markers of the verb phrase, negation, and other morphologic features develop in the later preschool years. At the age of 3 years, children learning AAE have developed the use of well-formed multiword constructions, simple declaratives, and questions, with subject, verb, and object complements and a few complex utterances also appearing (Stockman, 1986a). Elaborated sentences with embedded object complements, negative sentences, and the formation of tag questions appear before the age of 4 years. As children develop through the preschool years, a variety of complex sentences and complex semantic relations are used, including coordinated, subordinate, and relative clause sentences and complex *wh-* question forms (Craig & Washington, 1995; Washington & Craig, 1994). Thus, through the early preschool years, there is little difference in the development of morphologic and syntactic forms between children learning AAE and those learning GAE. This implies that the linguistic forms of children acquiring GAE and of children acquiring AAE cannot be distinguished until the children reach approximately 3 years of age (Steffensen, 1974).

The features that contrast AAE and GAE generally involve the later-developing forms, which begin to evolve at approximately 4 years of age. Like the continuum of development of GAE forms, it appears that AAE rules are also learned in a developmental sequence and that the frequency with which these rules are used increases with age (Cole, 1980; Reveron, 1978). Social class differences become most pronounced after the age of 4 years (Craig & Washington, 1994; Kovac, 1980; Reveron, 1978; Stockman, 1986a).

Cole (1980) found that AAE-speaking children exhibit the AAE rules for regular past tense, third-person singular, present tense copula, and remote past *(been)* at the age of 3 years. The AAE features of indefinite article regularization and multiple negation were observed in 4-year-old children. The features of reflexive and pronominal regularization occurred when the children were 5 years of age. Because Cole analyzed only the speech of 3-, 4-, and 5-year-old African American children, it can be assumed that other AAE features do not emerge until after the age of 5 years. If this is the case, it would make identification of language disorders within AAE-speaking children by conventional standardized tests extremely difficult (Stockman, 1986b). AAE forms not used until after 5 years of age include the use of *at* in questions (e.g., "Where my coat at?"), the *go* copula (e.g., "There go my coat."), distributive *be*, first-person future, embedded questions, past tense copula, present copula, and second-person pronouns. Features such as the habitual *be* (e.g., "She be working.") and the use of *what* to mark the relative clause (e.g., "He the one what broke it.") develop at much later ages than the other forms (Cole, 1980). Among the later-emerging contrastive AAE forms is the use of *had* to mark the simple past (e.g., "We had went to the store."), *steady* to mark an intensified continuative marker (e.g., "He steady be mockin' me."), and *come* to express indignation about an event or action (e.g., "He come hollering at me.").

Variables in the required use of certain linguistic forms can cause difficulty in distinguishing development from disorders or delays in morphologic development in AAE. For example, although speakers of AAE are required to use the form of *be* in statements such as "yes, he is," it is not obligatory in "John a boy" (Seymour, 1995; Seymour & Roeper, 1999). The expression of habitual *be* (e.g., "he be working"), as opposed to a temporary condition (e.g., "he working"), does not appear in GAE. The feature is not likely to be observed by speech-language pathologists assessing the development of morphologic features using GAE standards.

In summarizing the study on developmental trends in the language of African American child research, Stockman (2010, p. 26) reported that "African American children are neither nonverbal nor verbally impoverished. Their maternal caregivers use a child-directed speech register to simplify the linguistic input to young children in ways that have been described for speakers of other languages."

Phonological Development

Research suggests that the consonants in AAE develop in the same order and at about the same ages as in GAE (Stockman, 2007). As with speakers of other dialects, the number of accurately produced speech sounds by children using AAE increases with age. Because GAE and AAE are dialects of the same language, several phonological features are shared and are thus noncontrastive. Like the early development of morphology and syntax, the early phoneme development of children learning AAE is not different from that of children learning GAE (Seymour & Ralabate, 1985; Seymour & Seymour, 1981; Steffensen, 1974). By the age of 2 years, their speech sound repertoire consists of 15 frequently occurring English consonants that form the minimal core of word-initial consonants produced by African American children: /m/n/p/b/t/d/k/g/w/j/s/h/l/r/ (Bland-Stewart, 2003; Stockman, 2006, 2008). By their third birthday, AAE-speaking children also produce eight or nine word-initial consonant clusters, and by the age of 5 to 6 years, they are using fricatives such as /z/, /sh/, and /ts/ in one or more word positions. Thus, the early phonological development of AAE speakers is not unlike that of speakers of other dialects of English (Stockman, 2006, 2007, 2008, 2010).

The features that contrast AAE and GAE involve sounds and phonological features that develop after the age of 4 or 5 years. These features include final consonant deletion or weakening, final cluster reduction, unstressed syllable deletion, and interdental fricative substitution involving the final /th/ (Bland-Stewart, 2003; Haynes & Moran, 1989; Moran 1993; Seymour & Seymour, 1981; Stockman, 1995, 2006, 2008, 2010; Stockman & Settle, 1991; Vaughn-Cooke, 1986; Wolfram & Fasold, 1974).

Because standard articulation tests vary in the number of items related to AAE, they have limited usefulness in determining the phonological performance of children learning AAE (Cole & Taylor, 1990; Washington & Craig, 1992). Care must be taken to distinguish between those features that are contrastive and those that are not contrastive between AAE and GAE. According to Bleile and Wallach (1992) and Seymour and associates (2005), the following features are not contrastive between AAE and GAE and can thus be useful in distinguishing between normal disordered or delayed phonological development in children learning AAE:

- The use of more than one or two stop errors
- Initial word position errors (with the exception of /b/ for /v/)
- Glide errors in children older than 4 years of age

- More than a few cluster errors (with the exception of final clusters)
- Fricative errors other than /th/

The primary indicators of whether a child who speaks AAE is having difficulty in phonological development are the ability of those familiar with the dialect to understand the child at 5 years of age and the determination of whether the child is considerably more difficult to understand than his or her age and dialect peers.

Pragmatic Development

Communicative intent and semantic-linguistic functions in children learning AAE develop along the same lines as in children learning GAE. AAE-speaking children use language to accomplish basic interpersonal communication intent before the age of 2 years. They take turns, seek attention, identify objects and persons in their perceptual field, and request objects at similar ages and styles as their GAE peers (Stockman, 2010). Children between the ages of 18 months and 2 years develop the same functions as children learning other languages. These functions include informative, requestive, regulative, imaginative, affective, participative, and attentive functions (Blake, 1984, 1993; Bridgeforth, 1984; Stockman, 1986a). Their conversations begin to resemble narrative to include a variety of forms and genres between ages 2 and 3 years (Champion, 1998) and continue to develop to include the basic elements of introductions, endings, and plots through age 4 to 5 years (Price et al., 2006). Conversational structure and respect for conversational rules and routines emerges between the ages of 3 and 4 years. AAE-speaking children make comments, ask and answer questions, request objects, and request clarification using the same types of strategies used by speakers of GAE (Stockman et al., 2008). According to Vaughn-Cooke and Wright-Harp (1992), the similarity in the development of linguistic function appears to continue through the preschool years.

Because of the apparent lack of assessment tools that distinguish between normally developing AAE and true disorders, children developing AAE are often assessed using tools that fail to take into account the normal development of the dialect. It is essential that the normal development of features in AAE be considered in distinguishing between the least competent child considered to have normal development and the child considered to have delayed learning of AAE (Stockman, 1996b).

African American English and Literacy

Performance of speakers of AAE on the National Assessment of Educational Progress (2007) has prompted interest in the relationship between AAE and literacy. There is a well-documented disparity in the assessment of reading performance between African American children and their European American counterparts (Connor & Craig, 2006; National Center for Educational Statistics, 2010). The reports, however, do not specify whether the children were users of AAE but rather only specify the race of the children. Connor and Craig (2006) reviewed student performance on literacy tasks related to density of their use of features of AAE. They found that the students who used AAE features with greater or lesser frequency demonstrated stronger sentence imitation, letter work recognition, and phonological awareness skills than did preschool children who used AAE features with moderate frequency, when vocabulary was controlled. The children also used fewer AAE features during a sentence imitation task than they did during an oral elicitation task with specific expectations for GAE.

Recent studies have also looked at the use of AAE grammatical forms between oral and written language and literacy. Early research has shown that the features of AAE occur in the writing of children who are speakers of the dialect (Collins, 1981; Smitherman, 1993). The features frequently found in the writings of children who speak AAE include absence of third-person singular -s (e.g., she go), plural -s absence (e.g., four mile), possessive -s absence (e.g., John hat), copula is and are absence (e.g., We going), and -ed absence resulting in cluster reduction (e.g., They miss) (Ivy & Masterson, 2011). Features that occur infrequently in the writing of AAE speakers compared with their incidence in spoken language include multiple negation, the use of ain't, and the use of habitual be.

REDUCING BIAS IN THE CLINICAL MANAGEMENT OF AFRICAN AMERICANS

Nonbiased clinical management is the process of establishing a client's native language, dialect, and culture as the basis on which speech-language and hearing evaluations are conducted and results are interpreted and for which treatment is prescribed. For nonbiased management to occur with an individual client, the speech-language pathologist must discover the normal language patterns and cultural views of that client. Because of the complexity of cultural variables that can affect service delivery, reducing bias in clinical management must go beyond the administration of specific tests and procedures. Instead, it must be an entire process emanating from respect of a client's culture and language. See Chapter 12 for a further discussion of assessment.

CARIBBEAN AMERICANS

Although many persons with African heritage were brought to the Caribbean as a part of the transatlantic slave trade and European colonization, many were not immediately brought to the United States. Rather, they stayed in the Caribbean and continued to live in the regions colonized by the

European countries, eventually gaining independence even before slavery was abolished in the United States. The residents gained and maintained national identity according to the country where they and their ancestors lived (Arthur, 2005).

A small segment of African Americans or blacks in America are recent immigrants from the Caribbean and African continent. Many people with roots in the Caribbean immigrated to the United States and Canada in search of educational and economic opportunities and freedom from political oppression. According to the 2009 U.S. Department of Homeland Security, between 1990 and 2000 there was a 67% increase in the number of residents of the United States who identify themselves as Caribbean-born. There are 7.9 million persons living in the United States who immigrated from the Caribbean. According to the 2000 U.S. Census, 4% of persons identifying themselves as black were born in the Caribbean. Cuba accounted for the most Caribbean immigrants, followed by the Dominican Republic, Haiti, and Jamaica. According to Camarota (2007), director of the Center for Immigration Studies, Cuba is the country of origin for nearly 1 million Caribbean-born persons in the United States; the Dominican Republic, 695,000; Jamaica, 607,000; and Haiti, 570,000. Although most settled in Florida (47%), many have also settled in the northeastern states of New York and New Jersey (27%). Between 2000 and 2009, 100,000 persons from the Caribbean obtained permanent resident status. After the 2010 earthquake in Haiti, nearly 9000 Haitians arrived in the United States, the same number that arrived in the years before the earthquake. Approximately 7000 settled in Miami, with the others settling in New York (U.S. Border Protection Agency, 2011).

Many Caribbean Americans share a common ancestry with African Americans, having been brought to the region through the transatlantic slave trade. As many as 80% of the inhabitants of the Caribbean countries of Jamaica, Haiti, the Dominican Republic, the Bahamas, and Barbados descended from countries in West Africa. Although they share the common history of slavery, they took on the cultural roots of the British, Dutch, French, and Spanish, who controlled the various parts of the Caribbean area during the period of slavery.

The language used by immigrants from the Caribbean does not share the features of AAE. Most languages spoken in the Caribbean belong to one of four major Indo-European language families: English, Spanish, French, or Dutch. Of the 38 million persons in the Caribbean, 62% speak Spanish, 20% speak French, 15% speak English, and 0.7% speak Dutch. Other languages spoken include those spoken by persons migrating to the region from Asia, including Chinese and Indian languages. In addition, several Creole languages developed from influence of European and other countries during the colonial period. For example, although English is the official language of Jamaica, Jamaican Creole or Patois is based on influence by West African languages, British English, Scotch, and Hiberno English, with much of its lexicon deriving from Spanish, Portuguese, Hindi, Arawak, and African languages as well as Irish. Jamaican pronunciation, grammar, and vocabulary are different from English despite the heavy use of English words or derivatives (Harry, 2006). Because Jamaican Patois is a nonstandard language, there is no standard or official way of writing it.

Haitian Creole is derived from the influence of Spanish and a form of 17th to 20th century French, some African languages, including Arabic, and Spanish, Taino, and English (Gordon, 2008). It is the official language of Haiti along with French. Haitian Creole is widely used by Haitians who have immigrated to other countries, particularly the United States, especially central and south Florida, New York, and Boston, and Canada, especially Montreal. It is the second most spoken language in Cuba, where more than 300,000 Haitian immigrants speak it. Haitian Creole grammar differs from French and is more analytical. For example, verbs are not inflected for tense or person, and there is no grammatical gender.

Many Haitians who left their country in the 1980s and 1990s did not speak English or French. Very few non-Haitians knew the language, and most Haitians did not understand another language, even French. More recent Haitian immigrants who left their country after the earthquake are well educated and speak English, French, and Haitian Creole, having attended private schools in the country.

PERSONS FROM THE AFRICAN CONTINENT

Recent immigrants to the United States are distinguished from descendants of those who came to the country through the transatlantic slave trade and those who came from the Caribbean region. The immigration of persons from Africa did not begin in earnest until the later part of the 20th century. The number of African immigrants into the United States grew 40-fold between 1960 and 2007 to 1.4 million persons. There was a 167% increase in immigrants from Africa between 1990 and 2000. According to the U.S. Census, there were 1.4 million persons born in Africa residing in the United States in 2007. In 2009, 127,000 persons born in Africa obtained permanent residence in the United States (U.S. Department of Homeland Security, 2009). Approximately 3.7% of foreign-born persons in the United States were born in one of the countries of Africa. The leading countries of origin of African born are from West Africa, with most coming from Nigeria (13.1%), Egypt (9.6%), Ethiopia (9.5%), Ghana (7.4%), and Kenya (5.7%). Most immigrants from Africa settled in New York, New Jersey, Massachusetts, California, Texas, Maryland, and Virginia.

Most Africans came to the United States seeking an education or specialized training to advance themselves for service or work in their home country. However, there has been an increase in the number of persons who seek permanent residence and do not desire to return to their home country. Immigrants from Africa have the highest educational attainment of any immigrant group to the United States. The descendants of recent immigrants from Africa are more likely to be college educated than any other immigrant group. In 2007, less than one in three immigrants from Africa had limited English proficiency. Nearly 47% aged 5 years and older reported speaking English only, whereas 24% reported speaking English very well. Only 29% reported speaking English less than "very well," in contrast to the 52% of all foreign-born immigrants who reported speaking less than very well. The immigrants from Africa who spoke English "less than very well" spoke one of five languages: Arabic (20.1%), Amharic/Ethiopian (15.6%), French (14.3%), Kru (13.6%), and Cushite/Beja/Somali (12.6%).

African immigrants tend to retain the culture of their home country once in the United States. Because of the diversity of the various countries in Africa, there is no single African immigrant identity. They practice a variety of religions, including Christianity, Islam, and various traditional African religions. They speak a variety of languages. Because the language used by persons from Africa does not share the features of AAE and there are no data to indicate whether the features of the language or dialect used follow the same development path as GAE or AAE, speech-language pathologists must use caution in identifying the presence of a disorder in assessment and intervention for black persons from Africa. Terrell and colleagues (1992), for example, described a criterion-referenced method of determining the presence of a disability in a preschool child from Nigeria whose parents spoke English that was influenced by their native Nigerian language.

CONCLUSION

The descendants of Africa in the African diaspora include African Americans, Caribbean Americans, and new African immigrants. They share a common genealogic root, but their history, culture, and languages are different. Through socialization, intermarriage, and other opportunities, the three groups live in proximity and share experiences. Making this distinction is necessary as speech-language pathologists and audiologists come to understand the cultural parameters associated with service delivery to blacks and persons in the African diaspora. It is important that the speech-language pathologist and audiologist identify the ancestral root of the client to determine the specific psychological, cultural, and linguistic variables that affect service delivery to that client.

REFERENCES

American Speech-Language-Hearing Association (1983, September). Social dialects. *ASHA, 25,* 23-27.

American Speech-Language-Hearing Association (2011). Communication manifestations of pediatric HIV/AIDS. Retrieved from http://www.asha.org/research/reports/hiv_aids.htm.

Apel, K., & Thomas-Tata, S. (2009). Morphological awareness of fourth-grade African American students. *Language, Speech, and Hearing Services in Schools, 40,* 312-324.

Arinze, F. (1986). Values of the family in African culture. *International Review of Natural Family Planning, 10* (3), 185-207.

Arthur, C. (2005). Eye on the Caribbean. Retrieved January 14, 2011 from http://www.cis.org.

Balcazar, F. E., Suarez-Balcazar, Y, Taylor-Ritzler, T., & Keys, C. B. (2010). *Race, culture and disability: Rehabilitation science and practice.* Boston: Jones and Bartlett Publishers:

Baugh, J. (1983). *Black street speech.* Austin, TX: University of Texas Press.

Blake, I. K. (1984). Language development in working-class black children: An examination of form, content, and use. Doctoral dissertation, Columbia University Teachers College.

Bland-Stewart, L. M. (2003). Phonetic inventories and phonological patterns of African American 2-year-olds: A preliminary investigation. *Communication Disorders Quarterly, 24,* 109-112.

Bleile, K., & Wallach, H. (1992). A sociolinguistic investigation of the speech of African American preschoolers. *American Journal of Speech-Language Pathology, 1* (2), 54-62.

Bloom, L., & Lahey, M. (1978). *Language development and language disorders.* New York: Wiley.

Bridgeforth, C. (1984). The development of language functions among black children from working class families. Paper presented at the pre-session of the 35th annual Georgetown University Round Table on Language and Linguistics, Georgetown University, Washington, DC.

Brown, R. (1973). *A first language.* Cambridge, MA: Harvard University Press.

Burns, F. A., Velleman, S. L., Green, L. J., & Roeper, T. (2010). New branches from old roots: Experts respond to questions about African American English development and language intervention. *Topics in Language Disorders, 30*(3), 253-264.

Burns, F. A., & Weddington, G. T. (2010). Forward. *Topics on Language Disorders, 30*(2), 101-102.

Camarota, S. (2007). *Immigrants in the United States in 2007: A profile of America's foreign-born population.* Washington, DC: Center for Immigration Studies.

Campbell, T., Needleman, H. L., Reiss, J. A., & Tobin, M. J. (1995, June). Bone lead level and language processing performance. Poster session presented at the annual meeting of the Symposium on Research in Child Language disorders, Madison, WI.

Champion, T. (1998). "Tell me somethin' good": A description of narrative structures among African American children. *Linguistics and Education, 9*(3), 251-286.

Champion, T., Seymour, H., & Camarata, S. (1995). Narrative discourse of African American children. *Journal of Narrative and Life History, 5,* 333-352.

Charity, A. H. (2008). African American English: An overview. *Perspectives on Communication Disorders in Sciences in Culturally and Linguistically Diverse Populations, 15,* 33-42.

Cole, L. (1980). Developmental analysis of social dialect features in the spontaneous language of preschool black children. Doctoral dissertation, Northwestern University.

Cole, P., & Taylor, O. (1990). Performance of working-class African American children on three tests of articulation. *Language, Speech, and Hearing Services in Schools, 24,* 171-176.

Collins, J. L. (1981). Spoken language and the development of writing abilities (Report No. CS 206 187). Retrieved from ERIC database. (ED 199187).

Collins, J. L. (1985). Some problems and purposes of narratives in educational research. *Journal of Educational Research, 167,* 57-68.

Conner, C. (2002). Preschool children and teachers talking together: The influence of child, family, teachers and classroom characteristics on children's developing literacy. *Dissertation Abstracts International.* 63(7), 2452 (UMI No. 3057929).

Conner, C. M., & Craig, H. K. (2006). African American preschoolers' language, emergent literacy skills and use of African American English: A complex relation. *Journal of Speech, Language, and Hearing Research, 49,* 771-792.

Craig, H. K., & Washington, J. A. (1994). The complex syntax skills of poor, urban, African American preschoolers at school entry. *Language, Speech, and Hearing Services in Schools, 25,* 181-190.

Craig, H. K., & Washington, J. A. (1995). African American English and linguistic complexity in preschool discourse: A second look. *Language, Speech, and Hearing Services in Schools, 26*(1), 87-93.

Craig, H. K., & Washington, J. A. (2004). Grade related change in the production of African-American preschoolers and kindergartners. *American Journal of Speech-Language Pathology, 11,* 59-70.

Craig, H. K., & Washington, J. A. (2006). *Malik goes to school: examining the language skills of African American students from pre-school to 5th grade.* Mahwah, NJ: Earlbaum.

Davis, P. N., Gentry, B., & Dancer, J. (2001). Sickle cell disease and communication disorders. *Perspectives on Communication Disorders and Sciences in Culturally and Linguistically Diverse Populations, 8,* 4-8.

Erickson, F. (1984). Rhetoric, anecdote, and rhapsody: Cohesion strategies in conversations among black American adolescents. In D. Tannen (Ed.), *Cohesion in spoken and written discourse* (pp. 81-154). Norwood, NJ: Ablex.

Gee, J. (1985). The narrativization of experience in the oral style. *Journal of Education, 167,* 9-35.

Gee, J. (1989). Two styles of narrative construction and their literacy and educational implications. *Discourse Processes, 12,* 263-265.

Gordon, R. G. (2008). Haitian Creole French. Retrieved January 14, 2011 from http://en.wikipedia.org/wiki/Haitian_Creole_language.

Green, L. J. (2002). *African American English.* New York, NY: Cambridge University Press.

Harry, O. G. (2006). Jamaican Creole. *Journal of the International Phonetic Association, 36*(1), 125-131.

Haynes, W., & Moran, M. (1989). A cross-sectional developmental study of final consonant production in Southern black children from preschool through the third grade. *Language, Speech, and Hearing Services in Schools, 20,* 400-406.

Heath, S. B. (1982). What no bedtime story means: Narrative skills at home, at school. *Language in Society, 11,* 49-76.

Heath, S. B. (1986). Taking a cross-cultural look at narratives. *Topics in Language Disorders, 7,* 84-94.

Hester, E. J. (1994). The relationship between narrative style, dialect, and reading ability of African American children. Doctoral dissertation, University of Maryland, Baltimore.

Hester, E. J. (1996). Narratives of young African American children. In A. Kamhi, K. E. Pollock, & J. Harris (Eds.), *Communication development and disorders in African American children* (pp. 227-245). Baltimore: Brookes Publishing.

Hicks, D. (1991). Kinds of narratives: Genre skills among first graders from two communities. In A. McCabe & C. Peterson (Eds.), *Developing narrative structure* (pp. 55-87). Hillsdale, NJ: Lawrence Erlbaum Associates.

Horton-Ikard, R., & Miller, J. (2004). It is not just the poor kids: The use of AAE forms by African American school-aged children from middle SES communities. *Journal of Communication Disorders, 37*(6), 467-487.

Hyon, S., & Sulzby, E. (1994). African American kindergartner's spoken narratives: Topic associating and topic centered styles. *Linguistics and Education, 6,* 121-152.

Hyter, Y., & Westby, C. (1996). Using oral narratives to assess communication competence. In A. Kamhi, K. Pollock, & J. Harris (Eds.), *Communication development and disorders in African American children: research, assessment, and intervention.* Baltimore, MD: Brookes Publishers.

Ivy, L. J., & Masterson, J. (2011). A comparison of oral and written English styles in African American students at different stages of writing development. *Language, Speech, and Hearing Services in Schools, 42,* 31-40.

Jackson, S. C., & Roberts, J. E. (2001). Complex syntax production of African American preschoolers. *Journal of Speech, Language and Hearing Research, 44,* 1083-1096.

Kosoko-Lasaki, S., Cook, C. T., & O'Brien, R. L. (2009). *Cultural proficiency in addressing health disparities.* Boston: Jones and Bartlett Publishers.

Kovac, C. (1980). Children's acquisition of variable features. Doctoral dissertation, Georgetown University, Washington, DC.

Labov, W. (1966). *The social stratification of English in New York City.* Washington, DC: Center for Applied Linguistics.

Lahey, M. (1988). *Language disorders and language development.* New York: Macmillan.

Michaels, S. (1981). Sharing time: Children's narrative style and differential access to literacy. *Language in Society, 10,* 423-442.

Michaels, S., & Collins, J. (1984). Oral discourse styles: Classroom interaction and the acquisition of literacy. In D. Tannen (Ed.), *Cohesion in written and spoken discourse* (pp. 219-244). Norwood, NJ: Ablex.

McAdoo, H. P. (Ed.) (2007). *Black families* (4th ed.) Thousand Oaks, CA: Sage Publications.

McNeilly, L. G. (2005, July-August). HIV and communication. *Journal of Communication Disorders, 38*(4), 303-310.

Moran, M. (1993). Final consonant deletion in African American children speaking Black English: A closer look. *Language, Speech, and Hearing Services in Schools, 24,* 161-166.

National Center of Educational Progress (2007, September) Status and trends in the education of racial and ethnic minorities. Retrieved April 20, 2010, from http://nces.ed.gov/pubs2007/minoritytrends/.

National Center for Educational Statistics (2010, July). Status and trends in the education of racial and ethnic groups. Retrieved from http://nces.ed.gov/pubsearch/pubsinfo.asp?pubid=2010015.

National Center for Health Statistics (2011). *Health United States, 2010, with special feature on death and dying.* Hyattsville, MD: U.S. Department of Health and Human Services.

Needleman, H., & Bellinger, D. (1991). Health effects of low level exposure to lead. *Annual Reviews of Public Health, 12,* 111-140.

Nichols, P. (1989). Storytellin' in Carolina: Continuities and contrasts. *Anthropology and Education, 20*(3), 232-245.

Oetting, J. B., & Newkirk, B. L. (2008). Subject relatives by children with and without SLI across different dialects of English. *Clinical Linguistics and Phonetics, 22*(2), 111-125.

Olson, D. (1977). From utterance to text: The bias of language in speech and writing. *Harvard Educational Review, 47*(3), 257-282.

Pearson, B. Z., Bryant, T. J., & Charko, T. (2009). Phonological milestones for African American English-speaking children learning mainstream American English as a second dialect. *Language, Speech, and Hearing Services in Schools, 40,* 229-244.

Peuschels, S. M., Linakis, S. G., & Anderson, A. C. (Eds.) (1996). *Lead poisoning in children.* Baltimore: Brookes Publishing Co.

Price, J. R., Roberts, J. E., & Jackson, S. C. (2006). Structural development of the fictional narratives of African American preschoolers. *Language, Speech, and Hearing Services in Schools, 37,* 178-190.

Reveron, W. W. (1978). The acquisition of four Black English morphological rules by black preschool children. Doctoral dissertation, Ohio State University, Columbus, OH.

Roseberry-McKibbin, C. (1995). *Multicultural students with special language needs.* Oceanside, CA: Academic Communication Associates.

Ross, G. (2006). Minding the gap: access, availability, and service. Paper presented to National Leadership Summit on the Elimination of Ethnic Disparities in Health: Pre-Conference address on health care and wellness needs of women of color with disabilities. U.S. Department of Health and Human Services, Washington, DC.

Ross, S., Oetting, J. B., & Stapleton, B. (2004). Preterite had + v-ed: A developmental narrative structure on African American English, *American Speech, 79*(2), 167-193.

Seymour, H. (1995, December). Theory and practice in evaluating child African American English. Paper presented at the annual convention of the American Speech-Language-Hearing Association, Orlando, FL.

Seymour, H. N., Bland-Stewart, L., & Green, L. J. (1998). Difference versus deficit in child African American English. *Language, Speech, and Hearing Services in Schools, 29,* 96-108.

Seymour, H. N., deVilliers, J., & Roeper, T. (2000, November). A dialect-sensitive language screener. Paper presented at the annual convention of the American Speech-Language-Hearing Association, Washington, DC.

Seymour, H. N., & Roeper, T. (1999). Grammatical acquisition of African American English. In O. L. Taylor & L. Leonard (Eds.), *Language acquisition across North America: Cross-cultural and cross-linguistic perspectives.* San Diego: Singular Publishing Group.

Seymour, H., & Seymour, C. (1981). Black English and standard American contrasts in communication development of 4- and 5-year-old children. *Journal of Speech and Hearing Disorders, 46,* 276-280.

Seymour, H., & Ralabate, P. (1985). The acquisition of a phonological feature of Black English. *Journal of Communication Disorders, 18,* 139-148.

Seymour, H. N., Roeper, T. W., & DeVilliers, J. (2005). *Diagnostic evaluation of language variation: Criterion referenced test.* San Antonio, TX: Harcourt Assessment.

Sickle Cell Disease Association of America. (2005). A comprehensive guide to SCD and SCDAA services. Retrieved April 20, 2011 from www.aap.org/sections/hemonc/sicklecell/SCDPatient.htm.

Simpson, G. M. (2008). A qualitative perspective of family resources among low income: African American grandmother-caregivers. *Journal of Gerontological Social Work, 51*(1-2), 19-41.

Smitherman, G. (1977). *Talkin and testifyin: the language of Black Americans.* Boston: Houghton-Mifflin.

Smitherman, G. (1993). "The Blacker the Berry, the Sweeter the Juice": African American Student Writers and the National Assessment of Educational Progress. Paper presented at the Annual Meeting of the National Council of Teachers of English (83rd, Pittsburgh, PA, November 17-22, 1993).

Steffensen, M. (1974). The acquisition of Black English. Doctoral dissertation, University of Illinois, Chicago.

Stockman, I. J. (1984, September). The development of linguistic norms for nonmainstream populations. Paper presented at the National Conference for Concerns for Minority Groups in Communication Disorders, Nashville, TN.

Stockman, I. J. (1986a). Language acquisition in culturally diverse populations: The black child as a case study. In O. Taylor (Ed.), *Nature of communication disorders in culturally and linguistically diverse populations* (pp. 117-156). San Diego: College Hill.

Stockman, I. J. (1986b). The development of linguistic norms for nonmainstream populations. In F. H. Bess, B. S. Clark, & H. R. Mitchell (Eds.), *Concerns for minority groups in communication disorders* [ASHA reports 16] (pp. 101-110). Rockville, MD: ASHA.

Stockman, I. (1996a). Phonological development in African American children. In A. Kamhi, K. Pollock, & J. Harris (Eds.) *Communication development and disorders in African American children: Research, assessment and intervention* (pp. 117-153). Baltimore: Brookes.

Stockman, I. (1996b). The promises and pitfalls of language sample analysis as an assessment tool for linguistic minority children. *Language, Speech, and Hearing Services in Schools, 27,* 355-366.

Stockman, I. J. (2000). The new Peabody Picture Vocabulary Test-III: An illusion of unbiased assessment. *Language, Speech, and Hearing Services in Schools, 31,* 340-354.

Stockman, I. (2006). Evidence for a minimal competence core of consonant sounds in the speech of African American children: A preliminary study. *Clinical Linguistics and Phonetics, 20*(10), 723-749.

Stockman, I. (2007). African American English speech acquisition. In S. McLeod (Ed.). *International guide to speech acquisition* (pp. 148-168). Clifton Park, NY: Delmar Learning.

Stockman, I. (2008). Toward validation of a minimal competence phonetic core for African American children. *Journal of Speech, Language, Hearing Research, 51,* 1244-1262.

Stockman, I. (2010). A review of developmental and applied language research on African American children: From a deficit to difference perspective on dialect difference. *Language, Speech, and Hearing Services in Schools, 4,* 23-38.

Stockman, I., Guillory, B., Siebert, M., & Boult, J. (2009). Toward validation of a minimal competence grammatical core. Manuscript in preparation.

Stockman, I., Karasinski, L., & Guillory, B. (2008). The use of conversational repairs by African American preschoolers. *Language, Speech, and Hearing Services in Schools, 39,* 461-474.

Stockman, I. J., & Vaughn-Cooke, F. (1982). A re-examination of research on the language of black children: The need for a new framework. *Journal of Education, 164,* 157-172.

Stockman, I., & Vaughn-Cooke (1986). Implications of semantic theory research for the language assessment of nonstandard speakers. *Topics in Language Disorders, 6*(4), 15-25.

Stockman, I. J., & Settle, S. (1991, November). Initial consonants in young black children's conversational speech. Poster presented at the annual meeting of the American Speech-Language-Hearing Association, Atlanta.

Stone, J. H. (2005). *Culture and disability.* Thousand Oaks: Sage Publications.

Sue, D., & Sue, D. F. (1990). *Counseling the culturally different: Theory and practice.* New York: John Wiley & Sons.

Tannen, D. (1982). The oral-literate continuum in discourse. In D. Tannen (Ed.), *Spoken and written language: Exploring orality and literacy* (pp. 1-16). Norwood, NJ: Ablex.

Taylor, O. L. (1987). Clinical practice as a social occasion. In L. C. Cole & V. R. Deal (Eds.), *Communication disorders in multicultural populations.* Unpublished manuscript. Rockville, MD: American Speech-Language-Hearing Association.

Terrazas, A. (2009). *African immigrants in the United States.* Washington, DC: Migration Policy Institute.

Terrell, S., Arensberg, K., & Ross, M. (1992). Parent-child comparative analysis: A criterion-referenced method for the nondiscriminatory assessment of a child who spoke a relatively uncommon dialect of English. *Language, Speech, Hearing Services in Schools, 23,* 34-42.

Terrell, F., & Terrell, S. (1981). An inventory to measure cultural mistrust among blacks. *Western Journal of Black Studies, 5,* 180-185.

United Nations (2010). United Nation AIDS report on the global AIDS epidemic. Joint United Nations Program on HIV/AIDS, New York, NY. Retrieved January 12, 2011 from http://www.unaids.org/globalreport/Global_report.htm.

U.S. Census Bureau (2006). American community survey. In S. Ruggles, M. Sobek, & T. Alexander (Eds.), *Integrated pubic use microdata series* (version 3.0). Minneapolis: Minnesota Population Center, 2004.

U.S. Census Bureau (2008). *Statistical abstract of the United States national data book, U.S. Department of Commerce.* Washington, DC: U.S. Government Printing Office.

U.S. Department of Health and Human Services (2005). National healthcare disparities report (AHRQ Publication No. 06-0017). Rockville, MD: Author.

U.S. Department of Homeland Security, Office of Immigration Statistics (2009). *Yearbook of immigration statistics.* Washington, DC: U.S. Government Printing Office.

Vaughn-Cooke, F. (1986). Lexical diffusion: Evidence from a decreolizing variety of Black English. In M. Montgomery & R. Bailey (Eds.), *Language variety in the South* (pp. 111-130). Tuscaloosa, AL: University of Alabama Press.

Vaughn-Cooke, F., & Wright-Harp, W. (1992). Lexical development in working-class black children. National Institutes of Health Grant #RR08005-23.

Velleman, S., Pearson, B., & Zurer, B. (2010). Differentiating speech sound disorders from phonological dialect and differences: implications of assessment and intervention. *Topics in Language Disorders, 30*(3), 176-188.

Washington, J., & Craig, H. (1992). Articulation test performance of low-income African American preschoolers with communication impairment. *Language, Speech, and Hearing Services in Schools, 22,* 203-207.

Washington, J. A., & Craig, H. K. (1994). Dialectal forms during discourse of urban African American preschoolers living in poverty. *Journal of Speech and Hearing Research, 37,* 816-823.

Washington, J. A., & Craig, H. K. (1998). Socioeconomic status and gender influences on children's dialectal variations. *Journal of Speech, Language, and Hearing Research, 41,* 618-626.

Westby, C. (1985). Learning to talk-talking to learn: Oral literate language differences. In C. Simon (Ed.), *Communication skills and classroom success* (pp. 181-212). San Diego: College Hill.

Williams, R., & Wolfram, W. (1976). *Social dialects: Differences versus disorders.* Rockville, MD: American Speech-Language-Hearing Association.

Wolfram, W., & Fasold, R. (1974). *The study of social dialects in American English.* Englewood Cliffs, NJ: Prentice Hall.

World FactBook (2010). Retrieved from https://www.cia.gov/library/publications/the-world-factbook/index.html.

World Health Organization (2004). Incidence of selected diseases by WHO region. Retrieved January 15, 2011 from http://www.who.int/healthinfo/global_burden_disease/GBD_report_2004update_part3.pdf.

Wyatt, T. (1991). Linguistic constraints on copula production in Black English child speech. Doctoral dissertation, University of Massachusetts, Worcester, MA.

Zuniga, J. (2010). *Communication disorders and HIV disease.* International Association of Physicians in AIDS Care. New York: Health Care Network.

RESOURCES

American Speech-Language-Hearing Association Office of Multicultural Affairs. Available at www.asha.org/practice/multicultural/.

National Black Association for Speech, Language and Hearing (NBASLH). Available at http://www.nbaslh.org.

Chapter 3

Asian and Pacific American Languages and Cultures

Li-Rong Lilly Cheng

The purpose of this chapter is to provide information on Asian and Hawaiian and other Pacific Island American (APA/PIA) cultures and languages for speech-language pathologists (SLPs) for assessment and intervention of communication disorders. Beginning with the 2000 census, "Asian" refers to people having origins in any of the original peoples of the Far East, Southeast Asia, or the Indian subcontinent. It includes people who indicated their race or races as "Asian Indian," "Chinese," "Filipino," "Korean," "Japanese," "Vietnamese," or "Other Asian," or wrote in entries such as Burmese, Hmong, Pakistani, or Thai (U.S. Census Bureau, 2000a). "Native Hawaiian and Other Pacific Islander" refers to people having origins in any of the original peoples of Hawaii, Guam, Samoa, or other Pacific Islands. It includes people who indicated their race or races as "Native Hawaiian," "Guamanian or Chamorro," "Samoan," or "Other Pacific Islander," or wrote in entries such as Tahitian, Mariana Islander, or Chuukese (U.S. Census Bureau, 2000a). Countries in the Middle East will be considered in Chapter 6 on Middle Eastern and Arab American Cultures.

APA/PIAs are fast becoming an influential presence in the United States socially, politically, and economically. In 2010, Gary Lock was U.S. Secretary of Commerce, Stephen Chu was U.S. Energy Secretary, and Eric Shinseki was U.S. Secretary of Veteran Affairs. All are APA/PIAs. The 1990 Immigration Act relaxed immigration restrictions, which facilitated the increase in immigration eligibility worldwide. The law created flexible and separate worldwide ceiling limits per country on family-based, employment-based, and diversity immigrant visas and a lottery-based immigration eligibility. Immediate relatives of U.S. citizens are exempted from this quota. As of 2008, there are 13.5 million individuals self-identified as Asian Americans, representing 4.5% of the total U.S. population, and the increase in the Asian population alone (26.8%) was three times more than the increase in the overall U.S. population (U.S. Census Bureau, 2008). It is projected that by 2050, the white population in this nation will decrease from 70% to less than 50%, whereas the Asian and Pacific and Hispanic or Latino population will continue to increase to above 50% (U.S. Census Bureau, 2000a). By the year 2020, Asian American children in U.S. schools are projected to total approximately 4.4 million. The largest number of Asian immigrants in the United States is the Chinese, second only to the immigrants from Mexico (U.S. Census, 2011). APA/PIAs are extremely diverse in all aspects of their ways of life, including language, culture, religion, attitudes toward education, child-rearing practices, and roles within the family. The Asian and Pacific Island cultures, however, have interacted with and influenced each other for many generations and therefore share many similarities. For example, historically, Korea and Vietnam were once considered part of the Han dynasty (108 BC and 111 BC). The Japanese traveled to China in the Tang Dynasty (618 to 907 AD) and learned the Chinese language and took it back to Japan. Buddhism, which originated in India, was spread to China through the work of Tang San Zang (602 to 664 AD) in the Tang Dynasty (Wriggins, 2004). Buddhism was spread to Japan in the Tang Dynasty. In the Ming Dynasty from 1405 to 1433 AD, General Cheng Ho traveled seven times from the port of Quanzhou (Zetong) to Southeast Asia and South Asia, and finally arrived in Africa (Suryadinata, 2005). The long history of foreign cultural exchanges with the West began with the Silk Road. It was an extensive interconnected network of trade routes across the Asian continent that expanded to Europe, with Chinese silk as the major primary commodity. Since its trade began in 206 BC, it led to the inflow of many Middle Easterners and Europeans to China. However, warfare drew cultures into conflicts. After the First Sino-Japanese War (1894 to 1895), the Qing Dynasty ceded Taiwan to Japan. In the 20th century, Japan invaded China in 1938, and the war lasted 8 years until 1945 when Japan surrendered. Although the exchange of cultures through trade, politics, and religion resulted in many similarities that we observe today, it is important to also remember that each of these groups is different in its own way. The following information is presented to provide an understanding of APA/PIAs to assist the SPL in providing services to the culturally and linguistically diverse APA/PIA people.

OVERVIEW OF ASIAN AND PACIFIC AMERICAN PEOPLE

APA/PIAs have been immigrating to the United States for more than two centuries, with the first records of arrival of Chinese dating from 1785. Since that time, more than 20 Asian groups have immigrated to the United States. As of the 2000 census, the most numerous APA/PIAs have origins in India, China, Taiwan, Hong Kong, the Philippines, Korea, and Vietnam (U.S. Census Bureau, 2000a). Between 1975 and 2002, more than 1 million refugees from Southeast Asia settled in the United States (Jiobu, 1996; U.S. Census Bureau, 2000a). Each of the countries in Asia and the Pacific represents an individual and distinct culture with unique values, beliefs, and world views. Each has its own languages and dialects, communication behaviors, and styles. Within each of the countries, there are many different ethnic groups as well. For example, in China, there are 56 ethnic groups with many different languages and dialects. Han Chinese represents 91.6% of the population, with 55 other nationalities or ethnic groups also present throughout the country. It is critical that clinicians recognize the heterogeneity of the APA/PIA people and consider the unique characteristic of each subgroup as well as the uniqueness of individuals within the group.

In general, APA/PIA populations practice the collectivist culture in contrast to the Western individualistic culture. The collectivist culture is more interdependent, whereas the individualist culture is more independent (Buszynski, 2004; Cheng, 2010; Gudykunst, 2001). Unlike the earlier immigrants from East Asia, the Southeast Asian immigrants, who came through the three waves of immigration between 1975 and 1980, represented a diverse group from Vietnam, Kampuchea, and Laos known as "the boat people." In addition, most of the Hmong people came from the mountains of Laos. Later immigrants since 1970 came from Hong Kong, China, India, Pakistan, Malaysia, Indonesia, and other Pacific Rim and Pacific Basin areas. After the attack on the United States on September 11, 2001, fewer immigrants came from Pakistan and Afghanistan because of immigration restrictions on persons from the Middle East.

Refugees and immigrants from Asia and the Pacific Islands come from a variety of historical, socioeconomic, educational, and political backgrounds. Like many other refugees, APA/PIA refugees are often victims of civil wars and poverty. In recent years, many Chinese entered the United States illegally and paid thousands of dollars to persons often known as "snake heads" to bring them over. They often work in squalid conditions to pay off their debts and eventually find their "American Dream." APA/PIAs bring a variety of financial profiles, languages, folk beliefs, world views, religious beliefs, child-rearing practices, and attitudes toward education, all of which have a profound impact on speech-language pathology services.

Descendents of Immigrants

In general, the second generation of immigrants hears the mother tongue at home and may attend weekend schools to keep up the home language. The third generation tends to speak English in most environments and may have little knowledge of the home language of their grandparents. The Southeast Asian refugees who came in the 1970s and 1980s have their second and third generation families here in the United States. Just like the Japanese and the Chinese Americans, the third generation speaks English fluently, and most do not speak another language at home.

Definitions of Impairments: Role of Culture

A cultural definition of what constitutes an impairment or disorder is dependent on the values of each cultural group. APA/PIA folklore is full of the belief system and spiritualism. The treatment of birth defects, disorders, and disabilities is influenced by cultural beliefs and by the socioeconomic status of the individual and the family within a given group (Cheng, 1999, 2009; Gollnick & Chinn, 2005; Strauss, 1990). For example, in the Chinese language, the term for *deaf* is generally linked with *mute;* the term for deaf and mute is one term. Another Chinese term, *handicap,* is a combination of "broken" and "disease." In all cultures, attitudes toward disabilities can be traced in part to folk beliefs and superstitions. Many Asian Pacific cultures define the cause of a health-related problem in spiritual terms (Cheng, 1999, 2007; Meyerson, 1990; Strauss, 1990).

Many Eastern cultures view a disabling condition as the result of wrongdoing of the individuals' ancestors, resulting in guilt and shame. The cause of disabilities is explained through a variety of spiritual or cultural beliefs, or both, such as imbalance of inner forces, also known as *Qi,* which means steam or energy, bad wind, spoiled foods, gods, demons or spirits, hot or cold forces, or fright. For example, the Chamorro culture views a disability as a gift from God and believes that the person with a disability belongs to everyone in the community and is in the extended family. The person with the disability is thus protected and sheltered by the family. For example, many Chinese believe disability is caused by karma (fate). Pakistanis may view individuals with a visible disability as a curse and ostracize them from society (Cheng, 1989, 2007; Trueba et al., 1993). Attitudes toward disabilities are a reflection of current and historical beliefs about the nature of disabilities. All over the world, people use different methods to treat illnesses and diseases, including consulting with a priest, barefoot doctor, herbalist, Qi-Gong specialist, clansman, shaman, elder, or physician. Among the Hmong, for example, surgical intervention is viewed as invasive and harmful. The Hmong believe that spirits may leave the body once the body is cut open, causing death (Fadiman, 1997). Treatment procedures also vary, ranging from surgical intervention or therapy to acupuncture, message, cao (coin rubbing), gat gio (pinching), giac (placing a very hot cup on the exposed area), steam inhalation, balm application, herbs, inhaling smoke or ashes from burnt incense, or the ingestion of hot or cold foods (Cheng, 1995a).

Child-Rearing Practices

Child-rearing practices and expectations from children vary widely from culture to culture (Cheng, 2009; Hammer & Weiss, 2000; Heath, 1983; Van Kleeck, 1994; Westby, 1990, 2009). With the single-child policy in China, many children are considered "spoiled" and are pampered by their parents and grandparents (Cheng, 2010). There are differences in how parents respond to their children's language, how and who interacts with children, and how parents and families encourage children to initiate and continue a verbal interaction. Differences in what are considered the best educational practices must be taken into account as well. Some families understand and support bilingual education; others believe that schools know best about how to educate their children and that English should be used in schools. Among families there is also variation about attitudes toward the first and second language and culture, various levels of formal education in the first or second language, or both, and expectation for their children (Butler & Cheng, 1996; Cheng, 1998; Heibert, 1991). In many Eastern cultures, education is considered a combination of teaching and nurturing.

Language

The hundreds of different languages and dialects that are spoken in East and Southeast Asia and the Pacific Islands can be classified into five major families: (1) Malayo-Polynesian (Austronesian), including Chamorro, Ilo-cano, Hawaiian, and Tagalog; (2) Sino-Tibetan, including Thai, Yao, Mandarin, and Cantonese; (3) Austroasiatic, including Khmer, Vietnamese, and Hmong; (4) Papuan, including New Guinean; and (5) Altaic, including Japanese and Korean. Additionally, there are 15 major languages in India from four language families: (1) Indo-Aryan, (2) Dravidian, (3) Austroasiatic, and (4) Tibeto-Burman (Shekar & Hegde, 1995). Many Asians are polyglots and can speak multiple languages; for example, the people from the Philippines can speak English, Tagalog, Ilocano, and a number of dialects.

Folk Beliefs, Religions, and Philosophical Views

The Asian and Pacific populations hold a variety of religious and philosophical beliefs. Major religions and philosophies include Buddhism, Catholicism, Christianity, Confucianism, Taoism, Shintoism, Animism, and Islam. In addition, because of Western influence, Christianity is practiced. There are many Catholic churches in the Philippines and across the Pacific Islands. Many Pacific Islanders consider the Bible a major source of inspiration. There are many different Asian and Pacific folk beliefs. Folk beliefs are generally passed down informally through oral history from generation to generation, whereas religious beliefs are generally archived and passed down formally. People vary in their reactions to folk beliefs because of their diverse experience in different levels of education and exposure to Western education cultures. In addition to folk beliefs, many APA/PIAs practice faith healing; other methods of healing include exercises such as Qi-Gong, over-the-counter drugs, prescription drugs, herbs, acupuncture, acupressure, cupping, or a combination of methods. The use of non-Western methods of healing may be difficult for Western physicians to manage in their overall treatment of patients because they are not always familiar with such methods.

Collectivism versus Individualism

In general, Western cultural patterns pertain to minimal context orientation and convey information in a precise, linear, and straightforward manner (Cheng, 1993, 1995a). This logical manner is very different from the circular mode of orientation generally practiced by the Eastern culture. Another important part of the Asian culture is the practice of collectivism, which is different from individualism, and treating clients from an individualistic culture is therefore very different from treating clients from a collectivist culture. The Asian culture practices the collectivist view, in which family is the most important. Family can be a distant relative, an adopted child, a neighbor, a member of a clan, village, or town, a person who shares the same last name, or a good friend.

Individualism is respectful of personal space and privacy. Personal information may not be willingly shared even with members of the immediate family. Independence is preferred over interdependence.

Eastern and Western Definitions of Education

Western education tends to draw out wisdom in a horizontal manner. The emphasis is on critical thinking, creativity, and problem solving. The Chinese term for education is made up of two characters: teaching and nurturing. This definition emphasizes the vertical relation of teaching to nurture. Eastern education tends to center on teaching, nurturing, and providing knowledge, which emphasizes the vertical relationship between teacher and student, or parent and child. In comparison, the English word *education* is derived from the Latin verb *educere,* which means to lead, draw, and bring out. The Latin origin appears to emphasize the horizontal "drawing out" of wisdom into vision.

The prevailing views toward education in most Asian and Pacific cultures present challenges for American educators and SPLs. People from China, Korea, Japan, and Vietnam often view education as the most important goal one can achieve in life. This is largely a result of the influence of the teachings and principles of Confucius (Cheng, 1993, 2010). APA/PIAs often have different approaches to learning, and these approaches have implications for the strategies Asian students use to learn. The selected examples in Table 3-1 are representative of some Asian attitudes toward education and their educational implications. The relative importance of each of the attitudes differs from culture to culture.

As shown in Table 3-1, there are incongruities between Asian students' learning styles and American teachers' teaching styles. These differences can lead to teachers' misconceptions of students and students' confusion over the "proper" way of schooling, particularly with the naturalistic, whole-language approach to intervention used especially with preschool and early elementary school children. Again, the relative importance of each of the concepts varies with cultural group and among individuals within the group. Educators need to be sensitive to cultural tendencies of various APA/PIA groups. These tendencies, however, should not be viewed as static cultural rules. Generalizations must be avoided, and predictions should not be made based on a superficial survey of the culture. With the advancement of science and technology, the cyber-generation has access to the Internet, the World Wide Web, and social networks; these students share many commonalities because of their linkages in cyberspace.

CULTURAL CHARACTERISTICS OF ASIAN AND PACIFIC PEOPLES

All APA/PIA groups and the individuals in these groups present a common background as immigrants or descendants of immigrants. However, each may have a very different story to tell. Such diverse personal and group experiences must be taken into consideration when working with these individuals.

Clearly, intragroup and intergroup differences exist among the Asian and Pacific Islander immigrant and refugee groups. Refugees are generally not prepared for emigration and often leave their country of origin suddenly because of political turmoil there. Immigrants leave their country of origin willingly and go through long periods of application and petition to the new country, and they are generally prepared for emigration. As stated earlier, caution should be taken to avoid overgeneralization of this information in relation to a particular client or family because the APA/PIA clients and their families represent diverse social, cultural, and linguistic backgrounds.

The Chinese

Immigration History

Since the end of World War II, Chinese have been immigrating to the United States mainly from Taiwan and Hong Kong to study, to join their families, or for business purposes. After President Nixon's diplomacy in the 1970s, more Chinese from the People's Republic of China entered the United States. Between the 1980 U.S. Census and 2006, the number of Chinese immigrants increased nearly fivefold, and about one fourth of these immigrants arrived in 2000 or later, making them the largest APA/PIA immigrant group in the United States. Immigrants from the People's Republic of China constituted one of the largest groups of immigrants. In addition to large populations settling in New York and California, increasing Chinese immigrant populations are found in other states such as Nebraska, Tennessee, South Dakota, and Idaho.

Some political history on the relationships between China, the People's Republic of China (PRC), and Taiwan, Republic of China (ROC) is worth covering here because clinicians should be aware of the sensitivity toward the cultural terminology associated with the political tension. In 1949 after the Chinese civil war, Chairman Mao of the Communist party took over mainland China. Chiang Kai-shek and the Kuomintang party went to Formosa and established Taiwan, ROC. Postwar political tension between the two coasts persisted. The situation was exacerbated in 1971 when the General Assembly Resolution 2758 expelled Taiwan from the United Nations and was replaced by the PRC in all United Nation organs. Political controversy between the PRC and ROC continued for decades regarding Taiwan

TABLE 3-1 Asian Attitudes toward Learning

Asian Cultural Themes	Educational Implications
Education is formal.	Teachers are formal and are expected to lecture.
Teachers are to be highly respected.	Teachers are not to be interrupted. Students are reluctant to ask questions.
Humility is an important virtue.	Students are not to "show off" or volunteer information.
Reading of factual information is studying.	Fiction is not considered serious reading.
It is important to have order and to be obedient.	Students are to sit quietly and listen attentively.
One learns by observation and by memorization.	Rote memory is considered an effective teaching tool.
Pattern practice and rote learning are studying.	Homework in pattern practice is important and is expected.

independence and distinctive political cultures. Today, the political tension is somewhat abated. Direct travel between Taiwan and China is permitted. Still, many individuals from Taiwan may consider themselves as "Taiwanese" rather than "Mainland Chinese" because of this political history, and clinicians should avoid making a reference to this national identity instead of the ethnic identity as Han Chinese. Despite the political tension, people from mainland China and Taiwan share the same official language of Mandarin and have generally similar cultural patterns (Olson, 2010).

Religion and Values

The 56 ethnic groups in China practice a variety of religions, including Buddhism, Taoism, Catholicism and other forms of Christianity, and Islam. They also believe in ancestral worship and Confucianism. One of the most important ideals of the Chinese culture is the pursuit and maintenance of harmony. Value is placed on outward calmness and on control of undesirable emotions such as anger, jealousy, hostility, aggression, and self-pity. Open expression of emotion and confrontation is viewed as undesirable. The three least desirable characteristics in Buddhism are greed, anger, and ignorance.

The Family

Chinese culture places a heavy emphasis on respect for elders and the strength of the family as a unit. Confucianism is practiced in China in which each member of the family has a role that is clearly defined through an intricate kinship system. Traditionally, the father was responsible for all decisions, with the mother having direct responsibility for caring for the elders and with the oldest son or daughter having responsibility for the care of his or her younger siblings. Parents taught their children to behave according to strict rules. In recent decades, however, the changing role of women and China's zero-population-growth policy have had a significant impact on the roles of women and children in the family. Most families have only one child, and these children may be called "little emperor" or "little empress." This phenomenon of the single-child policy is being studied by scholars to see whether there are adverse effects.

Education

The Chinese traditionally believe that education is extremely important. Chinese Americans work hard to remove any linguistic and cultural barriers to obtain a good education. Most traditional Chinese families expect their children to do well in school. Teachers are highly respected. If a child is successful in school, the entire family receives credit. Parents do not praise their children readily, even when they excel, because excellence is generally expected. If a child does poorly in school or needs special education,

the parents often feel ashamed, perceiving the difficulties as a sign of their own failure. Many Chinese American parents take their children to a Chinese language school on weekends and expect them to learn Chinese and maintain the culture.

Chinese students who have gone to school in the PRC do reasonably well in American schools because they have had a competitive education similar to that in the United States. The terms *model minority, invisible minority,* and *silent minority* have been used to describe the success of Chinese students. Their communicative disorders may be overlooked because they are quiet and often invisible. Also, Chinese students from the PRC have been coming to the United States in large numbers in the past two decades. In fact, they rank number 1 in foreign student populations on U.S. campuses. Many choose to stay in the United States after their graduation. Many sponsor their family members to come to the United States. These new immigrants tend to settle in large cities, including Los Angeles, San Francisco, Houston, New York, and Chicago. For example, Hacienda Heights and Monterey Park are two enclaves where the new Chinese immigrants gather. In addition, Queens in New York is the new "China Town." In these concentrated areas, Mandarin is the language of communication and commerce. Many new immigrants do not speak English, and they may have difficulties owing to communication breakdown at school when their children need English as a Second Language (ESL) courses or special education services. Lo (2009) provided case studies of the challenges in service delivery when parents do not speak English.

Language

(For language characteristics, please see Box 3-1.)

The Koreans

Immigration History

Since World War II, South Korea and North Korea have been politically divided. In 2000, the two governments finally attempted diplomatic affairs. However, since 2000, political tension has increased between the two Koreas. Information about North Korea is still limited; for more than 60 years, North Korea has kept its door closed. What we have learned is sketchy at best. We know that there are many people suffering from starvation and that the country is very poor. On the contrary, South Korea has a booming economy, and there are Korean Americans in major cities in the United States. Some are in politics. For example, Michelle Park Steel is a Korean American who is on the Board of Equalization in the State of California.

Korean immigration to the United States began in the early 20th century when Korean laborers went to Hawaii to work in the pineapple and sugarcane plantations and later

BOX 3-1 Chinese Language (Mandarin/Cantonese)

- More than 80 languages and hundreds of dialects are spoken in China.
- Some dialects are closely related, whereas others are mutually unintelligible, even though their words are graphically represented by the same characters (Cheng, 1993).
- In China proper:
  - Up to 94% are reported to speak Han (a Sino-Tibetan language) and its dialects Mandarin, Wu, Yue (Cantonese), Xiang, Gan, Kejia, and Min.
  - More than two thirds of Han speakers speak the Mandarin dialect.
- Two main dialects spoken by the Chinese in the United States are Mandarin (i.e., the national language of Taiwan and of the People's Republic of China) and Cantonese.
- There are 56 ethnic groups in China, and the main groups are Han, Manchurian, Mongolian, Huei, Tibetan, Miao (Hmong), and Yao.
- Dialects come from five broad language groupings: (1) Sino-Tibetan, (2) Altaic, (3) Malayo-Polynesian, (4) Austroasiatic, and (5) Indo-European.

Phonological Characteristics

- No consonant clusters in Mandarin and Cantonese
- Tonal language (Li & Thompson, 1981)
  - Each syllable has one tone marked
  - Mandarin tones:
    /ma/ with a high tone: "mother"
    /ma/ with a rising-falling tone: "horse"
    /ma/ with a rising tone: "scold"
    /ma/ with a falling tone: "numbness" or "canvas".
- Limited final consonants
  - Mandarin: /n/ and /ŋ/
  - Cantonese: /m/, /n/, /h/, /p/, /t/, /k/, and glottal stop /ʔ/
- Characteristics of English learners
  - Final consonant omission/deletion

- Difficulty with double and triple consonant clusters (e.g., /spl/, /str/)
- Sounds of substitution
  - Substitute /s/ and /ʃ/ to similar phonemes in Chinese.
  - Vowels: /e/ for /ɛ/; /æ/ and /i/ for /ɪ/; /ou/ for /ɔ/ (e.g., "boat" for bought), or /u/ for /ʌ/ (e.g., "roof" for rough)

Morphosyntactic Characteristics

- A noninflectional language
  - No plural markers, tense markers, copulas, the verb have, the auxiliary do, articles, the or a
- Different rules for the use of prepositions, pronouns, negatives (e.g., "me no like it" instead of "I don't like it"

Orthography

- One character is one syllable for one free morpheme (e.g., the Mandarin word, "child," is made of two morphemes or Chinese characters, /haɪ/ and /tsɪ/.

Pragmatic Differences

- Turn-taking: generally do not interrupt a speaker to ask questions
- Politeness:
  - Generally taught to be humble
  - Generally embarrassed when praised.
- Social or power distance: determined by age, class, and marital status
- Expression of emotions:
  - In the past, hugging, kissing, and touching were not frequently observed.
  - Today, more are willing to express their emotions readily.

Other nonverbal signs may also be interpreted differently (e.g., a giggle can be used as a sign of embarrassment rather than a sign of disrespect).

---

went to the mainland. Before World War II, however, the Korean community in the United States was not visible because of its small population. Most Korean Americans emigrated from South Korea in the past three decades. The population increased about 27-fold between 1970 and 2000 from approximately 38,000 to 1.41 million (U.S. Census Bureau, 2000a). Koreans are the seventh largest immigrant group in the United States (Migration Institute Policy, 2003).

Religion

Korean immigrants are primarily Christians. Historically, Korean Americans have had a very strong fundamentalist and conservative Christian heritage. Between 70% and 80% identify themselves as Christian; 40% of those are immigrants who were not Christians at the time of their arrival in

the United States. Many Christian churches in Korean communities conduct services in the Korean language. These churches also provide social and emotional support and informational help and serve as acculturation agents (Suh, 2004).

The Family

As with persons from other Asian cultures, Koreans value the extended family, which typically includes three generations (Kim, 1978). Additionally, Korean values of social relations share their common influence by Confucianism with the Chinese (Keum, 2000; Yao, 2000). Traditionally, the father is the head of the family and represents the family honor. He is responsible for the welfare of the family and is typically the sole provider. The father or other men in the Korean family do not typically help with household chores

(Kim, 1984). The Korean mother, who centers her work on the home, usually represents the family in dealing with the school. The elderly family members previously received a great deal of respect from younger family members.

Parent-child conflicts based on language and cultural differences have increased between immigrant children and their parents. Because of economic pressures, the size of the Korean family has decreased in the United States. Children have begun to question the traditional role of the father and to challenge his authority. According to Moon (2006), there has been a rapid decline in commitment and practice of filial piety and elder care. Particularly, most Korean American elders and caregivers do not believe that it violates filial piety to place an elderly parent in a nursing home, nor should the children live with their elderly parents who have functional limitations that require extensive care. Additionally, they prefer to move into an assisted living facility, rather than becoming a burden to family. However, most Korean American elders prefer independent living.

Education

Since 1945, the educational system in South Korea has been patterned after the American educational system of elementary school, junior high, and senior high, followed by 2 years of junior college or 4 years at a university (Kim, 1978). Teachers have a great deal of authority. Korean

classrooms are orderly. Korean children are socialized into an environment in which going to the best schools is highly valued. They are accustomed to working extremely hard to obtain high scores on college entrance examinations to get into the best colleges. They are directed from the very beginning into specific fields such as business, science, medicine, or engineering and are not typically encouraged to go into fine arts and human services. There is little room for other alternatives or for students who are not capable of high achievement. On the other hand, disability is viewed as misfortune or punishment, and families of children with a disability may experience self-blame. It is important that clinicians acknowledge family interdependence and avoid stereotypes and labeling (Kim-Rupnow, 2005).

Language

(For language characteristics, please see Box 3-2.)

The Japanese

Immigration History

The Japanese have had a history of immigrating to the United States since 1860. They have assimilated well and participate in social, business, civic, political, and religious groups outside Japanese American communities. However,

---

BOX 3-2 Korean Language

- Altaic family
- Koreans in North and South Korea speak the same language
- Various regional dialects, but mutually intelligible
- Until 1443, the Koreans used the Chinese written system.
- After that time, current orthography uses the Hangul system.

Phonological Characteristics
- No word stress
- Nineteen consonants and eight vowels
- No labiodental, interdental, or palatal fricatives
- Limited final consonants
  - No fricatives and affricates
- Characteristics of English learners
  - Final consonant omission/deletion
  - Final stops are often nasalized when they occur before a nasal sound (e.g., "banman" instead of "batman")
  - Difficulty with double and triple consonant clusters (e.g., /spl/, /str/)
  - Can sound monotonous and have difficulty with interrogative intonation
- Sounds of substitution
  - Substitute /b/ for /v/, /p/ for /v/, /s/ for /ʃ/, /s/ for /z/, /tʃ/ for /tʃ/, or /dz/ for /θ/.
  - Because [r] and [l] belong to the same phonetic category, they may be used interchangeably (e.g., r/l and l/r) (Chu, 1999)

- Korean does not have vowel distinction, so the following vowels are problematic: /i/, /ɪ/, /u/, /ʌ/, and /au/.

Morphosyntactic Characteristics
- No gender agreement, articles, no verb inflection for tense and number, and relative pronouns

Pragmatic Differences
- Chinese influence
  - Emphasis on harmony, filial piety, social order, fairness, reverence for elders, and the maintenance of human relationships.
- Seven levels of speech on a continuum of the most formal and polite form (addressing the Bible) to impolite forms (close friends)
  - Korean children acquire the basic rules of honorifics by the time they enter elementary school (Chu, 1999).
  - The choice of words and grammar denote the relationship between the communicators and the importance of that relationship (Chu, 1990).
- Nonverbal communication:
  - Taciturnity reduces the amount of verbal interchange.
  - Silence is a much more important part of communication for the Korean speaker than for the English speaker (Chu, 1990).

the ban of immigration by the Immigration Act of 1924 limited Japanese immigrants. With Japan and the United States in opposition during World War II, Japanese Americans were put into internment camps because of their ancestry. When the war ended, they returned to their communities and since then have continued to integrate into predominantly white residential neighborhoods. Japanese Americans are the third largest Asian group in the United States. In the 2000 census, the largest Japanese American communities were in California, Hawaii, Washington, New York, and Illinois. Each year, about 7000 Japanese people immigrate to the United States (U.S. Census Bureau, 2000a). Many Japanese are active in the political arena, including Congressman Mike Honda, Norman Mineta, and Senator Inoue.

Religion

Shintoism, a form of Buddhism, is the dominant religion in Japan today, although Christianity has been adopted by a large proportion of its population. In the United States, many Japanese Americans are Christians. The Japanese are the largest ethnic group in Hawaii, and many are practicing Christians. In many ways, owing to the long-standing nature of Buddhist and Shinto practices in Japanese society, many of the cultural values commonly associated with Japanese tradition have been strongly influenced by these religions.

The Family

Japanese Americans are primarily U.S.-born, second (nisei)-, third (sansei)-, and fourth (yonsei)-generation citizens. Japanese families generally value obedience, dependence on the family, formality in interpersonal relationships, and restraint in the expression of emotions. As in other Asian families, Japanese family members have well-defined roles and positions of power. Japanese children are expected to maintain emotional bonds with and dependence on their parents and only secondarily develop self-reliance (Ima & Labovitz, 1990). Japanese parents, wanting children to be receptive to adult expectations, continually refer to duty and obligation and invoke fear of ridicule and shame to control their children's lives. Many Japanese American families are fifth or higher generation in the United States. They have become one of the most assimilated of all Asian American groups. Perhaps as a direct result of this, they also have one of the highest interracial marriage rates of all Asian Americans. As more Japanese Americans intermarry, the less likely their children are to identify themselves as Japanese Americans.

Education

The teaching profession is one of the most highly regarded professions to the Japanese. To the Japanese, education is of prime importance. The Japanese student is expected to

be attentive, work cooperatively, and be willing to accept the teacher's word as significant (Ima & Labovitz, 1990). Japanese American students are often sent to after-school classes or to private tutors to ensure academic success. This contributes significantly to the pressures placed on children to be successful. On the contrary, disability, considered not conforming to the society, is often treated as a strictly private, family matter (Brightman, 2005). The adverse effect may be the family's reluctance to seek professional remediation, and the practitioner should be mindful of this possibility and seek a nonconfrontational approach. However, this cultural attitude may diminish in strength from one generation to the next.

There are distinct cultural differences between the Japanese and Americans in classroom interaction. For example, group behavior and cooperation, important cultural concepts in Japanese society, are taught and learned in preschool: going to school in Japan is primarily training in group life, or shudan seikatsu (Peak, 1991). Lewis (1995) asserts that Japanese students do not just work in groups, they work as groups. Teachers create groups and group activities to help children enhance one another's strengths and overcome one another's weaknesses. Japanese children in the United States may still be expected to behave this way because of parental influence (Westby, 2009).

Language

(For language characteristics, please see Box 3-3.)

The Southeast Asians

Southeast Asia comprises Vietnam, Thailand, Laos, Kampuchea (Cambodia), and Myamar (Burma). These countries have similar foods and are similar in geography and climate but have differences in culture and religion. Because the Burmese and Thai are few in number in the United States, these groups are not discussed in this chapter. This section will focus on the Vietnamese, Lao, Khmer, and Hmong groups.

Immigration History

Before 1975, there were few Southeast Asians in the United States. After 1975, however, more than 1 million Southeast Asians fled their countries because of Communist control. The Vietnamese Americans have settled in many parts of the United States. The children of the refugee families that came in the 1970s are now grown; many have achieved in a variety of professions, and their success stories are often reported in the media. The following is a short account of their past history.

The first wave of Southeast Asian immigrants (refugees), who arrived in the United States in 1975, were Vietnamese who were well educated and had some previous exposure to

BOX 3-3 Japanese Language

- Altaic language family

Phonological Characteristics:

- Not a tonal language
- Words are polysyllabic, with every syllable produced with an equal stress
- Eighteen consonants (/k/, /s/, /t/, /n/, /h/, /m/, /y/, /r/, /w/, /g/, /d/, /b/, /z/, /p/, /tʃ/, /ʃ/, and /j/)
- Five vowels (/a/, /i/, /u/, /e/, and /o/) and vary in duration
- The /h/ and /f/ are actually a vowel-less bilateral fricative [/ɸ/] made by holding the lips together loosely and blowing air through them.
- Double consonants occur (e.g., /kk/ and /pp/)
- One final consonant: /n/
- Characteristics of English learners
  - Add vowels to syllabify words containing consonant clusters and final consonants (kurepu/crepe, desuku/desk, miruku/milk)
  - Approximations of phonemes (/f/ phoneme is pronounced between /f/ and /h/, resulting in /food/hood/)
- Sounds of substitution
  - Substitutes /r/ for /l/ and vice versa, /s/ for /θ/, /z/ for /ð/, /j/ for /dʒ/ and /ʒ/, and /b/ for /v/ (Whitenack & Kikunaga, 1999)

Morphosyntactic Characteristics

- Elaborated inflectional system
- Canonical order is subject-object-verb
- A pronoun-drop language (personal pronouns are often omitted because they are inferred from the context)
- No gender agreement, plurals or singularity, articles, no verb inflection for number, and relative pronouns
- Case markers indicate the grammatical role of the lexicon in relations to the verb (e.g., *wo* for direct object, *ga* for topic marking)

Orthography

- Three writing scripts: Kana (Katakana and Hiragana) and Kanji
- Kanji: characters adopted from the Chinese system. The Japanese modified the Chinese symbols for phonetic purposes, organizing a syllabary called *Kana* in which each symbol represents one syllable (Cheng, 1991).

Pragmatic Differences

- Honorific and humble forms of speech levels, as marked by word choice and inflections on verbs
- Children may speak succinctly about collections of experiences rather than elaborating on any one experience in particular (Minami & McCabe, 1991).
- Mothers may:
  - Request proportionally fewer descriptions from their children
  - Pay more verbal attention to boys than to girls
  - Give fewer evaluations
  - Show more verbal attention than parents in North America
- Rapport and empathy (omoiyari): children are expected to anticipate what will be asked of them and to do it without being asked directly.

Western ideology and culture. The second wave of Southeast Asian refugees arrived between 1979 and 1982. This group included Vietnamese, Cambodians, Laotians, Hmong, and ethnic Chinese who emigrated from Southeast Asia, having escaped after considerable hardship. Consequently, these immigrants were less well educated, less likely to have had contact with Western culture, and likely to have spent a long period of time in refugee camps before immigrating. The third wave of refugees came in 1982. The main purpose of this program was to allow Amerasians, elders, and unaccompanied minors to immigrate to the United States. Some of these refugees were preliterate or illiterate.

Many of the refugees took advantage of the numerous programs established to assist in their resettlement. For some, life was stable and prosperous; their children had educational and employment opportunities. Other refugees did not adjust well, did not learn English, are underemployed, and feel a sense of loss and isolation. The problems of cultural and linguistic isolation are particularly serious for women who, because of staying at home to care for the children, have not had opportunities to learn English or adapt to their new surroundings (Ima & Keogh, 1995). Today, those refugees are aging and require home health care

and rehabilitation, and there are only a handful of bilingual SLPs to help them. Recently, many Vietnamese Americans have returned to Vietnam to establish businesses and visit their families.

According to the 2000 U.S. Census, more than 1.8 million Southeast Asian Americans reside in the United States, including 1,223,736 Vietnamese, 186,310 Hmong, 206,052 Cambodians, and 198,203 Laotians (not including Hmong) (U.S. Census Bureau, 2000b). California, Massachusetts, Pennsylvania, and the State of Washington have the highest Cambodian populations; California, Minnesota, and Wisconsin have the highest Hmong populations; Lao populations are highest in California, Wisconsin, and Texas; and Vietnamese populations are highest in California and Texas.

The Vietnamese

After 1975, when the Vietnam War ended, many Vietnamese immigrated to the United States as refugee "boat people" fleeing from Communist persecution. Today, Vietnamese Americans have one of the highest rates of naturalization, with 72% of foreign-born naturalized, which makes up 82% of total naturalizations (U.S. Census

Bureau, 2006). Most are either first or second generation Americans; however, as many as 1 million Vietnamese who are 5 years and older speak Vietnamese at home, making it the seventh most spoken language in the United States (Cornwell, 2006).

Most Vietnamese people practice Buddhism; however, Taoism, Catholicism, Christianity, and Confucianism are also followed. The teachings from these religions form the foundation of all Vietnamese traditions, customs, and manners.

The Family

Vietnamese names usually consist of three parts, which occur in the following order: family or clan name, middle name, and given name. Common middle names are Van in men and Thi in women. Common family names include Nguyen, Tran, and Le (Chhim et al., 1987). In the Vietnamese culture, the family is paternally oriented and is the chief source of social identity for the individual. The family members live and work together and look first to one another in times of crisis. The family usually consists of multiple generations who live under one roof and includes the husband and wife, their unmarried children, the husband's parents, and their sons' wives and children. Both parents share in disciplining the children. Discipline is usually of a soft, verbal type, with no corporal punishment and no extensive limits on behavior. Often, the responsibility for the children is given to older siblings.

Language

(For language characteristics, please see Box 3-4.)

The Hmong

Immigration History

Originally from China, the Hmong (also spelled *Miao, Mung, Muong, H'mong, Hmoob,* and *Hmuoung*) moved to the mountainous area of Southeast Asia, primarily Laos, centuries ago. In 2000, approximately 170,000 Hmong Americans were of full Hmong ancestry. Approximately 171,000 ethnic Hmong live in the United States (Pfeifer, 2009). The Hmong population is dispersed throughout the United States, and California, Minnesota, and Wisconsin are home to some of the largest Hmong populations (U.S. Census Bureau, 2000a). The first generation may have never been outside their mountain homeland before their immigration to the United States and thus may not have experiences of the modern world. The immense social and psychological upheaval the older Hmong experienced has left them physically and financially dependent on their children, physically and psychologically isolated, lacking in self-esteem, and with few of the skills that are necessary for life in American mainstream society. The elderly Hmong in the United States continue to practice folk medicine and perform indigenous religious rituals. Clint Eastwood's film,

---

BOX 3-4 Vietnamese Language

Phonological Characteristics
- A monosyllabic tonal language
- There are generally six tones in the Northern dialect.
- Large vowel system that has single vowels, diphthongs, and triphthongs
- Limited final consonants: /p/, /t/, /k/, /m/, /n/, and /ŋ/ (Te, 1987)

Morphosyntactic Characteristics
- Generally a subject-verb-object word order
- A pronoun-drop language (personal pronouns are often omitted because they are inferred from the context)
- No marking of case, gender, number, or tense (and, as a result, has no finite/nonfinite distinction)

Lexicon
- Many words derived from English, French, Malay, and Chinese.

Orthography
- Diacritical marks are used to signify the tone of each word.

Pragmatic Differences
- Proficient and educated speakers speak two forms of Vietnamese: the high (formal) form and the vernacular (informal) form (Chuong, 1990).
- Language pronouns are used to maintain proper social distance and interpersonal relationships and show the intensity of respect or disrespect (Chuong, 1990).

The Grand Torino, tells a touching story about the Hmong community in the United States.

Education

The Hmong view of education is different from that of other Asian refugee groups in that they have not had a long tradition of literacy and formal schooling. Oral tradition is much more important to the Hmong people, and their history is passed down from generation to generation by storytelling and rituals. The statistics on educational achievement of Hmong may reflect that many who immigrated as adults or young adults had little or no access to education before their immigration (U.S. Census Bureau, 2000b). Newer generations of the Hmong American youth go to school and are part of the larger community. Approximately 60% of all Hmong older than 24 years have a high school or equivalent level education, with about 7% holding a bachelor's degree or higher. With better access to higher education and employment than that of their parents, Hmong American children who are born in the United States can attain better economic opportunities than their parents.

In her 1997 book, *The Spirit Catches You and You Fall Down,* Anne Fadiman detailed the story of a Hmong girl,

Le, who had epilepsy and was treated by both folk medicine and Western medicine. The breakdown in communication and cultural misunderstanding resulted in permanent brain damage and left Le in a vegetative state.

Language

(For language characteristics, please see Box 3-5.)

The Khmers (Cambodians)

Immigration History

Khmer Americans are one of the youngest ethnic groups in the United States. At the time of the 2000 U.S. Census, the median age of people of Khmer ancestry was approximately 22 years, compared with 35.1 for Americans overall (Niedzwiecki & Duong, 2004). Almost half of the Khmer Americans counted in that Census year were younger than 20 years. Khmer Americans also live in larger households than other Americans. The average number per household was 5.03, compared with an average of 3.06 in white American and 3.48 in black American households. These statistics reflect that, small as their numbers are, Khmer will continue to grow as a proportion of American society.

When Cambodia fell into the hands of the communist Khmer Rouge in 1975, there was a complete devastation of the economic, social, and educational systems. Many of the 7 million Cambodians escaped the communist takeover, in the face of horrible brutalities, including torture, robbery, and rape. Upon settling in America, cultural adjustment has been difficult, especially for those who came from rural areas and have few relevant job skills and little U.S. cultural familiarity (Bankston, n.d.). Cultural identity remains an issue between and within generations: older adults see themselves as Cambodians and may be linguistically isolated from the American culture, and the youths, who were either born in the United States or have no memory of Cambodia, consider themselves entirely American.

Religion

Approximately 85% of the population in Cambodia adheres to Buddhism, the official religion. The temple was the place of worship and was traditionally located in the center of each rural community (Chhim et al., 1987). However, some Cambodian Americans converted to Christianity, either in the refugee camps, or after arriving in the United States; they often were influenced by the tragedies of recent Cambodian history, the desire to assimilate into the American mainstream, and limited access to their traditional religion (Bankston, n.d.).

Education

Cambodians born after the intellectual purge during the Khmer Rouge in 1975 have most likely had no formal education. The movie, *The Killing Field*, tells a vivid story about the Khmer Rouge era. Within the Khmer American community, a cultural mismatch was observed between high parental aspiration for the child's academic success and minimal parental involvement (Akiba, 2010). Traditionally, teachers in Cambodia are viewed as figures of authority of utmost respect. Parents, as a result, generally

---

BOX 3-5 Hmong Language

Two dialects: white (Hmoob Dawb) and green (Hmoob Ntsuab)

Phonological Characteristics
- A polysyllabic tonal language with seven tones
- Fifty-six initial consonants and one final consonant /ŋ/
- Sixteen vowel phonemes
- Four series of stopped consonants: voiced/voiceless fricatives, nasals, liquids, and a single voiced glide
- Aspirated and unaspirated forms (e.g., /p/, /r/, and /t/)
  - The form /r/ is a stop rather than a liquid
  - Produced in the midpalatal area and may sound like /t/ when aspirated or /d/ when unaspirated
- Word-initial consonant clusters only:
  - Single, double, triple, and quadruple clusters (e.g., nasals + stops (/np/ and /nt/) and nasals + stops + /l/ (/npl/)
- Characteristics of English learners
  - Pronunciation problems: Hmong consonantal sound transfers that correspond directly with English, mainly due to the correct places and the manners of articulation.
  - Students may have problems with phonemic awareness and the pronunciation of certain sounds in English.

- Difficulty with final consonants, particularly final consonant clusters
- Pronouncing polysyllabic words with correct primary and secondary stress is fairly easy, once the syllables are thought of as individual words with tones.
- May place too much importance on the vowel sound in unaccented syllables, not understanding that in English these vowels are often *schwa* sounds.

Morphosyntactic Characteristics
- Generally a subject-verb-object word order
- Noninflectional
- Characteristic of English learners:
  - Difficulty with tenses, using infinitives and gerunds, stringing several verbs together, and using adjectives after nouns

Orthography
- Tones are indicated by final letters using Roman alphabets.
- A typical word consists of a consonant, vowel, and tone marker (e.g., in "kuv," k is the consonant; u, the vowel; and v, the tone marker).

expect the teachers to exert parental roles as guidance in the child's academic growth. However, foreign-born Khmer Americans who experienced the Khmer Rouge may view academic success negatively. Further, many Khmer Americans hold the Buddhist belief in following fate to guide human development, which discourages parents from playing active roles to facilitate the child toward academic success. Many Cambodian youths are plagued by identity problems and often confront racism from classmates. The Cambodian culture values courtesy and avoidance of direct confrontation; however, this may be stereotyped as passivity.

Language

(For language characteristics, please see Box 3-6.)

The Laotians

Immigration History

Laotian immigration to the United States peaked after the Vietnam War. By the year 2000, although with somewhat a diminished growth rate compared with during the 1980s, the population increased to 167,792, and in 2008, more than 240,000 Laotian Americans resided throughout the United States, with large communities concentrated in Ohio, Oklahoma, Iowa, Florida, Pennsylvania, and Louisiana (Bankston & Hidalgo, 2007).

Religion

The Laotian refugees brought many customs and beliefs to the United States. Most Laotians are Theravada Buddhists. Most Laotian men are required to spend 2 or 3 weeks as monks before they marry. Many believe in the practice of folk medicine and the ritual of Baci. In the belief that every human being has 32 souls, many Laotians ask a sorcerer to perform the ritual of Baci to call back the soul outside of one's body of a person who is sick to bring about that person's recovery (Lewis & Luangpraseut, 1989).

Education

Many Laotian refugees lacked basic literacy skills in their native language and found it difficult to learn English. The main focus of Laotian education is the Pagoda, which teaches how to read the sacred Buddhist texts. It takes great effort for Laotian parents to convince their children to continue their education beyond high school. Students work for prestige or community recognition, but education in itself is not seen as a requirement. Few Laotian American youths attend college, which may be attributed to the families' economic disadvantages. In 1990, only 26% of Laotian

---

BOX 3-6 Khmer (Cambodian) Language

- Austroasiatic family
- Approximately 90% of Cambodians speak Khmer, although many other languages such as Thai, Lao, and Cham are also spoken (Ouk et al., 1988)
- A homogeneous language with very little dialectal variation from one region to the next
- Standard Khmer is the form of the national language
- Four different forms of Khmer exist: the language of the ordinary people, formal language, language of the clergy, and royal language.

Phonological Characteristics

- A nontonal language
- Usually monosyllabic or disyllabic, with stress always on the second syllable
- Eighty-five initial consonant clusters in Khmer (e.g., *Mty*ul and *Sd*ap)
- No final clusters
- Many English consonants overlap with Khmer, but not vice versa
- Fifty vowels and diphthong sounds
- Stops /p/, /t/, /k/, /ʔ/, and /d/ are aspirated and unaspirated.
- Two fricatives
- Characteristics of English learners
  - Add vowels to syllabify words containing consonant clusters and final consonants (kurepu/crepe, desuku/desk, miruku/milk)
  - Approximations of phonemes (/f/ phoneme is pronounced between /f/ and /h/, resulting in /food/hood/
- Sounds of substitution
  - Substitutes /k/ for /g/, /v/ for /w/, /f/ for /b/, /tʃ/ for /ʃ/, /s/ for /θ/, and /t/ for /θ/.
  - The /r/ is approximated as a trill r.
  - Many final consonants such as /r/, /d/, /g/, /s/, /b/, and /z/ are omitted.
  - The /b/ and /d/ are implosive, and there are possible vowel distortions of /ɛ/, /i/, /u/, and /æ/.

Morphosyntactic Characteristics

- Noninflectional
- Canonical order is subject-object-verb.
- English learner characteristics:
  - Difficulty with forms of the verb to be, including copula and auxiliary verbs and progressive and future tense markers
  - May experience difficulty with placement of negative markers

Lexicon

- The few polysyllabic words are compound words or derived from other languages such as French (e.g., particularly technical terms such as aeroplane, café, and poste ["stamp"])

Americans (excluding the Hmong) between the ages of 18 and 24 years attended college, compared with 39% of white Americans and 28% of African Americans. Laotian American youths also had relatively above-average dropout rates, at 12% between 16 and 19 years of age in 1990, compared with 10% of white Americans and 14% of African Americans (Bankston & Hidalgo, 2007).

Language

(For language characteristics, please see Box 3-7.)

The Indians

Immigration History

India is one of the most populous countries in the world, with a population of more than 1.1 billion. It is projected that India's population will surpass China's population in 20 years. It is the largest country on the Indian subcontinent, which includes India, Bangladesh, Nepal, Pakistan, Sri Lanka, and Bhutan. In the 1980s and 1990s, more Indians came to the United States than all of the years before combined. According to the 2000 U.S. Census, Indian Americans represent 16% of the APA/PIAs, which is the third largest group in the Asian American population after the Chinese Americans and Filipino Americans. About 1 million Indian Americans are foreign born. Between 1990 and 2000, the growth rate of Indians in America was 130%.

Since 2000, the Indian American growth rate has continued to be higher than 100% (U.S. Census Bureau, 2004).

Religion

India is the birthplace of many religions, including Hinduism, Jainism, Buddhism, and Sikhism. Most Indians believe in a God, but there may be a few atheists. All Hindus believe in the doctrine of karma or predestination. The caste system is another unique feature of Hindu life. The Brahmins have the highest place as the priestly clan, Kshatriyas are the warrior class, Vaisyas are the cultivators and merchants, and Sudras are the menials and are found only in some remote parts of India. Postindependence reform abolished the caste system legally, but, in practice, it still lingers. Most Indians in the United States came from the Brahmin group. As such, they represent a people of considerable wealth who place a very high value on education and professional careers, particularly those in science and medicine.

The Family

Families in India are typically very large and include extended families. All members, including three or four generations, often live under the same roof or in close proximity to one another. In the United States, family structure is changing, and nuclear families are quite prevalent. In contrast, immigrant Indian families in the United States are

---

BOX 3-7 Laotian Language

Phonological Characteristics
- A tonal language with six tones (Chhim et al., 1987)
- Most words are monosyllabic, with some compound and polysyllabic words borrowed from Indian languages
- Individual words also have tonemes
- No final consonants
- No word stress
- Characteristics of English learners
  - Distortions (e.g., /c + ʃ/ for /tʃ/)
  - Substitutions (e.g., s/ʃ and s/tʃ)
  - Final consonant omission
  - Stress on words

Morphosyntactic Characteristics
- Generally a subject-verb-object word order
- Subjects can be omitted.
- Adjectives follow nouns.
- Plurality and possession are expressed with different combinations of words rather than morphologic markers.
- No verb morphology (e.g., "I go," "you go," "he go"), articles, and to be verb for predicate adjectives (e.g., "food good," "dress beautiful")
- Interrogatives are marked by placing *bo* at the end of the sentence

- Characteristics of English learners
  - Difficulty with tenses, using articles, and using adjectives before nouns

Pragmatics
- Contrasting sets of lexical items are used in conversations with people of different social status.
- Seven different words may be used by the speaker to refer to himself or herself, depending on the partner's social rank before having a conversation.
- If the rank is unclear, Laotians are uneasy about responding (Lewis & Luangpraseut, 1989).
- Students may not say "I don't know," believing it is a sign of disrespect.
- Similarly, they may rarely say "no," believing it is a sign of rejection.

Orthography
- There are more symbols than there are sounds.
- A typical word consists of a consonant, vowel, and tone marker (e.g., in "kuv," k is the consonant; u, the vowel; and v, the tone marker).

smaller in size. Although the traditional caste system is no longer promoted and intercaste marriages are becoming quite common, individuals from different castes still do not come into contact with each other. The "untouchables" are still considered the lowest in the social stratum and are found only in some rural areas and among the uneducated. Marriage is a necessity for Hindus on religious grounds. Among the Hindus, a male child is more desirable because eventually he will become the head of the household.

Education

The educational system in India is based on the British system. English language is taught in the schools. The educated are bilingual or multilingual; however, the illiteracy rate is the highest in India of any nations, owing to the large number of people living in extreme poverty (National Sample Survey Office, 2008; Shekar & Hegde, 1995). Immigrants to the United States, however, have achieved high academic success and are, in general, well educated. Most are college educated and are fluent English speakers. Indian immigrants have the highest educational attainment of all ethnic groups in the United States (U.S. Department Commerce, 1993a, 1993b). They tend to hold technical, managerial, professional, and sales positions. They also have higher income than the general U.S. population (Shekar & Hegde, 1995). According to the Indian American Education Foundation (2008), disability is traditionally viewed as a stigma, leaving those with disability a marginalized population of the society. Specifically, this has adverse effects on education of children with disability. Kumar (2004) wrote

that 36 million of 90 million children with disability worldwide are Indian but that these children are denied the access to mainstream education.

Languages

(For language characteristics, please see Box 3-8.)

The Filipinos

Immigration History

Because of its history of trade and repeated colonization, the Filipino culture is a mosaic, with influence from Spanish, American, Chinese, Malay, Indian, and other cultures. Filipino immigration to the United States began after the onset of American rule because of an unstable political climate, poverty, the search for better economic and educational opportunities, and reunion with family members.

The Filipinos came to the United States in three major waves. The first wave, which began in 1903, consisted of a highly select group of young men seeking a college education. These students returned to the Philippines after completion of their education and encouraged other young men and women to seek education in the United States (Melendy, 1977). In the second wave of immigration, between 1906 and the 1930s, Filipinos settled in Hawaii, seeking agricultural employment in pineapple and sugarcane plantations. The third wave of Filipino immigration, which began in 1965, included many well-educated families with

---

BOX 3-8 Indian Language

- Includes 845 dialects and 225 distinct languages
- The constitution of India recognizes 21 major languages, including Sanskrit and English.
- Hindi, the national language, is spoken or understood by 40% of the population.
- Most of the immigrants from South Asia to the United States speak a language of the Indic or Dravidian family, and many speak English very well.

Phonological Characteristics
- Hindi and Kannada: a similar vowel system (Shekar and Hegde, 1995)
  - Each has five short vowels /i/, /e/, /u/, /o/, and /a/, and their long counterparts.
  - Five tense vowels /ɑ/, /e/, /i/, /o/, and /u/, and their lax counterparts
  - Vowel length is phonemic in Hindi and Kannada.
  - Hindi also has nasalized vowels.
- Hindi and Kannada consonants not found in English:
  - Voiced bilabials and velar aspirated stops

- Dental and retroflex consonants
- Voiced and voiceless palatal affricates
- Palatal nasal
- Approximated consonants: English vs. Hindi
  - English /v/ is a labiodental fricative; Hindi /v/ phoneme is a bilabial fricative.
  - English /w/ is an allophonic variation of the Hindi phoneme /v/.
- Characteristics of English learners
  - Distortions (e.g., /c + ʃ/ for /tʃ/)
  - Substitutions:
    Alveolar series /t, d, l, r, n, s, z/ with their retroflex counterparts
    /f/ with a voiceless bilabial fricative, /ɸ/
    /v/ with a labiodental approximate, /ʋ/
    Or, /θ, ð/ with dental stops /t̪/ and /d̪/ (Wells, 1982)
  - Distinct stress and intonation patterns may negatively affect intelligibility (Bansal, 1978, 1990).

school-aged children, many of whom were seeking to unite with their families.

Between 1980 and 1990, the Filipino population in the United States increased by 81.6% to 1.5 million people. Estimates from the American Community Survey in 2007 showed the size of the Filipino American community in 2007 to be 4 million or 1.5% of the U.S. population (U.S. Census Bureau, 2007).

The Family

The Filipino people practice a bilateral system of family responsibility, by which they are obligated to both sides of the family. The extended family is common. The Filipino culture places importance on specific roles and responsibilities that are hierarchically defined. The specific roles remain in effect even after children reach adulthood. The child is not viewed as an individual but rather as an extension of many generations of the family. Families tend to be large with frequent contact of immediate and extended members.

Education

Public education is compulsory through the elementary level in the Philippines, although this is not enforced by the authorities. The Filipino people are status conscious and view education as a key measure of status and the key to success. As a result, parents are eager for their children to do well in school and to perfect their English language skills (Monzon, 1984). More recently, Filipino Americans have some of the highest educational attainment rates in the United States with 47.9% of all Filipino Americans older than 25 years having a bachelor's degree, which correlates with rates observed in other Asian American subgroups (U.S. Census Bureau, 2004). These statistics also reflect the increase in Filipino professionals filling the education, health care, and information technology shortages in the United States.

The attitude on disability has a spiritual component. Families cope with disability by showing deep concerns, seeking assistance in various ways, and adjusting their roles and lives to the needs of the family member with disability (Shapiro, 2005).

Languages

(For language characteristics, please see Box 3-9.)

The Pacific Islanders

The Pacific Islands are grouped into three clusters: Polynesia including Hawaii (many islands), Melanesia (black islands), and Micronesia (small islands). The Pacific Islanders have different views and ways of life based on their experiences, although they may share commonalities. According to the 2000 U.S. Census, there are 861,000 Pacific Islanders residing in the United States and its territories (thus considered U.S. citizens or permanent residents), which is 0.3% of the nation's population, and they are most concentrated in Hawaii, Alaska, and the West Coast, especially in California (U.S. Census Bureau, 2000b). Owing to the small proportion of this population (0.3% of the U.S. population), this section will generally discuss the population as a whole and highlight pertinent group-specific information. It should also be noted that until the 2000 census, the Pacific Islander population had been clustered with all Asians, and thus the patterns and trends specific to their population are masked. The three largest groups within the Pacific Islanders including the U.S. territories are the native Hawaiians (approximately 38%), Samoans (about 22%), and Guamanians (15%), which make up about 75% of the Pacific Islander population. Of note, the Pacific Islander group is relatively young, with a median age of 28 years, compared with the nation's median age of 35 years, and there is a higher percentage of married household at 79%, compared with the nation's at 68%. Foreign-born Pacific Islanders are primarily Guamanians, Fijian, and other Pacific Islanders; they make up about 50% of the Pacific Islander population as a whole. The language use may reflect a bilingual trend in this population. Although 44% of the Pacific Islanders reported that they speak another language besides English at home, 82% reported that they speak English very well (U.S. Census Bureau, 2000b).

Religion and Folk Beliefs

Many religions are practiced in the Pacific Islands. As a result of contact with people from the United States, Pacific Islanders practice various forms of Christianity, including Catholicism, Mormonism, and Protestantism. In addition, many have combined Western religions with indigenous folk beliefs. Suruhana and Surahano (practitioners of folk medicine) are often consulted for treatment in a case of illness.

The Pacific Islanders also treasure and value collective behaviors (i.e., the reliance of existence on the group rather than on the individual). In the school environment, children read, chant, and practice in unison. The American tradition of individualism and focus on individual achievement violates the Pacific Islanders' principles of collective work and community-oriented achievement and education.

The Family

Families in the Pacific Islands are usually extended and can include three generations living in the same house. Islanders' families place heavy emphasis on authority and expect children to comply with the wishes of elders and authority figures. The primacy of parents corresponds to the apparent

BOX 3-9 Filipino Language

- Malayo-Polynesian family
- Authorities disagree on the exact number of Filipino languages, with an estimate of 75
- Major languages are Tagalog (the national language), Ilocano, and Visayan
- Tagalog is the native language of approximately 25% of Filipinos and is the first or second language of more than half of all Filipinos.
- Many from the Philippines speak English, the language of most education and business.

Phonological Characteristics

- A polysyllabic language with its own dialectal variations
- Twenty-seven phonemes
- Sixteen consonants, including the significant glottal stop
- Five single vowels and six diphthongs
- Characteristics of English learners
  - Nine English phonemes do not occur in Tagalog: /v/, /z/, /t/, /ð/, /dz/, /f/, /ʃ/, /tʃ/, and /θ/.
  - Substitution: /p/ for /f/, /b/ for /v/, /s/ for /z/, and /t/ for /ð/
  - Differences in vowel boundaries influence the difficulty distinguishing (e.g., between "lift" and "left").

Morphosyntactic Characteristics

- Generally an object-verb-subject word order (opposite of English)
- Most words consist of roots and affixes.
- The combination of the root and its affix or affixes determines the meaning of the word.
- Verbs do not indicate true time distinctions but characterize something as begun or not begun and, if begun, as completed or not completed.
- Verbs are not inflected for number and are the same form for singular and plural.

- Furthermore, Tagalog does not indicate gender in third-person singular pronouns.
- Plurality is marked by the word *onga* placed before the pluralized nominal (e.g., "onga bata" meaning children) or by another word carrying the concept of plurality (e.g., "dala wang bata" meaning two children).
- Plurality and possession are expressed with different combinations of words rather than morphologic markers.
- No verb morphology (e.g., "I go," "you go," "he go"), articles, and to be verb for predicate adjectives (e.g., "food good," "dress beautiful")
- Interrogatives are marked by placing *bo* at the end of the sentence.
- Characteristics of English learners:
  - Difficulty with plural morpheme -s, particularly when it is redundant in the context (e.g., many friends).

Pragmatics

- Filipinos are comfortable in one-on-one conversations that begin with small talk.
- In greeting, Filipinos enjoy a strong and longer handshake: placing the freehand on top of the hand being shaken and patting or placing the free hand on the shoulder of the person being greeted is a common practice.
- It can be expected that Filipinos will be a few minutes late in keeping appointments.
- Early arrival indicates overeagerness and is usually avoided.
- Nonverbal communication to express ideas, especially if they do not believe the listener understands what they are saying
- May point with tightly closed lips rather than the finger
- May clench fist with the thumb hidden and palm turned upward to indicate consent

---

lack of concern over the individual and the focus on the well-being of the family.

Education

Formal education was not part of Pacific Islander history until the Europeans came in the 1900s. Much of their educational tradition is based on oral learning. Learning style is usually passive, with rote memorization being preferred (Cheng, 1989). Teachers are respected, and children go to great lengths to please their teachers. Studies of Hawaiian, Tahitian, and Samoan children have suggested that they are likely to be unaccustomed to interacting with adults on a one-on-one basis because they are often in situations in which direct communication is with other children and not adults. In addition, absenteeism is common, reflecting not only the more relaxed style of the Islanders but also a different emphasis on academic expectancies, such as being on time and completing projects. The U.S.

educational emphases on the individual, individual excellence, and creativity contradicts the Pacific Islanders' learning style, and it basically undermines their sense of well-being (the aloha spirit) because their identity is tied to the group and is not individualistic. As a group, the Pacific Islanders perform at much lower levels in school than their Hispanic and African American counterparts (Ima & Labovitz, 1990).

Particularly, statistics since 2000 revealed that the college graduation rate for Pacific Islanders is well below the average (U.S. Census Bureau, 2000b). Particularly, teachers' stereotypical expectations of the Samoan youths reflected the dissociation between academic success and Samoan identity. Consequently, the Samoan youths experience the stigmatized "othering"—that choosing one implied forfeiting the other (Stewart, 2005). According to Takeuchi and Hune (2008), statistics showed that in Washington State, children of API descent are often less engaged in school with high rates of absences, at risk for failing to graduate high school, and more likely to score below academic standards on state-wide standardize test.

Languages

Among the 5 million inhabitants of the Pacific Islands, more than 1200 indigenous languages are spoken. The lingua francas used by the Pacific Islanders are Chamorro, French, English, Pidgin, Spanish, and Bahasa Indonesian. Languages are heavily influenced by multicultural sources. Pidgin (meaning the language of business), or Hawaiian Creole English (HCE) , is an important part of the communication system among Pacific Islanders, including Hawaiians. Those who speak Pacific Island languages represent approximately 90,000 or 7.9% of those in Hawaii (U.S. Census Bureau, 2000b). Although looked down upon by some, it is the mode of communication that was first established by plantation workers who came from many different backgrounds as a way to understand each other. At the time of the 2000 census, 73.4% of Hawaiians who were 5 years or older spoke only English at home (U.S. Census Bureau, 2000b). Many local residents speak the Hawaiian pidgin and children may come to school speaking pidgin as well as English. Clinicians need to be aware of the possible bilingual background and not consider this form of discourse a disorder.

The diversity that exists among Pacific Islanders and persons from other Asian groups is challenging and interesting. The previous sections have provided a glimpse of this diversity. For SPLs and audiologists, the diversity among people in the Pacific Islands offers the beginning of a long quest for cross-cultural communicative competence. The following section offers guiding principles on assessment and intervention of APA/PIA populations.

ASSESSMENT AND INTERVENTION

Assessment Strategies

Chapter 13 focuses on assessment. This section offers brief principles and guidelines specific for the APA/PIA population.

APA/PIAs learning English as a second language with communication disorders face tremendous challenges in meeting the demands of school and acculturating into the American mainstream. To provide quality clinical services to children and adults with possible speech-language and hearing disorders, linguistically and culturally appropriate assessment is necessary. The purpose of assessment is to identify strengths and weaknesses of the individual so that appropriate clinical intervention can be provided, if necessary. As in all assessment, it is necessary to distinguish between language differences and disorders. This is particularly challenging in the assessment of communication in children who may still be in the process of developing

language. It is also challenging because of the many cultures, languages, and dialects of the APA/PIA people, the amount of exposure to English, and the difficulty in identifying clinicians competent to make an assessment in the first language of the client.

APA/PIA children and adults who are in need of speech, language, and hearing services often are underserved owing to a lack of trained bilingual professionals and understanding of the life history of the clients. The number of SPLs and audiologists in the United States who speak Vietnamese, Laotian, Khmer, Chamorro, Tagalog, Hmong, or Korean is minuscule. Only a few SPLs speak some of the other more widely used Asian languages, such as Mandarin and Japanese. Consequently, speech-language disorders in APA/PIA children and adults are sometimes not identified, and language differences are identified incorrectly as language disorders. According to the Individuals with Disabilities Education Act (IDEA), assessment of the abilities of all children in the United States and its territories with limited English proficiency must be conducted in their native language as mandated under Section 300.304 for evaluation procedures (U.S. Department of Education, 2004). Family involvement as mandated by the IDEA may pose a challenge because of cultural differences in the perception of the family's role in education. This may necessitate seeking the assistance of interpreters. (For additional information on the use of interpreters in assessment, see Chapter 13.)

Clients have diverse linguistic, paralinguistic, stylistic, and discourse backgrounds and experiences. It is important that clinicians determine the degree to which the communication behaviors observed are due to cultural and linguistic differences, rather than to a disorder. As indicated earlier, Asian and Pacific Islanders have many different values and beliefs. An awareness of the particular cultural and linguistic values of the particular population to which the individual client belongs is an essential tool for the SLP. The clinician must not assume the characteristics of the client's language and culture. It is essential that the clinician regard each individual client as an individual with unique cultural and linguistic characteristics and a unique degree of assimilation and acculturation. Because of the uniqueness and heterogeneity of APA/PIA clients, the traditional mode of assessment may not be appropriate.

Traditional Approach to Assessment

Traditional assessment approaches that use standardized formal tests designed to measure discrete areas of language are not able to effectively account for cultural and linguistic diversities. When incongruities between the native culture and the mainstream American culture exist, clients, particularly children, tend to experience confusion. The translation of standardized tests into other languages to accommodate the needs of culturally and linguistically diverse students is inappropriate. There are many words that cannot be translated from one language into another language without losing meaning. Also, words or concepts that may be considered common in English may not be common in the language of the APA/PIA being tested. According to Cheng (1991, 2009), these may include names of household objects (e.g., broiler oven), clothing (e.g., pea coat), sports (e.g., American football), musical instruments (e.g., tuba), professions, historically related events and holidays, games, values, and stories. Thus, formal assessment instruments, translated tests, and their interpretive scores are inappropriate for this population.

Recommended Assessment Procedures

The following guidelines for assessment are often referred to as the RIOT procedure (Cheng, 1995b). They are adapted here for APA/PIA populations:

1. **R**eview. Review all pertinent documents and background information. Many Asian and Pacific Island countries do not keep cumulative school records. When available, the records may not be in English. The academic subjects on the records may not match those of the traditional American curriculum. Oral reports are sometimes unreliable, yet they may be the only way to find the necessary information. Parents may be reluctant to discuss social and family background. An interpreter may be needed to obtain this information because of the lack of English language proficiency of the parents or guardians. Medical records may also be difficult to obtain. Pregnancy and delivery records might not have been kept, especially if the birth was a home birth or in a refugee camp. The client may be reluctant to share personal information. Medical care may have been provided by a family member or other person who would not have kept records. Records, if available, may not be provided in English. Interpreters may need to be used to get background information about pregnancy and birth history.

2. **I**nterview. Interview teachers, peers, family members, and other informants to collect data regarding the client and the home environment. The family can provide valuable information about the communicative competence of the client at home and in the community, as well as historical and comparative data on the client's language skills. The clinician needs information regarding the client's proficiency in the home languages and English. A description of the home environment and any cultural differences must also be discovered. The languages used in the home, proficiency of family members in different languages, patterns of language use, and ways the family spends time together are some areas for investigation. It is important to determine the family concerns and priorities. Teachers and other professionals can provide information about the child's communication behavior in relation to classmates, attempts to communicate, and attempts to revise and clarify communication failure. Interview questions are available from multiple sources (Cheng, 1990, 1991; Langdon & Saenz, 1996). Questions should focus on obtaining information on how the client functions in his or her natural environment in relation to age peers who have had the same or similar exposure to language or to English. Questions about comparing behavior with playmates or a play group might reveal useful data.

3. **O**bserve. Observe the client over time in multiple contexts with multiple communication partners. Observe interactions at school, inside and outside the classroom, and at home. This cognitive-ecological-functional model takes into account the fact that clients often behave differently in different settings. Clinicians determine how the client interacts with others, reacts to different situations and individuals, and adapts to social communication barriers. Direct observation of social behavior with multiple participants allows the clinician the opportunity to observe the ways the client communicates. Observe family dynamics with consideration given to the family role. Observe the proficiency of the parents in the native language and English. What languages do the parents and family members use in addressing the client? Do they use the same level of language in addressing the client as they do to his or her age peers?

4. **T**est. Test the client using informal dynamic assessment procedures in English and the home language. Use the portfolio approach by keeping records of the client's performance over time. Interact with the client, being sensitive to his or her need to create meaning based on what is perceived as important, the client's frame of reference, and his or her experiences. Describe the client during genuine communication in a naturalistic environment with low anxiety and high motivation. Assessment procedures should be culturally and pragmatically appropriate.

Collect narrative samples using wordless books, pictures, or other stimuli. Asking the client to describe familiar experiences, retell stories, predict future events, and solve problems provides rich data for analysis. Literature from the client's background or narratives can be used to assess skill in accounting (description of a present event), recounting (description of a past event), and event casting (description of a future event) (Heath, 1983). Stories translated into English may not be easily adapted to make them culturally appropriate. The clinician should then determine whether there are difficulties in communication owing to possible cultural and social mismatches between the two languages or to a true disorder.

In addition to the above recommended procedure, dynamic assessment procedure is highly recommended. Russian psychologist Lev Vygostky advocated the notion of Zone of Proximal Development, which led to the development of dynamic assessment. For more information, please refer to Vygostky's sociocultural theory (Johnson, 2004) and research on the methodology of dynamic assessments (Gutierrez-Clellen & Peña, 2001; Peña et al., 1992, 2001, 2006; Stubbe Kester et al., 2001).

SPECIAL CHALLENGES IN INTERVENTION

What clinicians learn from the assessment should be integrated into their intervention strategies. Intervention should be constructed based on what is most productive for promoting communication and should incorporate the client's personal and cultural experiences. Salient and relevant features of the client's culture should be highlighted to enhance and empower the client. Care should be taken not to consider differences in communication style as indicators of a communication disorder.

The following verbal and nonverbal communication behaviors can easily be misunderstood by clinicians working with APA/PIA clients:

Delay or hesitation in response

Frequent topic shifts and difficulty with topic maintenance

Differences in the meaning of facial expressions, such as a frown signaling concentration rather than displeasure

Short responses

Use of a soft-spoken voice

Lack of participation and lack of volunteering information

Different nonverbal messages, including eye contact, such as avoiding eye contact with adults, and body language, such as avoiding being hugged or kissed

Embarrassment over praise

Different greeting rituals, which may appear impolite, such as looking down when the clinician approaches

Use of Asian language–influenced English, such as the deletion of plural and past tense (Cheng, 1999)

APA/PIA clients may be fluent in English but use the discourse rules from their home culture, such as speaking softly to persons in authority, looking down or away, and avoiding close physical contact.

Surface analysis of linguistic and pragmatic functions is not sufficient to determine the communicative competence of children and might even misguide clinicians in their decision-making process. The home culture and discourse rules of the clients need to be explored by the clinicians, and discourse rules must be explained explicitly and modeled repeatedly before APA/PIA clients can make sense of the socialization process (Cheng, 1989, 1996). Cultural rules are not static but fluid. Children as well as adults learn to adjust to different languages and cultures by code switching and making necessary accommodation. It is difficult for adults to make the switches because their native culture is deeply ingrained. The acquisition of cultural competence is an important part of the training and education of SLPs. The topic of cultural competence has been discussed in many forums (Earley and Mosakowski, 2004; Lewis & Cheng, 2008).

Working with the Family

Sociologic and psychological difficulties may arise in the conflict of culture, language, and ideology between new-generation APA/PIAs, their parents, and the U.S. educational system. These difficulties can include the background of traditions, religions, and histories of the specific APA/PIA population; problems of acculturation; the understanding of societal rules; contrasting influences from home and the classroom or society; confusion regarding one's sense of identity relating to culture, society, and family; the definition of disability; and the implications of special education services.

Intervention activities and materials can be selected based on the client's family and cultural background using activities that are culturally and socially relevant. The concept of an optimal language learning experience and environment (OLLEE; Cheng, 2009, 2010) serves as the foundation of service provision. Alternative strategies should be offered when clients or caregivers are reluctant to accept the treatment program recommended by the clinician. Inviting the family to participate in special classes or speech and language sessions is a useful way to provide the needed information. Seeking assistance from community leaders and social service providers may also be necessary to ensure that services will be provided in a culturally appropriate manner and to convince the clients of the importance of therapy or recommended programs. The clients or caregivers may also be asked to talk with other persons in the community who have experiences with treatment programs. Other individuals can be effective in sharing their personal stories about their experiences with therapy. The clinician should be patient with the clients by letting them think through a problem and waiting for them to make the decision to participate in the treatment program. Several additional resources are provided in Chapter 13 to assist the clinician in providing culturally appropriate services.

Working with Other Professionals

Clinicians need support from other professionals in their attempts to examine the cultural dimensions of interaction between themselves and their clients. While trying to comprehend cultural differences, clinicians must also guard against stereotyping the clients.

OPTIMAL LANGUAGE LEARNING EXPERIENCE AND ENVIRONMENT

Creating an OLLEE is critical (Cheng, 2009). The following suggestions might be helpful:

1. Engage children in meaningful discourse
2. Read stories to children
3. Ask critical questions.
4. Ask hypothetical questions.
5. Provide a variety of reading materials.
6. Create a language-rich environment.
7. Create collective stories.
8. Engage in multicultural literacy.

Intervention

Activities that provide interesting content and natural opportunities for social interaction can provide a rich environment for language learning (Cheng, 2009, 2010; Goodman, 1986). The principles of experiential learning can be applied to speech-language intervention with the APA/PIA client, with the understanding that the approach is contrary to the teaching and learning styles of some cultural groups in which more direct instruction is the norm.

Johnston and associates (1984) provided therapy guidelines useful for pragmatic activities, some of which can be adapted for APA/PIA clients. For example, the conversation module includes talking on the telephone and asking for directions.

The following are specific guiding principles for all clinicians and other professionals to enrich language learning in real-life contexts for APA/PIA clients (Cheng, 1994, 2007, 2009, 2010):

1. Use language in multiple social contexts. Clients should be encouraged to participate in high-interest activities that are familiar to them. For example, Japanese clients could be encouraged to tell a native folk story. Chinese clients could be asked to demonstrate how to use chopsticks or to relate an event or story important to the culture.
2. Facilitate language learning in low-risk, low-cognitive-demand, and low-anxiety contexts. The clinician should get to know the client as an individual and not rely on general knowledge usually attributed to a cultural group. He or she should learn and understand interests, likes, and dislikes of the client. The clinician should attempt to determine the areas of strength and interest of the client and use those areas to form the context of the clinical intervention.
3. Use language activities that are experiential and relevant. When a clinician learns more about the clients and their experiences, the clients can be asked to share stories about experiences that are not only relevant but also meaningful to the client. Such activities can be a source of learning and bonding for everyone.

4. Encourage language interactions in comprehensible contexts, starting from the least demanding and proceeding to more cognitively challenging tasks. Art, music, and experiential activities with lower reliance on verbal language should be used before activities that require high verbal ability or high cultural knowledge, such as reading text on difficult topics. Contexts relevant to the client's interest and occupation serve as a support for learning new language skills.
5. Respect differences between home language discourse rules and discourse rules or expectation in English (Cheng, 1994). Clinicians need to make the effort to explain explicitly what is expected in discourse in the new language. Games and activities that are common and understood by American children may be unfamiliar to clients who have recently arrived in the country. The concepts of winning a game may also be new. Concepts in games such as Monopoly may be unfamiliar to clients unfamiliar with the American system of real estate and finance.
6. Seek natural support systems and allow clients to have self-selected cooperative groups. Clients should be allowed to select their own groups, seeking out peers with whom they are comfortable. Such an atmosphere provides the support they need to socialize.
7. Provide culturally familiar activities and unfamiliar activities. Most Asian newcomers do not know much about the Boy Scouts or Girls Scouts, the YMCA, YWCA, PTA, Boys and Girls Clubs, or the numerous other after-school programs that the schools and the community offer to the students and their families. Families should be encouraged to participate in some of these programs as appropriate. The schools, on the other hand, can invite family or community members to come into the schools and provide information on ethnic cultural activities from the various ethnic groups, thus providing the family and client the opportunity to show their peers the activities that they are familiar with and value. This exchange is mutually empowering and provides the school-home-child connection.
8. Use a "talk story" approach. Au and Jordan (1981) propose establishing contact with students first by chatting with them without any set agenda, capitalizing on the preexisting cognitive and linguistic experiences of the children. The approach allows the students to "talk story" (a major speech event in Hawaiian culture).

SPECIAL CLINICAL CONSIDERATIONS: ACCENT, STRESS, VOICE, AND TONES

Accent identifies a person as a member or nonmember of a particular linguistic community (Ainsfeld et al., 1962). Everyone speaks with an accent, ranging from a New York City accent to a Southern accent to a Cantonese accent. For tonal languages, tones are phonemic, and each syllable is assigned a specific tone. In English, intonation patterns are suprasegmental, and a variation of tones does not result in a completely different meaning. Individuals with tonal languages may apply their tonal patterns in their delivery of English, which makes their speech patterns distinct; hence, there are many versions of the English language, including French-influenced English, Hindi-influenced English, Tagalog-influenced English, Singaporean English, Australian English, British English, American English, and so on. Many of the distinct patterns and accents are not easy to change and can interfere with communication. Voice patterns also differ from culture to culture. A deep, soft voice indicates authority in Japan, but the same voice pattern may be viewed as a disorder in the United States. The aesthetics of voice also differ from culture to culture. For example, Chinese opera singers can use falsetto for performance, which sounds very pleasant to the audience; however, to the Western ear, Chinese opera may sound piercing and unpleasant. An easy way to understand this is to compare Chinese opera or Japanese opera with Western opera. An appreciation of the linguistic diversity of APA/PIAs will facilitate better communication between service providers and their APA/PIA clients. (For information on reducing accent in intervention, see Chapter 14.)

CONCLUSION

Providing speech-language and hearing services to individuals from Asia and Pacific Island countries is challenging. Preassessment information on the language, culture, and personal life history of the individual lays a solid foundation to further explore the client's strengths and weaknesses. Assessment procedures need to be guided by the general principles of being fair to the culture. Results of assessment should take into consideration the cultural and pragmatic variables of the individual. Intervention can be extremely rewarding when culturally relevant and appropriate approaches are used. The goals of intervention must include the enhancement of appropriate language and communication behaviors, home language, and literacy. Clinicians need to be creative and sensitive in their intervention to provide comfortable, productive, and enriching services for all clients.

REFERENCES

Akiba, D. (2010). Cambodian Americans and education: Understanding the intersections between cultural tradition and U.S. schooling. *The Educational Forum, 74*, 328-333.

Ainsfeld, M., Bogo, N., & Lambert, W. (1962). Evaluational reactions to accented English speech. *Journal of Abnormal Psychology, 65*, 223-231.

Au, K., & Jordan, K. (1981). Teaching reading to Hawaiian children: Finding a culturally appropriate solution. In H. Trueba, G. P. Guthrie, & K. Au (Eds.), *Culture and the bilingual classroom* (pp. 139-152). Rowley, MA: Newbury.

Bankston C. L. III (n.d.). Cambodian Americans. In *Countries and their cultures*. Retrieved October 18, 2010, from www.everyculture.com/multi/Bu-Dr/Cambodian-Americans.html.

Bankston C. L. III, & Hidalgo, D. A. (2007). Southeast Asia: Laos, Cambodia, Thailand. In M.C. Waters, R. Ueda, & H.B. Marrow (Eds.), *The new Americans: A guide to immigration since 1965* (pp. 625-640). Cambridge, MA: Harvard University Press.

Bansal, R. K. (1978). The phonology of Indian English. In R. Mohan (Ed.), *Indian writing in English* (pp. 101-114). Bombay, India: Orient Longman.

Bansal, R. K. (1990). The pronunciation of English in India. In S. Ramsaran (Ed.), *Studies in the pronunciation of English: A commemorative volume in honor of A.C. Gimson*. London: Routledge.

Brightman, J. D. (2005). AAPI culture brief: Japan. In *National Technical Assistance Center*. Retrieved October 12, 2010, from www.ntac.hawaii.edu/downloads/products/briefs/culture/pdf/ACB-Vol2-Iss6-Japan.pdf

Buszynski, L. (2004). *Asia Pacific security: Values and identity*. New York: Routledge Curzon.

Butler, K., & Cheng, L. L. (Eds.) (1996). Beyond bilingualism: Language acquisition and disorder. A global perspective. *Topics in Language Disorders, 16*, 1-6.

Cheng, L. L. (1989). Service delivery to Asian/Pacific LEP children: A cross-cultural framework. *Topics in Language Disorders, 9*, 1-14.

Cheng, L. L. (1990). The identification of communicative disorders in Asian-Pacific students. *Journal of Child Communicative Disorders, 13*, 113-119.

Cheng, L. L. (1991). *Assessing Asian language performance: Guidelines for evaluating LEP students* (2nd ed.). Oceanside, CA: Academic Communication Associates.

Cheng, L. L. (1993). Deafness: An Asian/Pacific Island perspective. In K. M. Christensen & G. L. Delgado (Eds.), *Multicultural issues in deafness* (pp. 113-126). White Plains, NY: Longman.

Cheng, L. L. (1994). Difficult discourse: An untold Asian story. In D. N. Ripich & N. A. Creaghead (Eds.), *School discourse problems* (2nd ed.) (pp. 155-170). San Diego: Singular.

Cheng, L. L. (1995a). *Integrating language and learning for inclusion: An Asian-Pacific focus*. San Diego: Singular.

Cheng, L. L. (1995b, July). The bilingual language-delayed child: Diagnosis and intervention with the older school-age bilingual child. Paper presented at the Israeli Speech and Hearing Association International Symposium on Bilingualism, Haifa, Israel.

Cheng, L. L. (1996). Beyond bilingualism: A quest for communicative competence. *Topics in Language Disorders, 16*, 9-21.

Cheng, L. L. (1998). Beyond multiculturalism: Cultural translators make it happen. In V. O. Pang & L. L. Cheng (Eds.), *Struggling to be heard* (pp. 105-122). Albany, NY: SUNY Press.

Cheng, L. L. (1999). Sociocultural adjustment of Chinese-American students. In C. C. Park & M. Chi (Eds.), *Asian-American education* (pp. 1-19). London: Bergin & Garvey.

Cheng, L. L. (2007). Cultural intelligence (CQ): A quest for cultural competence. *Communication Disorders Quarterly, 29*, 36-42.

Cheng, L. L. (2009, November). Working with multilingual/multicultural families: Implications for speech language pathologists. Symposium conducted at the meeting of the 3rd International Symposium on Communication Disorders in Multilingual Populations, Agros, Cyprus.

Cheng, L. L. (2010). The role of culture in language intervention. *Journal of the Speech-Language-Hearing Association of Taiwan, 25*, 79-90.

Chhim, S., Luangpraseut, K., & Te, H. D. (1987). *Introduction to Cambodian culture*. San Diego: San Diego State University Multifunctional Service Center.

Chu, H. (1990, September). The role of the Korean language on the bilingual programs in the United States. Paper presented at the Asian Language Conference, Hacienda Heights, CA.

Chu, H. (1999). Linguistic perspective on the education of Korean-American students. In C. C. Park & M. Chi (Eds.), *Asian-American education* (pp. 71-86). London: Bergin & Garvey.

Chuong, C. (1990, September). The speech island: A Vietnamese perspective. Paper presented at the Asian Language Conference, Hacienda Heights, CA.

Cornwell, D. D. F. (2006). Fact sheet. Naturalization rate estimates: Stock vs. flow. Department of Homeland Security. Retrieved October 11, 2010, from www.dhs.gov/xlibrary/assets/statistics/publications/ois_naturalizations_fs_2004.pdf.

Earley, P. C., & Mosakowski E. (2004). Cultural intelligence. *Harvard Business Review, 82*, 139-46, 158.

Fadiman, A. (1997). *The spirit catches you and you fall down: A Hmong child, her American doctors, and the collision of two cultures*. New York: Farrar, Straus & Giroux.

Gollnick, D. M., & Chinn, P. C. (2005). *Multicultural education in a pluralistic society* (7th ed.). New York: Merrill-Macmillan.

Goodman, K. (1986). *What's the whole in whole language?* Portsmouth, NH: Heinemann.

Gudykunst, W. (2001). *Asian American ethnicity and communication*. California: Sage.

Gutierrez-Clellen, V. F., & Peña, E. (2001). Dynamic assessment of diverse children: A tutorial. *Speech-Language-Hearing Services in Schools, 32*, 212-224.

Hammer, C. S., & Weiss, A. L. (2000). African-American mothers' views of their infants' language development and language learning environment. *American Journal of Speech-Language Pathology, 9*, 126-140.

Heath, S. B. (1983). *Ways with words*. New York: Cambridge.

Heibert, E. H. (Ed.). (1991). *Literacy for a diverse society: Perspective, practices and policies*. New York: Teachers College, Columbia University.

Ima, K., & Keogh, P-E. (1995). "The crying father" and "my father doesn't love me": Selected observations and reflections on Southeast Asians and special education. In L. L. Cheng (Ed.), *Integrating language and learning for inclusion: An Asian-Pacific focus* (pp. 149-177). San Diego: Singular.

Ima, K., & Labovitz, E. M. (1990, March). Changing ethnic/racial student composition and test performances: Taking account of increasing student diversity. Paper presented at the annual meeting of the Pacific Sociological Association, Santa Ana, CA.

Indian American Education Foundation (2008). Indian American Education Foundation. Retrieved November 27, 2010, from www.iaefseattle.org/.

Jiobu, R. M. (1996). Recent Asian Pacific immigrants: The Asian Pacific background. In B. O. Hing & R. Lee (Eds.), *The state of Asian Pacific America: Reframing the immigration debate* (pp. 59-126). Los Angeles: UCLA Asian American Studies Center.

Johnson, M. (2004). *A philosophy of second language acquisition*. Binghamton, NY: Vail Ballou Press.

Johnston, E. B., Weinrich, B. D., & Johnson, A. R. (1984). *A sourcebook of pragmatic activities*. Tucson, AZ: Communication Skill Builders.

Keum, C-T. (2000). *Confucianism and Korean thoughts*. Korea: Jimoondang Pub. Co.

Kim, E. C. (1984, April). Korean Americans in the United States: Problems and alternatives. Paper presented at the Annual Conference of Ethnic and Minority Studies, St. Louis.

Kim, R. H. (1978). *Understanding Korean people, language, and culture*. Sacramento, CA: California State Department of Education, Bilingual Education Resource Series.

Kim-Rupnow, W. S. (2005). AAPI Culture Brief: Korea. National Technical Assistance Center. Retrieved October 12, 2010, from www.ntac.hawaii.edu/downloads/products/briefs/culture/pdf/ACB-Vol2-Iss1-Korea.pdf.

Kumar, P. (2004). India's invisible minority: The handicapped children. *The Global Child Journal, 1*, 6-9.

Langdon, H. W., & Saenz, T. I. (1996). *Language assessment and intervention with multicultural students: A guide for speech-language-hearing professionals*. Oceanside, CA: Academic Communication Associates.

Lewis, C. C. (1995). *Education hearts and minds: Reflections on Japanese preschool and elementary education*. New York: Cambridge University Press.

Lewis, J., & Luangpraseut, K. (1989). *Handbook for teaching Lao-speaking students*. Folsom, CA: Folsom Cordova.

Lewis, N. P., & Cheng, L. L. (2008). Cultural due diligence. Presentation at ASHA Convention, Miami.

Li, C. N., & Thompson, S. A. (1981). *Mandarin Chinese: A functional reference grammar*. Berkeley, CA: University of California Press.

Lo, L. (2009). Chinese American children, families, and special education. In Lin Zhan (Ed.), *Asian American voices: Engaging, empowering, enabling*. New York: National League for Nursing.

Melendy, H. B. (1977). *Asians in America: Filipinos, Koreans, and East Indians*. Boston: Twayne.

Meyerson, D. W. (1990). Cultural considerations in the treatment of Latinos with craniofacial malformations. *Cleft Palate Journal, 27*, 279-288.

Migration Institute Policy (2003). Immigration data hub. In Migration Institute Policy. Retrieved October 11, 2010, from www.migrationinformation.org/datahub/

Minami, M., & McCabe, A. (1991). Haiku as a discourse regulation device: A stanza analysis of Japanese children's personal narratives. *Language in Society, 20*, 577-599.

Monzon, R. I. (1984). The effects of the family environment on the academic performance of Filipino-American college students. Thesis, San Diego State University, San Diego.

Moon, A. (2006). Working with Korean American Families. In G. Yeo & D. Gallagher-Thompson (Eds.), *Ethnicity and dementias* (2nd ed.) (pp. 245-261). New York: Routledge.

National Sample Survey Office (2008). Education in India, 2007-2008: Participation and expenditure. Retrieved November 28, 2010, from http://mospi.gov.in/press_note_NSS_%20Report_no_532_19may10.pdf.

Nieddzwiecki, M. & Duong, T (2004). Southeast Asian American Statstical Profile.

Olson, L. (2010). "China as a global competitor: cultural patterns." Lecture at East China Normal University, SDSU summer program. Shanghai, China. 4 Jun.

Ouk, M., Huffman, F. E., & Lewis, J. (1988). *Handbook for teaching Khmer-speaking students*. Folsom, CA: Folsom Cordova Unified School District.

Peak, L. (1991). *Learning to go to school in Japan: The transition from home to preschool life*. Berkeley, CA: University of California Press.

Peña, E., Gillam, R., Malek, M., et al. (2006). Dynamic assessment of children from culturally diverse backgrounds: Applications to narrative assessment. *Journal of Speech, Language, Hearing Research, 49,* 1-21.

Peña, E., Iglesias, A., & Lidz, C. S. (2001). Reducing test bias through dynamic assessment of children's word learning ability. *American Journal of Speech Language Pathology, 10,* 138-154.

Peña, E., Quinn, R., & Iglesias, A. (1992). The application of dynamic methods to language assessment: A non-biased procedure. *Journal of Special Education, 26,* 269-280.

Pfeifer, M. E. (2009). Southeast Asian American Data 2006 American Community Survey. In Hmong Studies Internet Resource Center. Retrieved October 11, 2010, from www.hmongstudies.org/SEA2006ACS .html

Shapiro, M. E. (2005). AAPI cultural brief: Philippines. In National Technical Assistance Center. Retrieved October 27, 2010, from http:// www.ntac.hawaii.edu/downloads/products/briefs/culture/pdf/ACB-Vol2-Iss3-Philippines.pdf

Shekar, C., & Hegde, M. N. (1995). India: Its people, culture, and languages. In L. L. Cheng (Ed.), *Integrating language and learning for inclusion* (pp. 125-148). San Diego: Singular.

Stewart, J.Y. (2005). Data reveal hard truths for Islanders: No longer lumped in studies with immigrants from Asia, Samoans see a portrait of a troubled community. *Los Angeles Times,* September 26.

Strauss, R. P. (1990). Cultural considerations in the treatment of Latinos with craniofacial malformations. *Cleft Palate Journal, 27,* 275-278.

Stubbe Kester, E., Peña, E., & Gillam, R. (2001). Outcomes of dynamic assessment with culturally and linguistically diverse students: A comparison of three teaching methods. *Journal of Cognitive Education and Psychology, 2,* 42-59.

Suh, S. A. (2004). *Being Buddhist in a Christian world: Gender and community in a Korean American temple.* Seattle: University of Washington Press.

Suryadinata, L. (2005). *Admiral Zheng He and Southeast Asia.* Singapore: Institute of Southeast Asian Studies.

Takeuchi, D., & Hune, S. (2008). Growing presence, emerging voices: Pacific Islanders and academic achievement in Washington. Retrieved November 27, 2010, from http://www.capaa.wa.gov/documents/PI ExecutiveSummary.pdf.

Te, H. D. (1987). *Introduction to Vietnamese culture.* San Diego, CA: Multifunctional Center, San Diego State University.

Trueba, H. T., Cheng, L., & Ima, K. (1993). *Myth of reality: Adaptive strategies of Asian American in California.* Bristol, PA: Falmer Press.

U.S. Census Bureau (2011). Statistical abstract of the United States: 2010 (130th ed.) Washington, DC: Author.

U.S. Census Bureau (2000a). *Statistical abstract of the United States: 2000* (120th ed.). Washington, DC: Author.

U.S. Census Bureau (2000b). *We the people: Pacific Islanders in the United States.* Census 2000 Special Reports. Washington, DC: Author.

U.S. Census Bureau (2004). The American Community—Asians: 2004. In American Community Survey Reports. Retrieved October 19, 2010, from http://www.census.gov/prod/2007pubs/acs-05.pdf.

U.S. Census Bureau (2006). *2006 American community survey: Selected population.* Profiles in the United States. Washington, DC: Author.

U.S. Census Bureau (2007). *2007 American community survey: Selected population.* Profiles in the United States. Washington, DC: Author.

U.S. Census Bureau (2008). *2008 American community survey: Selected population.* Profiles in the United States. Washington, DC: Author.

U.S. Department of Commerce (1993a). *We, the American Asians.* Washington, DC: U.S. Department of Commerce.

U.S. Department of Commerce (1993b). *We, the Asian and Pacific Islander Americans.* Washington, DC: U.S. Department of Commerce.

U.S. Department of Education (2004). Individuals with Disabilities Education Act (IDEA). Retrieved November 28, 2010, from http://idea.ed.gov/explore/view/p/%2Croot%2Cregs%2C300%2CD%2C300%252E304%2C.

Van Kleeck, A. (1994). Potential bias in training parents as conversational partners with their children who have delays in language development. *American Journal of Speech-Language Pathology, 3,* 67-68.

Wells, J. C. (1982). *Accents of English 3: Beyond the British Isles.* Cambridge, UK: Cambridge University Press.

Westby, C. (1990). Ethnographic interviewing: Asking the right questions to the right people in the right way. *Journal of Childhood Communication Disorders, 13,* 101-111.

Westby, C. (2009). Considerations in working successfully with culturally/ linguistically diverse families in assessment and intervention of communication disorders. *Seminars in Speech and Language, 30,* 279-289.

Whitenack, D., & Kikunaga, K. (1999). Teaching English to native Japanese students: From linguistics to pedagogy. In C. C. Park & M. Chi (Eds.), *Asian-American education: Prospects and challenges.* London: Bergin & Garvey.

Wriggins, S. (2004). *The Silk Road journey with Xuanzhang.* Boulder, CO: Westview Press.

Yao, X-Z. (2000). *An introduction to Confucianism.* United Kingdom: Cambridge University Press.

ADDITIONAL RESOURCES

Chang, J. M., Lai, A., & Shimizu, W. (1995). LEP, LD, poor and missed learning opportunities: A case of inner city Chinese children. In L. Cheng (Ed.), *Integrating language and learning for inclusion* (pp. 265-290). San Diego: Singular Publishing Group.

Cheng, L., Chen, T., Tsubo, T., et al. (1997). Challenges of diversity: An Asian Pacific perspective. *Multicultures, 3,* 114-145.

Fadiman, A. (1997). *When the spirit catches you and you fall down.* New York: The Noonday Press.

Jen, G. (2010). *World and town.* New York: Knopf.

Kristof, N. D., & WuDunn, C. (1994). *China wakes: The struggle for the soul of a rising power.* New York: Times Books.

Liu, E. (1998). *The accidental Asian: Notes of a native speaker.* New York: Random House.

Ly-Heyslip, L., & Wurts, J. (1989). *When heaven and earth changed places* (1st ed.). New York: Doubleday.

Ma, L. J. (1985). Cultural diversity. In A. K. Dutt (Ed.), *Southeast Asia: Realm of contrast.* Boulder, CO: Westview Press.

Mura, D. (1991). *Becoming Japanese.* New York: Doubleday.

Puttnam, D. (Producer), Joffé, R. (Director): (1984). *The killing fields* [motion picture]. United Kingdom: Warner home video.

Stone, O., Milchan, A., & Kassar, M. (Producers), Oliver, O. (Director): (1993). *Heaven and earth* [motion picture]. United States, France: Le Studio Canal, Regency Enterprises, New Regency Productions, & Todd-AO.

Takaki, R. (1989). *Strangers from a different shore.* Boston: Little, Brown.

Tan, A. (1996). Mother tongue. In G. Hongo (Ed.), *Under Western eye* (pp. 313-320). New York: Doubleday.

Tan, A. (2001). *The bonesetter's daughter*. United States: Ballantine Books.

Trueba, H. T., & Bartolome, L. I. (Eds.). (2000). *Immigrant voices*. New York: Rowman & Littlefield.

Young, R. (1998). Finding one's roots in uncertain lands: How the Asian Pacific American child copes. In V. O. Pang & L. Cheng (Eds.), *Struggling to be heard* (pp. 62-73). New York: SUNY.

USEFUL ADDRESSES

Websites were accurate and active at the time of publication.

http://www.sil.org/ethnologue/top100.html

http://www.krysstal.com/langfams.html

http://www.travlang.com/languages/index.html

http://www.sil.org/ethnologue/countries/Sout.html

http://www.zompist.com/lang8.html

Chapter 4

Middle East and Arab American Cultures

Freda Campbell-Wilson

During the past two decades, the development of and access to speech-language pathology and audiology (SLP-A) services in the Middle East and among Arab American populations have increased tremendously. These remarkable improvements may be attributed to increased awareness of the significance of communication disorders in Arab and other multicultural populations, the globalization of the world, and the influence of a new world view. The term *world view* refers to a set of belief systems and principles by which individuals understand and make sense of the world and their places in it.

Oil wealth, rapid development, and modernization in the Middle East have resulted in a greater infusion of SLP-A services throughout the Middle East. In addition, increased awareness of the values and significance of the Arab world and its diaspora serves as a guiding principle that common sense about the Arab world involves, above all else, understanding past legacies, current events, environmental conditions, and ideas and attitudes that stimulate Arab people.

The preceding decades were characterized by consistent growth in the demand for and creation of SPL-A services in the Middle East and in Arab American communities. As a result of increased educational, social, medical, health, and related services, Arabs acquired the resources, information, and awareness necessary to launch a multiplicity of initiatives dedicated to the management of communication disorders. SPL-A clinicians from around the world were hired at the King Faisal Specialist Hospital, King Abdulaziz Hospital, and King Khalid Hospital in Saudi Arabia, as well as at governmental hospitals in other Middle Eastern countries, during the late 1980s to the present. These communication disorder specialists were recruited worldwide to various sectors of the Arab world. They were brought into Arab countries and partnered with peer Arab colleagues to create university training programs and service delivery and research facilities at hospitals and private centers. The end goal was to render International SLP-A Standard Services.

The eagerness of the Arab world to offer its citizens the best communication disorders services as rapidly as possible is a testimony to the high regard and reverence that Arabs place on human communication. Throughout the life cycle, people of Arab descent place high value on family, business, and social entities that are communication centered.

The development of the SPL-A professions in the world fostered growth in military, rehabilitative, and social services for the disabled, the medically challenged, and others with communication disorders.

The Arab world and Arab American communities exported and imported speech-language pathologists and audiologists from Canada, the United Kingdom, Sweden, Jordan, Egypt, the United States, and other countries to help foster the expansion of communication disorder services in multicultural populations.

THE NATURE AND SIGNIFICANCE OF THE ARAB WORLD

The *Arab world* is a descriptive moniker that emerged, and became amplified, as countries, peoples, and scholars became more unified. The 21st century Arab world has become widely familiar outside of its physical boundaries owing to its wealth, religion, politics, poverty, technology, greater interaction with other countries, and regions. In addition, the frequent illumination of the Arab people and their cultural values, mores, and media were significant factors. Simply put, Arabism has reached international levels of recognition with the assertion of an independent Arab personality.

People who are Arabs extend from the Atlantic shores of Northwest Africa to the Persian (Arab) Gulf opening on the

Indian Ocean, from the interior of Northern Africa to the whole Southern Mediterranean shore, and to the Southern border of Turkey. Furthermore, the Arab world embraces more than 5 million square miles, approximately one eleventh of the earth's land mass. The Arab world in the Middle East includes more than 285 million people, which amounts to nearly one thirtieth of the population of humankind.

Worldwide, the *Arab diaspora* outside of the Middle East is estimated at more than 30 to 50 million, with 12 million first-generation Arabs distributed across every continent and almost every country in the world. More than half of the non–Middle East Arabic diaspora is concentrated in Latin America. Other regions with high concentrations are Western Europe, Western Asia, and North America. According to the International Organization for Migration, persons of Arab descent make up 3% of the population in Brazil, 4.2% of the population in Chile, 1.4% of the population in Ecuador, and 0.65% of the population in Argentina. They are 2.2% of the population in Australia, 1.4% of the population in Canada, and 1.1% of the population in the United States.

A core identity factor, which plays a powerful role in characterizing all things, values, and peoples as Arab, is the fact that the vast region of the Arab world is desert, a geographic land space virtually devoid of water.

The area of the globe that is the Arab world, relative to population and land mass, is deceptive. The ratio appears to indicate a very low density per square mile. Traditional historical images, together with the desert character of much of the region, have generated the picture of Arabs as nomads wandering through vast desert ponds on camels. Although this archaic picture was at one time somewhat accurate, 21st century Arab visuals are more akin to an amazing blend of old and new, which includes high-rise buildings, sky scrapers, luxurious automobiles, and camels.

The Middle East is a vast area of the world stretching from the lands surrounding the eastern edge of the Mediterranean Sea to the areas of Southwest India. Although the U.S. Census Bureau (2001) identifies countries such as Iran and Iraq as Asian, this text considers them to be in the Middle East. The distinction was made on the basis of the cultural roots of the countries and the roots of the languages spoken, rather than any political issues.

People who practice Arab culture, speak Arabic natively, or have a solid kinship to the Arabic language and Islam can be categorized as Arabs. Although Arab originally referred to the nomadic tribes of the Arabian Peninsula in southwestern Asia, the nomadic nature of Arab people has resulted in considerable ethnic diversity. Hence, the label Arab does not denote a single race of people!

Arab Americans and Arab people throughout the world are proud of their long and prodigious history. Over the centuries, they created great empires and established powerful centers of civilization. The Arab region is the center of the development of major contributions to the arts and sciences. In addition, it is the birthplace of three great religions of the world: Christianity, Judaism, and Islam. Moreover, the Middle East, the cradle of the Arab civilization, has become one of the world's major melting points of humanity.

At the heart of the Arab world and at the forefront of its accomplishments is the Arabic language. With the emergence and development of Islam, the fastest growing religion in the world, the Arabic language has increased in importance and significance. In recent times, the Arabic language continues to maintain its noble status; however, complex social and cultural issues in the present-day Arab world directly impinge on the language and its users.

Although Arab Americans are heterogeneous in origin and culture, they share in negative stereotypes and discrimination, related to the recent political events involving the Arab nations, such as the Gulf War of the early 1990s (Suleiman, 2001) and the subsequent conflicts in Iraq and Afghanistan. Although Arab Americans are less visible than other ethnic groups, the anti-Arab representation in the media makes them more visible in a negative way. There is considerable misunderstanding about the Middle Eastern people, particularly involving the beliefs and practices of non-Christian religions. Holidays such as Ramadan (associated with Muslims) and Passover (associated with Judaism), modes of dress, prohibitions about food products, fasting, and other practices often result in misunderstanding and stereotypes that can have an impact on clinical practices. (For a more detailed discussion of religious practices, see the Intervention section in Chapter 14.)

Persons of Arab descent are found in countries throughout the world, including the United States, Brazil, and Canada. Immigration of Arabs to Brazil started in the late 19th century, most of them coming from Lebanon, Syria, Palestine, and Iraq. Arab immigration to Brazil grew in the 20th century, and was concentrated in the state of São Paulo but also extended to Mato Grosso do Sul, Minas Gerais, Goiás, Rio de Janeiro, and other parts of Brazil.

Most Arab immigrants in Brazil were Christians, the Muslims being a small minority in comparison. Intermarriage between Brazilians of Arab descent and other Brazilians, regardless of ethnic ancestry or religious affiliation, is very high; most Brazilians of Arab descent only have one parent of Arab origin. As a result of this, the new generations of Brazilians of Arab descent show marked *language shift* away from Arabic. Only a few speak any Arabic, and such knowledge is often limited to a few basic words. Instead, the majority, especially those of younger generations, speak Portuguese as a first language. In Brazil, there are 7 million people of Lebanese origin, 3 million of Syrian origin, and 2 million from various other Arab origins, most notably Palestinians, Iraqis, Egyptians, and Moroccans. Canadians of Arab origin make up one of the largest non-European ethnic group in Canada. In 2001, almost 350,000 people of Arab origin lived in Canada, representing 1.2% of the total Canadian population. Of the Arab Canadians,

14% have their origins in Lebanon, 12% in Egypt, 6% in Morocco, 6% in Iraq, 4% in Algeria, and 4% in Palestine.

Geographic Diversity

The land of the Arab world lies in northern Africa and southwestern Asia. It ranges from Mauritania in the west to Oman in the east. The Arab countries from Egypt and Sudan eastward represent the region of the world known as the Middle East. The Arab world throughout the ages has been an international crossroads. As a result, it has often come under foreign rule and influence. Vast deserts and mountainous terrain cover more than half of the Arab world, resulting in most Arabs living in selected areas. Owing to the shortage of water in the Arab world, most Arabs live in the Fertile Crescent valley of the Nile, Euphrates, and Tigris rivers or along the Mediterranean Sea.

Today's Arab world includes diverse countries from the Mediterranean area and northern Africa to southwestern Asia. The countries include the large cosmopolitan areas such as Cairo in Egypt, Jerusalem in Israel, Jeddah in Saudi Arabia, and Beirut in Lebanon. They also include the rich agricultural area of the Fertile Crescent as well as the vast rural areas of the deserts in which most Arabs continue to live. Countries of the Middle East include Egypt, Jordan, Syria, Lebanon, Iraq, Iran, Saudi Arabia, Sudan, Algeria, Morocco, Turkey, and Tunisia. Other Arab nations include Kuwait, Mauritania, Oman, Palestine, Israel, Qatar, Somalia, Sudan, United Arab Emirates, and Yemen (Hsourani, 1991; Shipler, 1987).

The Middle East contains four main geographic regions that cut across national and political divisions. These are the northern tier, the Fertile Crescent, the largely desert south, and the western area. The northern tier, which encompasses Turkey, northern Iraq, and semiarid plateaus, depends on irrigation and light rainfall to support agriculture. The major language groups in the northern tier include Arabic, Kurdish, Turkish, and Farsi (Isenberg, 1976). The primarily desert southern lands include the oil-rich United Arab Emirates, Oman, and the two Yemeni Republics (North and South). The Fertile Crescent consists of the Gulf States of Qatar, Saudi Arabia, and Jordan. The Fertile Crescent forms the southern border of the northern tier. It stretches northward through Israel and Lebanon and then arches across northern Syria to the valleys of the Euphrates and Tigris rivers in Iraq. The primary languages spoken in the Fertile Crescent and the southern sectors of the Middle East are Arabic, Hebrew, and dialects of Aramaic, Berber, and Nubian origin (Isenberg, 1976). Djibouti, Ethiopia, Sudan, and Egypt capsule the western areas of the Middle East. The languages of this vast area include French, Arabic, and Aramaic.

The Middle East is a predominately Arabic-speaking region that is populated primarily by Arabs. This notion requires clarification, however, because the term Arab itself is not strictly definable. In a purely semantic sense, no people can be classified as Arab because the word connotes a mixed population with widely varying ethnographic and racial origins. Some people of Negro, Berber, and Semitic origins identify themselves as Arab (Wilson, 1996). Hence, Arab is best used within a cultural context (Lamb, 1987). Arab countries are those in which the primary language is Arabic and the primary religion is Islam. Consequently, the Middle East makes up the greatest portion of the Arab world, a world that reflects one of Islam from an embryonic phenomenon into a vast sphere of influence and civilization.

According to Lamb (1987) and Mansfield (1992), approximately 200 million Arabs occupy the Arab world. The paradox of parallel modernization and political turmoil has influenced language, learning, and SLP-A services in the Middle East. The hugely increased revenue flowing into the oil-producing Arab countries has facilitated the early phases of the development of SLP-A services, whereas the turmoil of civil and regional wars has created populations of patients of all ages who need services to treat communication disorders.

Additionally, age-old traditions of consanguinity (blood relationships) contribute to a variety of communication problems among Arab speakers. Jaber and colleagues (1997) studied the frequency of speech disorders in Israeli Arab children and its association with parental consanguinity. Twenty-five percent of 1282 parents responding to a questionnaire indicated that their children had a speech and language disorder. After examination by a speech-language pathologist (SLP), rates of affected children of consanguineous and nonconsanguineous marriages were 31.0% and 22.4%, respectively ($P < .01$).

ARAB AMERICANS AND ARAB ORIGINS

Immigrants to the United States from the Arab nations came as early as the 1880s in search of opportunity and education. The early immigrants were from the countries of Ottoman-ruled Lebanon and Syria. More than 90% of the immigrants from the area at the time were Christians. Although the area was predominantly Muslim, the Muslims were hesitant to come to the United States for fear that they would not be able to practice their religion. The early immigrants, who were called "Turks," "Armenians," and "Moors," settled in the urban areas of Chicago and New York. They were very industrious and made strides in the business community such that they were able to support their families in their new home as well as their families in the home country. The early Arab Americans were fully assimilated when the second wave of Arab immigrants came to the United States.

The second major wave of Arab immigration began in the 1940s after World War II. They were primarily well-educated professional Muslims who, like their predecessors, sought the educational and financial opportunities in the United States. The new wave sparked a resurgence of ethnic pride among descendants of the early immigrants. Since the mid-1960s, the number of Arabs living outside the Arab world has increased significantly. The United States, Germany, Brazil, Israel, England, France, Canada, and Sweden have among the largest populations of Arabs living outside the Middle East.

Current estimates of the number of Arab Americans living in the United States are about 3 to 5 million. Estimates vary because the U.S. Census Bureau does not use Arab American as a classification. In addition, recent immigrants from some Arab or Middle Eastern countries are reluctant to give personal and confidential information to the government because of the sociopolitical issues of the past decade. Officially, as shown in Table 4-1, according to extrapolated U.S. Census data, there are an estimated 1.5 million Arab Americans living in the United States. There are approximately 200,000 persons from Lebanon, 179,000 persons of Egyptian ancestry, and 149,000 Americans of Syrian ancestry.

Persons of Arab descent in the United States today are as diverse as the many countries of the origin of their descendants. They represent a variety of religions, values, and degrees of acculturation and assimilation. Because the major waves of immigration of persons from the Middle East occurred in the first half of the 19th century, 82% of Arab Americans are U.S. citizens, and 63% were born in the United States. As a cultural group, they are well educated, with 62% having at least some college education (compared with 45% of the non-Arab U.S. population) and twice as many as in the non-Arab U.S. population having a master's degree or higher.

More than 60% of Arab Americans hold white-collar or professional occupations, 12% are self-employed, and 20% are in retail trade business. Most reside in the urban areas of Detroit, New York City, Washington DC, Los Angeles, Chicago, Boston, Cleveland, and New Jersey (Immigration and Naturalization Service, 1998).

Arab American Families and Arab Lifestyles

Family life, religion, and harmony are important to nearly all Arab and Middle Eastern families. The family is the centerpiece of society in Arab states. All other establishments evolve from this basic unit. Most Arab American families are large. It is not uncommon for several generations to live together as an extended family, with the oldest man being the head of each family; the families are patriarchal, being based around the father, his sons, their wives, and their children. Although separated from their natal family, ties between women and their blood relatives are continued. Women frequently consult their natal families if there are problems with the children or other problems. Clinicians need to respect the sanctity of the nuclear and extended family and the role of elders within the family (Schwartz, 1999). Inviting the family to participate in assessment and intervention can be useful in helping the family understand the needs of the individual. In most Muslim families, the women are responsible for instilling the proper cultural values in children through child-rearing practices.

The concept of honor is very important in the lives of Arabs and Middle Eastern society. Fear of scandal is a major consideration in their daily lives. Upholding the honor of the family is vital. Because Arabs are very sensitive to public criticism, clinicians should express concerns to Arab American families in a way that prevents the "loss of face" (Adeed & Smith, 1997; Jackson, 1995, 1997).

Women in Middle Eastern Culture

Islam stresses the concept of public morality, which is to be enforced collectively. It is believed that women are to be separated from men so that they are not overly sexually appealing. Young women must be modestly dressed, which has evolved into the tradition of veiling. In the past, women were seen as the weak link to the family's dignity. More modern trends, however, have led more women to work outside the home, particularly in the fields of medicine, education, and the social sciences. A woman's household duties with regard to the children are not reduced when she gains employment outside of the home.

In this age of globalization, Arab women are entangled in the simultaneous movements of contraction and expansion whereby people of all cultures grapple with the global economy and debate universal values. The restrictions that many Arab women face are often like mirrors of the primordial ties

TABLE 4-1 Population by Selected Arab Ancestry Group in the United States, 2008

Population	No.
Total Arab	1,549,725
Egyptian	179,592
Iraqi	69,277
Jordanian	59,233
Lebanese	501,907
Moroccan	77,468
Palestinian	85,745
Syrian	149,541
Saudi Arabian	260,427
Other Arab	189,300

From U.S. Census Bureau (2008). American Community Survey, B04006: People reporting ancestry. Retrieved March 2010 from http://www .census.gov/acs/www/.

of Arab ethnicity, language, and religions. Consequently, Arab women are subjected to conditions and challenges in the Arab world that vary in intensity from one Arab country to another. Such conditions and challenges include populations in which as many as one in three is younger than 14 years of age; inadequate or underdeveloped education systems (especially educational entities for females); economies struggling to create and maintain competitive 21st century employment structures; limited water resources; limited or nonexistent political rights; societies grappling to define the role of women; and the crisis of identity (the most fundamental measure of who and what a person or society is).

The Arab region has some of the world's lowest adult literacy rates, with only 62.2% of the region's population 15 years and older able to read and write in 2000 to 2004, well below the world average of 84% and the developing countries' average of 76.4%. Great variations exist among the Arab states in their literacy rates for the group aged 15 years and older. The most recent data reveal that literacy rates range from 80% and higher in nine countries (Jordan, United Arab Emirates, Bahrain, Saudi Arabia, Syria, Kuwait, Lebanon, Qatar, and Libya), which are relatively small states with the exception of Saudi Arabia, to less than 75% in nine other countries with large populations, with Iraq, Mauritania, and Yemen standing as low as 40%, 41.2%, and 49%, respectively. There is considerable disparity between the education of girls and that of boys in the Arab world and also across countries. In some countries, nearly 20% of girls between the ages of 6 and 11 years do not attend school (Hammond, 2006). Female literacy rates of those aged 15 years and older in the Arab world today range from 24% in Iraq to 85.9% in Jordan. Although improvements have been made in education of women in recent years, high rates of illiteracy among women persist in most of the Arab countries; indeed, women today account for two thirds of the region's illiterate population, and according to the Arab Human Development Report of 2002 (p. 52), this rate is not expected to disappear *until 2040* (Daniel, 2005, p. 6) (Table 4-2).

TABLE 4-2 Improvement of Female Illiteracy in the Arab Countries

Age Group	Illiteracy Rate		
	1980	1990	2000
Women 15 to 24 years of age	44.9%	29.9%	19.4%
Women >15 years of age	64.9%	51.9%	40.2%

From Hammoud, R. (2001). *Non-formal education for girls* (p. 20). Beirut, UNESCO.

Religion in Arab Life

Religion is very important to Arab and Arab American families. Although most are Muslim, many follow the Christian beliefs of their ancestors from the early wave of immigration. Some Muslim Arab American families send their children to private Muslim schools so that they can receive education consistent with the religious beliefs of the family (Zehr, 1999). Some families opt to send their children to public schools. As the number of Arab American children in the public schools increases, many schools have adapted their programs and practices to accommodate the religious needs of the children. This includes adapting school menus to have alternatives to pork, which is not consumed by Muslims; allowing a place for prayer at the noon hour; and adapting the school lunch programs to allow for the fasting, required during Ramadan. Many school programs are reducing the emphasis on celebration of Christian holidays to relieve Muslim students from the stresses of participating in Christian and Judaic religious practices. Clinical materials and tests are being modified to remove items that may be specific to a particular Christian religion, such as items related to the celebration of Christmas. Clinicians should be sensitive to the religious beliefs of clients in selecting items for assessment and intervention.

Many Arabs continue to follow traditional ways, although modernization is rapidly changing their lifestyles. Historically, Arab cities, villages, and nomadic groups have remained interdependent. People in cities produce finished goods, villagers provide agricultural produce, and nomads supply animals that transport these products among the three kinds of communities. Owing to the uniformity of these lifestyles, Arabs are especially unique in their ability to maintain their cultural identity wherever they are located. Although most immigrants have their roots in the urban areas, some are from a more traditional rural community with less exposure to more modern European American traditions.

Most persons in the Middle East are farmers or laborers, although a great deal of the land space in the Middle East is unfit for agricultural use (Hitti, 1985). Because the oil wealth of the Middle East has benefited only a fraction of the Arab population, many inhabitants of the Arab world have speech, language, and hearing problems owing to lack of medical, educational, and human resources services. These inhabitants are often born into communities that do not systematically provide these services. According to Isenberg (1976), the reality of limited natural resources in most of the Middle East explains why the Arab world must be considered among the underdeveloped sectors of the world. Limited resources, too few trained professionals, and lack of access to services negatively influence speech, language, and hearing integrity among large populations of Arab speakers. For persons seeking assistance from SLPs trained in the Middle East in the major cities such as

Cairo, Jeddah, and Amman, the supply of clinicians is considerably below the demand for services. When the civil and regional political turmoil is considered, access to available services in the Middle East becomes even more restricted.

ARABIC LANGUAGE

Ethnic Diversity among Arab American Speakers

The Arab world, owing to its ancient and current history, remains a diverse melting pot of humanity, largely a result of Islamic pilgrimages. Because national languages and SLP-A dynamics are influenced by histories of invasions, conquests, slavery, and most importantly, the onset of Islam, the inhabitants of the Arab world represent a multiplicity of subgroups, all struggling to coexist in a collision of cultures. Perhaps the most useful method for classifying persons from the Middle East is according to the language they speak, religions they embrace, and traditions they honor (Mansfield, 1992). This categorization allows for four major national groups: the Turks, Iranians, Israelis, and Arabs. The extremely close relationships and overlapping of linguistic, cultural, racial, and sociologic factors of all these groups foster many of the chronic problems of Middle Eastern society.

The Arabic Languages

The languages of Arabs are divided among three very different language families: the Hamito-Semitic, the Altaic, and the Indo-European. Language is one of the major ways by which people from the Arabic world distinguish themselves and define their national identities and political allegiances. The most widely spoken language in the Arab world and among Arab Americans is Arabic, which is the sister language to Hebrew; however, Arabs from Pakistan, India, and Iran speak Urdu, Hindi, and Farsi, respectively. Israelis and Palestinians speak Hebrew and Yiddish.

Arabic belongs to the Semitic subdivision of the Hamito-Semitic language family. Globally, Arabic ranks as the sixth most common first language. It is the "mother tongue" or chief language in more than 18 countries in the Middle East and North Africa, with the exception of Israel, Iran, and Turkey.

Turkish, Persian (Farsi), and Kurdish are three other widely spoken languages in the Middle East and adjacent regions. The Turkish group of languages is a part of the Altaic language family. Consequently, Turkish is the predominant language in Turkey. Variations of Turkish are spoken in most of the countries in central Asia.

Persian, which is also referred to as Farsi, belongs to the Indo-European language group. It is the third most widely spoken language in the Middle East. Persian is widely spoken in Iran, Afghanistan, Tajikistan, Pakistan, and Uzbekistan and to some extent in Armenia, Turkmenistan, Azerbaijan, and Bahrain. Modern Persian has a kinship to Arabic because it uses a modified Arabic script, which makes it seem the same as Arabic, although the languages are different. There are nevertheless, many Arabic words used in Farsi. The word order in Persian is subject + object + verb.

Kurdish, which is the language of large populations in Iran, Iraq, Turkey, and Syria, is also a common language of Arab American refugees from the Gulf and Afghanistan wars. Hebrew, Armenian, Assyrian, and Greek are other major languages spoken by large groups of people in the Middle East and adjacent locations.

There is a significant distinction between spoken colloquial Arabic and written Arabic. Classical written Arabic, which is the language of the Holy Koran, is the religious and literary language of most of the Arab world. Classical Arabic serves as a bond throughout the Arab world and is the lingua franca that links educated Arabs worldwide.

The Arabic language has 29 letters, all of which, except the first, are consonants. They are written from right to left. The most consistent word order in Arabic grammar is verb + subject + object; however, one also may find the subject put first.

Arab Dialects

Two hundred million people speak Arabic or dialects of Arabic. The dialects are grouped into five geographic categories: (1) North African (Moroccan, Algerian, Tunisian, Libyan, and Mauritanian), (2) Egyptian/Sudanese, (3) Syrian or Levantine (Lebanese, Syrian, Jordanian, and Palestinian), (4) Arabian Peninsular (Saudi, Yemeni, Qatari, Kuwaiti, Gulf, and Omani), and (5) Iraqi (Wilson, 1996). North African dialects were influenced by the Berbers and the language of the colonists from other North African countries. The Egyptian/Sudanese dialect is understood by most Arabs because it is the dialect used in Egyptian movies, television, and radio that are seen and heard throughout the Arab world. Arabian Peninsular dialects, spoken in Saudi Arabia, Yemen, Qatar, Kuwait, Gulf, and Oman, are considered the closest to Classical Arabic. They are the dialects closest to the language of the Koran (i.e., the holy book of Islam) and are considered by Arabs to be the most prestigious of the dialects. Egyptian, Syrian or Levantine, and Arabian Peninsular dialects are mutually comprehensible. North African, Iraqi, and Gulf dialects are difficult for others to understand (Almaney & Alwan, 1982; Wilson, 1996).

Written Arabic is different from spoken Arabic. Written Arabic, or Classical Arabic, is the language of the Koran. It is more complex, grammatically more difficult, and has a considerably larger lexicon than spoken Arabic (Wilson, 1996). To be truly literate in Classical Arabic requires many years of study. Even after 5 or 6 years of study, the average Arab may be functionally illiterate in Classical Arabic (Wilson, 1996). Because of its difficulty, good command of Classical Arabic is admired in the Arab culture. Because the dialects have no prestige, a person who does not know Classical Arabic may be thought not to know Arabic, even if he or she is able to speak the local dialect well (Ferguson, 1971).

Arabic Phonology

Wilson (1996) and Swan and Smith (1987) describe several features of Arabic phonology that influence the speech of Arabic-speaking learners of English. Because of the various dialects of Arabic, there is some variation in the classification or description of the Arabic phonemes. Arabic has 8 vowels and 32 consonants. Short vowels have little significance in Arabic; they are often omitted or confused when Arabic speakers attempt to learn English. Frequent confusions include /ĭ/ for /ĕ/ (bit for bet), /ă/ for /ĕ/ (raid for red), and /ō/ for /a/ (hope for hop).

The consonants /p/, /v/, /n/, and /r/ do not have equivalents in Arabic. Several phonemes (/p/ and /b/, /f/ and /v/) are allophonic in Arabic. In addition, /tʃ/ and /ʃ/, /s/ and /z/, /d/ and /dʒ/ for /th/ unvoiced and voiced, respectively. In addition, /t/, /n/ is often produced as /n + n/. Because in Arabic, /r/ is a voiced flap, Arabic speakers often overproduce the postvocalic /r/. Finally, many English two- and three-element consonant clusters do not occur in Arabic; therefore, Arabic speakers learning English often insert short vowels into the cluster (e.g., sipring for spring).

Among the other features of Arabic that influence production of English are exaggerated articulation with equal stress on all syllables, fewer clearly articulated vowels giving a staccato effect, and the use of glottal stops before initial vowels. In Arabic, spelling is phonetic. Arabic speakers, therefore, tend to produce English words phonetically, including all consonants, even those that are not pronounced in English (Wilson, 1996). McLeod (2007) provides one of the few published accounts of speech acquisition in Arab languages including Jordanian Arabic and Lebanese Arabic.

Arabic Syntax and Morphology

Arabic syntax and morphology are patterned and predictable (Wilson, 1996). The irregularities of English, therefore, pose particular difficulty for speakers of Arabic who are learning English. The verb is often placed before the subject noun. Negatives are formed by placing an article before the verb. Adjectives follow their nouns. Because plurals are formed by internal vowel changes in Arabic, plural morphemes are frequently omitted when Arabic speakers are learning English. Arabic verb structure uses a simple present tense form for the English simple and present progressive tenses. There are no copula verbs, auxiliary "do," future tense, modal verbs, gerunds, or infinitive forms in Arabic. There are no indefinite articles.

Arabic Semantics

There is very little information on the development of semantics by Arab-speaking children published in English. Ferguson (1971) includes some information on early language development, including the use of child-directed talk or baby-talk in Syrian Arabic. Adults are reported to use baby-talk freely, with little concern that the use of baby-talk may inhibit the acquisition of adult language. Semantic fields in early language development include areas similar to those of children learning English (i.e., family names, food, body parts, and animals). Learning English vocabulary is particularly difficult for Arab speakers because there is little crossover between the languages. Some words that have been imported from Arabic include many words beginning with "al" (e.g., *algebra, alfalfa, alcove, alcohol, algorithm,* and *almanac*) and some foods (e.g., *coffee, sherbet, sesame, apricot, ginger, saffron, carob*), as well as *cotton, magazine, zenith,* and *tariff.* The following English words sound similar to vulgar words in Arabic and should be avoided, if possible*: zip, zipper, air, tease, kiss, cuss, nick, unique,* and *Biz* (Wilson, 1996).

Arabic Language and Religion

Arabs and Arab Americans place a high value on religion. Except for a small, aged generation of Jews and a small handful of Christians, religious minorities do not exist. Between 90% and 94% of the people are Muslims, and most speak or read Arabic.

Throughout the history of the Middle East, religion has probably been the most important bond and source of conflict dividing the inhabitants (Davidson, 1991; Hitti, 1985). The majority religion of the Middle East is Islam; the largest minority religion is Christianity. Both religions have played an important role in shaping the Middle East. The Arabic language has had a tremendous influence on the shaping and development of the modern Middle East. This is largely because the language of the Holy Koran is Arabic. Many links exist between Islam and Arabic. Arabic is the only official vessel for the transmission of Islam. Therefore, the purity and sanctity of Islam as a religion are strongly correlated with maintaining purity of linguistic integrity within the Arabic language. It is significant that Arabic is the medium of familial, societal, and national communication.

More than 95% of Arabic speakers in the Middle East and persons of Arabic origin are Muslim, and their standards for spoken and written Arabic are extremely high. Some are strict orthodox Muslims (Hitti, 1985), whereas others are more liberal. All regard their religion in a way that is difficult for the Western mind to grasp. The Arabic language is revered by Arabs as divine or holy because the Prophet Mohammed revealed the Word of God in the Holy Koran in Arabic.

Arabic Speakers and Culture

Arabic speakers typically use "national" versions of contemporary modern Arabic (CMA) in their everyday communication. Most Arabic speakers have formal and informal vernaculars that reflect social class, ethnographic background, and nationality. Typically, dialectal variations among native Arabic speakers reflect socioeconomic status, educational level, and nationality. French, English, and Turkish, as well as Spanish to a lesser extent, are language groups that have infiltrated CMA. The languages of northern India, Turkey, Iran, Portugal, and Spain are full of words of Arabic origin.

Socially, Arabic speakers use formal versions of CMA in business, academic, and religious settings. Typically, informal or colloquial Arabic is only used in informal communicative events that occur within family communication events. Because traditional Arab culture restricts interactions between nonrelated men and women, the use of informal Arabic is generally limited to family settings or intimate communication. Traditional Arab culture requires that "good" communicators use standard CMA (Lamb, 1987). Standard CMA refers to the hypothetical reference point for natural primary level (spoken) and standard secondary level (written) Arabic used by literate Arabic speakers. Standard CMA is derived from the Arabic of the Holy Koran and is spoken by the educated elite. In addition, native Arabic speakers are required to use formal or standard Arabic with their elders, authority figures, and religious leaders.

According to cultural mores, native Arabic speakers engage in lively interactive episodes of verbal communication that strongly adhere to highly stylized linguistic forms and rituals. Arab speakers across and within various national and language groups integrate Islamic and Arabic influences in all aspects of their communication. Younger communicators are expected to defer to their elders but are never excluded from participating in communication events. Typically, Arabic speakers engage in intense, interactive, communicative dialogues that allow several speakers to talk at one time.

Because Arab speakers strive to speak eloquently and to use their language creatively, a communication disorder may be perceived as having a greater social penalty for Arab speakers than it does for English speakers (Wilson, 1996).

LINGUISTIC AND CULTURAL ISSUES OF ARABS IN THE DIASPORA

Because the Arab world consists of a number of diverse countries, immigrants and political refugees from the Arabic-speaking diaspora (United States, Canada, Europe, Sweden, and other countries) represent a myriad of dialect and cultural variations. Thus, the Arab speakers that SLPs, audiologists, and educators encounter in schools, hospitals, and other settings are likely to be diverse in linguistic and cultural backgrounds. Moreover, Arab speakers from Jordan, United Arab Emirates, Saudi Arabia, Syria, Kuwait, Lebanon, Qatar, and Libya are likely to have levels of literacy of 80% or higher in their native national language (i.e., Arabic or Farsi), as well as more English proficiency than other Arab speakers from less well-developed countries such as Iraq, Mauritania, and Yemen, where literacy rates are 40%, 41.2%, and 49%, respectively (Hammond, 2006). However, in the oil-rich countries with low literacy rates, there also are people with high levels of literacy who are dependent on their ability to profit from the vast wealth of the oil industries.

Wherever Arab speakers are found in the Arab diaspora, the Arabic language is more than a medium of communication; it is an object of worship—an almost metaphysical phenomenon that bonds men and women to their God. Arabs, however, also view the mastery of other languages such as English and French to be important to economic prosperity. Therefore, Arab Americans and those in the diaspora usually demand that their children be bilingual and that Arabic or their national language be the dominant language, regardless of where they live. Naturally, this position poses problems for some children who may have psycholinguistic deficits or differences that can negatively influence bilingualism. Therefore, careful, culturally and linguistically fair assessment and treatment services must be rendered based on comprehensive probes into the cultural and linguistic backgrounds of the clients. The family, or appropriately informed family representatives, must team with the SLP, audiologist, or educator and work with an Arab speaker to facilitate maximal appropriate cultural input.

Communication Disorders among Arabs and Arab Americans

There is a high rate of disability in the Middle East, although it is difficult to obtain an exact incidence or prevalence rate because lack of national registers, biased reporting, variation in reporting methods, lack of uniform screening programs, and variability in consanguinity rates. For example, in recording the rate of cleft lip and palate in Saudi Arabia, the data vary from 0.3 to 2.19 per 1000 live births, nearly a seven-fold difference. Data also vary with the country and by racial or ethnic group within the country. For example, in Israel, cleft lip and palate is reported to occur in 0.37 per 1000 live births for Jews, but in 1.56 per 1000 live births for Arabs.

Children born in the Middle East have double the prevalence of deafness at birth, compared with their

U.S. counterparts. For example, Mustafa (2011) reported that in Egypt nearly 8 in 1000 children are born with a nonsyndromic hearing loss, compared with a rate of 1 in 1000 children in the rest of the world.

The World Bank (2005) reported that the most common disabilities in the Middle East and North Africa are job-related injuries, including spinal injuries and head injuries related to motor vehicle crashes, and disabilities related to poverty and poor maternal health. They report that the rate of disabilities in the region could be reduced by genetic counseling, improved maternal care, immunization of preventable diseases such as rubella, and the wearing of seat belts and helmets. They also report that although the region has areas of great wealth owing to oil production, only 1% to 2% of the population have access to rehabilitation services when there is a disability.

Although the prevalence of disability for various racial and ethnic groups has been documented, little attention has been paid to Arab Americans in the United States. This may be because most data do not identify Arab Americans as a group, and they are usually included with Caucasians for data collection. Dallo and associates (2009), however, used data from more than 4000 individuals 65 years and older identified as having Arab ancestry in 2000. Of these, 2280 were foreign-born and 1945 were U.S.-born Arab Americans. After adjusting for age and sex, the investigators found that the prevalence of having a physical disability was 31.2% for foreign-born and 23.4% for U.S.-born older Arab Americans, and the age- and sex-adjusted prevalence of having a self-care disability was 13.5% for foreign-born and 6.8% for U.S.-born Arab Americans. The foreign-born Arab Americans were more likely to report a physical disability than the U.S.-born Arab Americans. When adjusting for English language ability, the odds of having a physical disability for foreign-born Arab Americans was protective compared with U.S.-born Arab Americans. Foreign-born Arab Americans were 1.82 times more likely to report a self-care disability than U.S.-born Arab Americans.

Educational and Clinical Implications

Because there are only approximately 100 Arab speech-language and hearing professionals worldwide (Wilson, 1993), those with communication disorders in the Arab world (i.e., the Middle East and other locations where significant numbers of Arabs live, such as Europe, Canada, and the United States) face a dearth of services. Collectively, these professionals include native Arabic, Hindi, Urdu, Farsi, and French speakers. Approximately 66% of Arab SLPs and audiologists reside in the Middle East, particularly in Egypt, Israel, Jordan, Turkey, and Saudi Arabia, whereas the other 33% live in the Arab diaspora (Wilson, 1993). Consequently, only these Arab and other non-Arab SLPs, audiologists, and educators are available

to work with Arab speakers who have communication and educational problems. This professional pool must meet the formidable challenge of not only providing the services but also generating culturally and linguistically appropriate clinical and educational materials for a large number of Arab speakers who have communication disorders.

Linguistic, social, cultural, national, gender, and educational issues contribute to the constellation of variables that influence the management of the communication of native Arab speakers. These variables must be dealt with in a timely fashion to facilitate better speech-language, hearing, and educational services for Arab speakers. Therefore, considerable research, materials development, and SLP and audiologist personnel training are needed to improve the availability and quality of speech-language and hearing services to Arabs.

IMPLICATIONS FOR SERVICE DELIVERY

A significant percentage of speech-language-impaired and hearing-impaired individuals of Arab descent live in metropolitan areas worldwide. In the United States and the Arab diaspora, families continue to engage in connubial practices based on strict tribal or family lineage. Consequently, it is thought that intermarriage is linked to a large number of communication disorders found in Arab communities. Economic disparity, limited access to service, lack of trained native Arab SLPs and audiologists, and limited educational support systems result in large numbers of underserved, communicatively impaired individuals in the Arab world. To increase the variety and range of SLP and audiologist services to those in the Arab world and the Arab diaspora, the needs of the communicatively impaired must be examined from a worldwide perspective.

SPEECH-LANGUAGE PATHOLOGY AND AUDIOLOGY PRACTICE IN THE MIDDLE EAST AND ARAB AMERICA

Hospitals, rehabilitation facilities, skilled nursing facilities, home health agencies, outpatient clinics, private practice, specialty hospitals (i.e., pediatric hospitals, oncology hospitals, women's hospitals), schools, and research centers have special and unique characteristics that require SLPs and audiologists to achieve high standards of professional training and competence.

Health care changes in the Middle East and Arab American populations, in keeping with the Middle East thrust to achieve international health care status in the 21st century, have resulted in a new vision of the health care workplace for SLP-A clinicians in terms of demographics, case loads, opportunities, and challenges.

SPEECH-LANGUAGE PATHOLOGY AND AUDIOLOGY PRACTICE NEEDS IN THE MIDDLE EAST AND ARAB AMERICAN COMMUNITIES

Demands for up-to-date, quality SLP-A services in the Middle East and the Arab diaspora are high. The following are a few of the most critical needs:

1. Providing appropriate services that meet the needs of all sectors of the Middle East and Arab American populations
2. Achieving international SLP-A service standards and compliance across and within practice and professional domain with the Middle East and Arab American populations
3. Achieving quality and quantity of SLP-A service outcomes and performance improvement required by the Middle East and Arab American populations
4. Providing critically needed advocacy and educational campaigns, necessary to enlighten all aspects of the Arab world to SLP-A as a profession and a critical health care service
5. Promoting and marketing SLP-A professional services both internally and externally to all Middle Eastern countries
6. Using technology and telemedicine tools to increase access and delivery of services
7. Establishing competitive international standards for reimbursement and payment for SLP-A services
8. Providing SLP-A services to neonatal intensive care units
9. Establishing communicative wellness and effectiveness as a human right
10. Developing literacy services: SLPs and audiologists help parents, educators, physicians, and others lay the foundations for reading and writing by helping to build early speech, language, and hearing skills to prevent later reading and writing skills
11. Providing upper aerodigestive services: aeromechanical events related to communication, respiration, and swallowing (i.e., speaking valve selection, respiratory retraining for paradoxical vocal fold motion, stomal stenosis management, and insufflation testing after total laryngectomy)
12. Using telepractice for fostering SLP-A outreach services to the Arab world
13. Increasing the quality and quantity of culturally competent services as the cultural, linguistic, and ethnic makeup of the Arab world continues to expand and diversify
14. Providing geriatric SLP-A services
15. Developing Arab language and culturally competent SLP-A clinical tests, treatment materials, and other relevant resources
16. Creating of Arabic language–specific, evidenced-based practice tools and outcome strategies that are culturally competent
17. Developing SLP-A specialty services

CURRENT TRENDS IN SPEECH-LANGUAGE PATHOLOGY AND AUDIOLOGY IN THE MIDDLE EAST AND ARAB AMERICAN COMMUNITIES

As "Arabism" has matured and become more integrated into the global market, the citizens of the Middle East and Arab American communities have increased their demand for international best practice services in SLP-A.

The growth factors and increased demands for multiculturally and linguistically fair SLP-A services in the Arab world were the result of a variety of factors, including the following:

1. Changing population demographics
2. Increased awareness of communication health care–related disorders and their impact on the standard of living of children, adults, and senior citizens
3. Scientific and technologic advances
4. An expanding scope of SLP-A practices

Current governmental demographics indicate that approximately 1000 audiologists and SLPs work in a variety of sectors in the middle east. Audiologists and SLPs currently work in a variety of settings in the Middle East and in Arab American communities, including hospitals, rehabilitation centers, facilities for persons with disabilities, public and private schools, private practice, research centers, ministries of health and education, health care companies, home health care, university and medical settings, and other related industries.

ARAB WORLD VIEW AND COMMUNICATION DISORDERS

Limited knowledge about speech, language, and hearing often interferes with effective clinical service delivery in the Arab world and the Arab diaspora. World view refers to a set of belief systems and principles by which individuals understand and make sense of the world and their places in it. If clinicians are to effectively serve communicatively impaired Arabs, fundamental differences between the belief systems of those of Arab descent and those of non-Arab culture must be acknowledged.

Mansfield (1992) observed that the Western world is characterized by reductionism and enriched by the expansiveness of modern technology. Conversely, the Arab world view focuses on knowledge of the world and application of a lifestyle that is undergirded by the doctrines and influences of Islam. That is, Arab world sensibilities are driven by Islam, the Arabic language, family lineage, and a collective family-based culture. Another salient difference in world view is reflected in Arab versus non-Arab values. For example, those of Arab descent typically value extended family, groupism, collectivism versus individualism, present time, holistic thinking, and religious roots (frequently Islamic-based doctrines). Each of these values must be viewed as a part of the Arab mosaic that has meaning only as a sum total. At the core of the Arab's world view is the belief that all aspects of life are integrated or related to spirituality, even the secular aspects of everyday life activities.

Because belief systems extend beyond systems of thinking to integrate traditional knowledge, professionals who engage in service delivery to Arabs must incorporate culturally appropriate tribal and traditional mores into the constructs of their treatment models. For example, traditional Arab stories, proverbs, songs, and literature should be incorporated into treatment materials regardless of the language of treatment. Useful and common sources of Arab literature known to most Arabs, Muslims, or non-Muslims are stories or conversations that report the actions or sayings of the Prophet Mohammed.

CLINICAL INTERVENTION FOR ARAB AMERICANS AND MIDDLE EASTERN AMERICANS

Historically, Arabs in the Middle East and the Arab diaspora have been expected to maintain their Arab culture regardless of where they reside. When those of Arab descent leave their cultural communities, they face particularly difficult cultural conflicts. In addition, levels of acculturation vary significantly among parents, children, and communities. SLPs must consider the unique cultural background of the client and the family to avoid the stress associated with cultural conflict. The communicatively impaired client of Arab descent without culturally appropriate services may experience coercive assimilation (Alireza, 1991) or, more simply, cultural collisions. Coercive assimilation unmanaged leads to issues of alienation and cultural identity confusion. Naturally, cultural alienation in the treatment process makes successful communicative management difficult. Acculturation stress and its subsequent alienation disturb cultural exchanges and the mediation of information exchange essential to good clinical management. When acculturation stress issues exist in the clinical process, a body of information is at risk. Acculturation-related stressors may be significant factors that interfere with successful management of the communicatively impaired Arab population.

The range of levels of cultural maintenance is extremely wide among communicatively impaired Arabs. The SLP or audiologist who treats communicatively impaired Arabs must recognize that some choice exists in current levels of acculturation for any Arab person or family. Variation in acculturation among those of Arab descent is typically influenced by lifestyle choices, geography, marriage patterns, and native-language retention, loss, or bilingualism. Cole (1989) reported acculturation variability as a spectrum of family systems, including the traditional, neotraditional, bicultural, and acculturated. Specifically, this variability is grounded in changes in modality behaviors, which include language, tribal lineage, folk practices, and religious-based mores.

Families with Middle Eastern Roots

Because of the diversity in Arab American culture and, hence, Arab American clients, when providing clinical services for persons of Arab descent it is essential that clinicians understand the sociopolitical background of the client and family. A general guideline for providing service to clients and families with Arab roots follows:

1. Gather information about the extent of the family's support system. Are members of the extended family present? What are some of the role divisions in the family? What is the relative status of the father and the mother in the family? Are there any fellow countrymen in the neighborhood who can or do help?

2. Establish direct communication contact with the mother, but never discount the father or his role. Whenever possible, use a nonbiased interpreter to communicate information to the mother so that the information she receives related to the child and the intervention program are not filtered through the father.

3. Use informal, personalized forms of communication with Middle Eastern families rather than direct, assertive communication. Establish rapport and confidence before moving ahead with the intervention, keeping in mind that it is far more effective to come into the family as a friend who wants to help than as an authority figure.

4. Use tactful inquiry to be sure that the family has clearly understood the message and to learn whether they accept it. Politeness requires that the family members show agreement even though they may disagree; however, once the interventionist departs, the parents may continue their preferred practice. The inquiry should be gentle and carefully worded to avoid putting family members on the spot or pointing out disagreement within the family.

Role of Parents

The extended family is very important in the Arab world; often, three generations live together in one household (Sharifzadeh, 1998). Because of the emphasis placed on strong Arab families in the Middle East and the Arab diaspora, parent involvement in the clinical service program is critical. The relationships, role, and scope of Arab parents in the program must be clearly defined and continuous. Arab children are greatly cherished, and their education, growth, and personal development are of great importance to all segments of their nuclear and extended families. Typically, the parents and family members of communicatively impaired Arab patients go to great lengths to provide their family members with any necessary medical, educational, and rehabilitative services. Arab families may be uncomfortable using clinical services provided by non-Arabs, however. They may perceive social organization as attempts to replace the traditional functions of the extended family (Wilson, 1996). The family may also hold a stigma and discrimination against a person with a disability within the family. This may result in social exclusion of the individual and the denial of a disability or failure to seek services that may be available. They may be unwilling to talk about a disorder or disability, resulting in difficulty in obtaining an accurate or complete case history (Sharifzadeh, 1998; Wilson, 1996). If an Arab family member has a communication disorder, the family will likely seek help; however, because the family perceives its role as that of caring for the disabled family members, it may not accept a long-term intervention program (Wilson, 1996). A woman with a disability has a greater impact on the family because her expected role of caring for the children and the family may be diminished (World Bank, 2005).

Clinical intervention programs that involve clients or families of Arab descent must be sensitive to gender issues. Depending on fundamentalist religious beliefs, certain roles in the management of patients may only be assigned to men or women. For example, male clinicians may not be permitted to treat female clients without a male family member being present.

The more traditional family structure is patriarchal, with the man expecting to control all interactions between family and the clinician. The father or oldest male family member may make decisions regarding treatment, but the mother may be responsible for the child's development and for carrying out treatment suggestions (Wilson, 1996). Although Arab families expect their children to succeed in school, boys are expected to excel, whereas girls are only expected to receive a modest education (Wilson, 1996). Critical gender preferences must always be determined at the onset of the treatment process. Careful consideration of Arab cultural factors enhances the opportunities for successful cross-cultural communication management.

Cultural Variables in Assessment and Intervention

Because of the complexity and range of cultural differences among Arabs, clinicians must consider the culture of Arabs from the Middle East and the Arab diaspora during the evaluation. The speech-language and hearing assessment of Arab speakers requires alternative, culturally relevant models that acknowledge the differences in narrative socialization

and consider cultural factors that are fundamental to Arab culture (Guittierrez-Clellen & Quinn, 1993). For example, among Arab families, attachment and parent-child bonding are important. The families encourage interdependence among children and family members so that the mutual bonding necessary for adult life can occur. This may be in conflict with the frequent goal of independence in the intervention program often established in Western clinical programs (Wilson, 1996). In addition, language socialization practices may differ between American and Arab American children. Arab American children are discouraged from talking loudly and from talking during eating and meal times (Wilson, 1996). These have implications for expectations in the use of voice and expectations for discourse and conversation in intervention. Globally, the assessment of the speech, language, and hearing of Arab speakers must acknowledge all aspects of the speakers' language or languages within naturalistic environments (Damico, 1993).

Because clinicians have pursued information and cross-cultural research, systemic concerns must be addressed in language assessment and intervention. For instance, according to Wilson (1975), Butler (1989), and Damico (1991, 1993), the SLP who assessed the communication of the Arab Americans who speak Arabic must address critical factors such as normal second-language acquisition, dialectal influence, and cross-cultural interference. Thus, the successful assessment of the communication of Arab speakers poses some challenges for clinical services.

The core validity of virtually all existing tools and instruments is yet to be standardized for Arab speakers. Limited contemporary Arabic, Urdu, and other language tools and instruments exist. Of the instruments in existence, however, only a few have been standardized on Arabic speakers (Butler, 1989; Crago, 1990). Recently Wiig and El-Halees (2000) developed an objective and culturally and linguistically authentic Arabic language screening test for children. The test measures developmental delays in preschool children (3 to 6 years) and one for school-aged children (7 to 13 years). The development of the test was challenging because of the diversity among Arabic speakers, the diversity of Arab cultures, and the paucity of information on the speech and language development in Arabic-speaking children. The Arabic Receptive-Expressive Vocabulary Test (El-Halees & Wiig, 2000b) is also a culturally authentic test of Arabic vocabulary for children aged 3 to 13 years. The usefulness of the tests are limited because they were developed only for children in Jordan and Palestine. Scoring protocols and new standardizations will need to be developed if used for children in other regions of the Middle East or other Arab-speaking communities.

The most useful techniques and tools available for the communicative assessment of Arab speakers are naturalistic descriptive instruments (i.e., language sampling, narrative probes, and behavioral assessments). Speech-language screening in Jordan, for example, uses nonsubjective measures to evaluate whether a child follows an expected course of language development. Among the methods used is to ask the child to recite a prayer commonly taught to 3-year-old children and to judge the production for intelligibility and articulatory performance (Wiig & El-Halees, 2000). Estimates of normal development are made against the normative data used for speakers of English.

Any SLP or audiologist model of service delivery for persons of Arabic descent must consider the components of Arab culture important to the client and family as a central component of the clinical process. The assessment and intervention process must validate Arab culture, individual human potential, and the cultural and linguistic references of the Arab speakers, including consideration of influences from the national community or country (e.g., Arabic, Urdu, English). The service delivery model must be comprehensive and address the ecologies of home, school, community, and any other cultural factors that might be relevant to the individual client. For example, some persons from the Middle East place a greater emphasis on memorization in education than Americans. The children may sing songs or recite poetry or nursery rhymes in a language they do not speak or understand. Because many Arab children are accustomed to rote learning and drill, they may not be responsive to indirect or facilitated language intervention in a naturalistic environment (Wilson, 1996).

Clinicians serving Arab Americans should respect traditional Arab attitudes toward clinical services and Arab communication style in all interactions. Group services should be considered because they reflect the Arab value of collectivism. The group should be single gender. Clients may be reluctant to discuss personal information and personal feelings with unfamiliar persons. Respect for the privacy of the family should be considered in taking case history information. Certain information may not be provided until sufficient rapport has been established. The need for personal information and its relevance to the clinical situation should be explained. Because many Arab cultures maintain a close distance between communicators, Arab clients may be more comfortable sitting close to the clinician during interviews and other clinical interactions (Jackson, 1995).

The culturally appropriate service delivery model for the management of Arab speakers by SLPs and audiologists management must clearly validate Arab culture as a central component of the service delivery process. Wilson (1996) and Nydell (1997) have suggested several nonverbal and verbal cultural variables that should be observed and practiced when providing clinical services to those of Arab cultures. It is necessary to remember that the cultural variables important to a particular cultural group must be considered as individual to a client or family. The verbal and nonverbal variables cannot be applied across all groups without consideration of the specific preferences of the individual.

1. Sit with good posture to show respect. Do not lean against the wall or put your hands in your pockets.

2. Do not show the soles of your shoes when sitting with legs crossed. This is a sign of disrespect.

3. Arab men shake hands when greeting or parting. The handshake may appear to be prolonged according to Western practices. Some Arab men will not shake hands with a woman.

4. Greetings are long and formalized, with ritualized, predetermined expressions, and have a required response. Some formalized exchanges can last 5 or 10 minutes.

5. Formal dress is expected as an indication of professional respect. Women are not allowed to wear short skirts or pants in a formal situation.

6. Use of the left hand is considered rude. When handing objects, they should be placed directly in the right hand and not on a table or counter.

7. Some Arabs are frequently late for appointments or do not keep the appointment at all. Family needs may come before the need to keep to strict appointment times. However, among persons from Turkey, punctuality is important.

8. Arabs usually maintain a conversational distance of 2 feet between speaker and listener, in contrast to the usual American distance of 5 feet. Men frequently touch each other and use many gestures during conversation. Men do not usually touch women during conversations, especially women who are not close friends or family members.

9. During conversations, Arabs maintain steady eye contact with the listener.

10. A positive response ("yes") to a request may be an expression of goodwill, not an indication that the request will be carried out or agreement. Noncommittal answers usually mean "no."

The Arabic language is rich with forms of assertion, exaggeration, and rhetorical devices (e.g., metaphors, similes, and proverbs). Repeated words and overassertions are used in most routine exchanges for emphasis and to convince the listener that what is being said is actually meant. Emphasis and repetition should be used to stress meaning.

The ecologic approach, advocated by several researchers (Damico, 1993; Robinson and Cook, 1990; Wilson, 1975, 1990; Wilson, 1996), emphasizes the importance of bringing culture to the frontline in the delivery of services to Arab American speakers. An ecologic assessment system takes into account client culture, ethnicity, socioeconomic status, attitudes, self-concept, and learning style. This is critical to service delivery and management of Arab speakers. SLPs who serve speakers of Arab descent must develop new skills, including the following:

1. Use descriptive situational assessment and intervention techniques within the context of interactions between the Arab speaker's culture and the culture of the SLP or audiologist.

2. Incorporate literature and information characteristic of the Arab speaker's background into clinical intervention.

3. Apply the Arab speaker's culture to the diagnostic and treatment process.

4. Be aware of historical and political factors that may influence the delivery of services.

Finally, the ecologic and dynamic assessment methodologies propagated by several researchers (Butler, 1989; Crago, 1990; Taylor & Payne, 1983; Wilson, 1975; Wilson, 1996) offer valuable approaches to the culturally fair assessment and intervention of Arab speakers. These methodologies including the following:

1. Learn the history of immigration of the family and the client, including their political associations. This is particularly important, given the volatile political climate in the Middle East.

2. Identify roles and responsibilities within the family and the support system. Determine who is responsible for the intervention program and who makes decisions within the family. Take care not to discount the role of the father in decision making, even if the direct contact is with the mother.

3. Avoid touching without permission, especially areas around the head.

4. Respect religious beliefs and practices by avoiding taboo topics such as pigs, pork products, and Christian holidays for Muslim clients.

5. Avoid scheduling during the noon hour, which may be used for prayers and on Fridays, the Muslim Sabbath.

6. Respect concerns for services being provided by men to women or by younger clinicians to older clients.

CONCLUSION

Arabs in the Middle East, America, and the Arab diaspora are a composite of a changing society that is at once nostalgic about its past and eager to assume its role in the modern industrial world. It is a culture in which issues in male-female relations, dichotomies between urban-rural lifestyles, and conflicts between traditional conservative tribal culture and patriarchal authority contrast with the beneficiaries of the oil-rich land. The depiction of Arabs in America and the Arab diaspora has changed in the past 40 years. The challenge for the Middle East, Arab America, and the Arab diaspora is "how" to provide its constituents with the critical SLP-A services they need and deserve.

DISCUSSION QUESTIONS

1. What impact do the recent political events in the Middle East have on SPL-A services in the region?

2. The incidence of hearing loss and cleft palate in the Middle East is higher than in many other parts of the world. How would you develop a culturally appropriate program to prevent hearing loss in the Middle East?

3. The education of young girls has been improving in certain regions of the Middle East. What impact does the education of the mother have on the development of speech and language and the identification of speech-language problems in young children? How would you develop a culturally appropriate program to counteract the impact of this problem?

4. Many sectors in the Middle East have experienced political unrest for many years. What impact might such unrest have on speech, language, and hearing disorders in the region?

REFERENCES

Adeed, P., & Smith, G. P. (1997). Arab Americans: Concepts and materials. In J. A. Banks (Ed.), *Teaching strategies for ethnic studies*. Needham Heights, MA: Allyn & Bacon.

Alireza, M. (1991). At the drop of a veil. Boston: Houghton Mifflin.

Almaney, A. J., & Alwan, A. J. (1982). *Communicating with Arabs*. Prospect Heights, IL: Waveland Press.

Butler, K. G. (1989). From the editor, language assessment and intervention with LEP children: Implications from an Asian/Pacific perspective. *Topics in Language Disorders, 9,* iv-v.

Cole, L. (1989). E pluribus pluribus: Multicultural imperatives for the 1990s and beyond. *ASHA, 31,* 65-70.

Crago, M. B. (1990). The development of communicative competence in Inuit children of Northern Quebec: Implications for speech-language-pathology, *Journal of Childhood Communication Disorders, 13,* 54-71.

Dallo, F. J., Al-Snih, S., Ajrouch, K. J. (2009). Prevalence of disability among US- and foreign-born Arab Americans: Results from the 2000 US Census. *Gerontology, 55,* 153-161.

Damico, J. S. (1991). Descriptive assessment of communication ability in LEP students. In E. V. Hamayan & J. S. Damico (Eds.), *Limiting bias in the assessment of bilingual students* (pp. 157-218). Austin, TX: PRO-ED.

Damico, J. S. (1993). Clinical forum: Adolescent language. Language assessment in adolescents: Addressing critical issues. *Language, Speech and Hearing Services in Schools, 24,* 29-35.

Daniel, J. (2005, January 25). Education for all in the Arab world. UNESCO. Retrieved from http://www.portal.unesco.org/education/en/ev.

Davidson, E. (1991). *Islam, Israel and the last days*. Eugene, OR: Harvest House.

El-Halees, Y., & Wiig, E. (2000a). Arabic language screening test: Preschool and school age. Arlington, TX: Schema Press.

El-Halees, Y., & Wig, E. (2000b). Arabic receptive-expressive vocabulary test. Arlington, TX: Scheme Press.

Ferguson, C. A. (1971). *Language structure and language use*. Stanford, CA: Stanford University Press.

Guittierrez-Clellen, V. F., & Quinn, R. (1993). Assessing narratives of children from diverse cultural/linguistic groups. *Language, Speech and Hearing Services in Schools, 24,* 2-9.

Hammond, H. (2006). Illiteracy in the Arab world, adult education and development. 66 DVV International. Retrieved from http://www.iiz-dvv.de/index.php?article_id=208&clang=1.

Hitti, P. (1985). *The Arabs: A short history*. Chicago: The Gateway Edition, Regency Gateway.

Hsourani, A. (1991). *A history of Arab peoples*. Cambridge, MA: Belknap Press of Harvard University Press.

Immigration and Naturalization Service (1998). *Annual report: Statistical yearbook*. Washington, DC: U.S. Government Printing Office.

Isenberg, I. (1976). *The Arab world*. New York: Wilson.

Jaber, L., Nahamani, A., & Shohat, M. (1997). Speech disorders in Israeli Arab children. *Israel Journal of Medical Science, 33*, 663-665.

Jackson, M. L. (1995). Counseling youth of Arab Ancestry. In C. C. Lee (Ed.), *Counseling for diversity*. Needham Heights, MA: Allyn & Bacon.

Jackson, M. L. (1997). Counseling Arab Americans. In C. C. Lee (Ed.), *Multi-cultural issues in counseling* (2nd ed.) (pp. 333-352). Alexandria, VA: American Counseling Association.

Lamb, D. (1987). *The Arabs: Journeys beyond the mirage*. New York: Random.

Mansfield, P. (1992). *The Arabs*. New York: Penguin.

McLeod, S. (2007). The International Guide to Speech Acquisition. Clifton Park, NJ: Thomson Delmar Learning.

Mustafa, M. (2011). Prevalence of the connexin 26 mutation 35delG in nonsyndromic hearing loss in Egypt. Retrieved March 5, 2011 from http://webspace.webring.com/people/sr/ragerald/35delG-in-Egypt.pdf.

Nydell, M. K. (1997). *Understanding Arabs: A guide for Westerners*. Yarmouth, ME: Intercultural Press.

Robinson, C. A., & Cook, V. J. (1990). Alternative assessment: Ecological and dynamic. *NASP Communiqué, 18*, 28-29.

Sharifzaden, V. (1998). Families with Middle Eastern roots. In E. W. Lynch & M. J. Hansen (Eds.), *Developing cross-cultural competence: A guide for working with young children and their families*. Baltimore: Brookes.

Schwartz, W. (1999). Arab American students in public schools. *ERIC Digest* (Report No. 142). (ERIC Document Reproduction Service No. ED 429 144).

Shipler, D. K. (1987). Arab and Jew: *Wounded sprits in a promised land*. New York: Penguin.

Suleiman, M. (2001). Teaching about Arab Americans: What social studies teachers should know. *ERIC Digest* (ERIC Document Reproduction Service No. ED 442 714).

Swan, M., & Smith, B. (Eds). (1987). *Learner English: A teacher's guide to interference and other problems*. New York: Cambridge University Press.

Taylor, O. L., & Payne, K. (1983). Culturally valid testing: A proactive approach. *Topics in Language Disorders, 3*, 8-20.

U.S. Census Bureau (2001). *Statistical abstract of the United States* (120th ed.). Washington, DC: U.S. Department of Commerce.

Wiig, E. H., & El-Halees, Y. (2000). Developing a language screening test for Arabic-speaking children. *Folia Phoniatrica et Logopedica, 52*, 260-274.

Wilson, M. E. (1996). Arabic speakers: Language and culture, here and abroad. *Topics in Language Disorders, 16*, 65-80.

Wilson, W. F. (1975). Dialect-fair evaluation of the syntax of kindergarten children. *Doctoral thesis*, University of Illinois at Urbana-Champaign.

Wilson, W. F. (1990). Prevalence of communication disorders: A comparative survey. Paper presented at RCLMSS Seminar. Riyadh, Saudi Arabia: King Saudi University Press.

Wilson, W. F. (1993, November). The role of speech-language pathology and audiology in the management of handicapped children in Saudi Arabia. Paper presented at the First International Conference of the Saudi Benevolent Association for Handicapped Children. *Saudi Annals of Medicine*, Riyadh, Saudi Arabia.

Wilson, W. F. (2010, August). A rearview mirror and windshield view of communication disorders in the Arab World. Paper presented at the IALP, Athens, Greece.

World Bank (2005). Notes in disability services in the Middle East and North Africa. Retrieved from http://www.siteresources.worldbank.org/DISABILITY/. . ./MENA/MENADisabilities.doc.

Zehr, M. A. (1999). Guardians of the faith. *Education Week, 18*, 26-31.

ADDITIONAL RESOURCES

Naff, A. (1983). Arabs in America. In S. Abraham & N. Abraham (Eds.), *Arabs in the new world: Studies on Arab-American communities* (pp. 8-29). Detroit: Wayne State University Press.

Naff, A. (1998). *The Arab Americans*. New York: Chelsea House.

Nydell, M. K. (1997). Understanding Arabs: A guide for Westerners. Yarmouth, ME: Intercultural Press.

Sharifzadeh, V. (1998). Families with Middle Eastern roots. In E. W. Lynch & M. J. Hansen (Eds.), *Developing cross-cultural competence: A guide for working with young children and their families*. Baltimore: Brookes.

GENERAL ARABIC SPEECH AND LANGUAGE RESOURCES

Badry, F. (2009). Milestones in language development in Arabic. In *Encyclopedia of language and literacy development*. London, ON: Canadian Language and Literacy Research Network.

Badry, F. (2006). First language acquisition. In *Encyclopedia of Arabic language and literature* (vol. 2). Leiden: Brill.

Dyson, A., & Amaryeh, M. M. (2007). Jordanian Arabic speech acquisition. In S. McLeod (Ed.), *International guide to speech acquisition* (pp. 288-299). Clifton Park, NJ: Thomson Delmar Learning.

Chapter 5

Native American and Worldwide Indigenous Cultures

Carol Westby and Ella Inglebret

WHO ARE INDIGENOUS PEOPLE?

Definitions of Indigenous

UNESCO states that there are between 300 and 500 million indigenous peoples in more than 70 countries throughout the world, representing more than 5000 languages and cultures. There is not a universally accepted definition of *indigenous people*. In the Americas, Australia, and New Zealand, indigenous communities are those that occupied the land before the arrival of European settlers. In countries in Asia and Africa, many people consider themselves indigenous if they have achieved decolonization and self-determination from European colonial powers. In still other countries, people may consider themselves indigenous if they have endured domination from neighboring countries.

The United Nations uses the definition of indigenous peoples that was formulated by the International Labour Organization (ILO) (1989). The ILO defines indigenous peoples in two ways:

- Tribal peoples in independent countries whose social, cultural, and economic conditions distinguish them from other sections of the national community
- Peoples in independent countries who are regarded as indigenous on account of their descent from the populations that inhabited the country, or a geographical region to which the country belongs, at the time of conquest or colonization or the establishment of present state boundaries and who retain some or all of their own social, economic, cultural, and political institutions

Self-identification as indigenous is also regarded as a fundamental element in this working definition. On an individual basis, an indigenous person is one who belongs to an indigenous group through self-identification and is recognized and accepted by the group as one of its members.

The ILO uses both the terms indigenous peoples and *tribal peoples* because there are tribal peoples who are not indigenous in the literal sense in the countries in which they live, such as the San or Maasai peoples in Africa, who may not have lived in a region they inhabit longer than other population groups. The World Bank uses the term indigenous peoples in a broader way, relying on three variables: language, self-perception, and geographic concentration. The World Bank's definition is not exclusive to groups who have suffered colonization. These three variables are used in different combinations and given different priorities depending on the country. In Bolivia and Peru, language was the most important criterion; in Guatemala, self-identification or self-perception was most important; whereas in Mexico, language and geographic concentration were foremost (Psacharopoulos & Patrinos, 1994).

Indigenous peoples of the world are very diverse (Bartlett, Madariaga, O'Neil, & Kuhnlein, 2007). They live in all countries and form a spectrum of humanity ranging from hunter-gatherers and subsistence farmers to professionals. In some countries, such as Bolivia and Peru, they form the majority of the population, whereas in many others they comprise small minorities. Some seek to preserve traditional lifestyles while others seek to adapt to a country's mainstream. Despite extensive diversity in indigenous communities, all indigenous peoples (as defined by the ILO) have one thing in common: they all share a history of injustice and historical trauma. For many indigenous peoples, this historical trauma is cumulative emotional wounding across generations. It includes trauma from one's own lifespan and trauma that emanates from massive group ordeals such as massacres, boarding school abuses, and intergenerational transfer of traumatic responses (Evans-Campbell, 2008). Indigenous peoples are the victims of violent crime more often than national averages (Greenfield & Smith, 1999) and experience overt and covert instances of racism. The historical trauma response is in reaction to intergenerational traumatic history. Of the 17,000 Cherokees forced to leave their ancestral homes in North Carolina and relocate in Oklahoma, 8000 died (Churchill, 1996). Both the Creek and Seminole nations suffered approximately 50% mortality in their relocations as well (Foreman, 1989). Nearly every tribe in the United States has its own story of relocation and warfare. Even as late as the 1950s, American Indians were relocated—this relocation moving them from traditional lands to urban areas. Australian Aborigines had similar experiences. In Australia, under a government policy that ran from 1910 to 1971, as many as 1 in 10 of all Aboriginal children were removed from their families and placed in orphanages or foster homes in an effort to "civilize" them by assimilation into white society. Boarding schools had an especially negative impact on the quality of indigenous parenting and the development of domestic violence in indigenous families. Parents who were traumatized as children often pass on trauma response patterns to their offspring, including violence. Gender roles and relationships were also impaired as indigenous children were taught values that women and children were the property of men and that the corporal punishment of children was acceptable. People who have been traumatized tend to pass on the trauma.

In this chapter, we use the ILO definition of indigenous that involves experience with conquest or colonialism. We focus on indigenous populations in Hawaii, North America, Australia, and New Zealand. Indigenous populations in these areas have had somewhat similar experiences with colonization, and there are services for persons with communication disorders.

Countries vary in terms of how they identify and refer to indigenous peoples. Canada uses the term *aboriginal* or *indigenous* to describe three groups that make up their indigenous populations: First Nations, Inuit, and Metis (born out of relations between Indian women and European men in west-central Canada). The indigenous peoples of the Arctic or circumpolar north include American Alaska Natives; the Inuit in Alaska, Canada, and Greenland; the Saami in Scandinavia; and the Chukchi and Nenets in Siberia. Australia refers to its indigenous people as Aboriginal Australians, Aborigines, or indigenous Australians. New Zealand's indigenous people are commonly called Maori, but they prefer the term Tangata Whenua (people of the land).

In Latin America and the Caribbean, indigenous peoples make up 8% of the population. In Bolivia, they make up about 81% of the population, whereas in Argentina, they are a very small minority. In many of the countries, the groups are referred to by their self-identified names. In Brazil, the dominant culture refers to many of the indigenous groups as *indios*. In many of the Latin countries, a sizeable portion of the population identify themselves as mestizo (mixed European/Amerindian). In Mexico, 75% of the population are of mixed Indian and non-Indian heritage (mestizo), 20% full-blooded Indians, and 5% white; only those who speak native languages are considered indios. (Note: Because in Mexico the term *mestizo* has taken on myriad meanings, being used by mixed-race persons with no Amerindian or Spanish heritage, the designation mestizo is not used in official census counts.) Mestizos typically do not follow traditional ways of life (clothing, customs, language) but have adopted European dress, customs, and language.

Identifying indigenous groups in Asia is more difficult. The government of India officially recognizes many tribes as Scheduled Tribes. The Scheduled Tribes are a sizeable minority of India's population and spread across numerous states. They are assumed to be the oldest ethnic groups, but they are not always easily identified. The numbers vary from 250 to 593. China officially recognizes 56 ethnic minority groups, the largest being the Han, which constitute more than 90% of the ethnic minorities. China's ethnic minority groups, such as the Han, fit the World Bank's definition of indigenous peoples as social groups with a cultural identity distinct from the dominant society that makes them vulnerable to being disadvantaged.

The concept of indigenous peoples is particularly problematic in Africa, where the majority of Africans claim indigeneity compared with white colonists. Despite this, there are more than 14.2 million self-identifying Indigenous Peoples in Africa categorized into three groups: hunter-gatherers (e.g., Pygmy people of central Africa and the San of southern Africa), fisher people, and pastoralists (e.g., Maasai of Kenya and Tanzania).

In the United States, indigenous groups include Native Hawaiians and American Indians/Alaska Natives. (The term *Native American* is used interchangeably with *American Indian*.) The American Indian population consists of Indians, Inuit, Yupic, and Aleuts. Specifically, "Who is an Indian?" in the United States, however, is a difficult question to answer because no single federal or tribal definition is used to determine membership in this population. Three definition categories have been applied: biological, administrative, and mystical. Biological definitions are usually based on some minimum "blood quantum" or percentage of "Indian blood" (e.g., one fourth, one eighth). Each Native American group has always had a name for itself, which often translates to something like "The People." Official names have often been applied by outsiders, and often these names are now used by the Indians themselves. For example, the group known as Sioux is actually a number of related groups, including Ogala, Hunkpapa, and Yanktonia. The word *Sioux* comes from a French translation for a term applied to the group by their enemies, the Blackfoot, and means something like, "those who crawl in the grass like snakes." The Creek got their name from English settlers describing the location of their settlements next to creeks. Those called Native American or American Indian often prefer to identify themselves using terms specific to their native groups, such as Nee-me-poo (Nez Perce) or Dineh or Diné (Navajo). Native Americans of one nation were and are as different from Native Americans of another nation as the English are from the Spanish or the Swedes are from Italians (Heinrich, 1991).

The population figures for indigenous peoples of the Americas before the 1492 voyage of Christopher Columbus have proved difficult to establish. Most scholars writing at the end of the 19th century estimated the pre-Columbian population at about 10 million; by the end of the 20th century, the scholarly consensus had shifted to about 50 million (Taylor, 2002). There is general agreement that a very large percentage of these peoples succumbed to diseases introduced by Europeans. As of July 1, 2008, the estimated population of American Indians and Alaska Natives was 4.9 million, including those of more than one race. They made up 1.6% of the total population (www .infoplease.com/spot/aihmcensus1.html#axzz0zzsJFDCu.)

Native Americans reside in every state of the United States. About three fourths of the population is found in the West and upper Midwest. In the East, New York, North Carolina, and Florida have sizeable indigenous populations. In the 2000 census, the Cherokee tribe was the largest with 729,533 members. The Navajo had the second largest population with 298,197 members. The next largest tribe was the Sioux with a population of 153,360. Although most of the Indian population reside off their reservations, about one third live on reservations (U.S. Census Bureau, 2000). Of 279 recognized reservations, only 18 had populations of 5000 or more in 2000. Reservations vary in size from almost 16 million acres of land on the Navajo Reservation to less than 100 acres on smaller reservations. Some reservations are occupied primarily by tribal members, whereas others are inhabited by a high percentage of non-Indian land owners (Bureau of Indian Affairs, 1991). The Mountain States (Arizona, Colorado, Idaho, Montana, Nevada, New Mexico, and Utah) have the largest number of reservations in the United States. These reservations are relatively isolated and distant from urban centers. Given this remoteness, residents of these reservations intermarry less with non-Indians than do residents of other reservations—a fact reflected in the small share of American Indians reporting a multiracial heritage.

Multiethnicity and Ganma

In today's world, the lives of most indigenous peoples have been influenced by persons who have acted as colonizers. In recent years, it has been acknowledged that people frequently cannot be identified with one culture. Increasing numbers of interracial marriages and cross-cultural adoptions are resulting in multiethnic individuals and families (McCubbin et al., 2010). A great deal of diversity exists both within the American Indian and Alaska Native population and among the children of these groups. Some of these children live within a tightly knit circle of family, clan, and tribal members situated in remote reservations. Others live in cities distant from their family's reservation and have only limited contact with their families or tribe. Some of this heterogeneity is manifest in the "mark all that apply" option for racial identification in the 2000 U.S. Census. About 2.5 million people were identified as nothing other than "American Indian" or "Alaska Native" in the 2000 U.S. Census. But another 1.6 million people were identified

as American Indian or Alaska Native along with one or more other races, making a total of 4.1 million people who claim some connection with an American Indian or Alaska Native heritage. During recent years, many Native Americans have shifted from reservation to urban residences. Thus, exposure to the dominant culture and the associated adoption of dominant culture values varies widely.

Multiethnicity is not limited to those exposed to other cultures just through marriage or adoption. In this diverse world, many persons living in diverse environments develop multiethnic identities. Indigenous peoples are likely to have multiple identities that have been influenced by contact with multiple cultures. In a number of instances, there may have been more than one colonizer. For example, indigenous peoples in eastern Canada were influenced by the French and then later the English. In the Southwest United States, the colonizers were the Spanish in the 1500s, then in the 1800s, English-speaking persons became the colonizers over both the Spanish and indigenous populations. Cultural exposures can affect peoples' identities in different ways in different aspects of their lives.

To understand the cultural diversity of indigenous persons, one must recognize their multiethnicity. Indigenous lifestyles involve behaviors and beliefs regarding language, kin structure, religion, views of the land, and health (Red Horse, 1988). Each of these areas of beliefs and behaviors may be influenced in varying degrees related to the cultures encountered and whether the persons live on a reservation or ancestral lands versus an urban area. Some indigenous persons may maintain a traditional lifestyle in all aspects of their lives, whereas others may operate primarily within and identify with the dominant culture. In practice, many indigenous persons exhibit different cultures or different ethnicities or identities in different aspects of their lives.

Families with primarily a traditional identity adhere to culturally defined styles of living. Parents and grandparents speak primarily the Native language in the home (although they may speak the mainstream language outside of the home). Elders have respected roles because of their accumulated wisdom and have primary roles in child rearing. All family members are active in ritual ceremonies, and depending on the tribal or village customs, they maintain bonds through clan relationships and activities such as ritual naming ceremonies.

Families with bicultural identities maintain some aspects of indigenous beliefs and behaviors, but have adopted much of the dominant culture's lifestyle. Parents often understand the Native language but prefer to speak the language of the dominant culture. They do not teach the Native language to their children nor transmit traditional knowledge. Although they have acquired many characteristics of mainstream society, they are not totally socially integrated. They prefer relationships with other indigenous persons and often replicate traditional extended kin systems by incorporating nonkin friends into traditional roles. Their child-rearing practices

are likely to   ˙˙n values, although they may not
be able to artic   ˙lues explicitly (Miller &
Schoenfield, 1975). ˙ı.   ˙ powwows in urban
areas or social dances in ne...

Some families' identities ma˛   ˙˙d to the
dominant cultures—they speak only tu.   ˙˙
and use mainstream cultural child-rearing ⌐
have nonindigenous religions and no linkages to ı...
Ethnic identity is not static, however. Some persons
identify primarily with the dominant culture may at some
time experience a pan-renaissance—they may attempt to
redefine and reconfirm previously lost cultural lifestyles.
They and their parents may have identified with dominant
cultural values and behaviors, but they are now seeking
to regain their lost heritage. They speak the dominant language but, when possible, attempt to learn the indigenous
language, reestablish clan connections, and participate in
cultural activities.

It is important to realize that any one individual might
show differing ethnic identities across different behaviors.
That is, a person may retain traditional views about health
and religion, yet speak the mainstream language and have
no knowledge of his or her Native language (even when it
may be used by elders in the community). Individuals' ethnic identities will determine how each indigenous person
fits in to both indigenous and nonindigenous (dominant)
cultures. Each indigenous individual can have differing
values, beliefs, and worldviews, depending on the types and
degrees of exposures they have had to other cultures.

The Australian aboriginal concept of *ganma* provides a
means for addressing the effects of multiple cultures coming together in a more positive way than the concept of
acculturation. The ganma metaphor describes a situation in
which water from the sea (Western knowledge) and a river
of water from the land (Aboriginal knowledge) mutually
engulf each other upon flowing into a common lagoon and
becoming one (Pyrch & Castillo, 2001). In coming together, the streams of water mix across the two currents,
and foam is created. The foam represents a new kind of
knowledge. Essentially, ganma is the place where knowledge is created. One culture does not overwhelm another;
rather a third culture arises at the point of intersection.
Similarly, the collaboration of professionals from dominant
cultures with indigenous parties results in unique services
and training programs.

The ganma metaphor can serve as a foundation for
clinical interactions in educational and health care systems.
By employing the concept of ganma, one does not create
marginalized groups that exist alongside a dominant culture, but rather one recognizes the primacy of all groups'
backgrounds and experiences. There is no one dominant
culture enforcing a particular reality. If the two cultures
(waters) can be kept in balance, in what Cazden (2000)
called the "ganma space," the nutrients that come together
with the mix of waters nourish richly diverse forms of life.

INDIGENOUS LANGUAGES

Language Loss

Every 14 days, a language dies. By 2100, more than half of
the more than 7000 languages spoken on Earth—many of
them not yet recorded—may disappear, taking with them
a wealth of knowledge about history, culture, natural environment, and the human brain (http://www.nationalgeographic
.com/mission/enduringvoices/.) In many cases, indigenous languages are spoken by relatively few persons and are not supported (and are even discouraged) by the dominant culture. As a
result, indigenous languages are at high risk for being lost.

Indigenous languages vary greatly in the number of
speakers, from Quechua, Aymara, Guarani, and Nahuatl (in
Latin America) with millions of active speakers to a number
of languages with only a handful of elderly speakers. Of the
approximately 300 indigenous languages spoken in North
America before the arrival of Columbus and the 250 spoken
in Australia before the arrival of Europeans, more than half
are extinct, and many are near extinction (Krauss, 1998;
Walsh, 1991). In the United States, only about 20 languages
are still spoken by people of all ages and are thus fully vital
(Reyhner & Tennant, 1995). Some of these languages are
spoken by only a few individuals, and others, such as
Cherokee, Navajo, and Teton Sioux/Dakota, are spoken by
thousands (Estes, 1999). The Navajo language is the most
frequently spoken indigenous language in the United States,
with 148,530 speakers.

Language defines a culture. Many endangered languages
have rich oral cultures with stories, songs, and histories
passed on to younger generations, but no written forms.
Words that describe a particular cultural practice or idea
may not translate precisely into another language. With the
extinction of a language, an entire culture is lost. The
National Geographic Society's Enduring Voices Project
(www.nationalgeographic.com/mission/enduringvoices/)
and the Living Tongues Institute for Endangered Languages
(www.livingtongues.org/) both seek to document and, when
possible, to maintain or revitalize languages. By using
appropriate written materials, video, still photography, audio
recorders, and computers with language software, as well as
access through the Internet where possible, these projects
help empower communities to preserve ancient traditions
with modern technology. The National Geographic Society
has identified the most endangered language hotspots in the
world—places where no children and few adults speak the
indigenous language. Table 5-1 shows the eight most frequently spoken indigenous languages in the United States
(www.aaanativearts.com/article592.html.)

Indigenous groups in Hawaii, Australia, New Zealand,
and North America have also experienced severe language
loss. Latin America has large numbers of peoples who continue to speak indigenous languages. Mexico's Mesoamerica
region encompassed a large number of early civilizations,

TABLE 5-1 Most Frequently Spoken American Indian Languages

Language	Locations	Speakers
Navajo	AZ, NM, UT	148,530
Cree	MT, Canada	60,000
Objiwa	MN, ND, MT, MI, Canada	51,000
Cherokee	OK, NC	22,500
Dakota	NE, ND, SD, MN, MT, Canada	20,000
Apache	NM, AZ, OK	15,000
Blackfoot	MT, Canada	10,000
Choctaw	OK, MS, LA	9, 211

From www.cogsci.indiana.edu/farg/rehling/nativeAm/ling.html.

including the Olmec, Teotihuacan, Maya, and Aztec, before the arrival of Europeans. The region is now home to many of Mexico's indigenous groups, which continue to speak ancestral languages despite cultural pressure to speak Spanish. The Andes Mountains of Peru and the Amazon Basin of Brazil have high language diversity, but there is little documentation of remaining indigenous languages. Spanish, Portuguese (in Brazil), and more dominant indigenous languages are replacing smaller ones. Speakers of small indigenous languages are shifting to Spanish or larger indigenous languages, such as Guaraní.

Language Policy and Revitalization

Historically, Canada, the United States, and Australia sought to eliminate indigenous languages. Australia has relatively recently acknowledged the loss of Australian aboriginal languages in the National Indigenous Languages Survey (NILS) Report of 2005 (Australian Institute of Aboriginal and Torres Strait Islander Studies, 2005). Of the 145 languages that are still spoken, 110 are critically endangered. The Australian government is attempting to develop a national approach to preserve the languages. In 2009 to 2010, $9.3 million was invested in 65 projects around Australia to support the revival and maintenance of aboriginal languages.

Since the 1960s, in Canada, indigenous languages have increasingly been taught in schools (Assembly of First Nations, 1990; Burnaby, 2008; Kirkness & Bowman, 1992). In addition, indigenous languages have been the medium of instruction up to the third grade in some schools in the territories and Quebec, where the children begin school speaking only or mainly their indigenous language. Indigenous language immersion programs have begun in several communities, where the children start school speaking only or

mainly an official language (English or French). Nine indigenous languages have been made official languages in the Northwest Territories together with English and French. The new territory of Nunavut has declared Inuktitut, Inuinaqtun, French, and English as official languages and is actively developing policies for extensive use of these languages in many domains.

In the United States, the Native American Languages Act of 1990 recognized the importance of traditional indigenous languages to the survival of Native American cultural identity and ensured that the U.S. government would act together with Native Americans in preserving and promoting the use of Native languages. Despite this stated support for Native languages in the United States, in practice, use of the language in educational settings has had minimal support or has been actively discouraged by other laws or educational requirements. Sixteen states have passed English-only laws.

The latter 20th century has witnessed indigenous language revival efforts in Australia, New Zealand, Hawaii, North America, and the circumpolar north (Cantoni, 2008; King, 2009; Reyhner & Lockard, 2009). In the 21st century, indigenous communities around the globe have been using modern technology to help maintain and even revitalize their threatened and dying languages and cultures (De Korne, 2009). Thousands of tribal communities, from the circumpolar north to the outback of Australia to the forests of the Northwest Pacific Coast, are creating educational programs to record the stories and oral traditions of their elderly last speakers. Using cameras, film, and audio, community members are creating powerful archives of material as well as elaborate word dictionaries. By fall 2011, 20 episodes of the Berenstain Bears animated cartoon series will be broadcast on South Dakota Public Television, with all dialogue dubbed in Lakota. A DVD will be released as well, complete with a Teachers' Guide. This Lakota Language Consortium project was initiated last year as part of its mission to promote the language outside of the schools (www.lakhota.org/html/BBprojectstart.html.)

Passing the knowledge along to the younger generation has become of paramount importance and urgency. Without younger generations speaking and understanding the words and stories of their ancestors, the language dies. And when the language dies, the culture dies. Fishman (2000) observed that successful language revitalization initiatives in many parts of the world are not just about reversing language loss. Rather, they are "about adhering to a notion of a complete, not necessarily unchanging, self-defining way of life" (p. 14). An indigenous language is a link to the past, that is, to the ancestors and a traditional way of life. If the language is lost, many of the cultural practices and events no longer have meaning. It is through language that one is able to participate fully in cultural events. Without language, traditions such as hunts, songs, and dances would lose their significance because embedded in the songs and stories are values such as cooperation, kinship, respect (e.g., for self, mother earth, animals), and responsibility. The sense of place, belonging, identity, and values are expressed through language. The implications and consequences of attitudes toward language and its preservation and the resources available for language preservation and maintenance efforts are complex issues and affect progress across and within communities.

Indigenous English

In some indigenous groups, characteristics of the indigenous language have been transferred to the dominant language spoken in an area. The influences of indigenous languages on English have been documented for American Indians (Leap, 1993), Canadian First Nations (Ball & Bernhardt, 2008), Australian Aborigines (Butcher, 2008), and Maori (Bell, 2000; Holmes, 1997). There are several ways that indigenous languages influence English. Some of these influences include (1) retention of the phonemic and phonological characteristics of the indigenous language, (2) indigenous language syntactic rules taking priority over English syntactic rules, (3) word formation and grammar markings from the indigenous language influencing the English dialect, and (4) constructions found in other nonstandard variations of English also being found in indigenous English. Even when there has been no contact with the indigenous language for many generations, the indigenous language may strongly influence the present English dialect. For example, Wolfram (2000) has described and traced the roots of the Lumbee Indians in North Carolina. Although the Lumbee are not a recognized tribe, they are ethnically and culturally Native American. The Lumbee lost their language many generations ago. The Lumbee dialect shows the influence of early colonization by the English, Scots, and Scots-Irish, but Lumbee speech is distinctly different from its Anglo-American and African American neighbors. For example, Lumbee speakers may use the finite bes (e.g., "I hope it bes a little girl"; "It bes really crowded"; "The train bes running") and the perfective I'm (e.g., "I'm went down there"). African American and European American natives do not use these patterns, even when they grow up practically next door to the Lumbees who do (Dannenberg & Wolfram, 1998).

In the Southwest, where Native languages continue to be spoken by many tribes, influences of these first languages can be observed in the English language of both adults and children. In Navajo, Apache, and the Pueblo languages, words generally begin with consonants and end with vowels. When speaking English, these indigenous speakers are likely to devoice final consonants or substitute a glottal, which is the most common consonant in the languages. If an English word begins with a vowel, speakers may add an initial glottal. Voice onset time differs between these Native languages and English. These languages do not have the voiced-voiceless distinction present in the

plosives b/p, d/t, and g/k. Instead, there are single plosives with voice onsets between /p/ and /b/, /t/ and /d/, and /k/ and /g/. As a result, children are slow to distinguish between these phonemes in English.

These Southwest Indian languages have an SOV (subject-object-verb) sentence structure. Verbs are highly inflected. There are no gender pronouns or pronouns for "it." As a consequence, both children and adults may use gender pronouns incorrectly when speaking English. Pronominal prefixes on verbs code the relationships of subjects and objects to the verbs (possessor, agent, patient, benefactee) and person (first, second, third, fourth [passive]). Number is coded in the verb as one, two, and more than two. Location (coded by prepositions in English) is coded in the verb and is influenced by the characteristics of the objects (see example in Box 5-1). Size comparisons are made on the basis of volume and plane in space (vertical or horizontal). Hence, there are no generic words for big and little. As a consequence, preschool children may be confused when confronted by tasks of classifying objects as "big" or "little." One cannot use the same word to talk about a "big snake" and a "big elephant."

Valiquette (1990) noted that in Keres (spoken in five Pueblo groups), infinitives are rare, and dependent clauses (which in English use connective words such as when, while, until, because, before, after, although, if) are used but appear to be related to age privilege differences, not to age developmental differences. That is, as one matures and gains stature in the community, one uses dependent clauses with increasing frequency and a wider variety of purposes. A form of "and" is used as the connective in many dependent clauses. Valiquette (1990) suggested that this is the result of the frequent use of "and" ("y") in English and Spanish. It may, however, also be a reflection of how Native Americans perceive the temporal and causal relationships coded in dependent clauses (Hall, 1983). Time is not viewed as linear, and cause goes beyond physical principles (Cajete, 2000).

Speech-language pathologists (SLPs) must be alert to the varieties of indigenous English and how they may affect children's performance on speech-language tests. Silver and Miller (1997) have documented the basics of grammar in 160 Native languages, along with discourse genres (language functions) and relationships between language and worldview. Mithun (2001) provides information on the sound, syllable, and syntactic patterns of all the indigenous languages of North America. In addition, she provides some discussion of "baby talk," narrative, and ceremonial language use by some of the indigenous groups. Dixon (2007) provides linguistic descriptions of Australian Aboriginal languages, and Harlow (2007) provides this for Maori. An understanding of the characteristics of the indigenous language can enable SLPs to identify the characteristics of indigenous-influenced English in particular groups.

BOX 5-1 What does a Keres speaker say when told, "Place this object(s) on the table . . . ?"

To know what to say, the Keres speaker must know how to categorize the objects. The Keres words in bold print would all be translated as "put on" or "place on." To know which verb form to use, persons must understand the Keres categorization system. Notice how the objects are grouped by their characteristics. Preschool Keres-speaking children know how to classify objects to use the appropriate verb form.

pishidiicha (enclosed in a covntainer)	**picha** (singular)	**piguya** (mass)	**pit'cha** (wide flat shape of container)
purse	pen	trash can	basket
bag or popcorn	newsletter	chair	plate of cookies
sack of corn	cup	washing machine	basket of corn
groceries	ruler	TV	platter of chicken
carton of eggs	comb	apple	laundry
box of paper	scarf	10-gallon hat	
	computer disk		
	spoon		
	coat		
	pencil		
	empty mug		
	magazine		

piwaisht'i (liquid in bowl)	**piisha** (plural)	**piy'aat'a** (plural)	**pisht'icha**
bowl of posole	group of papers	3 chairs	(liquid in it)
	gloves		cup with water
			pot of coffee
			pitcher of milk

WORLDVIEWS AND CULTURAL VALUES

A worldview is a way of seeing the world. The worldviews of indigenous cultures contrast with worldviews of dominant cultures. Although there is considerable variation in values and beliefs among indigenous cultures, there are some similarities in their worldviews (Hart, 2010). Knudtson and Suzuki (1992) described the indigenous worldview as reflected in the stories and traditions from 22 different indigenous cultures around the world. They contrast the indigenous mind with the scientific mind. The worldviews of indigenous peoples have a spiritual orientation that is embedded in all elements of the world and cosmos. Indigenous peoples believe that humans live in harmony with the world. The resources of nature are viewed as gifts; and nature is honored through spiritual practices. Time is measured by the daily, monthly, and yearly cycles of nature. In contrast, dominant cultures typically view time as linear and document it in terms of a chronology of human activities.

To interpret assessment data and provide appropriate and acceptable interventions for indigenous peoples, clinicians must have an understanding not only of the ways of knowing of the group but also of the cultural values and beliefs that underlie their ways of knowing. A variety of approaches have been used to study cultural variations in values and beliefs among people (Hall, 1976; Hofstede, 1980; Kluckhohn & Strodtbeck, 1961; Triandis, 1995). Cultures can differ along several dimensions. Although there is considerable variation among indigenous cultures, there are some ways in which indigenous cultures are more similar to one another than they are to dominant cultures.

Individualism versus Collectivism

All societies must strike a balance between independence and interdependence—between individuals and the group (Greenfield, 1994). Dominant cultures of northern European heritage are strongly individualistic, whereas indigenous groups are generally collective. Individualistic cultures emphasize the individual's goals, whereas collectivistic cultures stress that group goals have precedence over the individual's goals. In individualistic cultures, people look after themselves and their immediate family only, whereas in collectivistic cultures, people look after members of their in-groups or collectives in exchange for loyalty (Triandis, 1995). Collectivistic cultures emphasize goals, needs, and views of the in-group over those of the individual; the social norms of the in-group, rather than individual pleasure; shared in-group beliefs, rather than unique individual beliefs; and a value on cooperation with in-group members, rather than maximizing individual outcomes. Perhaps a better term in indigenous cultures is "relatedness" (Martin, 2008). There is a depth of relatedness among all people within the group. In some indigenous cultures, relatedness is reflected by persons introducing themselves by first identifying the clans or extended families to which they belong rather than by their given names. In a YouTube video Terry Teller, a Navajo, introduces himself: "I'm from the Water Flows Together Clan (mother's clan). I'm from the Coyote Pass People (father's clan). My maternal grandparents are from the Sleeping Rock Clan. My paternal grandparents are from the One Who Walks Around Clan" (www.youtube.com/watch?v=ZbZBX2lgWUg0.) Aunts and uncles may be referred to as mother and father and cousins as brother and sister.

The collectivist nature of the indigenous cultures can influence assessment and intervention. Children in a collective culture are more likely to provide assistance to others, even in ways that mainstream teachers consider cheating. Although indigenous communities function collectively in terms of having responsibilities for one another, there is also respect for individuality. Everyone is viewed as fulfilling a purpose, and as a consequence, no one has power to impose values on others. Autonomy is highly valued, and children are expected to make their own decisions and operate semi-independently at an early age. They may be left alone to tend sheep or watch younger siblings at young ages. Children are allowed choices and freedom to experience the natural consequences of their choices. Despite the children's freedom to make choices, the impact of their choices on others is also emphasized (LaFromboise & Low, 1989). Mainstream service providers have sometimes misinterpreted this early independence as an indication of neglectful or uninvolved parents.

Doing versus Being or Being-in-Becoming

Cultures of northern European heritage epitomize the doing orientation in which there is "a demand for the kind of activity that results in accomplishments that are measurable by standards conceived to be external to the acting individual" (Kluckholn & Strodtbeck, 1961, p. 17). Persons seek to be in control, to be in charge. In contrast, indigenous cultures represent being and being-in-becoming cultures. The being orientation is concerned with who one is, not what one can do or has accomplished. One is valued simply for being. One's worth is not decreased if one has a disability or as one ages and becomes less physically able. The focus on human activity in the being-in-becoming orientation is on striving for an integrated whole in the development of self. Therefore, there is no need to compete and prove one better than others. As a result, indigenous children do not need to strive to be better or to stand out from others. A number of researchers, in fact, report that indigenous children may actively avoid being singled out even to be praised for good performance. Praise in front of a group may bring a sense of shame (Boggs, 1985, Hawaiian; Eriks-Brophy & Crago, 2003, Inuit; Deyhle, 1987, Navajo; Gould, 2008a, Australian Aboriginal).

Relationship to Nature

In indigenous cultures, the concept of relatedness applies not only to people but also to everything else in the world—indigenous peoples are related not only to one another but also to animals, plants, land, sky, and waterways. No one element is better than or less than another. Mainstream culture maintains a mastery-over-nature orientation, involving the perspective that all natural forces can and should be overcome or put to use by humans. With this value system, mainstream families may think about the significance

of a disability for the future. They may ask, "When will she learn to talk?" "Will therapy correct the problem?" or "When can he return to work?" They express concern regarding what persons cannot do, what they will be able to do, and when they will be able to do it. Parents, spouses, or clients take responsibility for alleviating the disability. Persons with these mainstream values seek treatment for disabilities and are co-participants in their therapy.

Indigenous peoples, in contrast, maintain a harmony-with-nature orientation that makes no distinction between or among human life, nature, and the supernatural. With their being-in-becoming and harmony with nature orientations, indigenous peoples tend to have a greater tolerance for variation, and they may feel less need to "fix things," focusing instead on learning how to accept and cope with their circumstances. Families may recognize that a family member is different but accept that difference as being who the person is. Because of such viewpoints and values, they may be less likely to seek out evaluation and treatment services. When they do become involved, it is important to include the extended family in decisions. According to Benally (1989), Navajo education focuses on preparing individuals to reach a state of *hozho*—a state achieved through a balanced and harmonious life. All knowledge is viewed with respect to its ability to draw one closer to this spirit of harmony. Traditionally, individuals are taught the interrelationship and interdependence of all things and how they must harmonize with them to maintain balance and harmony.

Time Orientation

Orientation to human activity influences perceptions and use of time. Mainstream cultures are driven by "clock time," whereas indigenous cultures are more attuned to "event time" (Harris, 1998). Hall (1976) refers to these two orientations toward time as monochronic and polychronic. Monochronic time emphasizes schedules, segmentation, and promptness. With the exception of birth and death, all important activities are scheduled. Polychronic time systems are characterized by several things happening at once. They stress involvement of people and completion of transactions rather than adherence to present schedules. Nothing seems firm; changes in the important events occur right up to the last minute, creating frustration for those who may value promptness and sticking to well-organized plans and schedules. Indigenous peoples believe in the cyclical nature of time—days, months (in terms of moons), and years (in terms of seasons or winters). Many cultures developed elaborate ways to track time. For example, the Anasazi, ancestors of the present Southwest Pueblo Indian groups, were highly attuned to time. At Fajado Butte in New Mexico, they arranged boulders and carvings in the rock mesa that mark the sun's solstices and equinoxes and the 11-year cycle of the moon (Sofaer, 2007; Sofaer & Ihde, 1983). The "sun dagger" of Fajado Butte is considered the Stonehenge of the New World.

Scollon and Scollon (1980) reported that Athabaskan Indians believe it is inappropriate to speak of plans or to anticipate the future. Navajos believe that one should live a long life and not limit one's potential with a specific plan or timeline. They believe that if one sets a specific plan for future actions, one may limit all other possibilities for living a long life (Mike et al., 1989). Although Native Americans may not be consciously aware of the reasons for not planning, they may have grown up in environments where planning ahead was not done and time was not rigidly scheduled. Activities are done "when the time is right." Although one may be told that a dance or a chapter house meeting may begin at a particular time, this may only mean that the event will occur in the near future. The actual event may not begin for several hours. The idea of what constitutes "being late," then, differs in mainstream and Indian cultures. Children growing up in polychronic time systems are less likely to have experienced the pressure to perform quickly, and as a consequence, they may not perform well on timed tests.

Mainstream cultures value schedules and punctuality. Actions focus on the immediate and the future. Activities are bound to the imposed rhythms of work days, time clocks, overtime, saving time, and taking time out. "The ticking of the clock is more important than the beat of the human heart" (Bruchac, 1994, p. 11). Mainstream service providers sometimes think that indigenous clients have no sense of time because they may not honor imposed schedules (Hall, 1983).

Cultural systems that value traditions highly are said to have past orientations. The future orientation predominates where change is highly valued (e.g., mainstream U.S. culture). Living in a dominant culture will result in indigenous peoples having some focus on the future, but at the same time many will continue to value and maintain the traditions of the past. As a consequence, elders are respected and hold power and must often be included in any decisions made regarding interventions for persons with impairments or illnesses.

Human Nature

Native Americans acknowledge that the world is made up of both good and bad. They believe, however, that in the end, good people will triumph. This belief is reflected in the trickster tales that appear in stories of many indigenous groups. Coyote (Southwest), Raven (Northwest), Iktomi (Plains), Amagug the wolf (Inuit), and Bampana (Australian Aborigine) fool, trick, cheat, and take advantage of good people, but in the end, they usually lose.

COMMUNICATION PATTERNS

Conversation

Frequent miscommunication arises when indigenous persons and dominant-culture persons interact because their values and beliefs affect their styles of communication.

Australia has produced a document, *Aboriginal English in the Courts,* to explain the confusions that can occur when examining Aboriginals in the court system (Eades, 2000). Eades noted that long periods of silence are generally avoided in mainstream discourse except among intimate friends or relatives. In Aboriginal societies, on the other hand, lengthy periods of silence are the norm and are expected during conversation, particularly during information sharing or information seeking. Persons in the dominant culture may interpret a person's silence or lack of overt acknowledgment during questioning as unwillingness to participate or answer. Greater tolerance of silence in conversation has been reported for a number of indigenous groups, including Australian Aborigine (Mushin & Gardner, 2009), Apache (Basso, 1990), Navajo (Plank, 1994), Salish (Covarrubias, 2007), and Inuit (Crago, 1990).

Scollon and Scollon (1980) suggested that problems arise between mainstream speakers and Alaskan Athabaskan natives in three areas: (1) speakers' presentations of themselves, (2) organization of talk, and (3) contents of talk. Table 5-2 summarizes communication differences between persons from northern European heritage backgrounds and indigenous speakers that have been identified by a number of anthropologists and educators studying indigenous persons in North America (Basso, 1990; Hall, 1959; 1976; 1983; Philips, 1983; Saville-Troike, 1989; Scollon & Scollon, 1980).

Mainstream persons get to know others by talking; only when they know someone well do they think there is less need to talk. In contrast, many indigenous people prefer talking to those they know well; when they do not know someone well, or in cases in which people have been separated for some time, they prefer to watch and listen until they have gathered sufficient information about a person. Basso (1990) tells the story of Native American parents waiting at the trading post for their children to arrive home from boarding school where they have been for several months. The children got off the bus and piled into their parents' trucks. Unlike mainstream families, in which parents would question children about their activities over the past months, the Native children and parents spoke minimally. When Basso questioned parents about this, they reported, "We know that our children have been to the Whiteman's school. When they return to us, we do not know who they are. We must watch and listen until we know who they are."

The nature of communication that occurs in classrooms employing a Western education system may be unfamiliar, confusing, or threatening to indigenous children. The person in the dominant position (the teacher or clinician) asks questions and then listens to persons in the subordinate position (students) to show what they know. Mainstream children are expected to perform even if they are not sure or make a mistake. In contrast, indigenous children are expected to learn by watching, and they do not perform

TABLE 5-2 Cross-Cultural Perspectives of Speakers

Mainstream Perspective of Native American Speakers	Native American Perspective of Mainstream Speakers
Presentation of Self	
Talk very little	Talk too much
Do not initiate	Always talk first
Avoid situations requiring talking	Talk to people they do not know
Only want to talk to close acquaintances	Think they can predict the future
Play down their abilities	Brag about themselves
Act as if they expect things to be given to them	Do not help people even when they can
Deny planning	Talk about what's going to happen later
Distribution of Talk	
Avoid direct questions	Ask many questions
Never start a conversation	Always interrupt
Talk off topic	Talk only about their interests
Never say anything about themselves	Boast about themselves
Are slow to take a turn to talk	Do not give others a chance to talk
Contents of Talk	
Are too indirect and inexplicit	Are too direct; are not careful when they talk about people or things
Leave without saying anything	Have to say "goodbye" even when they can see you are leaving

Source: Reprinted with permission from Scollon R., & Scollon, S. B. (1980). *Interethnic communication.* Fairbanks, AK: Alaska Native Language Center.

until they have mastered the skill. When teachers ask indigenous children to display knowledge, the children may be silent or may appear to become unruly. To the children, teachers may appear incompetent because they are not doing most of the talking, yet they are acting superior (Scollon & Scollon, 1980).

In mainstream interactions, persons are expected to "put their best foot forward." They are expected to speak well of themselves and have high hopes for the future. In contrast, in many indigenous cultures, it is not only inappropriate, but also bad luck, to speak highly of one's self, highlight one's experiences, or talk about one's plans for the future. As a consequence, parents may be hesitant to respond when asked about their child's strengths or to talk about their future plans for the child.

Hall (1959; 1976; 1983) differentiated cultures on the basis of the communication style that predominates in the culture. A high-context communication or message is one in which "most of the information is either in the physical context or internalized in the person, while very little is in the coded, explicit, transmitted part of the message." A low-context communication or message, in contrast, is one in which "the mass of the information is vested in the explicit code" (Hall, 1976, p. 79). Although no culture exists at either end of the low- to high-context continuum, the cultures of mainstream Australia, New Zealand, Canada, and the United States are placed toward the lower end; indigenous cultures fall toward the high-context end of the continuum. When persons from high-context cultures communicate with persons from low-context cultures, they

are likely to experience miscommunication. The indirect, nonspecific style of high-context indigenous individuals appears vague to low-context mainstream individuals, and they are likely to suspect that the high-context individual is being intentionally evasive or uncooperative. The loud, explicit, direct style of low-context mainstream individuals appears impolite, rude, and disrespectful to high-context indigenous peoples.

Narrative Discourse

I will tell you something about stories, he said. They aren't just entertainment. Don't be fooled. They are all we have, you see all we have to fight off illness and death. You don't have anything if you don't have stories

(from p. 2 of *Ceremony* [1977] by Leslie Marmon Silko, a member of the Laguna Pueblo tribe).

Narratives maintain the foundations for indigenous cultures; they are the means for communicating cultural traditions, values, and beliefs as well as a vehicle for passing on information about history, science, government, and politics. All cultures have narratives, but these narratives vary in terms of their functions (why they are told), content, structure, who tells them, and how listeners are to respond (McCabe, 1995).

Many indigenous cultures have identified particular people to be storytellers for the community. Children may be apprenticed to storytellers. The ages at which children become storytellers vary in different cultures. In Inuit and Australian Aboriginal groups, young girls begin sharing stories with one another (Eickelkamp, 2008). Yup'ik girls in Alaska may tell story knife stories. The story knife is a traditional girl's toy used for sketching pictures on the ground or in the snow. Originally, the knives were wood, bone, or ivory; now girls use butter knives. The pictures show clothing, people, houses, animals, and events, and are drawn to illustrate a story or as a game in which others try to guess the artist's subject. Australian Aboriginal girls tell sand stories, using a milpa (twig), or a bent wire that they call "story wire." The story wire is used to beat a rhythm and draw shapes in the sand that represent meaning in a story. In both cultures, boys traditionally do not tell these types of stories.

Indigenous narratives vary in multiple ways from narratives of dominant European and North American cultures, but by the time children are 9 or 10 years of age, dominant culture schools expect them to be able to comprehend and produce complete episode narratives including a setting, initiating event, response, plan, attempts, consequences, and resolutions (Hedberg & Westby, 1993). Dominant culture stories typically offer explicit details regarding these story components—who was involved, where they were, what they were doing, why they were doing it, and what were the results on their actions. In contrast, stories from indigenous speakers often appear "minimalist" to persons from dominant cultures (Sharifian et al., 2004). The stories do not appear to have the types of plots expected by dominant Western cultures. For example, Worth and Adair (1975) observed that Navajos devoted more attention to background and setting information than to the initiating events and consequences. In most Navajo stories, the storytellers spend much of their time describing walking, the landscape, and the places they pass, talking only briefly about what to us are the plot lines. Highwater (1981) proposed that Native American narratives represent a different view of space, time, and motion than narratives of people from Western cultures. The listener must be able to fill in the details of the stories from their own knowledge of the situation.

Indigenous narratives tend to have a different purpose than many mainstream narratives. This difference in purpose was exemplified in an episode of the television show, "Northern Exposure," in which a Native American medicine man attempted to understand white persons' stories. The Native American character reflected that Indian stories have a great healing power. They reflect on everyday life values and are told to influence people to change their life in some way. In contrast, he observed that white persons' stories tended to talk about mishaps and to put people down and did not appear to have any value in changing persons' lives. Basso (1990) noted this function of Native American stories to affect persons' lives. He discussed Apache historical tales that focus on persons who suffer misfortune as a consequence of actions that violate Apache standards for acceptable social behavior. Like arrows, these stories are shot at persons to warn them to change their ways. When using stories for assessment purposes, evaluators may need to establish a purpose for telling stories.

Stories produced by persons of European heritage tend to have a linear, temporal structure. In contrast, stories produced by Australian Aborigines and North American indigenous cultures are known to have a nonlinear structure. Australian Aborigines may not rely much on chronologic sequencing of events in their narratives. Instead, they may order events according to their salience in the schemas evoked in the mind of the speaker (Sharifian, 2002). This structure may be related to the Aboriginal worldviews of the Dreaming in which time is not sharply partitioned into past, present, and future. Benally (personal communication, 1989), a Navajo educator, described the structure of Navajo narratives as like Indian fry bread (a circular piece of dough fried in oil) with "an idea bubbling up here, another idea bubbling up over there." Lutz (1989) discussed the circle as a philosophical and structural concept in Native American narratives. The plots of Native American and Euro-American stories are affected by these circular and linear orientations and by cultural values. In stories of European and dominant North American cultures, a returning adventurer brings a happy ending with power, honor, respect, and material possessions for the individual. In Native American plots, the ensuing happiness and harmony that result from a person returning from a quest involve all persons within the circle affected, such as bringing rain clouds that affect the total environment rather than money for an individual. The cultural contrast in plots is a contrast between a community, tribal, circular mode and an individualist, materialist, and linear mode (Lutz, 1989).

The structure of the indigenous language can influence narrative organization and focus, even if the storyteller is telling the story in the language of the dominant culture. Lewis (1992) had Ute and Anglo children in first through sixth grade retell a favorite movie. She noted that non-Indian students' narratives had story themes and linear sequences of beginnings, middles, and ends. In contrast, the Ute students' narratives were event focused, characterized by unconnected events and unexplained descriptions. The non-Indian students presented the listener with some direction for the story; in contrast, the Indian students tended to jump directly into the storytelling without providing the listeners with background information or reasons for the story. The nature of the Ute students' narratives called into play a participatory speaker-listener engagement which is a guiding principle of Ute oral discourse (Leap, 1991). Ute storytellers assumed shared knowledge between the speaker and listener and expected that it was the listeners' responsibility to infer the meaning of the story or to question the storyteller. Crago and colleagues (1997) reported that Algonquin children tended to tell stories that ended at the high point, leaving the listeners to resolve the story. To listeners from European heritage cultures, such stories are deficient and unsatisfying. This expectation for listener participation in story comprehension can generate problems for students in classroom environments in which teachers expect predictable stories that stand alone.

A similar narrative discourse pattern was noted in beginning Navajo college students (Gregory, 1993). Gregory and other instructors who taught basic English to secondary and beginning college students were able to blindly identify essays written by Navajo students. Gregory observed that the structure and language choice in the Navajo essays was determined by interaction of the topic and audience. In contrast, the structure of the mainstream students' essays was determined by their genre or purpose. The Navajo students tried to make connections with the audience more so than the mainstream students. In oral language, Navajo students relied heavily on interaction to maintain clarity; they appeared to assume that readers have the same responsibility in reading their written language. Navajo writers were more likely to directly address the audience (using I, you, and we in their writings) than the mainstream writers, and they expected the audience to assume responsibility for interpretation. This personalized approach to written discourse may present particular difficulties as students are expected to comprehend and produce increasingly decontextualized expository texts in science and social studies classes in school.

Worldviews and familiarity with cultural events and schemas can affect the ways that persons comprehend narratives they hear or read. When indigenous narratives are told to persons who do not share the cultural schemas of the storyteller, listeners are likely to misinterpret the stories. When Australian non-Aboriginal educators were asked to retell narratives told by Aboriginal students, they partially recalled, distorted, and reinterpreted ideas and added ideas from their own schema knowledge (Sharifian et al., 2004). Indigenous persons experience similar difficulties when comprehending and retelling stories from the dominant culture. Indigenous students had more difficulty than Euro-American students in identifying the themes of short stories (with Euro-American themes), even though they were matched for reading skills (Bock, 2006).

HEALTH AND DISABILITIES

Types of Disabilities

Around the world, indigenous peoples (the Saami in Norway and Sweden; the Maori in New Zealand, the Inuit of the circumpolar north; the Aborigines of Australia; Native Hawaiians, Alaska Natives, and Native Americans in the United States; and First Nations people of Canada) have less education, higher poverty levels, and more physical and psychological health problems than persons in their countries from dominant cultures (Barnes et al., 2010; Faircloth & Tippeconnic, 2010; United Nations, 2009).

Indigenous peoples in North America, Australia, and New Zealand have the highest mortality rate of all ethnic groups in their countries and the highest rates of infant mortality (Bramley et al., 2004; Maternal and Child Health Section, 2008).

Otitis media (OM) is the most frequently identified disease of indigenous children in Australia, New Zealand, Canada, and the United States (Bowd, 2005; Giles, & O'Brien, 1991; Hunter et al., 2007; Morris et al., 2009; Thomson, 1994). OM occurs more frequently and is typically more severe in these populations. OM includes not only fluctuating hearing loss but also severe complications resulting in hearing impairment of a more permanent nature (Moore, 1999). Racial, anatomic, and familial variables are associated with the incidence of OM (Todd & Bowerman, 1985). Inuit children are at particularly high risk for OM and its complications (Bowd, 2005; Moore, 1999). Following an extensive literature review, Stewart (1986) concluded that occurrence of OM in indigenous people was influenced by (1) ethnic origin, (2) eustachian tube placement and insufficient middle ear aeration, (3) relative inefficiency of the immune system. Recent research is providing support for the theory that deficiencies in the immune systems of indigenous persons explain their susceptibility to OM (Wiertsema & Leach, 2009).

Diabetes and diabetic-related complications such as heart disease, retinopathies resulting in vision loss, circulatory problems that can result in amputations, and stroke are also high in indigenous populations in industrialized countries and are increasing (Si et al., 2010). Native Americans experience low rates of amputation but high rates of stroke. On average, American Indians and Alaska Natives are 2.3 times as likely to have diabetes as non-Hispanic whites of similar age in the United States. In Canada, prevalence of diabetes among First Nations peoples is at least 3 times the national average, and First Nations peoples with diabetes are 3 to 4 times more likely to suffer from heart disease and stroke. Maori and Pacific Island people in New Zealand have nearly 3 times higher prevalence of diabetes, and their mortality rates from diabetes in the 40- to 65-year age group are nearly 10 times higher than for Europeans. Although Aboriginal and Torres Strait Islander people in Australia experience 3 to 4 times higher prevalence of diabetes than in the general population, their death rate associated with diabetes for the 35- to 54-year age group is 27 to 35 times that of nonindigenous Australians. In some indigenous groups in the United States, 25% or more of the population is diabetic by age 40 years. Native American children are exhibiting increasing rates of diabetes. There has been a sixfold increase in diabetes in some groups of Native American children between 1976 and 1996 (Fagot-Compagna et al., 2000).

The incidences of alcohol abuse and fetal alcohol spectrum disorders (FASD) have been documented to be higher in many indigenous groups compared with dominant culture groups in the same countries (Szlemko et al., 2006). FASD is a constellation of physical abnormalities related to the teratogenic effects of alcohol ingestion during pregnancy. It results in prenatal and postnatal growth deficiency, central nervous system dysfunction (tremors, microcephaly), craniofacial anomalies (cleft lip and palate, thin upper lip, and epicanthic folds) (Streissguth, 1997). Children with FASD exhibit gross and fine motor delays, speech and language delays and disorders, learning disabilities, attention-deficit/hyperactivity disorder, hearing impairments, mental retardation, and behavioral disorders (Carney & Chermak, 1991; Streissguth, 1997).

Bowker (1993) stresses the need for caution when interpreting these data on educational achievement and a variety of health issues in indigenous populations. Mainstream professionals should not conclude that the indigenous culture itself fosters high school dropout rates, alcoholism, and poor health. Bowker notes that these behaviors are all highly correlated with poverty, and indigenous populations are typically the most poverty-stricken group in a nation. In recent years, the poverty and health issues of indigenous peoples is being linked to their historical trauma (Brave Heart & DeBruyn, 1998). Understanding how historical trauma might influence the current health status of indigenous populations may provide new directions and insights for eliminating health disparities and providing effective educational interventions. Efforts to reduce educational and health disparities among indigenous peoples involve exploration of ways to use traditional ceremonies and healers in the healing and intervention processes.

Attitudes toward Disabilities

Words such as disability, impairment, handicap, and rehabilitation are not easily translated in indigenous languages. Many indigenous languages do not have words that could be translated for the concepts of learning disabilities or cognitive impairments; instead they may use words such as incomplete or slow (Locust, 1986). Some behaviors that may represent disabilities in the mainstream culture may not be recognized in an indigenous community. For example, at an assessment workshop conducted by the first author, a school psychologist described how she explained the concept of learning disabilities to a Navajo family, "Your child is having difficulty doing White man's things in school." This was a reasonable description. The child exhibited the disability only when doing "White man's things."

Cultures vary in the ways disabilities are explained. The Navajo people are instructed to live harmoniously with Mother Earth and Father Sky, as well as to demonstrate respect for the circle of life, which includes the environment, animals, plants, and humankind. They believe that violations of beliefs and values may not only disrupt the natural order of life but also cause disharmony, which may manifest itself as ill health. A holistic approach to health implies that all things in life are connected to one another and that people are connected in a spiritual and physical sense in this circle. Many families live in both the indigenous and dominant culture, seeking services and explanations in both.

Views about the origin of disabilities are unique for each culture. Interviews with Navajo elders revealed that the origin of disabilities is related to violation of moral virtues by the First People (Vining & Allison, 2000). They believe that disabilities are becoming more prevalent because people are no longer honoring traditional belief systems and teachings. Disabilities are often associated with violation of cultural beliefs and practices. The interviews with Navajo elders also revealed a positive perception of children with disabilities. They believe that people with disabilities are "images of the Holy People" and, as such, should be considered sacred. They believe that the Holy People intended for a family to have a child with a disability.

In many Native cultures, both expectant mothers and fathers need to be careful with what they see, hear, feel, smell, and eat. In Navajo belief, supernatural projection on a baby within the womb results in the infant taking on characteristics of the entity being projected and may affect the child's physical, emotional, mental, and spiritual development. Although it can be useful for interventionists to know how a family explains a disability of a child or elder, the mainstream professional must exercise care in asking for this information. Many of these explanations are tied to religious beliefs and are not to be shared with the mainstream world.

Different Native American societies hold different views about disabilities. Some types of disabilities have particular meanings. For example, in some Southwest tribes, epilepsy is considered a sign of sibling incest and harmful to the community. Typically, however, Native American groups are accepting of disabilities, and in some instances, a child with a disability is seen as a special messenger from the spiritual world. Unusual behaviors may not be judged as either positive or negative but simply as part of who the child is (Nichols & Keltner, 2005).

In some instances, it is the dominant culture beliefs and attitudes about disabilities that affect access to services. Brazil has the wealthiest economy in South America and has university academic programs that prepare special educators and SLPs. Services for children with disabilities, however, are not typically available in schools. Most services are private and must be paid for by families. The Brazilian culture as a whole is not accepting of persons with disabilities (Watson et al., 2000). In Brazil, individuals with developmental disabilities are often referred to as "the sick one" (doente) or "the crazy one" (o doido). Private and public schools continue to refuse children with physical, cognitive, or developmental disabilities, even though Article

8 of Public Law 7.853 from October 24, 1989 states that such exclusion is a punishable crime (Ministerio da Justica, 1996).

Bolivia has the highest indigenous population of any country in the western hemisphere and the poorest Latin American economy. There is limited training for special educators and no training programs in the country for SLPs or audiologists. There are no services for children with special needs in schools and very limited private services of any type. Many persons, both indigenous and nonindigenous, believe that disabilities are caused by something that someone did wrong, that the person is cursed, and that being around a person with disabilities may bring harm to them.

APPROACHES TO SPEECH AND LANGUAGE SERVICE DELIVERY

A Framework for Assessment and Intervention

The International Classification of Functioning, Disability, and Health (ICF; World Health Organization, 2001) provides a conceptual framework for comprehensively examining and describing an individual's health and communication status. Taking into account (1) body structures and functions, (2) activity and participation, and (3) contextual factors, including personal and environmental variables, the structure of the ICF can serve as a means for framing culturally responsive service delivery. Figure 5-1 provides a visual representation of the ICF as it interconnects with speech-language pathology practice for members of indigenous populations.

A structure of concentric circles is used to frame the ICF for guiding clinical and educational practice with indigenous community members. The core of the structure centers on internal contextual factors of a personal nature. These reflect what an individual brings to a clinical interaction, such as cultural identity or identities, languages spoken, gender, and age. External contextual factors provide the outer structure for the framework and include environmental influences, such as self-determination and tribal sovereignty, institutional leadership and policies, curriculum and pedagogy, professional service providers, attitudes, and racism. Nested within this framework are body structures and functions considered at the individual level that are then surrounded by activities and participation involving families and community dimensions. All levels influence and interact with one another.

Metaphors are commonly used to communicate ideas in indigenous communities (Bergstrom et al., 2003; LaFrance & Nichols, 2008). For example, the New Zealand Government Ministry of Education (1996) uses "a woven mat" *(Te Whariki)* as a metaphor characterizing its culturally based early learning curriculum policy. In parallel, the ICF model presented here can be viewed as a circular mat on which all participants stand. The weaving of the mat begins at the center with textures and colors that vary based on personal factors, including cultural beliefs and values. Strands are woven outward from the center to interlink with the external circle, representing contextual factors emanating back from the surrounding environment, such as policies and attitudes. Connections made between the inner and outer circles generate tension that can strengthen (act as a facilitator) or weaken (act as an obstacle) the mat's structure. The strands interconnecting personal and environmental factors form a foundation for weaving in connections, with the two nested circles representing levels of capacity (ability to do a task) in body structures and functions of the individual and levels of performance (actually doing the task) in activities and participation within families and communities. Consideration of relationships connecting all levels and dimensions of the ICF determines the overall strength of the framework.

The role that indigenous knowledge might play when providing speech and language service delivery will be used to illustrate application of the ICF model. Beginning at the level of personal factors, the clinician asks the question, "What does the individual bring to the clinical interaction?" Indigenous knowledge is inherent in the personal factors of cultural identity, indigenous languages, gender, and age. Kipuri (2009) describes traditional indigenous knowledge as "the complex bodies of systems of knowledge, know-how, practices and representations maintained and developed by indigenous peoples around the world, drawing on a wealth of experience and interaction with the natural environment and transmitted orally from one generation to the next" (p. 65). Kipuri goes on to point out that traditional knowledge is reflected in "stories, songs, beliefs, customary laws and artwork or scientific, agricultural, technical and ecological knowledge" (p. 65) and the indigenous language that is specific to a particular place. The manner in which indigenous knowledge manifests itself will depend on all aspects of the oral tradition, going beyond spoken language, to include nonverbal behaviors and all life processes (Archibald, 2008). Roles of community members vary depending on gender and age, with elders playing a key role as teachers in intergenerational educational processes (LaFrance & Nichols, 2008).

The next question that a clinician might ask is, "How might surrounding environmental factors influence service delivery?" First, recognition and validation of indigenous knowledge are embodied in the rights of indigenous peoples to self-determination and tribal sovereignty over their lifeways on a broad scale. As a further environmental factor, international leadership and policies recognize the rights of indigenous peoples to determine the content and practice of education, inclusive of special education. The Declaration on the Rights of Indigenous Peoples, adopted by the United Nations in 2007, recognized the rights of indigenous peoples to determine their own identities and to

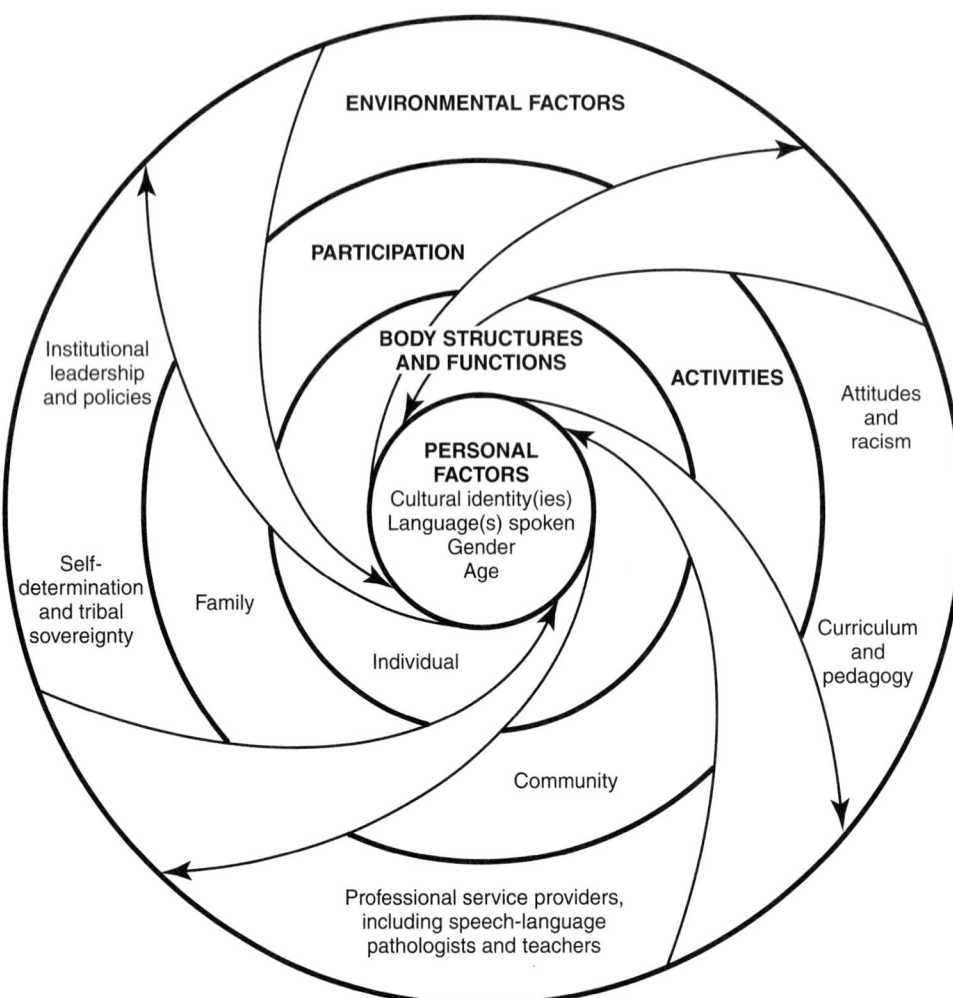

FIGURE 5-1 The International Classification of Functioning, Disability, and Health (ICF) and speech-language pathology practice with indigenous populations. *Adapted from: CHiXapkaid & Inglebret (2007); Inglebret, Brownfield, & CHiXapkaid (2008); and World Health Organization (2001).*

restore and pass on their traditional knowledge, languages and other cultural expressions, and histories. In addition, the Coolangatta Statement on Indigenous Peoples' Rights in Education (World Indigenous Peoples' Conference on Education, 1999) cites a variety of international policy statements that support the rights of indigenous peoples to self-determination as they strive to preserve and revitalize their heritage, languages, cultures, spirituality, and knowledge systems through education. Understanding the interweaving of indigenous knowledge across the personal and environmental contexts then leads to the question, "How might greater awareness of indigenous knowledge influence speech-language pathology practice in the ICF realms of body structures/functions and activities/participation?" Indigenous leaders and researchers in the United States (Goodluck, 2002; Kana'iaupuni, 2004; Research Agenda Working Group, Strang, & von Glatz, 2001), Canada (Canadian Council on Learning, 2007), and New Zealand (Rameka, 2007) have called for a paradigm shift that moves

away from focusing on deficits to examining and enhancing the health, well-being, and strengths of students. With this shift comes a focus on giving clients credit for the indigenous knowledge they bring to their learning. This may run contrary to practices that attempt to identify problems in body structures and functions through assessment of an individual's communication difficulties in a controlled environment and in isolation from the needs of everyday life. The design of the ICF is consistent with a shift away from just examining deficits in body structures and functions. By adding the dimension of activities (execution of tasks or actions) and participation (involvement in life situations), the ICF guides the clinician to examine communication skills and health in real-life settings as the individual relates to family and community members on a daily basis. Thus, indigenous knowledge reflected in these relationships is viewed as an asset. This also requires a shift away from a "professional as the authority" perspective to assume a reciprocal teacher-learner relationship, in which the professional service provider becomes a learner of what constitutes indigenous knowledge for a specific indigenous community.

The New Zealand Ministry of Education's (1996) early childhood curriculum policy statement entitled *Te Whariki* provides an example of ganma—it interweaves indigenous knowledge and Pakeha (Western) knowledge systems. It represents a reciprocal teacher-learner orientation, whereby students, family and community members, and professionals all learn from each other. The curriculum has developed four principles to guide assessment of student learning. These include (1) Whakamana (empowerment) —children's "sense of themselves as capable people and competent learners" is enhanced (p. 30); (2) Kotahitanga (holistic development)—"all dimensions of children's learning" are considered (p. 30); (c) Whanau Tangata (family and community)—families are active participants in assessment of children's learning; and (d) Nga Hononga (relationships)—"children learn through responsive and reciprocal relationships with people, places, and things" (p. 43).

These guiding principles exemplify the need to validate what children bring to the learning context and to go beyond examination of body structures and functions in a controlled situation to understand communication and learning within activities and participation in relationships with family and community members as well as with elements of a particular place (e.g., landscapes, plants, animals, foods, and medicines).

Assessment Issues

Indigenous children have frequently been inappropriately placed in special education classes; assessment approaches may violate client and family values; and disabilities related to learning, speech-language, and social-emotional difficulties may be misidentified or unidentified. Application of the ICF framework described previously can be used to illustrate both problematic and promising assessment practices.

Assessing Body Structures and Functions

One problematic practice may involve the use of standardized tools in the special education assessment process. For more than two decades, leaders in indigenous education in the United States have expressed concern regarding the use of standardized testing (Indian Nations at Risk Task Force, 1990; Nelson-Barber & Trumbull, 2007; Tippeconnic, 2003; White House Conference on Indian Education, 1992). This concern has been echoed by researchers in Canada (Ball & Janyst, 2008), Australia (Gould, 2008a, 2008b, 2008c; Klenowski, 2009), and New Zealand (Rameka, 2007). Standardized tests are generally restricted to assessing the level of capacity in body structures and functions in a controlled environment. The learner is typically required

to respond individually to "in the head" tasks for which contextual cues have been minimized or removed (Rameka, 2007). The standardized testing situation and associated response patterns become problematic because they often do not represent interactional patterns typical within indigenous communities. Gould (2008a) shares an example of Australian Aboriginal children feeling "shame" when the response expectations of a standardized testing situation are unfamiliar. The term is used when a person is silent, not answering a question, or avoiding eye contact. The Western professional is likely to interpret the behavioral response as shyness, but Aboriginal shame is much more than shyness. Aboriginal shame is a strong negative sense of stepping outside one's limits (Vallance & Tchacos, 2001). It does not have the same meaning as the European concept of shame. Aboriginal shame is associated with being singled out as the focus of attention, of losing face in a relationship, and a sense of being powerless and ineffectual. It involves deep feelings for which there are no words. This sense of shame in a testing situation can lead to a child's lack of response or reluctance to speak, reflecting a cultural norm that may be confused with a language disorder.

In an effort to identify language screening and assessment tools suitable for use with indigenous children, some research has been conducted with one of the largest tribes in Oklahoma, the Cherokee. Studies of nonreservation, English-speaking Cherokee Indian children indicated that standardized tests are of questionable use with this population (Long, 1998a). Long reasoned that Indian children who live, socialize, and are educated among whites would evidence the same type of language skills as the white children. Yet Long and Christensen (1997) found a significant difference in the linguistic and social-communication language skills between these two groups. When compared with 3- to 4-year-old white children, Cherokee Indian children performed less well on linguistic and social-communication skills. In a further study comparing the performance of Native American and white 5-year-old Head Start children on the Test of Pragmatic Skills (Shulman, 1986), Native American children obtained significantly lower scores than white children (Long, 1998b). Although research has shown that the use of standardized language instruments is questionable even with English-speaking Native American children, the practice of diagnosing speech-language disorders using standardized instruments continues to be frequently used in assessments and evaluations (National Research Council, 2002).

In an effort to evaluate bilingual, bicultural Native American children, service providers have attempted to translate various assessment tools. Parts of speech-language tests, for example, have been translated from English to several Native languages to evaluate students' verbal processing, syntactic (grammar and syntax), and semantic (meaning of words) abilities. Assessors and translators need to be aware that vocabulary words may not be equivalent.

For example, there is not a single word in Navajo that can be translated for the word *construction*. The concept is translated as "there is a man hitting a board with a hammer." Clearly, this sentence is not as complex as the word construction. The phonological and syntactic structures of Native languages are so markedly different from English that translation of articulation and syntactic tests is inappropriate and unrealistic (Allison & Vining, 1999).

Potential problems also exist when using untrained individuals to interpret from English to an indigenous language and vice versa. Interpreters may know a particular language but may not be accepted and respected within the family, community, or culture. Many concepts and words, especially medical jargon, are not easily interpreted or translated into other languages. It is essential that interpreters receive training in confidentiality, medical terminology and concepts, cultural beliefs and practices with respect to disability, and culturally appropriate ways to explain sensitive information.

Assessing Activities and Participation

Appropriate assessment of the communication and health status of indigenous persons requires the clinician to move beyond a focus on capacity of body structures and functions in controlled tasks to examine performance of activities and extent of participation in daily life, including family, community, and school contexts. Data regarding real-life functioning might be gathered by obtaining a case history, interviewing communication partners, observing a student in a natural environment, teacher or parent report, or home language questionnaires. Behavioral inventories, criterion-referenced testing, and work samples such as portfolios can serve as effective means to evaluate cognitive and linguistic abilities as well as linguistic, cultural, and environmental influences that affect learning. Of particular note are the assessment strategies of naturalistic language sampling, ongoing documentation of learning stories, and dynamic assessment.

Language sampling in natural settings provides a means to examine communication skills in daily life, inclusive of both indigenous and other languages. Gould (2008a) compared the use of three language sampling techniques with Australian Aboriginal children who spoke Aboriginal English (AE). These techniques included (1) minimally structured storytelling, (2) elicited story generation, and (3) story retelling. Her findings indicated that the length and complexity of children's language samples varied based on three conversational features: (1) participants, (2) topic, and (3) setting. The most effective strategies involved interactions with adult speakers of AE from the child's community, topics related to local Aboriginal stories and movies, and remaining in a quiet area of a classroom setting versus being pulled out into another room. Language sampling during free play in an AE-speaking classroom or in a home or community setting also resulted in longer and more complex utterances. The least effective language sampling strategies were story retelling, eliciting narratives based on photographs or picture stimuli, and one-to-one conversations with a non-Aboriginal examiner about general topics or objects. It was important that the children had a clear understanding of the communicative expectations and were comfortable in the assessment setting so that a sense of shame could be avoided.

The ongoing documentation of "learning stories" serves as another means to examine health and communication development over time within real-life contexts. Learning stories are narratives or stories that are less clinical. The language used in the telling is understandable to parents and other family members. Learning stories allow two-way learning—from the professional to family and from family to professional. For older children, the stories might include the child's own account of an event. Carr (2001) describes the use of learning stories in an early learning program enrolling Maori children in New Zealand. In this setting, learning opportunities target five domains: (1) well-being (Are the child's needs met with care and sensitivity?), (2) belonging (Are the child's and family's interests and abilities appreciated and understood?), (3) communication (Are the child's efforts to communicate responded to, and is the child invited to communicate?), (4) contribution (Is the child encouraged and assisted in participating with others?), and (5) exploration (Is the child offered appropriate challenges to extend his or her world?). Learning stories are recorded to provide a series of vignettes portraying each child's longitudinal development in the target domains. They focus on documenting the increasing complexity of children's activities and the resources and means used to participate in the learning process. Learning stories are developed from multiple perspectives—service providers and family and community members—allowing for a holistic assessment of the child's development. Rameka (2007) provides an example of a learning story composed by a staff member regarding a 1-year, 8-month-old boy who was participating in a bilingual early learning program in south Auckland. The story describes the child's attempts to problem-solve methods to retrieve a toy thrown over a barrier. After finding a method that worked, the learning story goes on to describe and interpret the child's affective response in relation to the previously described guiding principle of Whakamana (empowerment). "George displays wonderful perseverance and determination to retrieve his toy. Kaitoro—George takes a risk and succeeds in his chosen task. Tumeke (fantastic) George!!"

Dynamic assessment procedures are used with culturally and linguistically diverse students to differentiate children with learning differences from those with learning disorders (Lidz & Peña, 1996; Hwa-Froelich & Vigil, 2004; Peña, 1996; Peña et al., 1992). Dynamic assessment yields information on the process of how students learn. The test-teach-retest methodology used in dynamic assessment rules out lack of experience with test stimuli and tasks. Dynamic assessment tasks involve active teaching by adults who carefully "mediate" the child's learning (Feuerstein et al., 1987). Thus, dynamic assessment provides a means to examine communication at the level of activities and participation in functional social interactions.

Most dynamic assessment tasks have focused on learning noun labels, but label learning may not be the most discriminating task for children from some backgrounds. Ukrainetz and colleagues (2000), working with Arapahoe and Shoshone Head Start children, initially attempted to use dynamic assessment procedures to measure their ability to learn labels for objects. This approach, however, did not differentiate between children developing language typically and those exhibiting language learning difficulties. Observation of the Head Start curriculum the children were exposed to revealed that they had been explicitly taught to label. Ukrainetz then taught category identification (food, clothes, transportation, animals) because the Native American children were observed not to express categorical labels. This dynamic assessment strategy significantly differentiated children judged to be stronger or weaker language learners based on teacher report and examiner observation.

More recently, use of dynamic assessment to evaluate oral narrative abilities of indigenous children has been explored. Using the Dynamic Assessment and Intervention (DAI) tool (Miller et al., 2001), a test-teach-retest strategy was implemented with third-grade children enrolled in a school on the Samson Cree Nation Reserve in Alberta, Canada (Kramer et al., 2009). The modifiability of oral narrative responses to wordless picture books was compared for two groups: (1) children considered to be normal language learners (NLL) and (2) children with possible language learning difficulties (PLLD). Both groups were observed to benefit from adult mediation associated with the teaching phase. However, the NLL group displayed greater linguistic growth and generalization to nontargeted narrative features. High levels of sensitivity and specificity in using the DAI supported the use of dynamic assessment to discriminate language difference associated with culture from language learning difficulties for this particular population.

Intervention

A holistic approach to assessment that is guided by the ICF model will lead to an intervention approach that addresses body structures and functions as they intersect with the broader context of a person's activities and participation with family and community members in authentic life situations. This requires the professional to identify means for bridging the communication expectations of home and community with the expectations of school. Historically, SLPs

have facilitated the development of verbal language skills in oral and gestural modes. More recently, the connections between oral and written language have been recognized, and as a consequence, SLPs are actively involved in facilitating both language and literacy. As SLPs serve persons from indigenous backgrounds, a need to rethink the concept of literacy emerges.

A multiliteracies framework was recently proposed as a guide for teachers and SLPs serving members of culturally and linguistically diverse communities (Healy, 2008; Westby, 2010). The concept of multiliteracies grew out of a need to recognize that what is considered literacy varies across cultures and that rapid technological advances are changing the way communication takes place locally and globally (New London Group, 1996). The concept of literacy is no longer limited to reading and writing of traditional texts. As SLPs serve members of indigenous populations, the concept of multiliteracies becomes particularly salient. Indigenous knowledge has traditionally been grounded in the oral tradition (Archibald, 2008; Dunn, 2001). A view of literacy focused on the printed word misses other ways in which knowledge is represented in indigenous communities. The multiliteracies framework brings recognition to the multiple modes that can be used in comprehending and interpreting information. Using the multiliteracies approach, SLPs and teachers maintain a focus on the linguistic mode and add other modes, including visual, audio, gestural, spatial, and spiritual, associated with cultural and linguistic diversity to the process of facilitating literacy development (Cope & Kalantzis, 2009; Healy, 2008; Kress, 2003; LaFrance & Nichols, 2008; Westby, 2010). The dimensions of these multiple modes and examples of associated culturally based and multimedia literacies are presented in Table 5-3.

The multiliteracies framework can serve as an interface between indigenous and nonindigenous worlds. Martin (2008) explains that when Australian Aboriginal and non-Aboriginal literacies come together in the learning processes of school, home, and community, the points of interaction become sites of "much action and agency, and equally, tension and confusion" (p. 75). Just as with the concept of ganma, new types of knowledge can be generated at these sites. However, it requires that teachers and SLPs be cognizant of their roles as designers of the learning environment and mediators who make the learning process explicit. Educational personnel can create opportunities to generate knowledge through multiple modes, including visual, audio, gestural, spatial, and spiritual, as well as linguistic, associated with both past and present technology. In addition, they can facilitate the development of students' metalanguage pertaining to the associated multiple forms of literacy.

The process of enacting a multiliteracies pedagogy is guided by the four components of: (a) situated practices, (b) overt instruction, (c) critical framing, and (d) transformed

TABLE 5-3 Multiple Design Modes for Comprehending and Interpreting Information

Mode	Dimensions	Examples of Culturally Based and Multimedia Literacies
Visual	Size, shape, color, still or moving image, sculpture, scene, perspective, page layouts, screen formats	Creating video documentaries: use of camera angles, zooming, and composition of foreground and background, uploading images; creating various forms of art, such as glasswork, pottery, sculpture, carving, drawing, painting, weaving of blankets, clothing, and baskets
Audio	Music, ambient sounds, noises, alerts, voice	Playing a drum, chanting or singing a song, generating sound effects for a video
Gestural	Body language, movements of the hands and arms, expressions of the face, eye movements and gaze, gait, clothing, regalia, hair style	Producing or acting out a story, participating in a powwow or in traditional games and sports, performing a traditional dance, using sign language
Spatial	Landscape, ecosystem, graphic design, interpersonal distance, architecture/building	Understanding the ecosystem of a particular place (animals, plants, water, land, air, climate), using geographic information systems (GIS) as a tool for mapping landscape attributes, researching traditional place names and food sources, traditional tracking and hunting
Spiritual	Daily life activities, holistic worldview focused on balance among mind, body, spirit, and environment	Learning indigenous stories of creation and relatedness to ancestors, viewing of language as sacred expression, learning through visions and dreams, understanding that ceremonies often reflect private knowledge not be shared with outsiders
Linguistic	Content (meaning), form (phonology, morphology, syntax), and use (pragmatics), oral and written, coherence, diverse languages	Expressing humor, learning and teaching an indigenous language, learning about the history of a particular group of people through various text forms, including books, Internet sites, oral speeches or stories, interviews with elders, poetry, petroglyphs, pictographs

Adapted from Cope & Kalantzis (2009); Healy (2008); and Kress (2003).

practice (Healy, 2008; New London Group, 1996). Situated practice starts with knowledge bases and worldviews that students bring to learning and then links new learning to these. Overt instruction recognizes that it is often necessary for students of culturally and linguistically diverse backgrounds to translate between knowledge bases of home and community and knowledge bases common to schools. This translation process must be made explicit. Critical framing involves stepping back from the immediate situation to examine and address real needs of particular communities from multiple perspectives. Assumptions underlying learning are brought to the surface. In transformed practice, students use what they have learned in new ways, for new purposes, and for different audiences. Overall, multiliteracies pedagogy requires the educators, SLPs, and students to shift between the roles of teacher and learner on an ongoing basis.

Early Learning

A key element of the multiliteracies framework is situated practice. In parallel with the level of activities and participation in the ICF model, involvement of family and community members in early learning provides a foundation for understanding the knowledge base that young children bring to their learning. U.S. federal legislation, Part C of the Individuals with Disabilities Education Act of 2004 (IDEA), requires that family needs and priorities be addressed in intervention for infants and toddlers. The need to connect with tribal and community entities in designing, implementing, and evaluating early intervention for indigenous children has been emphasized by researchers and educators in Canada (Ball, 2009), New Zealand (Cullen et al., 2009), Australia (Martin, 2008), and the United States (Banks-Joseph & McCubbin, 2006).

Educational practices of an intercultural early learning program in New Zealand (Cullen et al., 2009) are presented to illustrate situated practice, along with the other components of the multiliteracies framework. The Wycliffe Nga Tamariki Kindergarten, located in Napier Aotearoa, New Zealand, serves children and families from Maori, Samoan, and European backgrounds. The intent is to build English language skills while promoting the maintenance of a first language (Samoan) and revival of a heritage language (Maori). Thus, situated practice is grounded in symbols and stories representing each of these cultural and linguistic groups. Examples of cultural tools include names, songs, greetings, poetry, and photographs of local cultural events.

Books present stories of each cultural group and are available in three languages: Maori, Samoan, and English. Input into curriculum development is gained from families through their ongoing program involvement and through periodic focus groups held with community members. Overt instruction bridges the languages and cultures of the children's homes with academic language and learning tools. For example, working together, children and adults use multiple design modes along with contemporary technology to construct Power Point stories. On a daily basis, children and adults take digital photographs of learning activities. These images are downloaded, and associated text is written. A child might take the lead in writing the text, with scaffolding provided by a peer or an adult. As another option, a child and an adult may co-construct the written text. Children may code-switch as they draw from their home or heritage language orally during the process of composing the written story in English. Critical framing occurs as the children experience and select from various text types, technologies, languages, and cultural resources to construct the stories of their everyday experiences. In addition, stories can be framed to represent multiple perspectives. Transformed practice is reflected as children learn through the symbols and stories of their own culture and language and transfer associated meaning to learning through another child's culture and language. In addition, the knowledge that each child brings to the learning process is respected and validated so that reciprocal educator-child teaching and learning takes place. Thus, children use what they have learned in family and community contexts in a new way—to teach educators.

School Age

The Shadow of the Salmon curriculum (Northwest Indian Fisheries Commission, 2009) developed in the United States is well suited to serve as a structure for implementation of the multiliteracies framework for school-aged children. The curriculum was developed for use with eighth-grade classes and consists of a video docudrama accompanied by a curriculum resource guide. In addition, the curriculum has been aligned with Washington State standards in eight content areas (Inglebret & CHiXapkaid, 2009). All materials are readily available at no cost through the Internet. The docudrama portrays the story of Cody Ohitika, an adolescent boy of Lakota Sioux and Salish heritage who visits his Coast Salish relatives in the Northwest. Cody has the opportunity to learn about issues of relevance to the survival of the salmon through traditional Coast Salish educational experiences. These experiences illustrate a variety of traditional indigenous modes for promoting the comprehension of information and portray intersections with Western knowledge bases. Thus, the concept of ganma comes into play as students grapple with multiple ways of knowing and communicating about their surroundings. The following description demonstrates how the multiliteracies framework can be enacted using the Shadow of the Salmon curriculum. Box 5-2 shows types of activities associated with each multiliteracy component.

Situated Practice

Through presentation of culturally based communication and learning activities, the Shadow of the Salmon docudrama situates practice by drawing on the background that

---

BOX 5-2 Multiliteracy in a Native American Curriculum

Situated Practice
- Share experiences about salmon and canoes
- Participate in a canoe journey
- Watch the video, "Shadow of the Salmon"
- Tribal representatives share indigenous perspectives on salmon
- Read/listen to stories related to the ecosystem of which salmon is a part (e.g., "Salmon Woman and Her Children")

Critical Framing
- Examine multiple perspectives of natural resource management practices developed to revitalize the salmon population
- Explore multiple websites
- Analyze multiple solutions for saving salmon
- Compare Native and Western scientific solutions
- Determine whether conclusions of statistical studies reported in media are reasonable

Overt Instruction
- Do KWL (what I know; what I want to know; what I learned)
- Discuss values/beliefs/customs depicted in video/stories
- Facilitate the use of metalanguage to make explicit text design elements and comprehension strategies
  - Discuss the parts/structure of the video
  - Discuss how the words/video depict important concepts/concerns

Transformed Practice
- Write a letter to editor of local newspaper presenting a persuasive argument relating historical events, such as treaties between the U.S. government and American Indian tribes, and the current status of the salmon
- Apply scientific and Native knowledge to develop a solution to the loss of salmon

Adapted from Inglebret, CHiXapkaid, & Lehr (2008) and Northwest Indian Fisheries Commission (2009).

many indigenous students in the Northwest United States bring from their homes and communities. Educational activities build on intergenerational relationships through observation, listening, hands-on experiences, and humor shared among youth, elders, relatives, and community members. The accompanying resource guide provides materials to use in initiating discussion regarding the variety of ways in which people communicate, including storytelling, music, dance, art, and the First Salmon Ceremony. A selection of stories related to the ecosystem of which the salmon is a part, such as "Salmon Woman and Her Children," is provided along with suggested discussion questions and activities. The importance of contacting local tribes and bringing in representatives who can share indigenous perspectives on the salmon is highlighted.

Overt Instruction

Overt instruction involves the use of metalanguage to make explicit various text design elements and comprehension strategies as well as their interrelationships. For instance, teachers and SLPs might facilitate use of a metacognitive learning strategy, such as an adaptation of the KWL process (Henderson, 2008). Use of this strategy involves three stages: K—students identify what they know and how they know it, W—students identify what they want to know and how they will come to know it, and L—learning occurs to generate new knowledge. Overt instruction focuses on the first two phases, K and W. As an example, in the K phase, pairs of students might identify what they currently know about the salmon and the text design modes (i.e., visual, audio, gestural, spatial, spiritual, and linguistic) they used to gain this knowledge. Next, the students move into the W phase and identify what they wish to know about the salmon and the modes they can use to gain this knowledge. To carry out the W phase, students might invite experts representing tribal and state government perspectives in natural resources management to share information on the current status of the salmon. These guest presentations would provide an opportunity to examine different modes used by the speakers to communicate. Through the K and W processes, the knowledge and ways of learning that students bring from their homes and communities is recognized and validated.

Critical Framing

Critical framing might take the form of examining multiple perspectives of natural resource management practices developed to revitalize the salmon population. As was previously mentioned, guest speakers from tribal and state government can present a range of perspectives that are framed by cultural, economic, political, or ecological issues. In addition, students can examine the salmon using different design modes associated with particular academic content areas, such as those associated with state education standards (e.g., communication, reading, writing, science, mathematics, social studies, health and fitness, and arts). Inglebret and CHiXapkaid (2009) have identified various learning activities associated with the Shadow of the Salmon curriculum that align with these academic content areas. Critical framing aligns with the L phase of the KWL metacognitive strategy when students reflect back on the overall learning process and the new knowledge generated.

Transformed Practice

Educational practice is transformed as students use the knowledge they have generated in new ways, with new purposes, and with different audiences. Inglebret, CHiXapkaid, and Lehr (2008) describe a variety of means for extending language and literacy learning through use of the Shadow of the Salmon curriculum. For example, students might build on their new knowledge by further investigating the salmon life cycle using various forms of technology (e.g., searching the Internet or sharing written stories on blogs). They might make connections between the oral stories of the salmon told by an elder and current salmon management techniques used by tribes and the state and federal governments. Students might write a letter to the editor of a local newspaper presenting a persuasive argument relating historical events, such as treaties between the U.S. government and American Indian tribes, and the current status of the salmon. In this way, the knowledge that students bring to the classroom is validated, and the ICF domain of activity and participation involving families and local community members becomes a focal point of the intervention process.

CONCLUSION

Indigenous peoples around the world continue to record their history and pass it on orally through stories as they have done for centuries. They face an uncertain future, however, because of the tremendous outside influences and pressures that are eroding their languages and cultural ways of life. Educators and SLPs serving these populations need to employ the principles of ganma, respecting and valuing the indigenous culture as they make available the knowledge and skills of the dominant culture. When employing ganma, professionals must work in a 3rd space (Barrera & Corso, 2003). To work in a 3rd space, professionals must understand the values, beliefs, and behaviors of the indigenous children and families with whom they are working; they also must have a conscious awareness of their own values, beliefs, and behaviors and how they differ from those of the indigenous family. The professionals then reframe the contradictions they experience between their own ideas of the situation and the families' ideas. They shift their perspective from a we-they framework to a mindset that integrates the complementary aspects of the diverse values, behaviors, and beliefs of themselves and the family into a new whole (a third space). The cultures of the family and professionals are each respected and maintained, and (as in the ganma metaphor) a third culture arises at the intersections of the two cultures. It is in this third space that assessment and intervention are provided.

ACKNOWLEDGMENT

The second author would like to acknowledge CHiXapkaid (D. Michael Pavel), tradition bearer for the Southern Puget Salish peoples and Professor of Native American Studies in Education, University of Oregon, for his mentorship over the past 15 years. His guidance provided a foundation for contributions to this chapter.

REFLECTIVE QUESTIONS

1. Describe efforts that indigenous communities are making to revitalize their ancestral languages. How might an indigenous language program be linked to speech-language service delivery?
2. Describe characteristics of indigenous languages that may be transferred to the dominant language spoken in a particular area. How might these characteristics affect speech and language assessment results?
3. Explain how indigenous worldviews and cultural values might affect the speech-language assessment and intervention process.
4. Apply the ICF framework to speech-language service delivery for a particular indigenous group.
5. Explain how the multiliteracies framework might be applied in speech-language intervention for a child of indigenous background.

REFERENCES

Allison, S. R., & Vining, C. B. (1999). Native American culture and language considerations in service delivery. In T. V. Fletcher & C. S. Bos (Eds.), *Helping individuals with disabilities and their families: Mexican and U.S. perspectives* (pp. 193-206). Tempe, AZ: Bilingual Review Press.

Archibald, J. (2008). *Indigenous storywork: Educating the heart, mind, body, and spirit.* Vancouver, BC: University of British Columbia Press.

Assembly of First Nations (1990). Towards Linguistic Justice for First Nations, Education Secretariat, Assembly of First Nations, Ottawa.

Australian Institute of Aboriginal and Torres Strait Islander Studies (2005). *National Indigenous Languages Survey Report.* Available from www.arts.gov.au/__data/assets/pdf_file/0006/35637/nils-report-2005.pdf.

Ball, J. (2009). Supporting young Indigenous children's language development in Canada: A review of research on needs and promising practices. *Canadian Modern Language Review, 66,* 19-47.

Ball, J., & Bernhardt, B. M. (2008). First Nations English dialects in Canada: Implications for speech-language pathology. *Clinical Linguistics and Phonetics, 22,* 570-588.

Ball, J., & Janyst, P. (2008, November). Screening and assessment of Indigenous children: Community-university partnered research findings. Policy Brief presented at the Early Years Policy Forum, Vancouver.

Banks-Joseph, S. R., & McCubbin, L. (2006). American Indian and Alaska Native early childhood family involvement: A review of the literature. *Proceedings of the Rural Early Childhood Forum on American Indian and Alaska Native Early Learning* (pp. 132-143). Little Rock, AR: Mississippi State University.

Barnes, P. M., Adams, P. F., & Powell-Griner, E. (2010, March 9). Health characteristics of the American Indian or Alaska Native adult population: United States, 2004-2008. *National Health Statistics Report,* 1-22.

Bartlett, J. G., Madariaga-Vignudo, L., O'Neil, J., & Kuhnlein, H. V. (2007). Identifying indigenous peoples for health research in a global context: A review of perspectives and challenges. *International Journal of Circumpolar Health, 66,* 4.

Barrera, I., & Corso, R. M. (2003). *Skilled dialogue: Strategies for responding to cultural diversity in early childhood.* Baltimore, MD: Brookes.

Basso, K. H. (1990). *Western Apache language and culture.* Tucson: University of Arizona Press.

Bell, A. (2000). Maori and Pakeha English. A case study. In A. Bell & K. Kaiper (Eds.), *New Zealand English* (pp. 221-248). Wellington, NZ: Victoria University of Wellington.

Benally, L. (1989). Personal communication.

Bergstrom, A., Cleary, L. M., & Peacock, T. D. (2003). *The seventh generation: Native students speak about finding the good path.* Charleston, WV: ERIC Clearinghouse on Rural Education and Small Schools.

Bock, T. (2006). A consideration of culture in moral theme comprehension: Comparing Native and European American students. *Journal of Moral Education, 35,* 71-87.

Boggs, S. T. (1985). *Speaking relating and learning: A study of Hawaiian children at home and school.* Norwood, NJ: Ablex.

Bowd, A. S. (2005). Otitis media: Health and social consequences for aboriginal youth in Canada's north. *International Journal of Circumpolar Health, 64,* 5-15.

Bowker, A. C. (1993). *Sisters in the blood: The education of women in Native America.* Bozeman, MT: Center for Bilingual/Multicultural Education.

Bramley, D., Hebert, P., Jackson, R., & Chassin, M. (2004). Indigenous disparities in disease-specific mortality, a crosscountry comparison: New Zealand, Australia, Canada, and the United States. *New Zealand Medical Journal, 1201,* 1-16. Retrieved from www.nzma.org.nz/journal/117-1207/1215/.

Brave Heart, M. Y. B., & DeBruyn, L. M. (1998). The American Indian Holocaust: Healing historical unresolved grief. *American Indian and Alaska Native Mental Health Research, 8,* 56-78.

Bruchac, J. (1994). The circle of stories. In M. A. Lindquist & M. Zanger (Eds.), *Buried roots and indestructible seeds: The survival of American Indian life in story, history, and spirit.* Madison, WI: University of Wisconsin Press.

Bureau of Indian Affairs (1991). *American Indians today.* Washington, DC: BIA.

Burnaby, B. (2008). Language policy and education in Canada. In S. May & N. H. Horberger (Eds.), *Encyclopedia of Language and Education* (2nd ed., Vol. 1). *Language policy and political issues in education* (pp. 331-341). New York: Springer.

Butcher, A. R. (2008). Linguistic aspects of Australian Aboriginal English. *Clinical Linguistics and Phonetics, 22,* 625-642.

Cajete, G. A. (2000). *Native science: Natural laws of interdependence.* Santa Fe, NM: Clear Light Publishers.

Canadian Council on Learning (2007). Redefining how success is measured in First Nations, Inuit, and Metis learning. *Report on learning in Canada 2007.* Ottawa, ON: Author.

Cantoni, G. (Ed.) (2007). *Stabilizing indigenous languages.* Flagstaff, AZ: Northern Arizona University.

Carney, L. J., & Chermak, G. D. (1991). Performance of American Indian children with fetal alcohol syndrome on the Test of Language Development. *Journal of Communication Disorders, 24,* 123-134.

Carr, M. (2001). *Assessment in early childhood settings: Learning stories.* London: Paul Chapman.

Cazden, C. (2000). Four innovative programmes: A postscript from Alice Springs. In B. Cope & M. Kalantzis (Eds.), *Multiliteracies: Literacy learning and the design of social futures.* London: Routledge.

CHiXapkaid (Pavel, D. M., & Inglebret, E.) (2007). *The American Indian and Alaska Native student's guide to college success.* Westport, CT: Greenwood Press.

Churchill, W. (1996). Like sand in the wind: The making of an American Indian diaspora in the United States. In L. Foerstel (Ed.), *Creating surplus populations: The effects of military and corporate policies on indigenous people* (pp. 19-52). Washington, DC: Maisonneuve Press.

Cope, B., & Kalantzis, M. (2009). Multiliteracies: New literacies, new learning. *Pedagogies: An International Journal, 4,* 164-195.

Covarrubias, P. (2007). (Un)biased in Western theory: Generative silence in American Indian communication. *Communication Monographs, 74,* 265-271.

Crago, M. (1990). Development of communicative competence in Inuit children: Implications for speech-language pathology. *Journal of Communicative Disorders, 13,* 73-83.

Crago, M. B., Eriks-Brophy, A., Pesco, D., & McAlpine, L. (1997). Culturally based miscommunication in classroom interaction. *Language, Speech, and Hearing Services in Schools, 28,* 245-254.

Cullen, J. L., Haworth, P. A., Simmons, H., et al. (2009). Teacher-researchers promoting cultural learning in an intercultural kindergarten in Aotearoa New Zealand. *Language, Culture, and Curriculum, 22,* 43-56.

Dannenberg, C., & Wolfram, W. (1998). Ethnic identity and grammatical restructuring: Be(s) in Lumbee English. *American Speech, 73,* 139-160.

De Korne, H. (2009). The pedagogical potential of multimedia dictionaries: Lessons from a community dictionary project. In J. Reyhner & L. Lockard (Eds.). (2009). *Indigenous language revitalization: Encouragement, guidance & lessons learned* (pp. 97-108, 141-153). Flagstaff, AZ: Northern Arizona University. Available at: http://jan.ucc.nau.edu/~jar/ILR/.

Deyhle, D. (1987). Learning failure: Tests as gatekeepers and the culturally different child. In H. T. Trueba (Ed.), *Success or failure: Learning and the language minority child* (pp. 85-108). New York: Newbury House.

Dixon, R. M. W. (2007). *Australian languages: Their nature and development.* New York: Cambridge University Press.

Dunn, M. (2001). Aboriginal literacy: Reading the tracks. *The Reading Teacher, 54,* 678-687.

Eades, D. (2000). *Aboriginal English in the courts: A handbook.* Brisbane, Australia: Dept. of Justice. Available at: www.courts.qld.gov.au/.

Eickelkamp, U. (2008). 'I don't talk story like that': On the social meaning of children's sand stories at Ernabella. In J. Simpson & G. Wigglesworth (Eds.), *Children's language and multilingualism: Indigenous language use at home and school* (pp. 79-99). New York: Continuum International Publishing Group.

Eriks-Brophy, A., & Crago, M. (2003). Variation in instructional discourse features: Cultural or linguistic? Evidence from Inuit and non-Inuit teachers of Nunavik. *Anthropology and Education Quarterly, 34,* 396-419.

Estes, J. (1999). *How many indigenous American languages are spoken in the United States? By how many speakers?* National Clearinghouse for Bilingual Education [On-line]. Available from www.ncbe.gwu.edu/askncbe/faqs/20natlang.htm.

Evans-Campbell, T. (2008). Historical trauma in American Indian/Native Alaska communities: A multilevel framework for exploring impacts on individuals, families, and communities. *Journal of Interpersonal Violence, 23,* 316-338.

Faircloth, S. C., & Tippeconnic, J. W. III. (2010). *The dropout/graduation rate crisis among American Indian and Alaska Native students: Failure to respond places the future of Native Peoples at risk.* Los Angeles: The Civil Rights Project/Proyecto Derechos Civiles at UCLA. Available at: www.civilrightsproject.ucla.edu.

Fagot-Campagna, A., Pettitt, D. J., Engelgau, M. M., et al. (2000). Type 2 diabetes among North American children and adolescents: An epidemiologic review and a public perspective. *Journal of Pediatrics, 136,* 664-672.

Feuerstein, R., Rand, Y., Jensen, M. R., et al. (1987). Prerequisites for assessment of learning potential: The LPAD Model. In C. S. Lidz (Ed.), *Dynamic assessment: An interactional approach to evaluating learning potential* (pp. 35-51). New York: Guilford Press.

Fishman, J. A. (2000). Reversing language shift: RLS theory and practice revisited. In G. E. Kindell & M. P. Lewis (Eds.), *Assessing ethnolinguistic vitality: Theory and practice, selected papers from the third international language assessment conference* (pp. 1-25). Dallas, TX: SIL International.

Foreman, G. (1989). *Indian removal: The emigration of the five civilized tribes of Indians.* Norman: University of Oklahoma Press.

Giles, M., & O'Brien, P. (1991). The prevalence of hearing impairment amongst Maori schoolchildren. *Clinical Otolaryngology Allied Science, 16,* 174-178.

Goodluck, C. (2002). *Native American children and youth well-being indicators: A strengths perspective.* Portland, OR: National Indian Child Welfare Association.

Gould, J. (2008a). Language difference or language disorder: Discourse sampling in speech pathology assessments for Indigenous children. In J. Simpson & G. Wigglesworth (Eds.), *Children's language and multilingualism: Indigenous language use at home and school* (pp. 194-215). New York: Continuum International Publishing Group.

Gould, J. (2008b). Non-standard assessment practices in the evaluation of communication in Australian Aboriginal children. *Clinical Linguistics & Phonetics, 22,* 643-657.

Gould, J. (2008c). The affects of language assessment policies in speech-language pathology on the educational experiences of Indigenous students. *Current Issues in Language Planning, 9,* 299-316.

Greenfield, P. M. (1994). Independence and interdependence as developmental scripts: Implications for theory, research, and practice. In P. M. Greenfield & R. R. Cocking (Eds.), *Cross-cultural roots of minority child development* (pp. 1-37). Hillsdale, NJ: Erlbaum.

Greenfield, L. A., & Smith, S. K. (1999). *American Indians and crime.* Washington, DC: U.S. Department of Justice.

Gregory, G. A. (1993). The texture of essays written by basic writers: Dine and Anglo. PhD dissertation, University of New Mexico.

Hall, E. T. (1959). *The silent language.* New York: Doubleday.

Hall, E. T. (1976). *Beyond culture.* New York: Doubleday.

Hall, E. T. (1983). *The dance of life.* New York: Doubleday.

Harlow, R. (2007). *Maori: A linguistic introduction.* Cambridge: Cambridge University Press.

Harris, G. A. (1998). American Indian cultures: A lesson in diversity. In D. E. Battle (Ed.), *Communication disorders in multicultural populations* (pp. 78-113). Boston: Butterworth-Heinemann.

Hart, M. A. (2010). Indigenous worldviews, knowledge, and research: The development of an indigenous research paradigm. *Journal of Indigenous Voices in Social Work, 1,* 1-6.

Healy, A. (2008). *Multiliteracies and diversity in education: New pedagogies for expanding landscapes.* South Melbourne, Victoria, Australia: Oxford University Press.

Hedberg, N., & Westby, C. E. (1993). *Analyzing storytelling skills: From theory to practice.* Tucson, AZ: Communication Skill Builders.

Heinrich, J. S. (1991). Native Americans: What not to teach. In *Rethinking Columbus* (p. 15). Milwaukee: Rethinking Schools.

Henderson, R. (2008). Mobilising multiliteracies: Pedagogy for mobile students. In A. Healy (Ed.), *Multiliteracies and diversity in education: New pedagogies for expanding landscapes* (pp. 168-200). South Melbourne, Victoria, Australia: Oxford University Press.

Highwater, J. (1981). *The primal mind: Vision and reality in Indian America.* New York: Harper & Row.

Hofstede, G. (1980). *Culture's consequences: International differences in work-related values.* Newbury Park, CA: Sage.

Holmes, J. (1997). Maori and Pakeha English: Some New Zealand social dialect data. *Language in Society, 26,* 65-101.

Hunter, L. L., Davey, C. S., Kohtz, A., & Daley, K. A. (2007). Hearing screening and middle ear measures in American Indian infants and toddlers. *Internal Journal of Pediatric Otorhinolaryngology, 71,* 1429-1438.

Hwa-Froelich, D., & Vigil, D. C. (2004). Three aspects of cultural influence on communication: A literature review. *Communication Disorders Quarterly, 25,* 107-118.

Indian Nations At Risk Task Force (1990). *Indian Nations at risk: An educational strategy for action.* Washington, DC: U.S. Department of Education (ERIC Document Reproduction Service No. ED 339578).

Inglebret, E., Brownfield, S., & CHiXapkaid (Pavel, D. M.) (2008). Elements of an effective government-to-government relationship between a tribe and a school. In CHiXapkaid (Pavel, D. M.), Banks-Joseph, S. R., Inglebret, E., et al., *From where the sun rises: Addressing the educational achievement of Native Americans in Washington State* (p. 123). Pullman, WA: Clearinghouse on Native Teaching and Learning.

Inglebret, E., & CHiXapkaid (Pavel, D. M.) (2009). *Meeting Washington State education standards using the Shadow of the Salmon curriculum: Examples for grade 8.* Pullman, WA: Clearinghouse on Native Teaching and Learning. Available at libarts.wsu.edu/speechhearing/overview/native-american.asp.

Inglebret, E., CHiXapkaid (Pavel, D. M.), & Lehr, T. (2008). Connecting with culture through middle school environmental curriculum. *Perspectives on Communication Disorders and Sciences in Culturally and Linguistically Diverse Populations, American Speech-Language-Hearing Association Division 14, 15,* 12-18.

International Labour Organization (1989). Convention 169. Retrieved December 13, 2010, from www.ilo.org.

Kana'iaupuni, S. M. (2004, December). Ka'akalai Ku Kanaka: A call for strengths-based approaches from a Native Hawaiian perspective. *Educational Researcher,* 26-32.

King, J. (2009). Language is life: The worldview of second language speakers of Maori. In J. Reyhner & L. Lockard (Eds.), *Indigenous language revitalization: Encouragement, guidance & lessons learned.* Flagstaff, AZ: Northern Arizona University. Available at http://jan.ucc.nau.edu/~jar/ILR/.

Kipuri, N. (2009). Culture. In United Nations. *State of the world's indigenous peoples* (pp. 52-81). New York: United Nations Department of Economic and Social Affairs, Division for Social Policy and Development, Secretariat of the Permanent Forum on Indigenous Issues.

Kirkness, V., & Bowman, S. (1992). *First nations and schools: Triumphs and struggles.* Toronto: Canadian Education Association/Association Canadienne d'éducation.

Klenowski, V. (2009). Australian Indigenous students: Addressing equity issues in assessment. *Teaching Education, 20,* 77-93.

Kluckhohn, F. & Strodtbeck, F. (1961). *Variations in value orientations.* New York: Row, Pederson.

Knudtson, P., & Suzuki, D. (1992). *Wisdom of the elders.* Toronto: Stoddart Publishing.

Kramer, K., Mallett, P., Schneider, P., & Hayward, D. (2009). Dynamic assessment of narratives with grade 3 children in a First Nations community. *Canadian Journal of Speech-Language Pathology and Audiology, 33,* 119-128.

Krauss, M. (1998). The condition of Native North American Languages: The need for realistic assessment and action. *International Journal of the Sociology of Language, 132,* 9-21.

Kress, G. (2003). *Literacy in the new media age.* London: Routledge.

LaFrance, J., & Nichols, F. (2008). *Indigenous evaluation framework: Telling our story in our place and time.* Alexandria, VA: American Indian Higher Education Consortium.

LaFromboise, T. D., & Low, K. G. (1989). American Indian children and adolescents. In J. T. Gibbs, L. N. Huang, & Associates (Eds.), *Children of color: Psychological interventions with minority youth* (pp. 114-147). San Francisco: Jossey-Bass.

Leap, W. (1993). *American Indian English.* Salt Lake City: University of Utah Press.

Leap, W. (1991). Pathways and barriers to literacy-building on the northern Ute reservation. *Anthropology & Education Quarterly, 22,* 21-41.

Lewis, J. M. (1992). The story telling strategies of Northern Ute elementary students. *Journal of Navajo Education, 9,* 24-32.

Lidz, C., & Peña, E. (1996). Dynamic assessment: The model, its relevance as a nonbiased approach, and its application to Latino preschool children. *Language, Speech, and Hearing Services in Schools, 27,* 367-372.

Locust, C. (1988). *American Indian belief systems concerning health and wellness.* Tucson, AZ: Native American Research and Training Center, University of Arizona.

Long, E. E. (1998a). Native American children's performance on the Preschool Language Scale-3. *Journal of Children's Communication Development, 19,* 43-47.

Long, E. E. (1998b). Pragmatic language skills of English-speaking Native American children. Paper presented at the ASHA annual convention, November, 1998, San Antonio.

Long, E. E., & Christensen, J. M. (1997). Indirect language assessment tool for English-speaking Cherokee Indian children. *Journal of American Indian Education, 38,* 1-14.

Lutz, H. (1989). The circle as philosophical and structural concept in Native American fiction today. In L. Coltell (Ed.), *Native American literatures.* Servizio Editoriale Universitario, Vicolo della Croce Rossa 5-56126 Pisa.

Martin, K. (2008). The intersection of Aboriginal knowledges, Aboriginal literacies, and new learning pedagogy for Aboriginal students. In A. Healy (Ed.), *Multiliteracies and diversity in education: New pedagogies for expanding landscapes* (pp. 58-81). South Melbourne, Victoria, Australia: Oxford University Press.

Maternal and Child Health Section (2008). *American Indian Infant Mortality Review Project: Minnesota 2005-2007.* Minneapolis, MN: Minnesota Department of Health.

McCabe, L. (1995). *Chameleon readers: Teaching children to appreciate all kinds of good stories.* New York: McGraw-Hill.

McCubbin, H., Ontai, K., Kehl, L., et al. (2010). *Multiethnicity and multiethnic families: Development, identity, and resilience.* Honolulu, HI: Le'a Publications.

Miller, L., Gillam, R., & Peña, E. (2001). *Dynamic assessment and intervention: Improving children's narrative abilities.* Austin, TX: Pro-Ed.

Miller, M., & Schoenfield, T. (1975). *The Native Americans.* Austin, TX: National Education Lab.

Mithun, M. (2001). *The languages of Native North America.* New York: Cambridge University Press.

Mike, E. H., Bidtah, L., & Thomas, V. (no date). Cultural conflict. Central Consolidated Schools, District 22, Title VII, Bilingual Education Program.

Ministerio da Justica (1996). *Os direitos das pessoas portadoras de deficiencia Lei 7.853/89, Decreto 914/93* [The rights of individuals with disabilities. Law 7.853/89, Section 914/93]. Brasilia: CORDE.

Moore, J. A. (1999). Comparison of risk of conductive hearing loss among three ethnic groups of Arctic audiology patients. *Journal of Speech, Language, and Hearing Research, 42,* 1311-1322.

Morris, P. S., Richmon, P., Lehmann, D., et al. (2009). New horizons: Otitis media research in Australia. *Medical Journal of Australia, 191,* 73-77.

Mushin, I., & Gardner, R. (2009). Silence is talk: Conversational silence in Aboriginal talk-in-interaction. *Journal of Pragmatics, 11,* 2033-2052.

National Indigenous Languages Survey Report (2005). Canberra, Australia: Australian Institute of Aboriginal and Torres Strait Islander Studies. Available at www.arts.gov.au/__data/assets/pdf_file/0006/35637/nils-report-2005.pdf.

National Research Council (2002). *Minority students in special and gifted education.* Committee on minority representation in special education, M. Suzanne Donovan & Christopher T. Cross, editors. Division of Behavioral and Social Sciences and Education, Washington, DC: National Academy Press.

Nelson-Barber, S., & Trumbull, E. (2007). Making assessment practices valid for Indigenous American students. *Journal of American Indian Education, 46,* 132-147.

New London Group (1996). A pedagogy of multiliteracies: Designing social futures. *Harvard Educational Review, 66,* 60-93.

New Zealand Government Ministry of Education (1996). *Te Whariki early childhood curriculum.* Wellington, NZ: Learning Media.

Nichols, L. A., & Keltner, B. (2005). Indian family adjustment to children with disabilities. American Indian & Alaskan Native Mental Health Research. *Journal of the National Center, 12,* 22-48.

Northwest Indian Fisheries Commission (2009). *Shadow of the Salmon.* Olympia, WA: Office of Superintendent of Public Instruction, Indian Education Office. Available at libarts.wsu.edu/speechhearing/overview/native-american.asp.

Peña, E. (1996). Dynamic assessment: The model and its language applications. In K. N. Cole, P. S. Dale, & D. J. Thal (Eds.), *Assessment of communication and language.* Baltimore: Brookes.

Peña, E., Quinn, R., & Iglesias, A. (1992). The application of dynamic methods to language assessment: A nonbiased process. *Journal of Special Education, 26,* 269-280.

Phillips, S. (1983). *The invisible culture: Communication in classroom and community on the Warm Springs Indian Reservation.* Long Grove, IL: Waveland Press.

Plank, G. A. (1994). What silence means for educators of American Indian children. *Journal of American Indian Education, 34,* 3-19.

Psacharopoulos, G., & Patrinos, H. A. (Eds.) (1994). *Indigenous people and poverty in Latin America: An empirical analysis.* Washington, DC: The World Bank.

Pyrch, T., & Castillo, M. T. (2001). The sights and sounds of indigenous knowledge In P. Reason & H. Bradbury (Eds.), *Handbook of action research: Participatory inquiry & practice* (pp. 379-385). Thousand Oaks, CA: Sage.

Rameka, L. (2007). Maori approaches to assessment. *Canadian Journal of Native Education, 30,* 126-146.

Red Horse, J. (1988). Cultural evolution of American Indian families. In C. Jacobs & D. Bowles (Eds.), *Ethnicity and race: Critical concept in social work* (pp. 186-199). Silver Spring, MD: National Association of Social Workers.

Research Agenda Working Group, Strang, W., & von Glatz, A. (2001). *American Indian and Alaska Native educational research agenda.* Washington, DC: U.S. Department of Education.

Reyhner, J., & Lockard, L. (Eds.). (2009). *Indigenous language revitalization: Encouragement, guidance and lessons learned.* Flagstaff, AZ: Northern Arizona University. Available at http://jan.ucc.nau.edu/~jar/ILR/.

Reyhner, J., & Tennant, E. (1995). Maintaining and renewing native languages. *Bilingual Research Journal, 19,* 279-304.

Saville-Troike, M. (1989). *The ethnography of communication* (2nd ed.). New York: Basil Blackwell.

Scollon, R., & Scollon, S. B. K. (1980). *Interethnic communication.* Fairbanks, AK: Alaska Native Language Center.

Silko, L. M. (1977). *Ceremony.* New York: Penguin.

Sharifian, F. (2002). Chaos in Aboriginal English discourse. In A. Kirkpatrick (Ed.), *Englishes in Asia: Communication, identity, power, and education* (pp. 125-141). Melbourne: Language Australia.

Sharifian, F., Rochecouste, J., & Malcolm, I. G. (2004). 'But it was all a bit confusing...': Comprehending Aboriginal English texts. *Language, Culture, and Curriculum, 17,* 203-226.

Shulman, B. B. (1986). *Test of Pragmatic Skills.* Tucson, AZ: Communication Skill Builders.

Si, D., Bailie, R., Wang, Z., & Weeramanthri, T. (2010). Comparison of diabetes management in five countries for general and indigenous populations: An internet-based review. *BMC Health Services Research, 10,* 169.

Silver S., & Miller, W. R. (1997). *American Indian languages: Cultural and social contexts.* Tucson, AZ: University of Arizona Press.

Sofaer, A. (2007). The primary architecture of the Chacoan culture: A cosmological expression. In S. Lekson (Ed.), *Architecture of Chaco Canyon, New Mexico* (pp. 225-254). Salt Lake City: University of Utah Press.

Sofaer, A., & Ihde, A. (1983). *The sun dagger.* Bethesda, MD: Atlas Video.

Stewart, J. (1986). Hearing disorders among the indigenous peoples of North America and the Pacific Basin. In O. Taylor (Ed.), *Nature of communication disorders in culturally and linguistically diverse populations* (pp. 237-276). San Diego: College-Hill Press.

Streissguth, A. (1997). *Fetal alcohol syndrome.* Baltimore: Brookes.

Szlemko, W. J., Wood, J. W., & Thurman, P. J. (2006). Native Americans and alcohol: Past, present, and future. *Journal of General Psychology, 13,* 435-451.

Taylor, A. (2002). *American colonies; Volume 1 of The Penguin history of the United States.* New York: Penguin.

Thomson, M. (1994). Otitis media: How are First Nations children affected? *Canadian Family Physician, 40,* 143-150.

Tippeconnic, J. W. (2003). The use of academic achievement tests and measurements with American Indian and Alaska Native students. ERIC Digest EDO-RC-O3-07.

Todd, N. W., & Bowerman, C. A. (1985). Otitis media in Canyon Day, Ariz., a 16-year follow-up in Apache Indians. *Archives of Otolaryngology, 111,* 606-608.

Triandis, H. C. (1995). *Individualism and collectivism.* Boulder, CO: Westview Press.

Ukrainetz, T. A., Harpell, S., Walsh, C., & Coyle, C. (2000). A preliminary investigation of dynamic assessment with Native American kindergartners. *Language, Speech, and Hearing Services in Schools, 31,* 142-154.

United Nations (2009). The state of the world's indigenous peoples. Available from www.un.org/esa/socdev/unpfii/documents/SOWIP_web.pdf.

U.S. Census Bureau (2000). *We the people: American Indians and Alaska Natives in the United States, Census 2000 special reports.* Available from www.census.gov/prod/2006pubs/censr-28.pdf.

Valiquette, H. P. (1990). *A study for a lexicon of Laguna Keresan.* Albuquerque, NM: University of New Mexico.

Vallance, R. J., & Tchacos, E. (2001). *Research: A cultural bridge.* Freemantle, Western Australia: Australian Association for Research in Education. Retrieved September 27, 2010, from www.aare.edu.au/01pap/val01102.htm.

Vining, C. B., & Allison, S. R. (2000). *Navajo perceptions of developmental disabilities: Project Na'nitin institute manual.* Albuquerque, NM: University of New Mexico.

Walsh, M. (1991). Overview of indigenous languages of Australia. In S. Romaine (Ed.), *Languages in Australia* (pp. 27-48). New York: Cambridge University Press.

Watson, S. R., Barreira, A. M., & Watson, T. (2000). Perspectives on quality of life: The Brazilian experience. In K. D. Keith & R. L. Schalock (Eds.), *Cross-cultural perspectives on quality of life* (pp. 59-71). Washington, DC: American Association Mental Retardation.

Westby, C. (2010). Multiliteracies: The changing world of communication. *Topics in Language Disorders, 30,* 64-71.

White House Conference on Indian Education (1992). *The final report of the White House Conference on Indian Education* (executive summary). Washington, DC: Author.

Wiertsema, S. P., & Leach, A. J. (2009). Theories of otitis media pathogenesis, with a focus on indigenous children. *Medical Journal of Australia, 191,* 5054.

Wolfram, W. (2000). *Indian by birth: The Lumbee dialect.* Raleigh, NC: North Carolina State University.

World Health Organization (2001). *International classification of functioning, disability, and health (ICF).* Geneva: Author.

World Indigenous Peoples' Conference on Education (1999). Coolangatta statement on peoples' rights in education. *Journal of American Indian Education, 39,* 52-64.

Worth, S., & Adair, J. (1972). *Through Navajo eyes.* Bloomington: University of Indiana Press.

ADDITIONAL RESOURCES

International Resources

Bernhardt, B. M. (2008). Acknowledgements, questions, and additional resources. *Clinical Linguistics & Phonetics, 22,* 671-677. [Resources for Canada, Australia, New Zealand, and international contexts].

The Declaration on the Rights of Indigenous Peoples. Available at: www.un.org/esa/socdev/unpfii/en/declaration.html.

International Network of Indigenous Health Knowledge and Development (INIHKD): www.iwri.org/inihkd.

Journal of International and Intercultural Communication: focuses on international, intercultural, and indigenous communication issues.

The Turtle Island Native Network. Available at: http://www.turtleisland.org/.

United States: American Speech-Language-Hearing Association, Native American Caucus. Available at: http://libarts.wsu.edu/speechhearing/overview/nap-caucus.asp.

United Nations (2009). *State of the world's indigenous peoples.* New York: Department of Economic and Social Affairs, Division for Social Policy and Development, Secretariat of the Permanent Forum on Indigenous Issues, United Nations.

United Nations Permanent Forum on Indigenous Issues (UNPFII). Available at: www.un.org/esa/socdev/unpfii/.

Culturally Based Early Childhood Materials

Connor, J. (2007). Dreaming stories: A springboard for learning. [Book and DVD containing Aboriginal Nations' animated short films]. *Research in Practice Series, 14,* 2. Available at: www.earlychildhoodaustralia.org.au.

Eaglecrest Books: set of primary-leveled books representing First Nations children. "Stories reflect experiences of First Nations children involved in cultural activities and in everyday life at home and school." Available at: www.eaglecrestbooks.com/home.htm.

Jones, G. W., & Moomaw, S. (2002). *Lessons from Turtle Island: Native curriculum in early childhood classrooms.* St. Paul, MN: Redleaf Press.

Mandolson, A., Ward, B., & Dodington, N. (1998). *You make the difference in helping your child learn: An Aboriginal adaptation developed in partnership with the Walpole Island First Nation community.* Toronto: The Hanen Centre.

Culturally Based School-Age Materials

Aboriginal Education: The Department of Education, Australia. Culturally-based curriculum resources and information on promoting aboriginal community involvement. Available at: www.det.wa.edu.au/aboriginal-education/detcms/portal/.

Alaska Native Knowledge Network. Publications, curriculum and cultural resources, cultural atlases and talking maps, native education associations. Available at: www.ankn.uaf.edu.

Culture card: A guide to build cultural awareness—American Indians and Alaska Natives. Available at: www.samhsa.gov/samhsanewsletter/volume_17_number_2/americanindianculture.aspx.

From where the sun rises: Addressing the educational achievement of Native Americans in Washington State. Report prepared for the Washington State Legislature, 2008. Appendix contains information on a variety of culturally based curriculum resources. Available at: http://education.wsu.edu/nativeclearinghouse/achievementgap/.

Indian education for all: Connecting cultures and classrooms K-12 curriculum guide: Language arts, science, social studies (2006). Montana Office of Public Instruction, Helena, MT. Available at: http://opi.mt.gov/pdf/indianed/ConnectingCultures.pdf.

Nga Whanaketanga Rumaki Maori. National Standards in Maori-medium education. Available at: www.minedu.govt.nz/NZEducation/EducationPolicies/MaoriEducation.aspx.

Chapter 6

Hispanic and Latino Cultures in the United States and Latin America

Hortencia Kayser

The term *Hispanic* has been used in the United States to describe Spanish speakers since 1990, when it was first used as part of the U.S. Census (U.S. Census Bureau, 1990). It is a term that has not been understood by many individuals— Spanish speakers and mainstream English speakers. When the federal government provides a descriptor of a subgroup population, that population may provide a term that is more acceptable to many of these individuals. Thus, came the term *Latino*. When is it appropriate to use Hispanic, or should we be using Latino? Hispanic and Latino are umbrella terms that encompass many facets of different cultures that have the similar root language, Spanish.

Hispanics or Latinos in the United States are heterogeneous in their language, their practice of religion, political leaning, educational and socioeconomic status, mores, and belief systems concerning health and disability. There is no one Latino culture. Instead, there are different cultures or ethnic groups who speak Spanish. The word *Hispanic* has been defined as an individual who comes from a Spanish-speaking background regardless of race (U.S. Census Bureau, 2008). It is a government-issued term. *Latino,* on the other hand, is the descriptor among people who see themselves as coming from a Spanish-speaking background. Each group, whether Mexican, Puerto Rican, or Cuban American, defines whether it is Latino or prefers a different ethnic marker. Individuals who are of Mexican or Spanish descent in New Mexico may prefer to be identified as American, Mexican American, Spanish American, or *Chicano* (a term used by individuals of Mexican descent who may not view themselves as American or Mexican). Whatever the ethnic group, Latinos are heterogeneous and are an increasing population within the United States. *Hispanic* is a term that will be used in U.S. government reports. *Latino* will likely be used by authors who recognize the need for identity by these groups. This chapter uses both terms, interchangeably.

Within each ethnic group are subgroups whose members identify with each other on the basis of geography, income,

religion, education, history, political beliefs, and so forth. Much like other societies, members of one subgroup may never interact with those of another subgroup for their own reasons, known or unknown, whether language use or societal. As an example, northern New Mexico was heavily settled by the Spaniards. New Mexico has two major groups of Hispanics: northern and southern New Mexicans. The persons in the southern region identify with Mexico, whereas, those in the Northern region see themselves as direct descendents of Spain. These two groups differ concerning historical beginnings, religious practices and beliefs, foods, and Spanish vocabulary. For example*, sopapilla is* fluffy fried bread served with the meal in northern New Mexico, but as a dessert with honey in southern New Mexico. A more serious example would be choosing a teacher for a school position. A principal in a school with a large Spanish-speaking student population in southern New Mexico would not hire a northern Spanish-speaking teacher because he believed the teacher used Spanish that would not be understood by the children in his school. The Spanish of the northern region has been described as archaic Spanish used by Spaniards settling in the region 500 years ago.

Pride and identity associated with where one comes from and how one uses Spanish can become a barrier or a welcome sign not only in New Mexico, but also in other states where there is a large population of Latino inhabitants. Understanding the backgrounds of these different groups will help the professional to understand the population's perspective on life, how they might perceive the English and Spanish language, and what they believe is important for their children to know about identity, culture, and language use.

The purpose of this chapter is to describe the Hispanic-Latino populations in the United States and in Latin America. The objectives for this chapter are as follows:

1. Describe the population and educational and immigration demographics for the 10 largest Latino groups in the United States.

2. Describe the focus of early education and literacy in Latin America and the United States.
3. Discuss the cultural perspectives of Latino populations.
4. Describe communication disorders in bilingual Spanish- and English-speaking populations.
5. Discuss implications for assessment and treatment of individuals with communication disorders.

LATINOS IN THE UNITED STATES

The Hispanic population can be described as an explosion of newcomers for all parts of the nation. According to the 2008 U.S. Census, Hispanics are the largest ethnic minority group in the United States at 42.7 million, 15.5% of the total U.S. population. The U.S. Census Bureau (2006) projected that the Hispanic population would increase to 102.6 million or make up 24.4% of the U.S. population by 2050.

Texas, Hawaii, New Mexico, and California have been designated as majority-minority states. This means that there are more Hispanics in these states than there are whites. The U.S. Census Bureau reports that the District of Columbia, Maryland, Mississippi, Georgia, New York, and Arizona are at the 40% mark and are expected to reach the same status as majority-minority states. California has the largest Hispanic population with 12.4 million persons as of 2008. New Mexico has the largest proportion of Hispanics for the total state population with 43% (Pew Hispanic Center, 2008a; U.S. Census, 2008).

Table 6-1 provides a description for each of the 10 largest Latino groups in the United States. The variables that are summarized include the following percentages: total Hispanic population; citizens, who report speaking English proficiently; and citizens who report speaking English less than proficiently. Median age and where the largest number of this ethnic group is reported to live are included. Let's examine the age variable. Mexicans are the youngest of the 10 ethnic groups, with a median age of 25 years. Guatemalans and Hondurans have a median age of 28 years. Puerto Ricans, Dominicans, and El Salvadorans have a median age of 29 years. Ecuadorians, Peruvians, and Colombians have median ages of 32, 35, and 36 years of age, respectively. Cubans have the oldest group, with a median age of 41 years. Age is an important factor when viewing the family's history, fertility rate, health history, and work experiences in the home country and in the United States. Younger individuals typically have children, have fewer health problems, and may have less work experiences. Thus, the Latino population is diverse in median age as well as other variables.

Table 6-2 summarizes the population and percentages of foreign born for the 10 largest Hispanic groups in the United States. Thirty-eight percent of all Hispanics in the United States are foreign born. Mexicans and Puerto Ricans are the two largest groups, with 66% and 9%, respectively.

Cubans, Salvadorans, and Dominicans each share 3% of the total Hispanic population in the United States. Seven of the groups have populations with more than 60% foreign born. Mexicans and Puerto Ricans have the lowest percentages of foreign born, 37% and 1.1%, respectively.

Newcomer Communities

The Hispanic populations of the United States have historically been located in the Latino centers of the Southwest, the Northeast, and Florida. In the past 10 years, however, there has been a migration to all parts of the United States. The Kaiser Commission (2006) reported that between 1996 and 2003, the Latino population doubled in new-growth communities. New-growth communities are defined as smaller urban and rural areas that previously had few Latinos but are now experiencing high rates of growth. This growth was evenly spread across the nation. Latinos are now living in small communities in states such as Arkansas, Georgia, and Tennessee. These new regions grew by 3.7 million, representing a 93% increase for these new areas. For example, Arkansas grew in Hispanic population from 2000 to 2006 by 60.9%. Georgia and South Carolina grew in Hispanic population by 59.4% and 57.4%, respectively. In comparison, the major Latino centers had only a 23% increase in Latino population. Although this growth is substantial for smaller communities, it only represents 5% of the population in these areas (U.S. Census Bureau, 2006).

Socioeconomic Status

Latino populations have made economic progress in the United States, with approximately 80% above the poverty level. In the United States, 12.7% of the general population lives in poverty. In comparison, about 20.7% of Latinos live in poverty in the United States. The poverty levels vary depending on the ethnic group. For example, Dominicans (23.2%), Puerto Ricans (22.6%), Mexicans (22.3%), Hondurans (21.5%), and Guatemalans (20.6%) have the highest poverty levels. Only the Colombians (11.0%) and Peruvians (9.5%) have lower poverty levels than the general U.S. population. Related to poverty is the availability of health insurance to a population. Insurance allows families to access health care and provide medication for illnesses that affect children's growth and development.

Insurance

A major concern for new growth communities is that 42% of Latinos are uninsured (Pew Hispanic Center, 2008b). States with new Latino communities limit access to public coverage such as Medicaid and State Children's Health Insurance Program (SCHIP) for the first 5 years new immigrants reside in the United States, whereas the major

TABLE 6-1 Description of Major Hispanic Ethnic Groups in the United States

Ethnic Group	Description
Mexico	Most immigrants from Mexico (63.4%) arrived in the U.S. in 1990 or later. Two in 10 of Mexican immigrants (22%) are U.S. citizens. A majority of Mexicans (61.6%) speak English proficiently. Some 38.4% of Mexicans aged 5 years and older report speaking English less than very well. They are younger than the U.S. population and Hispanics overall. The median age is 25 years; the median ages of the U.S. population and all Hispanics are 36 and 27, respectively. Some 36.7% live in California and 25.2% in Texas. About 22.3% live in poverty, higher than the rate for the general U.S. population (12.7%) and slightly higher than for all Hispanics (20.7%)
Puerto Rico	Most Puerto Ricans in the U.S. were born in the 50 states or the District of Columbia. One third of the Puerto Rican population in the U.S. was born in Puerto Rico. People born in Puerto Rico are considered native born because they are U.S. citizens by birth. About 80.5% speak English proficiently. Some 19.5% of Puerto Ricans aged 5 years and older report speaking English less than very well. The median age of Puerto Ricans is 29 years. A majority of Puerto Ricans (55.4%) live in the Northeast, mostly in New York (26.0%). Nearly 27.9% live in the South, primarily Florida (17.9%). Some 22.6% live in poverty.
Cuba	Some 60.1% of Cubans are foreign born. Most are immigrants from Cuba (57.2%) and arrived in the U.S. before 1990. About 58.2% are U.S. citizens. A majority of Cubans (58.3%) speak English proficiently. Some 41.7% of Cubans aged 5 years and older report speaking English less than very well. Cubans are older than the U.S. population with a median age of 41 years. They are geographically concentrated in Florida (68.5%). About 13.2% live in poverty, similar to the general U.S. population (12.7%).
Dominican Republic	Some 57.3% of Dominicans in the U.S. are foreign born. About 57.0% arrived in the U.S. in 1990 or later, and 47.4% are U.S. citizens. A majority (53.4%) speak English proficiently. Some 46.6% of Dominicans aged 5 years and older report speaking English less than very well. Dominicans are young, median age is 29 years. About 79.4% live in the Northeast and 50.6% live in New York. Roughly 23.2% live in poverty.
Colombia	Some 66.5% of Colombians in the U.S. are foreign born. Most immigrants from Colombia (58.7%) arrived in the U.S. in 1990 or later. About 48.8% are U.S. citizens. Roughly 57.5% of Colombians speak English proficiently. Some 42.5% of Colombians aged 5 years and older report speaking English less than very well. The median age is 36 years. Colombians are concentrated in the South (46.8%), mostly in Florida (31.9%), and in the Northeast (37.3%), mostly in New York (16.1%) and New Jersey (12.9%). About 11.0% live in poverty.
Ecuador	Some 66.4% of Ecuadorians are foreign born. About 66.2% arrived in the U.S. in 1990 or later, and 37.2% are U.S. citizens. Roughly 49.1% speak English proficiently. About 50.9% of Ecuadorians aged 5 years and older report speaking English less than very well. The median age of Ecuadorians is 32 years. About 68.0% live in the Northeast, and 42.5% live in New York. Nearly 13.5% live in poverty.
Guatemala	Some 69.4% of Guatemalans in the U.S. are foreign born. About 69.6% arrived in the U.S. in 1990 or later, and 23.8% are U.S. citizens. Roughly 39.1% speak English proficiently. Some 60.9% of Guatemalans aged 5 years and older report speaking English less than very well. The median age of Guatemalans is 28 years. About 40.2% live in the West, mostly California (33.9%), and 32.4% live in the South. Nearly 20.6% of Guatemalans live in poverty.
Honduras	About 68.6% of Hondurans in the U.S. are foreign born. Roughly 74% arrived in the U.S. in 1990 or later, and 21.5% are U.S. citizens. About 39.7% speak English proficiently. Some 60.3% of Hondurans aged 5 years and older report speaking English less than very well. Hondurans are young, with a median age of 28 years. A majority of Hondurans (54.9%) live in the South, mostly in Florida and Texas. About 12.9% live in California and in New York (12.5%). Nearly 21.5% live in poverty.
Peru	Some 69.3% of Peruvians in the U.S. are foreign born. About 66.1% arrived in the U.S. in 1990 or later, and 42.3% are U.S. citizens. Roughly 55.1% speak English proficiently. Some 44.9% of Peruvians aged 5 years and older report speaking English less than very well. The median age of Peruvians is 35 years. Peruvians are more geographically dispersed than other Hispanic origin groups. Nearly 19.8% live in Florida, 16.8% live in California, 12.9% live in New Jersey, and 12.3% live in New York. About 9.5% live in poverty.

Adapted from Pew Hispanic Center, April 22, 2010. Available at: http://pewhispanic.org/data/origins/.

Latino centers provide state-funded coverage programs for immigrants. Lack of insurance and language difference with health professionals and hospital staff are major barriers to health care for new immigrants (Kaiser Commission, 2006).

Education

There is a difference between the U.S. general population and Hispanics in educational attainment for individuals 25 years and older. Males and females in the general

TABLE 6-2 Population and Percentages of Foreign Born for Major Hispanic Groups in the United States

Country of Origin	Population* (%)	Foreign Born (%)
All Hispanics	46,822,000 (100)	38.1
Mexicans	30,746000 (66)	37.0
Puerto Ricans	4,151,000 (9)	1.1
Cubans	1,631,000 (3)	60.1
Salvadorans	1,560,000 (3)	64.7
Dominicans	1,334,000 (3)	57.3
Guatemalans	986,000 (2)	69.4
Colombians	882,000 (2)	66.5
Hondurans	608,000 (1)	66.6
Ecuadorians	591,000 (1)	66.4
Peruvians	519,000 (1)	69.3
Other Groups	(9)	

*Rounded to the nearest thousand.
Data from Pew Hispanic Center, 2010. http://pewhispanic.org/.

TABLE 6-3 Major Hispanic Groups in the United States and Their Educational Attainment

Group	Achieving High School Education (%)	Achieving College Education (%)
All Hispanics	26.0	12.9
Peruvians	29.7	29.8
Ecuadorians	29.0	18.2
Puerto Ricans	28.8	16.0
Cubans	26.7	25.1
Colombians	26.9	30.3
Dominicans	25.7	15.6
Mexicans	25.5	9.1
Salvadorans	23.4	8.4
Hondurans	22.3	10.3
Guatemalans	22.1	8.8

Adapted from Pew Hispanic Center, Country of Origin, 2010. http://pewhispanic.org/.

population complete high school education at rates of 83.5% and 84.6%, respectively, whereas Hispanic males and females complete high school education at rates of 58.7% and 61.7%, respectively. The completion rate of a bachelor's degree among the general U.S. population is reported by the U.S. Census Bureau at 27.9% for males and 26.2 for females. Hispanics complete a college education at rates of 11.5% for males and 13.1% for females (U.S. Census Bureau, 2006). Table 6-3 provides a description of the high school and college graduation rates for the 10 largest Hispanic ethnic groups in the United States.

One in four (26%) Hispanics will graduate with a high school diploma, whereas 12.9% will graduate from college. Colombians, Peruvians, and Cubans have the highest rates of college graduation at 30.3%, 29.8%, and 25.1%, respectively. The three groups with the lowest completion rates of a college education are Mexicans at 9.1%, Guatemalans at 8.8%, and Salvadorans at 8.4%. Heterogeneity is found in the completion of high school and college education for the 10 Hispanic groups in the United States. Professionals must not assume that all Latinos are not well educated.

Language Use

Tables 6-4 and 6-5 describe the English-speaking abilities of two age groups, 5 to 18 years and 18 years and older. Of Latino children between 5 and 18 years living in the United States, those who are of Caribbean descent are most likely (29.2%) to live in homes where only English is spoken. Mexican, Caribbean, and Central and South American populations have large percentages of children who speak

English very well. The South American population in the United States has the highest percentage of children who speak English very well, 66.8%. Only Mexican (43.1%) and Central American (41.0%) children aged 5 to 18 years living in the United States are reported to speak English less than very well.

Among adults aged 18 years and older living in the United States, those of Caribbean descent have the highest percentage of speakers who use only English in the home (32.8 %), whereas South Americans report 34.5% speaking English very well. Mexican and Central American adults are reported to have the highest percentages of adults who speak English less than very well, 76.5% and 69.9%, respectively.

In summary, the Hispanic population in the United States is growing in all regions of the country, and it is a young population (see Table 6-1), is less educated than the general U.S. population, with many living in poverty. The growth and needs of Latino populations has become a national debate and that is proving emotionally charged and difficult to resolve.

LATIN AMERICA

Latin America refers to territories in the Americas where the Spanish or Portuguese languages prevail: Mexico, most of Central and South America, and in the Caribbean, Cuba, the Dominican Republic, and Puerto Rico-in summary, Hispanic America and Brazil. Latin America is, therefore, defined as all those parts of the Americas that were once part of the Spanish and Portuguese Empires.

(Rangel, 1977)

TABLE 6-4 English-Speaking Ability, Ages 5 to 18 Years, and Region, 2008

Country of Origin	No. with Only English Spoken at Home (%)	No. with English Spoken Very Well (%)	No. with English Spoken Less Than Very Well (%)	Total No.
Mexico	23,893 (2.6)	497,910 (54.3)	395,620 (43.1)	917,423
Caribbean	54,347 (29.2)	80,344 (43.1)	51,740 (27.8)	186,431
Central America	19,256 (13.5)	64,972 (45.5)	58,529 (41.0)	142.747
South America	23,163 (12.7)	121,385 (66.8)	37,265 (20.5)	181,813

From U.S. Census Bureau (2006). *American Community Survey*. Washington, DC: Author.

TABLE 6-5 English-Speaking Ability, Ages 18 Years and Older, and Region, 2008

Country of Origin	No. with Only English Spoken at Home (%)	No. with English Spoken Very Well (%)	No. with English Spoken Less Than Very Well (%)	Total No.
Mexico	326,860 (3.1)	2,129,361 (20.4)	8,001,687 (76.5)	10,457,908
Caribbean	1,058,455 (32.8)	776,094 (24.0)	1,395,602 (43.2)	3,230,151
Central America	149,459 (5.8)	628,831 (24.3)	1,804,562 (69.9)	2,582,852
South America	378,087 (16.0)	815,322 (34.5)	1,169,299 (49.5)	2,362,708

From U.S. Census Bureau (2006). *American Community Survey*. Washington, DC: Author.

Latin America has a rich history. It began with the many indigenous peoples who lived in the deserts, coasts, mountains, jungles, and plains of Mexico, Caribbean, and Central and South America centuries before the Spaniards occupied the lands. The conquest of the indigenous groups by Spanish *conquistadores* brought a change in the regions through the dominance of the languages of Spanish and Portuguese and a new group developed as a result of intermarriage between Europeans and indigenous groups. The *mestizo*, European and indigenous mix, makes up the majority of the populations in Latin American. Other immigrant groups, such as the Germans, Japanese, Chinese and U.S. citizens, have settled in these lands but they are relatively new arrivals compared with the Spaniards.

We typically describe Latin America as the Spanish-speaking southern hemisphere. We usually do not perceive the United States as one of these Spanish-speaking countries. The populations of Latin America are as diverse as the Latino populations in the United States. Individuals in Mexico, Caribbean, Central and South America do not refer to themselves as Latinos. They identify themselves by their nationality (e.g., Chileans, Ecuadorians). When they arrive into the United States, their identities become blended into Latino or Hispanics. Hopefully, speech-language pathologists will encourage immigrant families to be proud of their heritage as children and parents become acculturated into American society.

Economics, political pressures, and culture in one Latin American country affect surrounding countries. For example, what happens in Colombia (e.g., violence from drug cartels) has an impact on the neighboring countries such as Ecuador and Peru with new immigrants. Children may be separated from their parents, or the children become orphans and are traumatized because of a violent death of a family member. I spent time with a child from Colombia while I visited Ecuador in the summer of 2010. This child was thought to be mute by staff at a children's center in an urban park in Quito. The girl eventually did speak to me and what she talked about was related to her mother's disappearance, her death, her father's murder, and how she now lived with a grandmother. This is a child who will need more than language development and socialization with other children. She may not be interested in learning in school, playing with other children, or talking to adults. A team of professionals will be needed to intervene for a child who has seen and experienced great loss.

Political corruption and unrest, boundary disputes, language contact, lack of funding for education, and less than stable economies all contribute to the perception that Latin America has a number of still developing countries where democracies struggle to maintain stable governments. Each country has its governmental system and attempts to provide the people with basic needs, but frequently, individuals choose to immigrate to the United States (Kayser, 2008).

Mestizo populations dominate in countries such as Colombia, Ecuador, El Salvador, Honduras, Nicaragua, Paraguay, and Peru. Argentina, Chile, Costa Rica, Uruguay, and Venezuela view themselves as primarily European in background. These countries also have African and indigenous languages that continue to be spoken in the rural regions, sea coasts, jungles, and mountains. Many of these countries have experienced large numbers of immigrants from Haiti since the earthquake of 2010. The Dominican Republic and Cuba report more mixed African and Spanish, called mullato.

Spanish is the dominant language in 15 countries in Latin America and 5 countries have multiple languages within their borders because of the variety of indigenous languages spoken within the countries. For example, Mexico has 65 different indigenous groups that continue to use their native languages. Spanish is learned when children enter schools at 5 or 6 years of age and are offered bilingual education. Spanish may be spoken by teachers and priests in Catholic schools, but the villagers may use only their native language for community events. Much like in the United States among Latinos, many parents and children maintain their native language at home and in their community but learn to speak Spanish through the educational systems. Children and adults become bilingual if there is a need to use the two languages.

Mexico, Panama, Ecuador, and Puerto Rico are countries that require English as part of the education of children and for completion of the university degree. Many public schools may offer a range from 1 to 5 hours per week of English classes. Private schools typically offer up to 2 hours per day of English lessons. Students who complete public school secondary education may have up to 6 years of English. The important variable is the instructor for English classes. Many of these teachers are second language learners of English and may not present English as it is spoken in the United States. As the countries develop their political strength, English is becoming the second language of these countries and is fast becoming an important part of the education of children in public and private schools (Kayser, 2008).

An Exception to the Rule

Guyana, Suriname, and French Guiana are interesting regions of South America. Guyana was under the United Kingdom's control until 1966 when it received its independence. It is the only officially English-speaking country in South America. Suriname was under Dutch control for more than 300 years until 1975 when it became an autonomous part of the Netherlands and gained independence. Dutch is the official language. French Guiana continues to be a territory of France, with French as the official language. French Guiana has representation in the French government (U.S. State Department, 2005).

Literacy

Table 6-6 lists the 10 highest U.S. Latin American immigrant countries and their literacy rates. The International Data Base of the Census Bureau defines literacy for these countries as the ability to read and write in anyone older than 15 years (U.S. Census Bureau, 2008; Kayser, 2008). The least literate nation in the Caribbean is Haiti, with an estimated 62.1% literacy rate. Cuba is the most literate Latin American country, with a 100% literacy rate.

Table 6-6 also provides the number of children who begin and complete the primary grades, or survival rate to

TABLE 6-6 Literacy and Survival Rate to Last Primary Grade (%), 2003 to 2008, for 10 Latin American Countries

Country of Origin	Youth (15 to 24 Years) Literacy Rate, 2003 to 2007		Survival Rate to Last Primary Grade (%), 2003 to 2008
	Male	Female	
Mexico	98	98	92
Puerto Rico	—	—	—
Cuba	100	100	97
El Salvador	95	96	69
Dominican Republic	95	97	61
Guatemala	88	83	62
Colombia	98	98	88
Honduras	88	93	61
Ecuador	96	97	76
Peru	99	97	85

Data from Huebler, F. (2008). Survival rate to the last grade of primary school. Executive Summary: The State of the World's Children. Paris: UNESCO Institute for Statistics.

the last primary grade. Cuba has the highest survival rate for male and female students, with Mexico following at 97% and 92%, respectively. El Salvador, the Dominican Republic, Guatemala, and Honduras have survival rates from 61% to 69%.

In summary, the people of Latin America are from diverse groups and backgrounds. The countries in Latin America have evolved over the past 500 years to develop their own identities. The use of English is growing in many of these nations, but Spanish will continue as a world language and will be one that U.S. citizens will develop in the coming decades. An important factor in the development of Latin America will be the education of children and these Latin American countries' efforts in alleviating the needs of children and adults that culminate in immigration to the United States.

IMMIGRATION

A 2008 Pew Hispanic Center Report stated that 12.7 million Mexican immigrants lived in the United States in 2008, a 17-fold increase since 1970 (Pew Hispanic Center, 2008a). Mexicans now account for 32% of all immigrants living in the United States. Filipinos are the second largest immigrant group and make up 5% of all immigrants in the United States. Persons from Mexico represent 59% of the estimated 11.9 million unauthorized immigrants in the United States and also make up the largest number of legal immigrants in the United States, 21%. No other country in the world has as many total immigrants from all countries as the United States has immigrants from Mexico alone. Eleven percent of everyone born in Mexico is currently living in the United States (U.S. Census Bureau, 2008).

The Pew Hispanic Center (2008c) reports a recent reversal in the growth of the Hispanic population in the United States. They report an overall reduction of 8% in the number of unauthorized immigrants currently living in the United States to 11.1 million in March 2009 from a peak of 12 million in March 2007. The most marked decline in the population of unauthorized immigrants comes from Latin American countries other than Mexico.

LATINO HEALTH IN THE UNITED STATES

With large Latino populations entering the United States, there are concerns that their presence is a burden to the health system. The Pew Hispanic Center (2010) reported that 15.5% of the general U.S. population does not have insurance compared with 42% of all Hispanics who do not have this benefit. This information provides a general description of how Latinos live in the United States but does not provide a day-to-day description of what families and children may have to accept as part of life, health, and disability.

Hispanic adults are younger than the general U.S. population, 27 years versus 35 years, respectively (U.S. Census Bureau, 2006). Thus, these young adults have a lower prevalence of many chronic health conditions reported by the U.S. adult population as a whole. Hispanics do have a higher prevalence of diabetes than non-Hispanic white adults and are more likely to be overweight, which puts them at risk for diabetes. When Hispanics are asked about why they lack a usual health provider, 41% of the respondents stated that the principal reason is that they are seldom sick. Hispanic adults also reported that their information about health and health care came from the media (83%), medical professionals (71%), and social networks (70%) (Pew Hispanic Center, 2008b). Salas-Provance and associates (2002) reported similar results within four generations of one family (40 people), who said that they sought medical resource information from their medical specialist and family, 87.5% and 62%, respectively.

These data indicate that Hispanic populations listen to the media and physicians for information on health and wellness. Speech-language pathologists and audiologists should increase the use of media and the medical community to provide information concerning communication and hearing disorders to the Spanish-speaking populations in the United States. An important finding is the use of social networks, family, and friends. Livingston and colleagues (2010) did not report whether this social network information is similar to what medical professionals may provide. It is known that Latinos depend on each other for health information as well as remedies for wellness (Perrone et al., 1989; Salas-Provance et al., 2002). The effectiveness of home remedies is yet to be determined.

HOME REMEDIES

Folk healing and home remedies are part of all cultures in some form, with some individuals given a title as part of this belief in keeping wellness in the community (Kayser, 2008; Maestas & Erickson, 1992; Salas-Provance et al., 2002). Among Latinos, there are a number of ailments that are "cured" by the use of specific herbs, teas, and ointments, along with prayer. Among Mexicans, *curanderismo* is practiced in Mexico and in large Hispanic regions of the United States, such as Los Angeles and Chicago, and along the U.S. and Mexican border (Kayser, 2002, 2008; Salas-Provance, 2002).

Curanderismo encompasses material, spiritual, and mental levels using objects and ritual in conjunction with the power of God to promote healing (Perrone at al., 1989). It is a method of healing for those who have historically had little access to medical specialists. Typically, this form has been used to heal illness, not disabilities or birth defects. The practice of *curanderismo* in some communities has been merged with modern medicine by Hispanic students in nursing school who also use the folk medicine that Mexican and other ethnic groups may use (Kayser, 2002, 2008; Perrone et al., 1989). For many Mexicans without access to health care, there is only the *curandera,* and if she cannot help, they believe the saying, "Lo que no se puede remediar, hay que aguantar" (What cannot be healed, has to be put up with) (Kayser, 2008; Salas-Provance et al., 2002).

Gunther and colleagues (2005) reported that herbal use is important for doctors (and other professionals) to understand and know about because of potential toxicity of certain herbs. There may be potential negative herb-drug interactions that patients and doctors may not recognize. These researchers suggested that families using *curanderismo* are willing to discuss the measures that have been taken before seeing the doctor. Guenther and colleagues stated that Mexican families will likely use folk healing as well as Western medicine to help their children.

An important consideration is that not all Latinos use folk healing. Salas-Provance and associates (2002) reported that family members may not use folk healing as individuals become more educated and have more experience with Western medicine. Older generations may adhere to folk healing. New generations immigrating into the United States who have not had access to Western medical systems may use folk healing. Cultures change with exposure to Western medicine and culture.

LATINO CHILDREN'S HEALTH IN THE UNITED STATES

The World Health Organization (WHO) defines health as "a state of complete physical, mental, and social well-being, and not merely the absence of disease or infirmity" (ChildStats, 2005). Data not available through the U.S. government include measures concerning disability, mental health, and child abuse and neglect. This section describes the health and well-being of Hispanic or Latino children and adolescents in the United States, primarily from data reported by ChildStats (2005) and the Centers for Disease Control and Prevention (CDC; 2005).

The WHO International Classification of Functioning, Disability, and Health (ICF) changed the perspective of disability from cause to impact on health conditions. This change in focus takes into account the social aspects of disability and does not see disability only as a "medical" or "biologic" dysfunction. By including contextual factors in which environmental factors are listed, ICF allows the clinician to record the impact of the environment on the client's functioning.

Among Latino children, there are three variables that have important effects on growth and development as well as health: the environment the children live in; smoking habits of adults they live with; and the amount of lead found in houses and surrounding grounds, particularly in low-income and urban areas. Environments that contain contaminants such as pollutants in the air, food, and drinking water, affect children with a number of different ailments and developmental growth difficulties. The Coalition of Hispanic Health and Human Services Organizations (1996) stated that reducing exposure to air pollution is a priority for Latino communities because 80% of Latinos live in areas that do not meet the U.S. Environmental Protection Agency ambient air quality standards. This affects the quality of life for Latinos with chronic respiratory conditions such as asthma.

Tobacco smoke is another environmental hazard for children. The adverse effects of secondhand smoke are infections of the lower respiratory tract, bronchitis, pneumonia, middle ear fluid, and sudden infant death syndrome. Environmental tobacco smoke can also exacerbate the symptoms of asthma. From 1999 to 2002, 84% of African American children aged 4 to 11 years had cotinine (a breakdown product of nicotine) in their blood, compared with 58% of white and 47% of Mexican American children (CDC, 2005). The CDC reported that Latinos are at a disadvantage in regard to smoking because of poor English skills, limited exposure to anti-smoking information, market targeting by the tobacco industry, and exposure to second hand smoke more often than the general population. With increased acculturation, the CDC (2005) reports that the rate of smoking for Latino persons increases and approaches that of the general population. This trend is of particular concern with regard to younger people. Children who live below the poverty level are more likely to have cotinine in their blood and live in homes where someone smokes.

Lead exposure is another environmental hazard to children. Children exposed to lead are likely to have learning problems, reduced intelligence, cognitive deficits, reading disability, and lower vocabularies. Children may also exhibit hyperactivity and distractibility. The main sources of exposure are dust contaminated by lead paint in older homes and soil containing lead. Young children are especially vulnerable because of hand-to-mouth activities. The CDC (2005) reported that children below the poverty level had greater blood lead levels than children above the poverty level. A blood lead level of 10 micrograms per deciliter or greater is considered elevated, but adverse effects have been found in lower levels in children.

Young Latino children are exposed to a variety of environmental hazards that may pose barriers to them becoming healthy young adults. Small and large Latino communities should receive health education concerning health risks within their environments and the impact on children's lives. Although the Kaiser Commission (2006) did not specifically report on children as a separate population, this subgroup is definitely affected by their parents' inability to communicate their children's health needs or to determine where access for health care may be available (Flores et al., 2002). Children living in areas with large Latino populations generally have access to health care and most likely have access to health care professionals who speak Spanish. Children living in new Latino communities are not as fortunate (Figs. 6-1 to 6-3). The children in Figures 6-1 to 6-3 have spent the day waiting to see the volunteer doctor who visits their village once a year.

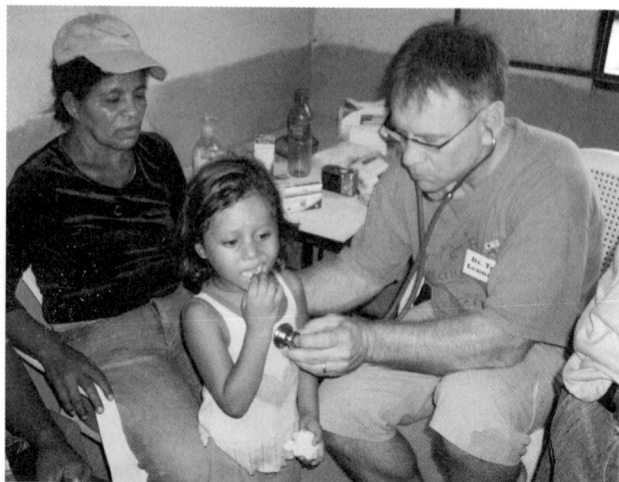

FIGURE 6-1   Mother and child are examined by a volunteer American doctor, Nicaragua, June 2010. *(Courtesy of Project Hope, Springfield, MO. Available at: www.PJHope.org.)*

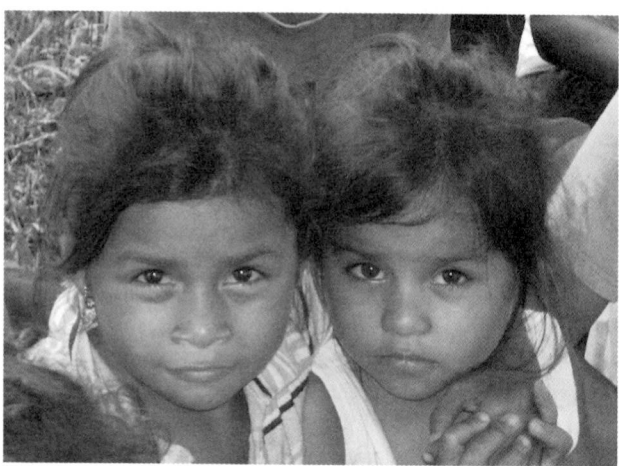

FIGURE 6-2   Two girls pose for the camera, Nicaragua, June 2010. *(Courtesy of Project Hope, Springfield, MO. Available at: www.PJHope.org.)*

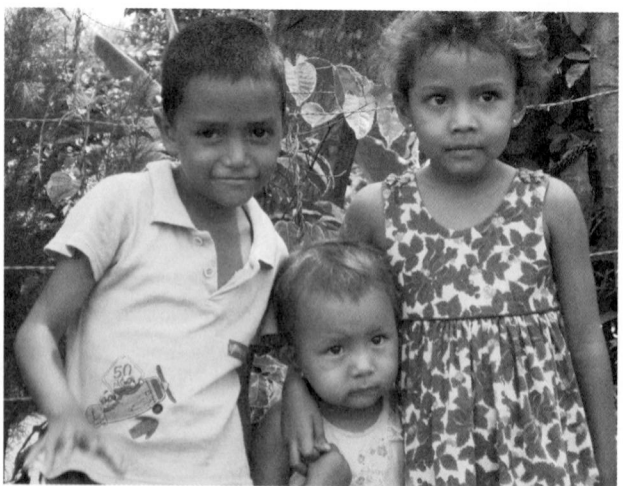

FIGURE 6-3   Children in front of their home, Nicaragua, June 2010. *(Courtesy of Project Hope, Springfield, MO. Available at: www.PJHope.org.)*

LATINOS: COLLECTIVISTIC GROUPS WITHIN AN INDIVIDUALISTIC SOCIETY

Cultural tendencies of Latinos have been described by numerous authors (Kayser, 1995, 2002, 2008; Iglesias, 2002; Goldstein, 2004; Langdon, 2009; and Roseberry-McKibbin, 2002). The focus has been on Mexican and Puerto Rican cultures mainly because of easier access for observation and research than other Latino groups. Cultures do change as immigrant individuals become assimilated or acculturated into mainstream America (Battle, 2002; Rodriguez & Olswang, 2003). Latinos in New York will not be like Latinos who live in Nebraska or Mississippi. Those in New York will be exposed to more than 100 different cultures and languages, and these individuals will either take on the belief systems of a dominant culture near them or isolate themselves to maintain the language and native culture. Those in Nebraska or Mississippi may take on some of the belief systems and behaviors of those mainstream Americans in contact with the new Latino communities. I grew up in Texas, and the Spanish speakers learned English with a Texas accent, and the next following generation began to use Spanish with an English Texas accent. The English dialect in the community is the model for these new Latino immigrants.

What may help professionals who work with Latinos is to understand that these groups may begin as collectivistic in their views of the world, but their worldview may change to reflect the individualistic culture of their American community. The specific practices of cultures may change, but certain characteristics within groups may persist.

Triandis and associates (1988) describe the mainstream English-speaking middle-class white person in the United States as primarily individualistic, that is, the individual has more importance than the group. One's own personal goals are more important than the needs of an identified group. This definition is, of course, on a continuum because many people in the United States have collectivistic values and are also mainstream English-speaking middle-class whites. In contrast, collectivistic societies are populations that defer individual needs to the needs of the group. Latino populations tend to be collectivistic. The values and belief systems within the family may be different for the first generation compared with the fourth generation of individuals who have immigrated to the United States. The following descriptions may help orient the professional to how collectivistic populations see the world.

Triandis and associates describe basic concepts that differentiate the two societies, individualist versus collectivistic. For each of these basic concepts, there can be numerous examples in the differences between the two groups. For example, time is not as critical in the events of life to collectivistic groups as it is among individualistic persons. Among individualistically oriented persons, a meeting begins at 8 A.M. sharp. The collectivistic group considers the event more important than the time that it takes place. Children may stay up late with their parents because this family time together is more important than the time children should go to bed, say, 8 P.M. Parents may use this event to talk about the day, plans for the next day, or family concerns. Family time together becomes more important than a specific bedtime that is likely to be more important for families with individualistic tendencies. Another example is the appointment to see the speech-language pathologist. The event is therapy, the time is not as critical. The mother knows that it's on Tuesday in the morning. She may have to take two or three busses to get to the clinic, but she'll get there because the event is important, not the exact time of the event.

Roles are important among Latinos. There is a specific way that a husband, wife, and children are to behave in public and at home. The mother may depend on the grandmother to help her in socializing the children so that when the family is at a public event, the children know their roles and expectations for appropriate behavior, such as to kiss and greet important family members and not to interrupt adult conversations. Girls have their role within the family. They may assume more responsibility around the house and may be responsible for younger children. Boys may not have as much responsibility and may not be expected to care for their own needs until much later than what is expected of girls. Parents see themselves as caregivers and teachers are professionals who have another role, teaching their children at school (Kayser, 2008; Langdon, 2009).

Group membership is important. The group defines who the person is and how he or she is thought of by the community. For example, children in classrooms know which children are accepted and which children are not accepted in the group. This is observed when children with speech-language disorders are not part of the group of Latino children who are "accepted" in the class. Group identity among Latinos is important. In family gatherings, men will interact with men, women with other women, and children with other children. Women will watch their children, but group membership can be observed during these gatherings (Langdon, 2009). In Figure 6-4 one child was asked to pose for a picture but insisted that his friends participate in the photo.

There is great respect for authority figures among collectivistic populations, whereas among individualistic groups, there is less of a vertical relationship between the employer and the employee, or the professor and the student, the mentor and the mentee. Collectivistic societies view these relationships as important, and the distance between the relationships are greater for them than for those in individualistic societies. There are social boundaries with the employer, the doctor, and the teachers in schools. Within Hispanic cultures, respect is extended to individuals who have specialized skills, such as a guitarist, a singer, or an artist. They are referred to as *maestros*, persons who mastered a

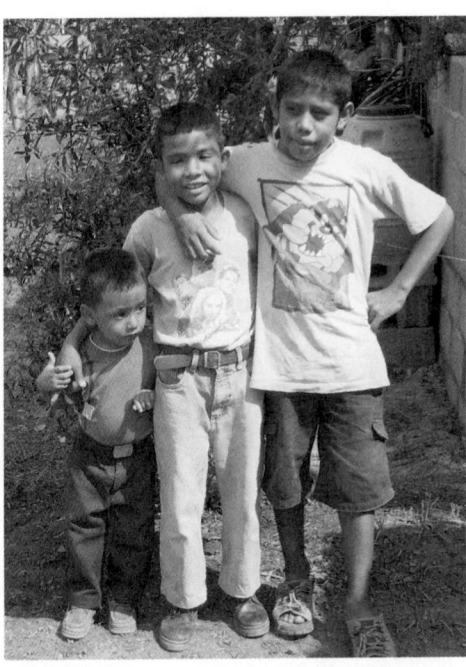

FIGURE 6-4 Friends for life, Nicaragua, June 2010. *(Courtesy of Project Hope, Springfield, MO. Available at: www.PJHope.org.)*

skill. One does not consider themselves an equal to one who has authority.

Among collectivistic groups, relationships are long term. A new friendship may be accepted by an individual, then the family is introduced, and finally the community will know the new friend. Within individualistic communities, a friendship may begin as part of a committee, but once the committee work is completed, the persons within the group may not speak to each other again for years. Friendship among collectivistic individuals will continue over years and in many cases for life. Discussions among family members may revolve around the whereabouts and activities of family and friends and how contacts can be made with these relationships. When a collectivistic or Latino individual wants your phone number and address, his or her expectation of friendship will be that of maintaining and nurturing the friendship. The term *familism* is used to describe the Hispanic's view of friendships that become part of the family (Harry, 1992; Kayser, 2002; Langdon, 2009; Zayas & Palleja, 1998). In Figure 6-5 a few children were invited to attend a puppet show, but a large crowd attended.

Formality is prevalent among collectivistic groups. First names are not used readily, but rather are used only gradually as the relationship is developed. Asking children to call an adult stranger by their first name is not appropriate. What the child may say is "Miss" or "teacher" as a form of respect rather than to use a first name or a name that may not be pronounceable to the child. First-name basis on the first meeting with a Latino parent would be inappropriate, especially if there is an older person present, such a grandmother. Persons who are older are referred to with the

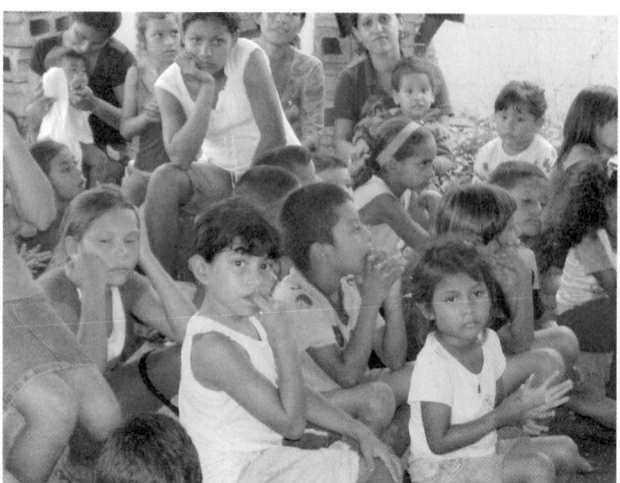

FIGURE 6-5 A puppet show in Nicaragua, June 2010. *(Courtesy of Project Hope, Springfield, MO. Available at: www.PJHope.org.)*

formal *usted* form rather than the informal *tu*. Thus, professionals should keep in mind that showing respect to another person requires formality in referencing (Harry, 1992; Kayser, 2008; Langdon, 2009).

Gift giving is important to collectivistic societies. A gift is given when a person is grateful for an action, service, or assistance, or because they are visiting. Gifts can also be items that the parent has handmade. When I was a beginning speech-language pathologist, I received gifts from mothers that included sugar cane, tortillas, and fruit. Gifts to the child are also important. Parents socialize the child to remember who has given the gift and will remind the child of who gave the gift when it is worn or used. When a child is asked, "who gave you this?" the child will be able to provide the name of the giver and when the gift was received. This is part of the child's socialization.

The need for privacy is not as strong among collectivistic groups as it is for individualistic societies. Children may grow up in a small home and share the same bedroom, use one bathroom, and take turns eating at a table with two chairs, when there are eight people in the family. Brothers, sisters, and cousins may never be alone. A very large industry in Latin America is language schools that provide language instruction and boarding houses to Americans, Asians, and Europeans who visit Latin America to learn Spanish. The important component of this industry is the host family. Many of these families may host dozens of foreigners in 1 year, and some of these visitors may stay 1 week to 1 year with the host family. Privacy for the family is not as critical as welcoming another person into their family.

Gender and age are very important among collectivistic societies. Men and women have their roles, and some attitudes of women in men's roles may be looked at with discomfort or disapproval. In many parts of Latin America, these roles are changing for young adults as they enter

Western corporations that indoctrinate Latino professionals to Western values. Age is definitely given respect, and the younger you are, the less likely your opinion will be accepted. Wisdom comes with age (Harry, 1992).

Collectivistic societies enjoy working in groups. Recognition for the group's work is preferred over individual praise. Latino children work well collaboratively in play and educational assignments. Bilingual children will help each other when they don't understand the classroom topic, the assignment, the task, the purpose, the goal, or whatever the teacher has instructed in the classroom. The group orientation keeps the individual child from making mistakes, protects the individual when confronted by enemies, and also provides a network for assistance when in need. Latino children may place higher value on cooperation than on individual competition.

Families are defined as the whole extended family; this includes the nuclear family, aunts, uncles, grandparents, cousins, godparents, and whoever else has been adopted into the "*familia*" (Harry, 1992; Kayser, 2002; Langdon, 2009; Zayas & Palleja, 1998). There is a strong tie for these large families, and reunions are common in Latin America and the United States. The child who needs to go to a second cousin's wedding views it as an important event in the life of the family. Leaving school for a month because there is a Christmas celebration with the family in Mexico is an important event for the family. Family and family events are central to the socialization of the child in collectivistic societies.

Triandis and colleagues provide a broad taxonomy that describes collectivistic and individualistic societies. This section described primarily collectivistic societal tendencies. The reader is cautioned that the dichotomy of collectivism and individualism is a continuum and that as Latinos become part of mainstream America, both individualistic and collectivistic behaviors may be evident. Figure 6-6 is an example of one child who wanted to be left alone.

COMMUNICATION DISORDERS IN BILINGUAL POPULATIONS

Goldstein (2004) reported that Latinos with speech-language impairment represent 12.7% of students between the ages of 6 and 21 years. He estimated that of the 6.8 million Latino students in the schools, there are approximately 870,000 Spanish-speaking children who exhibit some type of communication impairment in the native language. It is possible that there are a number of children who are not identified and provided services because of the lack of qualified bilingual personnel or personnel who do not have access to research that will assist in the assessment and intervention of bilingual populations. This section cannot summarize all the research that has been completed in the past 15 years concerning bilingual Spanish- and English-speaking children, in areas such as specific language impairment, late talkers, grammar,

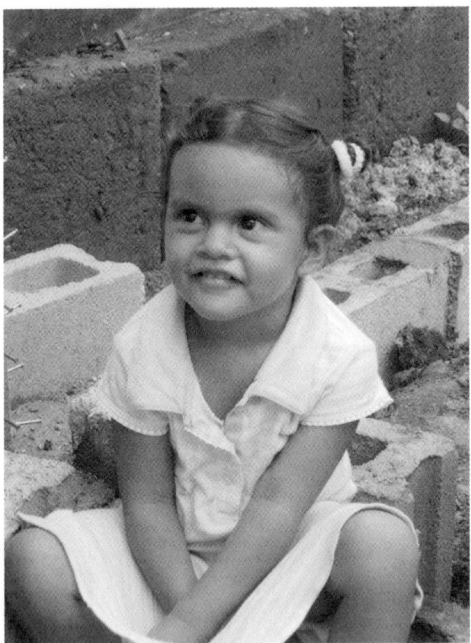

FIGURE 6-6 Young girl in Nicaragua, June 2010. *(Courtesy of Project Hope, Springfield, MO. Available at: www.PJHope.org.)*

morphology, phonology, narratives, literacy, alternative testing procedures (e.g., dynamic assessment and conceptual scoring), and test construction (i.e., validity and reliability). The research has provided insights into speech and language impairment in bilingual English- and Spanish-speaking children. The reader is referred to the resource section at the end of this chapter for further readings.

Differentiating a language disorder from a language difference in bilingual English- and Spanish-speaking children has been the goal for speech-language pathologists, special educators, psychologists, and researchers. The early literature in school psychology compared the bilingual student's performance with that of English speakers on psychological instruments developed for English monolingual children—a procedure that is not supported by current writers (DeLeon, 1995; Kayser & Lopez, 2008; Rhodes et al., 2000). Rhodes and coworkers (2000) and Battle (2002) reported that children from culturally different backgrounds experience a "double jeopardy," that is, these children may have environmental as well as biologic factors that influence their overall development. Children living in poverty are at high risk for environmental and biologic concerns. These factors include prenatal care, low birth weight, environmental toxins, poor nutrition, drugs, and limited access to medical care. The identification of a language or communication disorder in a bilingual child must begin with an understanding of the family history and the child's health and development.

Ortiz and Maldonado-Colon (1986) and Willig and Greenberg (1986) provided behavioral observations of typical English language learners who were referred for special education. Ortiz and Maldonado-Colon (1986) reported that Hispanic children were initially referred for speech and language services, but as they began the middle grades (grades 2 to 4), these same children were reassessed and determined to have a learning disability. Box 6-1 provides a list of typical English language learners' behaviors from the field of bilingual special education. The behaviors seen in second language learners do appear similar to those of children with learning disabilities. An English language learner who doesn't understand English may appear to have a short attention span, distractible, daydream, and so forth. A child in a preschool classroom learning English may also appear nervous, timid, and fearful and, at the extreme, appear autistic.

These same researchers described English language learners' communication behaviors. These are listed in Box 6-2. School adaptation is difficult for children with learning disabilities and may also be observed in second language learners. To briefly summarize these behaviors

---

BOX 6-1 Typical English Language Learner Behaviors*

Attention/Order	Person/Emotional
Short attention span	Difficulty in adjusting to new situations
Distractible	Nervous, anxious
Daydreams	Shy, timid
Demands immediate gratification	Poor self-confidence
Disorganized	Fearful
Unable to stay on task	

*Normal behavior characteristic—often referred because different from teacher's expectations.
Adapted from Ortiz & Maldonado-Colon (1986) and A.C. Willig and H. F. Greenberg (1986).

BOX 6-2 Typical and Atypical English Language Learner Behaviors

School Adaptation**	Language*
Does not complete assignments	Speaks infrequently
Cannot work independently	Uses gestures
Does not initiate	Refuses to answer questions
Exerts little effort	Comments inappropriately
Lacks interest; apathetic	Poor recall
Cannot manage time	Poor vocabulary
Lacks drive	Difficulty sequencing ideas
Disorganized	Difficulty sequencing events
Cannot plan	Unable to tell or retell stories
Unable to tolerate change	Confuses similar sounding words
	Poor pronunciation
Sporadic academic performances	Poor syntax and grammar
	Does not volunteer information
	Poor comprehension

*Normal behavior characteristic—often referred because different from teacher's expectations.
**Behavior characteristic frequently associated with learning disabilities.
Adapted from Ortiz & Maldonado-Colon (1986) and A.C. Willig and H.F. Greenberg (1986).

describe a child with learning disabilities who first does not complete assignments because of a variety of reasons, such as not managing time well, being disorganized, inability to plan, and inability to tolerate change. A second language learner may have difficulty with English comprehension and thus may refuse to answer questions, comment inappropriately, confuse similar sounding words, and so on. The characteristics that are listed may be observed in English language learners.

Although observations of classroom and communication behaviors are helpful in the identification of a language disorder, the speech-language pathologist must document the communication disorder with specific identifiers. Box 6-3 lists language characteristics described by investigators using form, content, and use as categories (Damico et al., 1983; Kayser, 1990, 1995, 2008; Langdon, 1993, 2008; Linares-Orama & Sanders, 1977; Mattes & Omark, 1991; Roseberry-McKibbin, 1995). These authors describe their observations of the articulation, phonology, syntax, morphology, semantics, and pragmatics in bilingual Spanish- and English-speaking children identified as language impaired. Speech-language pathologists began to observe the speech and language behaviors of Latino children and used terminology specific to the field. The descriptions listed in Box 6-3 are for English and Spanish.

Goldstein (2004) reported that the data available concerning bilingual English and Spanish speakers in the United States are from children aged 4 to 7 years. Box 6-4 provides a summary of research that describes the linguistic competency of English- and Spanish-speaking children. He states that the summary of the research available supports Grosjean's (1989) statement that the bilingual person is not two monolingual people in one but rather is a unique individual with communicative competence that is not like any other person. Each language has a different structure that appears to determine the development of each language feature, from phonology to grammar. What appears to be difficult for an English speaker may not be seen for the Spanish-speaking child.

IMPLICATIONS FOR ASSESSMENT AND INTERVENTION

The assessment of bilingual children requires time and effort by a team of professionals who regularly evaluate children who are becoming speakers of two languages. Leung (1995) describes the RIOT procedure that has a four-step process. **R**—review all information available concerning the child; **I**—interview all those informants who have contact with the child and would be able to discuss the child's communication abilities; **O**—observe the child in different contexts; and **T**—test the child, which should be the last step in the process of assessment. What may not be understood by professionals is that testing is not the first step for these children. The biased effects of English tests

---

BOX 6-3 Reported Characteristics of Bilingual English- and Spanish-Speaking Children with Language Learning Disability

Form

Does not express basic needs adequately

Does not associate sounds with objects or experiences

Does not discriminate tones, phonemes, and morphemes

Difficulty with who, what, where, and why questions

Difficulty with the following phonemes: /s/, /l/, /r/, and /rr/

May distort, substitute, or omit sounds

May use syllable deletion, coalesce or reverse order of sounds

Difficulty using: articles, pronouns, prepositions, copulas "ser" and "estar," auxiliary "estar," reflexive pronoun "se," plural endings, and conjunctions

May use incorrect word order, substitute schwa for articles, pronouns, and other morphemes

Difficulty with noun-verb and article-noun agreement and confuse verb tenses

Difficulty with correcting grammatical errors in sentence constructions

Content

Difficulty conveying thoughts in an organized, sequential manner that is understandable to listeners

Word finding difficulties that go beyond normal second language acquisition patterns

Failure to provide significant information to the listener, leaving the listener confused

Inappropriate verbal labels for common objects, actions, and persons

Difficulty with problem solving, making inferences, formulating hypotheses, and making predictions

Difficulty with figurative language

Difficulty following oral and written directions

Use

Nonverbal aspects of language that are culturally inappropriate

Replaces speech with gestures

Rarely initiates verbal interaction with peers

Responds inappropriately to peer-initiated conversation

Peers respond with difficulty in understanding the student

Poor topic maintenance

Difficulty with conversational turn-taking skills

Perseveration on a topic

Poor ability to clarify information

Difficulty with asking and answering questions appropriately

Echoing what child hears

Lacking dialogue and conversation with peers

Limited friendships

Difficulty with retelling stories or narrating personal experiences

---

Data from Damico, Oller, & Storey (1983); Kayser (1990, 1995, 2008); Langdon (1983, 2008); Linares-Orama & Sanders (1977); Mattes & Omark (1991); and Roseberry-McKibbin (1995); adapted by H. Kayser.

BOX 6-4 Linguistic Features of Bilingual English- and Spanish-Speaking Children with Language Impairments

- Bilingual children with grammar impairments do not necessarily exhibit same difficulties in each language.
- Spanish-speaking children with specific language impairment have difficulty with articles and clitic pronouns.
- Narratives for Spanish speakers are characterized by a lack of cohesion throughout the narrative, omission of referents for pronouns, and limited episodic information.
- Bilingual children have little transfer between languages in phonology and are more accurate on sounds shared between the two languages than on sounds unique to each language.
- Phonological development is similar but not identical to monolingual development in either language.
- Bilingualism does not cause stuttering.
- Removing one of the two languages does not improve the child's stuttering behaviors.
- No cases of stuttering occurring only in one language; it occurs in both languages.
- Structural differences between two languages may result in different severity ratings for each language.
- Code switching results in higher stuttering occurrences.
- Linguistic nonfluency is not stuttering; language formulation occurs in one language only.

From Goldstein, B. A. (2004). Bilingual language development and disorders in Spanish-English speakers. Baltimore: Paul H. Brookes. Adapted by H. Kayser, 2010.

have been documented over the years, and we should know that these tests provide an invalid and skewed view of a bilingual child's linguistic abilities of English. Tests in Spanish continue to be developed with the Spanish monolingual in mind, not the bilingual—the child with a unique linguistic system.

As the professional reviews information about the child, the birth history becomes an initial point of information; where the child was born, rural versus urban, may mean a birth in a village with no doctor versus birth in a hospital with medical attention. The number of visits for well-baby check-ups and doctor's visits when there are ear infections, fevers, and dehydration from bacterial infections should be documented. The typical practice of health maintenance, including herbal use and beliefs about maintenance of wellness, cannot be underestimated and should be part of the information-gathering process. A thorough case history is paramount for a successful evaluation of a child's birth, health, and development.

Latin American children born in the United States should also be viewed with a different perspective. Latino children may live in poverty. Their home environments may include poor housing conditions, lack of availability of food, and pollution should be considered as part of the evaluation. Children who are not physically well and do not see a physician for ear infections, chronic respiratory conditions, and lead elevation in the blood may be encountered in this population.

Language use, the number of languages spoken in the home, who uses each language and the level of proficiency, and the importance of each language to the family are variables to consider in the communicative environment of a child or adult. For example, a child may be born in Latin America to a family who speaks only Spanish. The family moves to Arkansas, where there is a small Latino community and Spanish is not used extensively in the school, community, or business. The child attends a school where English is the only language used for instruction and completes third grade in Arkansas. During the family's 8 years in Arkansas, the child has lost the ability to speak Spanish because the parents did not maintain Spanish in the home and wanted the child to learn English at school. The family then moves to Chicago to a large Spanish-speaking community. Education for children in this area is in English and Spanish because of the high numbers of Latino children from Spanish-speaking homes. The child must relearn Spanish to communicate within the bilingual education classroom, to develop friendships, and to communicate with community members. Business and community members speak Spanish. The child learned English, Spanish attrition occurred while in Arkansas, and then the child must relearn Spanish to function in the Chicago school and community. Families may move for better employment, for better opportunities for their children, or to be near family and friends.

Parents may need information about the evaluation process and the treatment for communication disorders. The information must be in their native language, Spanish, in written and oral form. The diagnostic process needs to be explained so that parents do not assume that we are "playing with the child" rather than collecting information about their communicative competence. This information must be available to parents throughout the diagnostic and intervention sessions. Parents must recognize the importance of what the speech-language pathologist and audiologist is doing and why this is important to the child's speech and language development. Information could be offered by CD or DVD so that parents can review the information at home. This extra time allows the family to come together to form questions to ask the professional.

Treatment should include the parents and siblings. Parent involvement in treatment strategies may be unusual or uncomfortable for the family; therefore, every effort must be made to use culturally relevant materials and sensitivity in treatment sessions. For example, using a preschool classroom as the therapy room may be a new environment for the child and parents. Playing with toys that are familiar to the child rather than toys that are part of an

American mainstream child's experience would provide a valid and productive treatment session. Kayser (2008) provides a list of questions that may be used to view the child's play behaviors. The extended family can be involved in treatment. Using group therapy with the family, siblings, or cousins may help the child respond positively to the language models of the extended family.

Time in scheduling should be flexible until parents are acculturated into the mainstream expectation of promptness for therapy. The family may have transportation difficulties to diagnostic and treatment sessions. A mother may have to take two or three buses to reach the destination. Professionals should keep in mind that therapy goals and objectives may need to be implemented with flexibility within the therapy session. For example, if the speech-language pathologist has three objectives for the session (e.g., activity 1 is scheduled for 10 minutes; activity 2 is scheduled for 20 minutes; activity 3 is scheduled for 20 minutes), the professional should consider that the child may want to complete activities on the basis of the child's interests rather than the timing of the clinician's scheduled objectives. The speech-language pathologist may shape the child's interests toward the clinician's objectives of time spent on each activity over the course of a few weeks. Children require some time to be accustomed to mainstream use of time.

FUTURE RESEARCH

Diagnostic and treatment protocols for Latino children require the collaboration of teacher, professional, and parents. The limited time in treatment programs that professionals provide with these children can be dramatically improved if teachers and parents are involved in the diagnostic and treatment programs.

Research is needed to understand the home backgrounds and how these affect the child's learning in school. How does urban versus rural living in Latin America determine the child's learning in school? Will parents from urban areas more readily involve themselves in parent and teacher programs in the schools? How does health and wellness in Latino communities affect the learning of Latino children in the schools? What is the best form of parent literacy program for Spanish-speaking families from Nicaragua versus Mexico? How can we best reach parents so that they understand that education is more than 6 years of schooling? How can we provide an excellent education to Spanish-speaking children when we only have English-speaking teachers and professionals in the schools? How can we incorporate culturally sensitive materials into our diagnostic and treatment sessions? There are many questions that can be asked for future researchers. An important question is how do we bring new research into the practice of bilingual and monolingual speech-language pathology?

CONCLUSION

Latinos are diverse in their understanding of the world, their health practices, how they must survive economically, politics, and language backgrounds. Latinos in Latin America and the United States are diverse in culture and language use. We cannot assume that Hispanic is an all-encompassing term that defines these ethnic groups.

The population growth of Latinos in the United States has not gone unnoticed by the majority of U.S. residents. It has become a political issue that has supporters for several possible solutions, but that may or may not be supported by Latinos living in the United States (Pew Hispanic Center, 2006). Immigration has become an emotional issue and one that is dividing communities across the United States. Laws have been enacted in states to create barriers for newcomers to work and receive health services.

Children and adults from Latin America come to this country with different experiences depending on their country's economic and governmental stability and ability to assist families in health and nutrition. Public and early education is perceived differently in each of these countries. Latino families come to the United States for various reasons and once here, have much to learn about this nation's culture, language, history, and educational opportunities for their children.

Information is the great resource for Latin America, and we need to do more outreach programs to these nations. Preparing teachers in Latin America by providing workshops to professionals in these countries would benefit children. The United States can be an outstanding resource to Latin American nations to assist children with special needs. We cannot go to countries thinking that we have all of answers and change their model of interventions, but we can go with an attitude of learning about the rich cultures, pride, language use, and methods of education that have been used with children. The goal is to learn how we can help. The Latin American nations know what they believe is most important to help their children, and our responsibility is to determine how we can help. Basic survival in some areas of Latin America is more important than whether the child is talking. Food and medicine for children may be more important to a mother than whether she is reading to her child. The mother may just want her child to live. Families know and understand their child, and we must look to parents to help professionals glean that information with a thorough case history. Parents must receive information concerning the educational system and how it works to benefit their child.

The professional can assist families and children by being an active advocate for families who are immigrants and help families by finding resources within the school. The professional can organize parent information sessions that may help parents understand the expectations for students in the school and how they can assist their child in making the transition to American ways of learning and teaching. The professional can show parents the importance of reading in our society and how they can help their child to succeed. Most important, children must receive affirmation concerning who they are, where they come from, and how they can contribute to our society. These children must learn to be proud of their identity within the family and community. These are important characteristics for Latinos.

DISCUSSION QUESTIONS

1. What have been your beliefs about Latin America's population? Have these beliefs changed? Why or why not?
2. How can you assist parents to recognize the importance of education in the United States?
3. How do you perceive and describe the socialization of the American English-speaking child, and how is this different from what you have learned about collectivistic societies?
4. How have the definitions of communication disorders in bilingual Spanish- and English-speaking children changed over the years?
5. What can be done to improve or expand the educational services to parents concerning speech and language disorders?

REFERENCES

Battle, D. (Ed.) (2002). *Communication disorders in multicultural populations* (3rd ed.). Boston: Butterworth-Heinemann.

Centers for Disease Control and Prevention (2005). National Center for Health Statistics, National Health Interview Survey. Retrieved May 18, 2011, from www.cdc.gov/nchs/nhis.htm.

ChildStats: Federal Interagency Forum on child and Family Statistics (2005). Health, America's children: Key national indicators of well-being 2005. Retrieved July 4, 2006, from http://childstats.gov/americaschildren/hea.asp.

Coalition of Hispanic Health and Human Service Organizations (1996). Hispanic environmental health: Ambient and indoor air pollution. *Otolaryngology Head and Neck Surgery, 114,* 256-264.

DeLeon, J. (1995). Intelligence testing of Hispanic students. In H. Kayser (Ed.), *Bilingual speech-language pathology: An Hispanic focus* (pp. 223-264). San Diego, CA: Singular Publishing Group.

Flores, G., Fuentes-Afflick, E., Barbot, O., et al. (2002). The health of Latino children: Urgent priorities, unanswered questions, and a research agenda. *Journal of the American Medical Association, 288,* 82-90.

Goldstein, B. A. (2004). *Bilingual language development and disorders in Spanish-English speakers*. Baltimore: Paul H. Brookes.

Guenther, E., Mendoza, J., Crouch, B., et al. (2005). Differences in herbal and dietary supplement use in the Hispanic and non-Hispanic pediatric populations. *Pediatric Emergency Care, 21,* 507-514.

Harry, B. (1992). *Cultural diversity, families, and the special education system: Communication and empowerment*. New York: Teachers, College Press.

Iglesias, A. (2002). Latino culture. In D. Battle (Ed.), *Communication disorders in multicultural populations* (3rd ed.) (pp. 179-204). Boston: Butterworth-Heinemann.

Kaiser Commission on Medicaid and the Uninsured (2006). *Health coverage and access to care for Hispanics in "New Growth Communities" and major Hispanic centers*. Washington, DC: Author.

Kayser, H. (1995). Intervention with children from linguistically and culturally diverse backgrounds. In M. E. Fey, J. Windsor, & S. F. Warren (Eds.), *Communication and language intervention series (Vol. 5). Language intervention: Preschool through the elementary years* (p. 315). Baltimore: Brookes.

Kayser, H. (2002). Bilingual language development and language disorders. In D. E. Battle (Ed.), *Communication disorders in multicultural populations* (3rd ed., pp. 205-232). Boston: Butterworth-Heinemann.

Kayser, H. (2008). *Educating Latino preschool children*. San Diego: Plural Publishing.

Kayser, H. & Lopez, E. (2008). Psychological and cognitive assessment of preschoolers. In H. Kayser (Ed.), *Educating Latino preschool children*. San Diego: Plural Publishing.

Langdon, H. W. (2009). Providing optimal special education services to Hispanic children and their families. *Communication Disorders Quarterly, 30,* 83-96.

Leung, B. (March, 1995). Non-biased assessment. Workshop presented for Alliance 2000, Monterey, CA.

Maestas, A. G., & Erickson, J. G. (1992). Mexican immigrant mothers' beliefs about disabilities. *American Journal of Speech Language Pathology, 1,* 5-10.

Ortiz, A., & Maldonado-Colon, A. (1986). Reducing inappropriate referrals of language minority students in special education. In A. C. Willig & H. F. Greenberg (Eds.), *Bilingualism and learning disabilities* (pp. 37-52). New York: American Library.

Perrone, B., Stockel, H., & Krueger, V. (1989). *Medicine women, curanderas, and women doctors*. Norman, OK and London: University of Oklahoma Press.

Pew Hispanic Center (2006). *America's Immigration Quandary*. Washington, DC: The Pew Research Center for the People and the Press.

Pew Hispanic Center (2008a). Statistical portrait of Hispanics in the United States, 2008. Retrieved April 22, 2010, from http://pewhispanic.org/data/origins/.

Pew Hispanic Center (2008b). Hispanics and health care in the United States: Access, information and knowledge. Retrieved September 8, 2010 from http://pewhispanic.org/reports/report.php?ReportID=91.

Pew Hispanic Center (2008c). Trends in unauthorized immigration. Retrieved September 8, 2010, from http://pewhispanic.org/reports/report.php?reportID=94.

Pew Hispanic Center (2010). U.S. unauthorized immigration flows are down sharply since mid-decade. Retrieved September 8, 2010, from http://pewhispanic.org/reports/report.php?ReportID=126.

Public Law 94-311, 29 U.S. Code, Section 8, June 16, 1976, 90 Stat. 688.

Rangel, C. (1977). *The Latin Americans: Their love-hate relationship with the United States*. New York: Harcourt Brace Jovanovich.

Rhodes, R. L., Kayser, H., & Hess, R. S. (2000). Neuropsychological differential diagnosis of Spanish-speaking preschool children. In E. Fletcher-Janzen, T. L. Strickland, & C. R. Reynolds, (Eds.), *Handbook of cross-cultural neuropsychology* (pp. 317-334). New York: Kluwer Academic/Plenum Publishers.

Rodriguez, B. L., & Olswang, L. B. (2003). Mexican-American and Anglo-American mothers' beliefs and values about child rearing, education, and language impairment. *American Journal of Speech-Language Pathology, 12,* 462-492.

Roseberry-McKibbin, C. (2002). *Multicultural students with special language needs* (2nd ed.). Oceanside, CA: Academic Communication Associates, Inc.

Salas-Provance, M. B., Erickson, J. G., & Reed, J. (2002). Disabilities as viewed by four generations of one Hispanic family. *American Journal of Speech Language Pathology, 11,* 151-152.

Triandis, H., Brislin, R., & Hui, C. H. (1988). Cross-cultural training across the individualistic-collectivistic divide. *International Journal of Intercultural Relations, 12,* 269-289.

Willig, A. C., & Greenberg, H. F. (Eds.) (1986). *Bilingualism and learning disabilities.* New York: American Library.

U.S. Census Bureau (1990). www.census.gov/prod/1/90dec/cph4/appdxe.pdf.

U.S. Census Bureau (2006). *American community survey.* Washington, DC: Author.

U.S. Census Bureau (2008). *International data base.* Washington, DC: Author.

U.S. Census Bureau (2010). *International data base.* Washington, DC: Author.

U.S. State Department (2005). www.state.gov/countries/.

Zayas, L. H., & Palleja, J. (1998). Puerto Rican families: Considerations for family therapy. *Family Relations, 37,* 260-264.

ADDITIONAL RESOURCES

Goldstein, B. A. (2004). *Bilingual language development & disorders in Spanish-English speakers.* Baltimore: Paul H. Brookes.

Kayser, H. (2008). *Educating Latino preschool children.* San Diego: Plural Publishing.

Kohnert, K. (2008). *Language disorders in bilingual children and adults.* San Diego: Plural Publishing.

Argentina
Asociación Argentina de Logopedia Foniatría y Audiología (ASALF)
E-mail: *asalfa@ciudad.com.ar*

Brazil
Sociedade Braseleira de Fonoaudiologica
E-mail: *directoria@sbfa.org.br www.sbfa.org.br*

Chile
Colegio de Fonoaudíologos de Chile
E-mail: *Colfono@colfono.tie.cl*

Costa Rica
Asociación Costarricense de Terapeutas del Lenguaje
E-mail: *Marce_MV@Yahoo.com*

Cuba
Asociación de Linguístas de Cuba

Mexico
Sociedad Mexicana de Audiología y Foniatría

Panama
Colegio Nacional de Fonoaudiólogas de Panamá
E-mail: *thelmaderocha@hotmail.com*

Puerto Rico
Organización Puertoriqueña de Patología de Habla, Lenguaje y Audiología (OPPHLA)
Website: http://opphla.org

Uruguay
Asociación de Fonoaudiología del Uruguay (A.deF.U.)
E-mail: *adefu@adinet.com.uy*

Venezuela
Federación Latino-Americana de Sociadades de Fonoitría Logopedia y audiología (FLASFLA)

Part II

Communication Disorders and Development in Multicultural Populations

Chapter 7

Multilingual Speech and Language Development and Disorders

Helen Grech and Sharynne McLeod

Most people in the world understand and speak more than one language. Multilingualism is supported by the media, mobility (both legal and illegal), international economics, global literacy initiatives, progress in information technology, the drive for lifelong learning, and many other factors. Within this chapter, different definitions of multilingualism are explained, particularly relating to concepts such as successive and sequential multilingualism and language proficiency. Reasons children are multilingual are discussed, with particular emphasis on international migration. Features of typical and atypical speech and language acquisition are contrasted, followed by a discussion of the challenges related to assessment and differential diagnosis to distinguish between difference and disorder in multilingual children. Intervention strategies, particularly regarding the language of instruction and whether instruction in one language is able to be generalized to another, are also discussed. Finally, recommendations for future research are provided.

DEFINING MULTILINGUALISM

Multilingual people understand and speak more than one language. This definition seems simple; however, the term *multilingualism* is controversial and is defined differently throughout the world. Parameters that characterize definitions of multilingualism include the following:

1. The number of languages known (e.g., bilingual, trilingual, polyglot, semilingual)
2. The age and timing of the acquisition of each language (e.g., simultaneous versus sequential acquisition)
3. Proficiency in each language (e.g., minimal skill, functional, proficient in daily life, or proficient in all contexts including educational, academic, and professional contexts)
4. Domains of language knowledge and use (e.g., perception and comprehension versus production)

5. Language output mode (e.g., oral versus signed versus written)
6. Languages spoken within the community (e.g., majority versus minority languages)

To demonstrate differences in use of the term multilingualism, three definitions of multilingualism are provided below from the most to least conservative. Definitions 2 and 3 are exemplified by their use in the context of speech-language pathology and audiology.

Definition 1. Multilingualism only applies to those who experience bilingual first language acquisition. This definition was used by Genesee and colleagues (2004, p. 6) when they stated: "When we refer to simultaneous bilingual children (or just bilingual children), we mean children who are exposed to and given opportunities to learn two languages from birth." They used the term *second language learners* for children who acquire their second language after 3 years of age.

Definition 2. Multilingualism applies to those who are functional in the use of more than one language. For example, Cruz-Ferreira (2010, p. 2) stated, " . . . multilinguals are people who use more than one language in their everyday lives." A similar definition is used by the American Speech-Language-Hearing Association (ASHA, 2004, p. 3) for speech-language pathologists (SLPs) or audiologists. They state that one aspect of the knowledge and skills needed by SLPs and audiologists to provide culturally and linguistically appropriate services is to have "Native or near-native proficiency in the language(s) spoken or signed by the client/patient."

Definition 3. Multilingualism is a continuum in which people can have different levels of proficiency in each of the languages they use. They may have minimal skill, be functional, or be proficient. For example, Valdés and Figueroa (1994, p. 115) suggest that bilingualism, "rather than being an absolute condition is a relative one. Bilingual individuals can be both slightly bilingual or very bilingual." This definition is used by the Royal College of Speech and Language Therapists (RCSLT) in the United Kingdom, which indicates that bilingual people are "individuals or groups of people who acquire communicative skills in more than one language. They acquire these skills with varying degrees of proficiency, in oral and/or written forms, in order to interact with speakers of one or more languages at home and in society. An individual should be regarded as bilingual regardless of the relative proficiency of the languages understood or used" (RCSLT, 2006, p. 268).

In this chapter, an inclusive definition of the term multilingual is used and is closest to definition 3. That is, a person who is multilingual is able to comprehend or produce two or more languages in oral, manual, or written form regardless of the level of proficiency or use and the age at which the languages were learned. In this chapter, multilingualism is used as an umbrella term for both bilingualism and multilingualism.

Throughout this chapter, research from different parts of the world is used to exemplify different aspects of multilingual speech and language acquisition. Therefore, it is important to remember that the wide range of terminology and the lack of specificity of meaning of terms makes comparative analyses difficult. For example, some research studies exclude data from people who have better language skills in one language than the other, so they may describe a partial view of multilingualism as defined in this chapter. The time individuals are exposed to each language and how often they use that language also are likely to affect the results of research. In addition, research data vary regarding languages explored, sample type, and methodologic approach, so it is not easy to compare findings. An appendix to this chapter is provided to demonstrate the diversity of studies of typical and atypical multilingual speech and language acquisition and to facilitate preliminary comparisons of key features.

SIMULTANEOUS VERSUS SEQUENTIAL LANGUAGE ACQUISITION

One important issue for understanding multilingual acquisition is the age of first exposure to each language. The terms *simultaneous acquisition* and *sequential acquisition* are most commonly used to differentiate the age of exposure.

Simultaneous Acquisition

Some people are regarded as simultaneous bilinguals because they acquired two or more languages at the same time, very early in their lives. Genesee and colleagues (2004) indicate that in order to be considered simultaneous bilinguals, people should learn two or more languages within

the first year of life, or at least by age 3 years. De Houwer (2009) differentiated two categories of simultaneous bilinguals. The first included children who have *bilingual first language acquisition* (BFLA) when there was no existing chronologic difference of the exposure of both languages; and the second included children who are *early second language learners* (ESLLs). ESLLs are exposed to a second language on a regular basis between 1;6-4;0 years of age. De Houwer clarified this as being exposed to a second language through day care, play schools, nurseries, or other group settings. For example, most of the children living in Malta are exposed to Maltese at home and English when they start attending preschool at 3 years of age; so they would be regarded as ESLLs by De Houwer (2009).

Sequential Acquisition

Some people are sequential bilinguals because they acquired one language, then learned the second (and subsequent) languages after their first language was (at least partially) established. Genesee and associates (2004) refer to second language learners as those whose exposure to the second language (L2) occurred after 3 years of age or after establishment of the first language (L1). Others have terms for acquiring subsequent languages upon or during formal schooling. For example, De Houwer (2009) refers to formal second language acquisition when children are introduced to a second language and literacy at about 5 years of age. Martin (2009) refers to learning English as a second language at school and not through exposure by interpersonal interaction with terms including *English as a second language* (ESL), *Second language acquisition* (SLA), and *English language learners* (ELLs). Equivalent terms would be used in non-English contexts, such as *Icelandic as a second language* in Iceland (cf. Másdóttir, 2011). Sequential acquisition can also refer to learning subsequent languages at any time during life, whether as a result of education, migration, family (e.g., marriage), occupation, personal interest, or any other reason.

Proficiency in First and Second Languages

Balanced bilinguals (people who are equally proficient in two languages) do not exist. Diversity in proficiency of the second (and subsequent) language exists even among individuals in the same family (Kayser, 1995). Like many adults, children may use the two languages for different reasons. The preference to use one of the two languages may be sociologically or culturally influenced and may also reflect changes in self-identity.

Children who acquire languages simultaneously are likely to differ from those who acquire their languages successively. Simultaneous versus sequential acquisition of languages will influence typical development. When children learn languages sequentially, there may be a delay in achieving language competence. Sequential multilingual children may take up to 2 years to start expressing themselves in their second language (Martin, 2009). Cummins (2003) classifies two phases of language proficiency for sequential learners. The first is called *basic interpersonal communication skill* (BICS) and the second is called *cognitive academic language proficiency* (CALP), which requires a command of L2 enabling children to follow the curriculum optimally. It may take a child 5 to 7 years to acquire CALP, and proficiency in both L1 and L2 increases throughout their lives.

LANGUAGE LEARNING CONTEXT

Different countries support differing levels of multilingualism. Some countries, such as the United States, have no official languages, yet the majority of people in this country speak English (with a large minority speaking Spanish). Some countries have one official language, and this is the language spoken by the majority of people (e.g., in Australia the majority language is English; in Nicaragua, Spanish; in Saudi Arabia, Arabic; in Turkey, Turkish; in Vietnam, Vietnamese). Some countries have two or three official languages, yet there is still a majority language used by most of the population. For example, New Zealand's official languages are English, Māori, and New Zealand Sign Language; however, the majority use English. Hong Kong's official languages are Cantonese, Putonghua (Mandarin), and English, and all these languages are taught in school; however, most children initially learn Cantonese. Other countries (e.g., Belgium, Canada, Switzerland) have a number of official languages, and these languages are routinely spoken both in official and daily contexts.

Another type of multilingual language learning context occurs when more than one language is extensively used, such as in countries that have numerous official languages (e.g., Afghanistan, India, South Africa, Zambia). In some of these countries, such as India, children speak many languages as a part of daily life. South Africa has 11 official languages and many other unofficial ones. In South Africa, English is the most commonly spoken language in official and commercial public life but is not the most commonly spoken home language (Jordaan et al., 2001). Singapore has four official languages: English, Malay, Chinese (Mandarin), and Tamil. However, it is acknowledged that more than 20 languages are spoken in Singapore (Gupta & Chandler, 1993). The Republic of Congo has French, Lingala, and Kituba as national languages, as well as other dialects, including Kikongo. In Sweden, Swedish is the main language, and Finnish, Meänkieli, Romani, Sami, and Yiddish are recognized as minority languages. The *Central Intelligence Agency World Factbook* provides an overview of languages spoken in different countries (https://www.cia.gov/library/publications/the-world-factbook/fields/2098.html).

The intersection between learning majority and minority languages with simultaneous and sequential bilingualism has been illustrated in a quadrant drawn by Genesee and colleagues (2004, p. 8). These authors indicate that the boundaries between the quadrants are not fixed but rather can be seen as a continuum.

Quadrant A consists of people who are simultaneous bilinguals who live in a majority ethnolinguistic group. This would include children who live in multilingual communities such as Québec, Canada, and learn both English and French from birth.

Quadrant B consists of people who are simultaneous bilinguals who live in a minority ethnolinguistic group. This would include children who live in a multilingual family; for example, children who live in the United States and learn both Spanish and English from birth (although in some parts of the country, such as in California and Florida, speakers of Spanish may be considered a majority ethnolinguistic group).

Quadrant C consists of people who are sequential bilinguals who live in a majority ethnolinguistic group. This would include children who live in Hong Kong and learn Cantonese from birth, then English and Putonghua (Mandarin) when they start school.

Quadrant D consists of people who are sequential bilinguals who live in a minority ethnolinguistic group. This would include children who live in Australia and learn Arabic from birth, then English when they start school.

Factors Influencing the Context of Multilingual Language Learning

Migration

Migration has a major impact on multilingualism and multiculturalism throughout the world. In 2005, there were nearly 200 million international migrants (9.2 million of whom were refugees) around the world, a significant increase from 82 million in 1970 (Global Commission on International Migration for the United Nations, 2005, http://www.gcim.org/en/). Sollors (2009) reported that there are 56 million migrants in Europe, 50 million in Asia, 40 million in North America, 16 million in Africa, 6 million in Latin America, and nearly 6 million in Australia (making up 18.7% of the total population of Australia). In Japan, the number of expatriate workers increased from 750,000 to 1.8 million between 1975 and 2001. With China and India gaining economic momentum, it is likely that there will be a large migratory flow to these countries also in the near future, which will create new forms of multilingualism (Sollors, 2009).

In the United States, 75% of population growth between 1995 and 2000 was the result of migration (Sollors, 2009). At the time of the 2007 U.S. Census, more than 55.4 million

(20%) people older than 5 years spoke languages other than English (Shin & Kominski, 2010). Although the predominant non-English language was Spanish (62% of those who spoke a language other than English), 19% spoke another Indo-European language (e.g., German, Italian), 15% spoke an Asian and Pacific Island language (e.g., Chinese, Tagalog, Vietnamese, Korean, Japanese), and 4% spoke another language (e.g., Haitian Creole). The majority of people in each of these language groups reported that they spoke the other language "very well" (Shin & Kominski, 2010). The uneven distribution of speakers of languages other than English in the United States reflects the continuous flow of non-native populations, with about 500,000 to 1 million migrants becoming U.S. citizens annually (U.S. Census Bureau, 2000). Sollors (2009) states that in this era of global migration and regional cultural and linguistic diversity, many countries are endorsing educational curricula that encourage the learning of languages other than the respective country's official one. This is a challenging goal because there is still a dearth of knowledge about multilingual speech and language acquisition, particularly regarding whether multilingual children show similar patterns of acquisition to those of monolingual speakers.

Although immigrants in a given country differ linguistically, culturally, and socioeconomically, many share common characteristics, such as insufficient knowledge of the languages, dialects, and accents spoken by the residents in their new country (Cheng, 2004). Cheng reports that immigrants often have different medical and social experiences as well as different educational backgrounds and home-language literacy skills compared with residents in their new country. In addition, immigrants may experience stress from immigration depending on the circumstance of the reason for migrating. Consequently, Cheng and Butler (1993) report that immigrants may experience tiers of adaptation in the country in which they land:

1. Migrants may initially reject the new culture and language in the hope of retaining their home language and culture.
2. Migrants may try to blend portions of the two cultures.
3. Migrants may become isolated as a result of refusing to maintain their native culture or to assimilate into the new culture.
4. Migrants may eventually try to accept both cultures but not blend in either, with the result that they may perceive marginalization and feel uncertain about which rules to follow.
5. The optimal and most gainful level involves the full involvement of both cultures, termed *biculturalism,* whereby migrants feel confident and secure blending both cultures. At this stage, such individuals often achieve proficiency in the language of the host country.

However, this level may lead to rejection of the use of their own native language and cultural rituals.

It seems that a core underlying issue of migrant dissatisfaction is difficulty communicating (Grech & Cheng, 2010). Different nations respond to multilingual issues relating to migration in different ways. European Union (EU) educational policies and strategies have attempted to address diverse cultural and linguistic characteristics by offering support services and expanding resources for optimal learning of all children, including those of ethnic and migrant communities. National curricula are increasingly endorsing two languages, particularly in many European bilingual contexts (Huguet & Lasagabater, 2007). For example, the 1995 White Paper (CEC, 1995) on teaching and learning proposed that EU citizens should be proficient in three European languages (i.e., mother tongue and two other EU community languages). Additionally, the European Commission (EC) is offering incentives to individuals with multilingual proficiency, including jobs (mobility opportunities) and opportunities for educational staff and student exchange. There is also a push toward multilingual educators and professionals. Lassagabaster and Huguet (2007) report the results of a transnational study among trainee or student teachers in nine bilingual areas/states in Europe, indicating that 70% of student teachers claimed to have high proficiency in a minority language; almost all of the student teachers reported high proficiency in the majority language. The multilingual areas/states involved in the study were Basque Country, Catalonia, Galicia, Valencian Community, Belgium, Friesland, Ireland, Malta, and Wales. Some of the student teachers were proficient in at least three languages (but this varied from one area/state to another; in some, more than 50% of the student teachers reported proficiency in at least three languages). The importance of multilingual educators (and SLPs) is reinforced by the fact that the course of language development in monolingual children may be different from that of bilingual children and that language acquisition is influenced by culture, attitudes, and beliefs.

International Adoption

Within many Western countries, another significant group of migrants are children who are adopted internationally. For example, in the United States in 2009, 12,753 international adoptions took place, with the majority of children coming from China, Ethiopia, Russia, South Korea, Guatemala, Ukraine, Vietnam, Haiti, Kazakhstan, and India (Child Welfare Information Gateway, 2010). In previous years, even more children were adopted by families in the United States. In 2004, 22,990 children were adopted internationally. In 2008, when 17,229 international adoptions took place, the majority (48%) were of children 1 to 4 years old, an additional 34% were of children younger than 1 year, and the remainder (18%) were of children 5 years and older (Child Welfare Information Gateway, 2008).

Children who are adopted internationally are often referred to as *second first language learners* because they are neither monolingual nor multilingual (Pollock, 2007). Typically children who are adopted internationally begin learning one language in their home country, then at the time of adoption, exposure to their first language ceases, and they begin to learn another language. A meta-analysis of language outcomes for children who were adopted internationally showed that they were more likely to have poorer language outcomes; however, there was great variation (Scott et al., 2011). One mediating factor was the age of adoption; there was a slight trend in favor of children who were adopted at younger age groups. Gauthier and Genesee (2011) also indicate that children adopted from China tended to have better language outcomes than children adopted from countries in which deprivation was more common.

MULTILINGUAL SPEECH AND LANGUAGE DEVELOPMENT

There are a number of theories regarding how culture and social relationships influence the acquisition of communication skills in children. For example, the information processing theory addressed in Bates and MacWhinney (1982, 1987) claims that language acquisition is motivated by the communicative intent of the child. Bruner (1986) emphasizes the contextual situation and communicative functions as the motivation for language acquisition. Snow (1981) refers to the social interaction theory, claiming that the child-caregiver interaction drives language development in the context of biologic and environmental influences. Martin (2009) supports the sociocultural approach to the study of multilingual children and emphasizes the importance of acknowledging cultural and linguistic diversity and not undermining the notion that language is an enabling tool for learning through social and cognitive means. Children of linguistically and culturally diverse families are therefore faced with a multitude of cultural values, beliefs, and social rules that influence their acquisition of language.

Appendix 7-1 provides a summary of a number of research studies (published in English) that have examined multilingual speech and language development in typical and atypical children. Much of the research that has been conducted in English has focused on Spanish-English speech and language development conducted in the United States. However, the appendix lists many additional language pairs. Readers are encouraged to access the original sources to learn more about typical and atypical acquisition of languages.

Historically, many studies of multilingual children's speech and language acquisition compared multilingual children's skills with those of monolingual children. For example, Hemsley and associates (2006) conducted a large-scale study of 101 11-year-old children speaking either Vietnamese-English, Samoan-English, or monolingual English. They examined their skills in English lexicon and nonword repetition and concluded that "despite six years of formal schooling in English, including focused ESL [English as a second language] support, bilingual students from both Vietnamese and Samoan cultural backgrounds perform less well than their [monolingual] peers in their understanding and use of the English lexicon" (Hemsley et al., 2006, p. 453). Although information such as this is valuable, it is also imperative that children's skills be examined in all of the languages they speak to fully understand their abilities. Indeed, subsequent longitudinal research published by the same authors described younger children's vocabulary acquisition in both Samoan and English (Hemsley et al., 2010). They found that if a composite score was created by adding words known by children in each language, the Samoan-English children's receptive (but not expressive) language scores were equivalent to their age-matched monolingual English peers. By considering both (or all languages) understood and spoken by children, an enriched (and more holistic) view of their abilities can be gained.

Positive and Negative Transfer, and Cross-Linguistic Differences in Multilingual Acquisition

When comparing typical speech and language acquisition of multilingual children with monolingual acquisition, SLPs should expect both positive and negative effects of multilingualism as well as cross-linguistic differences. In a recent review of research on multilingual speech acquisition, Goldstein and McLeod (2011, p. 1) indicated that "in comparison to monolingual children, multilingual children exhibit speech sound skills that are less advanced (i.e., negative transfer) and more advanced (i.e., positive transfer) than their monolingual peers. Moreover, results from those studies indicated that speech sound skills are not simply mirror images of each other in the two languages but are distributed somewhat differently in each constituent language, owing to the phonotactic properties of the languages being acquired."

Positive transfer occurs when children learning more than one language have enhanced skills compared with their monolingual peers. Examples of positive transfer have been found for children speaking Spanish-German (Kehoe et al., 2001; Lleó et al., 2003), and Maltese-English (Grech & Dodd, 2008) compared with their monolingual peers. Fabiano-Smith and Goldstein (2010) extended the definition of positive transfer to include when multilingual and monolingual children have similar skills. They found that typically developing 3-year-old Spanish-English speaking children acquired two speech sound systems in approximately the same amount of time that monolinguals acquired one system. Other studies have found similar skills between typically developing multilingual and monolingual children. For example, Gildersleeve-Neumann and Wright (2010) found a similar number of syllable-level errors between Russian-English (RE) bilingual children and monolingual English-speaking (E) children (ages 3;3-5;7). Specifically, they reported that "RE and E children did not differ in their overall production complexity, with similar final consonant deletion and cluster reduction error rates, similar phonetic inventories by age, and similar levels of phonetic complexity" (p. 429). Positive transfer has also been shown for children with speech sound disorder in Spanish-English (Goldstein, 2000), Mirpuri-English, Urdu-English (Holm et al., 1998), and Italian-English (Holm & Dodd, 1999b).

In contrast, there are also examples of negative transfer whereby speech and language acquisition of multilingual children is less advanced than that of monolingual children. Negative transfer has been shown in some aspects of speech acquisition by typically developing Spanish-English bilingual children (e.g., Fabiano-Smith & Goldstein, 2010; Gildersleeve et al., 1996; Gildersleeve-Neumann et al., 2008; Goldstein & Washington, 2001). For example, Holm and Dodd (1999a) described the phonological development of two children who had been exposed only to Cantonese until 3 years of age, when they began to attend a childcare center where only English was spoken. Disruption of the children's phonological acquisition in Cantonese was noticed on exposure to English and some established contrasts were lost. Both children's error patterns in English were atypical of monolingual English phonological acquisition. In this instance, early sequential bilingualism seemed to have disturbed phonological acquisition. Indeed, Kohnert and colleagues (2005) emphasize that it is important to continue to support acquisition of children's first language, particularly for children with language impairment. In contrast, bilingual first language acquisition (simultaneous bilingualism) might have different consequences for speech and language acquisition from that of sequential bilingualism (De Houwer, 2009).

Thus far, it has been shown that multilingual children exhibit positive and negative transfer between languages (and within some studies, such as by Fabiano-Smith and Goldstein, 2010, they experience both). However, children's skills in each of the constituent languages are not identical. For example, cross-linguistic differences in acquisition were found by Bunta and associates (2009), who examined the speech of 3-year-olds typically developing Spanish-English bilingual, monolingual Spanish, and monolingual English children. For Spanish, there were differences between monolingual and bilingual children for consonant accuracy, but not for whole word measures. For English, there were differences between monolingual and bilingual children for both measures. Cross-linguistic

differences have also been found for Spanish-English children with speech sound disorders (Goldstein et al., 2008) and for typically developing Cantonese-English children (Holm & Dodd, 2006).

The findings that speech (phonological) acquisition of multilingual children differs from that of monolingual children indicates that having two phonologies affects the course of acquisition of phonology. This is in line with the interactional dual-systems model for the mental organization of more than one language as proposed by Paradis (2001). The model asserts that bilingual children have two separate phonological systems but that those two systems can influence one another. The model fits with data from other studies of the phonology of typical and atypically developing multilingual children (e.g., Johnson & Lancaster, 1998 [Norwegian-English]; Holm & Dodd, 1999a, 1999b, 1999c [Cantonese-English, Italian-English and Punjabi-English, respectively]; Keshavarz & Ingram, 2002 [Farsi-English]; Salameh et al., 2003 [Swedish-Arabic]). On the other hand, Navarro and associates (1995) found no atypical phonological error patterns in the speech of 11 successive multilingual Spanish-English preschool children. These apparently conflicting findings may reflect differences between language pairs, or the timing and ages of exposure to the different languages.

Multilingual Speech Development

Phonological Development

In the late 1960s, Roman Jakobson offered the following statement regarding children's speech acquisition across the globe: "Whether it is a question of French or Scandinavian children, of English or Slavic, or Indian or German, or of Estonian, Dutch or Japanese children, every description based on careful observation repeatedly confirms the striking fact that the *relative chronological order of phonological acquisitions remains everywhere and at all times the same . . . the speed of this succession is, in contrast, exceedingly variable and individual . . .*" (Jakobson, 1968, p. 46, emphasis added). This statement, although appealing in its simplicity, has been proved on numerous occasions not to be true. A more current understanding is that children's speech acquisition is influenced by a complex interrelationship between phonetic complexity, functional load, and phonetic frequency and this varies by language (see Ingram, 2011, for an overview). Phonetic complexity or ease of production refers to the articulatory difficulty or ease producing a sound. For example, fricatives are said to be more complex than stops because they require finer motoric movements to produce, have lower acoustic saliency, occur less frequently in babbling, and so on. Functional load refers to how often a sound contrasts with other phonemes (Meyerstein, 1970). For example, in

English /ð/ (voiced *th*) has a low functional load (because it is in only a few words); however, in Greek it has a high functional load. Phonetic frequency refers to how often a sound occurs in spoken language. For example, in English /ð/ has high phonetic frequency because words such as *the*, *this*, and *that* are used frequently. Stokes and Surendran (2005) demonstrated the relationship between these three factors for different languages. They found that a child's age of emergence of sounds in Chinese was predicted by phonetic frequency, but in English it was best predicted by functional load. They found that accuracy of production was best predicted by phonetic complexity in English, but not in Dutch. Late acquisition of complex consonants was predicted by phonetic complexity in Arabic. It appears that, to date, one generalization can be made: "Phonemes with high functional load in a language will be acquired earlier by both typically developing children and by children with phonological deficits" (Ingram, 2011, p. 12). A comprehensive summary of monolingual speech acquisition for more than 20 languages is provided by McLeod (2010). However, little is known about the relative factors that influence multilingual speech acquisition for different languages, so SLPs need to constantly update their knowledge on this topic.

Multilingual Language Development

Lexical Acquisition

Multilingual and monolingual children typically have similar numbers of words in their lexicon; although the multilingual children's words are distributed across the languages that they speak (Peña et al., 2002). Some words are unique (termed *singlets*), whereas others overlap (termed *translation equivalents*) (e.g., a translation equivalent occurs if a child knows both the English and Spanish words for the same object: *pen* and *pluma*) (Hemsley et al., 2010). Perhaps unsurprisingly, 7-year-old French-English bilingual children were found to have more unique words (singlets) in their dominant language than their nondominant language (Paradis et al., 2003). It has been found that multilingual and monolingual children tend to use similar strategies for categorizing words (Peña et al., 2002) but will rely on context for words that they choose. For example, although most Spanish-English bilingual children said *cake* when asked to name foods at a party, when speaking Spanish children followed this by *arroz* (rice) and *frijoles* (beans), whereas when speaking English, they listed *hamburger* and *hotdog*.

CASE STUDY: Multilingual Speech Acquisition in Malta

The Maltese Islands are found in the middle of the Mediterranean Sea below Italy and Sicily. Immigrants from Malta are found around the world, but mostly in the United States, Canada, and Australia. There are two official languages in Malta: Maltese and English. Most children are bilingual in that they have some knowledge of both languages but one of the languages may be dominant. Parental report indicates that in some homes, one of the languages may be used consistently, whereas other families use both languages. This multilingual context was used in a large-scale project to study the effects of language exposure at home on the rate and course of phonological acquisition (Grech & Dodd, 2008). A total of 241 Maltese children aged 2.0 to 6.0 years, drawn randomly from the public registry of births, were assessed on a picture naming task to evaluate articulation, phonology, and consistency of word production. Ninety-three children (38.6%) were reported by parents to speak both Maltese and English at home, 137 (56.9%) were reported to speak Maltese, and 11 (4.7%) only English at home. During testing, children were allowed to choose which language they wanted to use (either Maltese or English). The data gained were analyzed for percentage of consonants and vowels correct, adult phonemes absent, developmental speech error patterns, number of English and Maltese words used, and percentage of children using translation equivalents. Results of the study indicated that children reported to be monolingual differed qualitatively and quantitatively from children reported to be bilingual in Maltese and English. The bilingual children had a faster rate of phonological acquisition in that they suppressed developmental error patterns more rapidly than those exposed only to Maltese. The two groups also exhibited different error patterns (developmental phonological processes) in specific ages, although some error patterns were also observed in all the participants. Children exposed to both Maltese and English at home appeared to perform better also on percentage consonant correct (PCC) and consistency compared with children exposed only to one language at home. Conclusions from this study were that early exposure to two languages might enhance phonological acquisition. The conclusion that children in a bilingual learning context may be at an advantage for spoken phonological acquisition (positive transfer) is supported by other researchers who looked at children exposed to more than one European language (e.g., Bialystok et al., 2005, for English-Spanish or Hebrew; Yavaş & Goldstein, 2006, for Spanish-English). The results indicate that children who are regularly exposed to more than one spoken language discriminate whether the language they hear spoken is worth their attention. Such children learn to distinguish between the two languages using phonological cues and consequently become aware of the constraints specific to each language's phonology and thus increase their phonological knowledge. Phonological knowledge is considered to be a marker of phonological ability (Gierut, 2004). Thus, children acquiring language in a bilingual community, like Malta, may have greater phonological knowledge than children in a monolingual community.

Morphosyntactical and Narrative Acquisition

To communicate effectively, multilingual children need to follow the grammatical rules for each language. When language mixing occurs, children typically mix nouns with nouns and verbs with verbs (Paradis et al., 2000). Nicholls and colleagues (2011) conducted a study of the acquisition of English morphological skills by 148 3-year-old children: 74 were multilingual, speaking over 31 different languages in addition to English, and were 74 monolingual children matched for age. The multilingual and monolingual groups showed a similar developmental progression in the acquisition of morphology, with the same grammatical skills being more difficult for both groups; however, the multilingual children had a slower rate of acquisition. In another study, Cleave and colleagues (2010) assessed 26 children with specific language impairment; almost half the children were monolingual speakers, whereas the other children were dual-language learners, with English being the dominant language. They found that the multilingual children achieved higher scores on the production of language from using narrative assessment, rather than using standardized tests of morphosyntax. However, all the children scored below average on measures from narrative samples for productivity, narrative structure, literate language, and language form. Bedore and colleagues (2010) similarly found the usefulness of eliciting narratives to determine 170 bilingual Spanish-English children's language abilities. They found that English mean length of utterance (MLU), as well as English and Spanish grammaticality, was the best predictors of language use in these bilingual children.

Language Mixing and Code Switching

Language mixing, or code switching, refers to the practice of moving back and forth between two languages or between two dialects or registers of the same language. Historically, it was believed that language mixing was a negative characteristic of multilingualism. For example, individuals who engaged in language mixing were seen as having a lack of proficiency in either language. Parents who language-mix were said to be providing a poor language model for their children because this was thought to reflect poor language competence (Kayser, 1995). However, Crystal (1997) indicated that there was no justification for claiming that children exposed to multilingualism are linguistically at risk. Indeed, Karrebæk (2003) stated that code switching is "the result of cognitive processes, of a multilingual competence." There are increasing reports (e.g., Martin et al., 2003; Stow & Dodd, 2003) indicating that language mixing, or code switching, indicates competence at sociolinguistic skill rather than reflecting psycholinguistic incompetence. This has also been the view of some authors such as Cheng and Butler (1989) who reported that SLPs have mistakenly viewed code switching as a cause for concern. Attrition in language mixing between 2 to 3 years of age has been reported for simultaneous bilingual development (e.g., Vihman, 1985). This pattern has been generally associated with increasing linguistic competence reflecting increasing competence in language selection (Deuchar & Quay, 2000) and of enhanced differentiation between languages (Lanza, 2004).

CASE STUDY: Language Mixing and Code Switching in Malta

Two studies conducted in Malta have provided insights into children's language mixing. Language mixing occurs frequently in Malta, both in typically developing children and adult native speakers. Bilingualism is widespread on the Maltese Islands, and substantial language mixing occurs on a national scale. Grech and Dodd (2008) reported findings on the use of language code and translation equivalents giving an indication of the children's knowledge of their community's languages. Language mixing did not show any negative affect on bilingual language acquisition. Adult-child interactions involved specific patterns of language contact, with child-directed speech (CDS) being characterized by English content words embedded in Maltese utterances. A typical example of CDS in the Maltese context would be "Poġġi d-dolly fuq il- bed" meaning "Place the doll on the bed." As a result, Maltese children acquire language in the context of mixed input in the home. Gatt (2010) described the development of lexical expression in typically developing

Maltese children aged between 12 and 30 months who were exposed primarily to Maltese language in their homes. The child-directed speech of caregivers included English-Maltese mixing in a Maltese dominant context. The children's vocabularies included mainly Maltese words, although between 14% and 30% of the words used across the 12- to 30-month age were English words. The children's use of English words diminished as they grew older and as their Maltese vocabulary expanded. Maltese-speaking children's use of English words could be considered as an example of lexical mixing. As the proportion of English word usage was decreasing, there was a growing use of translation equivalents and therefore a trend toward more balanced bilingual vocabulary development. Gatt (2010) claimed that this finding could be related to the input reflecting a single mixed language. She concluded that these young Maltese participants could be considered monolingual who subsequently became early sequential bilinguals.

ASSESSMENT OF MULTILINGUAL CHILDREN'S SPEECH AND LANGUAGE

Multilingualism is not a cause of speech and language impairment. Indeed, it may actually be the reverse because multilingualism is reported to be beneficial for speech and language development and a positive experience for children with speech and language deficits (Paradis et al., 2003). Because bilingualism is not thought to cause communication impairment, the percentage of children with speech and language difficulties should not differ for multilingual compared with monolingual children (Winter, 2001).

Multilingual children with speech or language impairment are those who exhibit impairment (delay or disorder) in both or all the languages they hear regularly (Holm et al., 1999). Some evidence to support this claim comes from case studies of Cantonese-English bilingual children (Holm & Dodd, 1999a) and Welsh-English bilingual children (Ball et al., 2006). Simultaneous multilingual children should understand both languages and speak at least one of the languages they are exposed to relatively early in their lives (De Houwer, 2009). Referral to an SLP should occur if this is not the case, or if children have concomitant sensory, structural, or neural difficulties such as hearing loss, cleft palate, or cerebral palsy.

Differential Diagnosis

Differential diagnosis of multilingual children is not always straightforward, particularly to differentiate typically developing multilingual children who are having difficulty learning one of their languages from multilingual children who are having difficulty in all of their languages. The distinction between language development, language difference, and language disorder presents a challenge to SLPs because of differences in terminology as well as limitations of resources to assess and diagnose multilingual individuals with communication impairment. Various case studies have been reported of typically developing bilingual children who have been incorrectly identified as having a speech or language disorder specifically because of their perceived underachievement, reflecting on their daily function and social interaction. For example, Murphy and Dodd (2010) describe the challenges of differential diagnosis for a 13-year-old child with hearing loss from a Vietnamese-English background living in Australia. They found that his language difficulties could not be attributed either to his hearing loss or multilingual background.

Meanwhile, typically developing children who are culturally or linguistically different from the majority of the population may be identified as having a speech and language impairment because of unclear definitions of subgroups of speech and language impairments as well as health and education policies regarding inclusion and exclusion criteria. For example, the identification of specific language impairment (SLI) may be based on the exclusion of global learning difficulties or cognitive impairment, neurologic or sensory deficits, and psychosocial and emotional factors. If the identification of a cognitive impairment is based on intelligence tests, this may mistakenly identify multilingual children who may obtain low scores because such tests may be linguistically and culturally biased. Multilingual children may be misdiagnosed as having educational learning difficulties specifically because of their perceived low proficiency in language skills, particularly their second language (e.g., Martin, 2009; Steege, 2006). The assessments used in education may not capture the demands of multilingual communication, and the child's learning skills may not be analyzed holistically.

Another criterion that is often used in the identification of multilingual children with SLI is their performance compared with development trajectories of typically developing monolingual children. Paradis (2005) compared the morphologic skills of typically developing children acquiring English as a second language with those of monolingual English-speaking children with specific language impairment. The results revealed similar accuracy rates and error types for both groups of children, indicating that multilingual children could easily be misdiagnosed as having a language impairment. Any conclusions based on developmental patterns of monolingual children (very often not even language specific) could therefore lead to misdiagnosis (Stow & Dodd, 2005). Multilingual speech and language acquisition may show a different path and rate of development compared with monolingual children.

The diagnosis of speech or language impairment should be considered with caution when referring to multilingual children. Leonard (1998) indicated that language impairment in bilingual children exists when their comprehension or expressive abilities are different from those of their bilingual peers and this interferes with communication. Comparing language proficiency with peers exposed to the same language is a useful way of differentiating difference from disorder. This implies that bilingual children's language proficiency should be compared with that of their bilingual peers and not monolinguals. However, this still poses the question of whether the specific bilingual norms are available.

Another issue related to the differential diagnosis of multilingual children is distinguishing between subgroups of impairment. Clinicians are often concerned about whether the classification they employ with monolingual children is applicable to multilingual children. (e.g., determining whether children have an articulatory or phonological delay, or atypical speech). Data regarding classification of speech and language impairment in bilingual children are limited. A few examples include data from Cantonese-English (Holm & Dodd, 1999a), Italian-English (Holm & Dodd, 1999b), and Punjabi-English (Holm & Dodd, 1999c).

It is claimed that a differential diagnosis reflecting different subgroups of speech disorders used with monolinguals (i.e., articulation disorder, delayed phonology, consistent or inconsistent phonological disorder, and developmental verbal dyspraxia) is also applicable to multilingual children (Holm & Dodd, 1999c).

The debate about whether monolingual children with language impairment have delayed or disordered development persists and has been extended to multilingual children (Leonard, 1998; Salameh et al., 2004). The latter observed bilingual language acquisition over a 12-month period in 10 Swedish-Arabic preschool children with severe language impairment and 10 control subjects matched for age, gender, and exposure to Swedish and Arabic. The results of repeated assessments in both languages (focusing on phonology, grammatical markers, and verbal comprehension) indicated that both groups developed grammatical structures in both languages in the same way, although the language-impaired group made slower progress in both languages.

Phases in the Assessment Process

There are two phases in the assessment of multilingual children's speech and language skills: preassessment and direct assessment. These are followed by analysis of the results, diagnosis, and undertaking intervention, if indicated.

Preassessment

Preassessment involves consideration of environmental and personal factors that are important for the child, family, and their social and educational context. During the preassessment, information should be gained about the following:

1. Language use and proficiency of children and their families, including length of time the language has been spoken, its frequency and context of use, proficiency in the language, a language history of the countries the child has lived in (and, if known, where they intend to live in the future), as well as child, parental, and community attitudes toward different languages spoken
2. Cultural heritage, including generalized sociocultural factors alongside individual beliefs and practices and families' cultural perspectives that will affect parent-child interactions, family acknowledgment of disability, and access to and engagement with SLP services
3. Parent- and teacher-reported concerns regarding children's speech and language skills in relation to the skills of their siblings and multilingual peers

The Alberta Language and Development Questionnaire (ALDeQ) (Paradis et al., 2010) is a valuable method for quantifying multilingual children's early milestones, language use, preferences, and family history. It is a psychometrically validated measure that is not specific to a particular language or cultural group. The ALDeQ has been normed on 139 typically developing Canadian children and 29 children with language impairment. The scoring criteria allow for consideration of children who have experienced war, trauma, or lack of funds. If a child scores less than 1.25 standard deviations below the mean, the score is more consistent with a child with language impairment than a typically developing child. Measures such as the ALDeQ provide SLPs with direction for the direct assessment.

Cheng (2006) suggested the use of SWOT (strengths, weaknesses, opportunities, and threats) and RIOT (review, interview, observation, and testing) approaches for evaluating bilingual children's language competence and planning clinical strategies (see Chapter 3). She suggested that only through such an holistic analysis would a clear profile of the child's communication skills be captured. All pertinent background information about children's language exposure and use needs to be reviewed. Stakeholders that may influence children's acquisition of communication skills should be interviewed, such as peers, grandparents, and educators. The children should be observed in the different domains with a variety of people. Finally, children's proficiency should be tested (possibly informally) in all the languages used.

A SWOT analysis involves taking information from the case history and clinical analysis and identifying internal (strengths and weaknesses) and external (opportunities and threats) factors. Case history needs to be thorough and should include aspects about family history of communication difficulties, any reported traumatic experience (such as in migration), attitude toward and proficiency of the second language of the parents and siblings, the extent of code switching, attitude of caregivers toward education and literacy development, and any other relevant personal development information that could reflect on the child's communication difficulties. The background history for each language exposure should also be taken into consideration. This includes the amount of input; onset of language exposure; level of proficiency of carers, educators, and siblings; and the attitudes to use of each language. The clinician should also become aware of the needs and priorities of the family.

Direct Assessment

Direct assessment of children's speech and language is a complex task. Assessment can include consideration of expressive and receptive language, speech production and perception, phonological awareness and preliteracy, hearing, and oromusculature. Assessment of each of these areas can be undertaken using formal and informal assessment procedures as well as dynamic assessment.

Formal or Norm-Referenced Assessments

In English-speaking countries such as the United States, many SLPs use English norm-referenced assessments or informal assessments when evaluating multilingual children (Caesar & Kohler, 2007; Kritikos, 2003; Skahan et al., 2007).

However, conducting SLP assessments in all languages spoken by children is often recommended as best practice. For example, guidelines from both the Royal College of Speech and Language Therapists (2006) and the International Association of Logopedics and Phoniatrics (2006) state that bilingual children should be assessed in both languages.

Currently there are few standardized assessments available for the evaluation of multilingual children's speech and language. Consequently, there are two primary barriers to appropriate assessment of multilingual children, and each barrier relates to the use of formal assessments (Bedore & Peña, 2008). The first barrier is the use of translated tests because they may miss particular diagnostic markers that are important in a language. Translation of tests, test items, or "making allowances" for bilingual children on tests devised for monolinguals can lead to inaccurate identification of impairment (e.g., Grech & Dodd, 2007; IALP, 2006; RCSLT, 2006). The original objectives of these tests would therefore not be addressed in the translated version because language structures are likely to be different, particularly morphology, phonology, and syntax. The validity of standardized assessment tools may be inappropriate for multilingual children. Children may not be familiar with some pictures, test items, or the task itself. Furthermore, developmental stages may be different cross-linguistically. It is likely that what is normal will differ according to which language combinations are learned, when they are learned, and which language was learned first. Multilingual language acquisition patterns vary (when each language is tested separately) compared with monolingual norms for the same languages (e.g., Hua & Dodd, 2006; Quinn, 2001). For example, Grech (1998) reported cross-linguistic differences in children's rate and type of phonological developmental error patterns for monolingual Maltese speakers and monolingual English speakers, and these patterns also differed for Maltese-English bilingual children (Grech & Dodd, 2008).

The second barrier to using formal assessments with multilingual children pertains to the difficulty of compiling test norms for multilingual children because cross-linguistic norms for monolingual children differ from norms for multilingual children. To date, most formal speech and language assessments are designed for and standardized on monolingual speakers and thus may not be appropriate for use with multilingual children (Bedore & Peña, 2008). For example, Crutchley and associates (1997) conducted a comparative study of a group of bilingual and monolingual children with specific language impairment. The monolingual children spoke English, and the bilingual children used English as one of their two languages. They administered a series of speech and language assessments that were standardized on monolingual speakers. Within this study, the bilingual children performed more poorly on the standardized tests compared with their monolingual peers. These results were interpreted in two ways: either that bilingualism could act as a compounding factor or that there existed differences between bilingual and monolingual language-impaired children. The authors concluded that it may be inappropriate to use tests that were standardized on monolingual children with bilingual children. Consequently, specific speech and language assessments for multilingual children need to be constructed.

Although there are numerous monolingual speech assessments available in languages other than English, including Arabic, Cantonese, Dutch, German, Spanish, and Turkish (McLeod, 2011a), there are few multilingual speech assessments. The multilingual speech assessments that are available are for Pakistani-heritage languages (Mirpuri, Punjabi, Urdu)–English (Stow & Pert, 1998; 2006a), Spanish-English (Peña et al., n.d.), German-Russian/Turkish (Wagner, 2008), and Maltese-English (Grech et al., n.d.). McLeod (2011b) provides guidance for the creation of cross-linguistic speech assessments, outlining both stages in the conceptualization and operationalization of assessments. A meta-analysis of Spanish-English language assessments was conducted by Dollaghan and Horner (2010). They listed 15 different index measures that included "parent reports, spontaneous and elicited expressive language production, novel word and morpheme learning" (p. 20), yet they found that there was "no single, widely agreed reference standard for diagnosing presence or absence of LI [language impairment] in bilingual Spanish-English children" (p. 22).

Criterion-Referenced Assessments

Criterion-referenced assessments outline identified criterion that should be met (e.g., intelligible speech, grammatically correct language). They may or may not also be norm-referenced; that is, enable comparison of an individuals' responses on the assessment with a normative sample. Criterion-referenced assessments are often suggested to be more adequate for identifying multilingual children with SLI than norm-referenced tests (Battle, 2002). However if criterion-referenced tests are based on English criteria, then criterion-referenced assessments could be inappropriate for children speaking other languages and more so for bilingual children (Martin, 2009). Theoretically, criterion-referenced tests examining motor speech and articulatory skills could be expected to be applicable cross-linguistically and for children exposed to more than one language because they are not linguistically based. However, there are some research data to indicate that even diadochokinetic performance (DDK) performance varies across languages as well as for monolingual and bilingual children (Grech & Dodd, 2008; Prathanee et al., 2003).

Observations

Observations can provide additional assessment information if they are undertaken meticulously and objectively. Records of behavior in multilingual children can assist clinicians with differential diagnosis (Omark, 1981). For example, it is recommended that both conceptual vocabulary (i.e., the total number of concepts known across the two languages) and total vocabulary (i.e., the total number of labels used for those concepts) be determined when assessing bilingual children. Miller (1984) observed that typically developing bilingual children may know a word in one language but not in the other (singlets versus translation equivalents). In these circumstances, children may try different routes to get their message across, such as by saying the word in the other language, circumlocuting, or using gestures. Clinicians should observe such communication strategies in bilingual children and compare them with their bilingual peers. The extent of language mixing and why this is done in the home is useful information to collect as a mixed language could very well be the typical home language and may therefore not necessarily reflect lack of proficiency of any of the child's languages.

Communicative interaction of multilingual children with language impairment and their typically developing peers should also provide useful information for diagnosis. For example, Kayser (1990) reported on the social communicative behavior of Mexican-American children with and without language impairment. She reported that typically developing bilingual peers may indicate nonverbally or verbally that they do not understand language-impaired bilingual children and rarely initiate conversation with these bilingual language-impaired children. Such observations may assist clinicians in differentiating language difference from language disorder.

Dynamic Assessment

Dynamic assessment identifies learning potential and focuses primarily on the engagement between the adult (practitioner, educator, caregiver) and the child so that there is gradual assistance and elicitation of language and conceptual learning. Roseberry-McKibbin and O'Hanlon (2005, p. 183) indicated, "When using this kind of assessment, the SLP does not necessarily ask what the student already knows; in other words, language knowledge is not assessed. Rather, he or she asks how the student learns. This circumvents the problem seen for so many ELL [English Language Learner] students: lack of prior knowledge of items presented on standardized tests." Dynamic assessment therefore facilitates diagnosis of speech and language impairment as well as planning of intervention. Various approaches are suggested in the literature toward this type of assessment. These include the baseline approach (test-teach-test), task/stimulus variability, and graduated prompting, whereby intervention overlaps with assessment (Laing & Kamhi, 2003). When working with multilingual children, Gutiérrez-Clellen and Peña (2001) recommend that the test-teach-test is better for differential diagnosis between difference and disorder. However, testing the limits and graduated prompting are best used for determining readiness for intervention progress. For example, Jacobs and Coufal (2001) created a dynamic

assessment to determine multilingual children's ability to learn grammatical elements of a new language (Kiswahili), using a computerized assessment.

INTERVENTION

The Language of Intervention with Multilingual Children

Once multilingual children are identified with speech or language difficulties, SLPs need to determine which language to use in intervention. There are (at least) three options to consider:
1. Intervention in the child's first language (L1)
2. Intervention in the child's second language (L2)
3. Multilingual intervention

The appropriateness of each option should be weighed by integrating the three aspects of evidence-based practice: external research evidence, individual clinical expertise, and client (family) preference (Dollaghan, 2007; Sackett et al., 1996), including consideration of whether there is an effect of intervention in one language on the other language. To date there is limited evidence regarding the generalization of intervention in one language to the other and the impact of different intervention methods. Thordardottir (2010, p. 523) recommended that for language intervention, "the few studies available to date uniformly suggest that interventions that include a focus on both languages are superior to those that focus on only one language." Case studies have shown that articulation therapy in English (e.g., production of /s/) has generalized to Cantonese; although the same did not apply for phonological intervention (Holm & Dodd, 2001; Holm et al., 1997). In another case study, core vocabulary intervention in English resulted in increased consonant accuracy in both English and Punjabi (Holm & Dodd, 1999c, 2001). In yet another case study, minimal contrast therapy (phonological intervention) in English that targeted final consonant deletion, gliding of liquids, and cluster reduction resulted in decreased occurrence of phonological error patterns and increased consonant accuracy in Hindi, Gujarati, and English (Ray, 2002). Larger-scale intervention studies need to be undertaken to better understand the impact of intervention in one language for multilingual children.

Intervention in the Child's First Language

For young children in the initial stages of language intervention, it is recommended that language intervention occur in the child's home language. If children do not develop their home language, there is "potential negative long-term consequences on the child's social, emotional, and academic development as well as on the family dynamics" (Kohnert et al., 2005, p. 253) because they will not be able to communicate effectively within their family, community, and social networks. Indeed Kohnert and associates (2005, p. 254) strongly assert: "it is crucial that SLPs and early childhood educators go beyond simply encouraging continued use of the home language by families of young children with LI [language impairment] to actively promote its development. Facilitating, rather than just maintaining, skills in the home language should be a fundamental objective of intervention programs with preschool-age children with LI."

Three reasons for conducting speech intervention in the child's home language were suggested by Gildersleeve-Neumann and Goldstein (2011, p. 13): "(a) the intervention is meaningful to the child, thus resulting in little resistance to it; (b) the intervention is meaningful to the family and family members are more likely to value and support the intervention being conducted; and (c) once stronger phonological and articulatory skills are achieved in the home language, it will be easier to transfer this knowledge and skill to the academic and community language."

Intervention in Child's Second Language

Although there have been a number of surveys to consider SLPs' assessment of multilingual children (Kritikos, 2003; Skahan et al., 2007), there have been fewer to consider SLPs' intervention with multilingual children. One international study surveyed intervention practices of 99 SLPs in 13 different countries (Jordaan, 2008). The majority of SLPs (74%) were monolingual, and 87% reported that they only used one language during intervention. This led the author to conclude, "many therapists were providing therapy in their own language rather than the languages of their clients" (Jordaan, 2008, p. 101). Thus, intervention undertaken in the primary language spoken by the SLP frequently results in intervention being undertaken in the child's second language (L2). Various justifications were given by the SLPs for the language used during intervention, such lack of knowledge of the child's L1, scarcity of interpreters, lack of availability of assessments, parental insistence, and that intervention was undertaken in the language of the school, community, therapist, or child.

Multilingual Intervention

Many people suggest that intervention be conducted both in the home language and the child's second language (e.g., Gutiérrez-Clellen, 2001; Thordardottir, 2010). A number of authors have suggested that intervention in L1 followed by intervention in L2 (sequential intervention) could give children the opportunity to acquire language components in both languages (Miller & Abudarham, 1984; Perozzi & Sanchez, 1992). For example, Roseberry-McKibbin (2002) suggested that children with language impairment ideally should receive bilingual language therapy to optimize the

maintenance and enhancement of their L1 skills while also assisting them to learn L2. She stated, "Students will learn faster and more thoroughly and experience less language loss if they learn in these ideal bilingual situations" (Roseberry-McKibbin, 2002, p. 205). Roseberry-McKibbin also urged parents to speak to their child in the language in which they are most comfortable. Simard (2011) recommends four different approaches to language choice during intervention: (1) *one person, one language,* in which the parent and SLP each use a different language; (2) *turn-taking,* in which a different language is used during each round of a game; (3) *context directed,* in which the language appropriate to a specific task is selected; and (4) *code switching,* in which the child selects the language and the adults follow the child's lead.

Culture and Intervention

Cultural and linguistic diversity affects attitudes, such as the need for referral to professional services, including speech-language pathology, the drive for education and literacy skills development, and the need to interact with other socioculturally and linguistically different groups. Simmons and Johnston (2007) conducted a written survey concerning child-rearing practices and beliefs, especially those about patterns of speech addressed to their preschool children, to identify differences in the beliefs and practices in approximately 100 Indian- and European-heritage mothers living in Canada. Results indicated cross-cultural variation. Cultural group membership could be predicted with a 96% accuracy rate for cross-cultural attitudes related to the importance of family, perceptions of language learning, and children's use of language in family and social interactions. Indian heritage immigrant families tended to favor later independence and achievement, and direct instruction was the preferred mode of input to children. The regard for cultural influences in child language assessment and intervention cannot be overstated.

CLINICAL CULTURAL COMPETENCE

Communication and culture are intertwined so that cultural differences, beliefs, and attitudes affect assessment, diagnosis, and intervention by SLPs (Battle, 2002). Respectful consideration of the perspectives of children, families, and communities is enhanced by SLPs' acknowledgment (self-assessment) of their own cultural perspectives and biases (ASHA, 2010). Professionals such as SLPs must understand culturally appropriate behaviors from many different cultures because they may otherwise misinterpret behaviors that could lead to misdiagnosis. For example, lack of turn-taking or avoidance of eye contact could be culturally appropriate (e.g., Johnson & Wong, 2002) yet could reflect negatively in assessment of pragmatic skills unless the professional knows the specific culture's norms. Such behavior may also be misinterpreted as socially unacceptable or disrespectful by service providers, with the consequence of having a breakdown in communication. Tester bias may also play a role in misdiagnosis of difference versus disorder. There is evidence indicating variation in inter-rater reliability for test administration subject to the amount of training that test administrators receive in relation to testing children with cultural and linguistic diversity (Pray, 2005). Overscoring or underscoring such children can lead to misdiagnosis.

Undertaking assessment and intervention with multilingual children is a challenge. It would be ideal if SLPs were native speakers of more than one language. However, many SLPs have limited or no proficiency in the languages spoken by their clients and their caregivers. ASHA (2009) reports that fewer than 5.1% of its members identify themselves as bilingual. Stow and Dodd (2003) report that only 5% of the undergraduate students in the United Kingdom are bilingual, in an area where the population is dominated by bilingual ethnic individuals. Only a few SLPs in England receive specialist training in multilingual intervention (Winter, 2001). This seems to be a worldwide challenge, and limited theoretical and practical training related to multicultural and multilingual settings is being offered to SLP students (Cheng et al., 2001; Raval et al., 1999). There is a call for professional organizations and academic training programs to support SLPs' acquisition of additional languages (Caesar & Kohler, 2007; IALP, 2010; Jordaan, 2008). The development and evaluation of modules for SLPs and practitioners on issues related to sociocultural and psycholinguistic aspects of multilingualism are recommended in educational institutions.

Interpreters are often used to translate during SLP sessions, and their professional skills are important for facilitating understanding of both the culture and language of children and their families. As Isaac (2007) identified, the role of the interpreter is complex: "while interpreters may describe their role as facilitating communication between the SLP and child (and/or child's family), SLPs may actually be asking interpreters to facilitate communication, facilitate the SLP's understanding of the child's background and cultural influences on the session, and facilitate their diagnosis by providing description of and commentary on the child's speech and language characteristics." For example, Roger and Code (2011) indicate that SLPs' requests to describe errors in a client's speech is outside of an accredited interpreter's code of ethics because typically it is their role to interpret, not comment on, a speaker's dialogue. Stow and Dodd (2003) suggest additional difficulties, including that the interpreter may not necessarily use or comprehend the dialect of the child's first language and that the session may take longer because interpretation and translation are time consuming.

When interpreters are not available, peers, friends of the family, or even older siblings could be employed to administer informal assessments under the guidance of the SLP so that information to evaluate the proficiency in all languages is gathered (RCSLT, 2006). However, family members may not necessarily be the appropriate interpreters for all aspects of SLP assessment and intervention, particularly sensitivities of discussing confidential information, including the diagnosis of impairment.

FUTURE RESEARCH DIRECTIONS

During the past three decades, many studies about children's speech and language acquisition and disorder have been published. Many of these studies are about monolingual children's speech and language development and disorder, in a vast array of languages (see McLeod, 2007, 2010, for summaries of speech data from more than 20 languages). However, there is increasing interest in studies of multilingual children's speech and language development and disorder (e.g., McLeod & Goldstein, 2011). Appendix 7-1 provides a sample of studies of multilingual speech and language that are published in English. Additionally, Hua and Dodd (2006) take a multilingual perspective on phonological acquisition and disorder, examining typical and atypical acquisition data from monolingual and bilingual children speaking 12 different languages. These data are useful for clinicians because the studies describe both typical and atypical acquisition, providing evidence relevant for clinical assessment and intervention of multilingual children with speech or language disorders.

Research describing children's multilingual speech and language acquisition is limited in terms of the language pairs studied and the language learning contexts investigated (see Appendix 7-1). Many studies written in English have focused on children acquiring languages (e.g., Cantonese, Punjabi heritage language, Spanish) in a predominantly English-speaking environment (e.g., United Kingdom, United States). That is, these children live in a minority ethnolinguistic community (akin to quadrants B and D outlined at the beginning of this chapter) For example, a child who lives in a Spanish-speaking family that migrates to an English-speaking community becomes bilingual because the family location has changed from one linguistic environment to another.

Multilingual children are becoming the focus of research on speech and language acquisition, but there is so much to learn about different language pairs and their effect on acquisition. Research on multilingual children's acquisition of language has often focused on children acquiring two languages from the same language family. For example,

English, Spanish, and French are Indo-European languages for which the predominant language structures are similar (Hua & Dodd, 2006). Less is known, however, about bilingual language acquisition involving different languages families (e.g., Cantonese [Sino-Tibetan] and English [Indo-European] [Yip & Matthews, 2007]; Maltese [Semitic] and English [Indo-European]).

The development of norms and appropriate assessment tools for specific multilingual populations is crucial considering the increase in international migration and the scarcity of assessment tools for identification of communication disorders in this population (Bedore & Peña, 2008; McLeod, 2011a). Research on bilingual children can also shed light on subgroups of speech and language disorder (Hua & Dodd, 2006) and provide reliable information regarding best clinical practice for multilingual children.

Research about multilingual children's speech and language acquisition will also contribute to the understanding of theoretical issues. For example, the study of multilingual language acquisition can clarify the relative contribution of biologic and language-specific factors to the pace and order of development. The issue of universality versus language specificity is better addressed in the multilingual context. Future research can also continue to unravel the effect of code switching on language acquisition and impairment and whether children have one underlying language system or separate systems for each language (cf. Paradis, 2001).

Another important issue that needs to be addressed in research on multilingualism is harmonization of terminology and data reporting. Available data are difficult to compare because terms (even relating to the definition of multilingualism) are not necessarily described in the publications, and research methodologies vary. Cross-linguistic comparison calls for an integrated approach for data collection and reporting.

To plan appropriate SLP services for culturally and linguistically diverse populations, researchers also should access national census data and other large-scale health and education databases regarding language use in the home and the proficiency of spoken and written languages. In some countries, such as the United States and Australia, these data are commonly aggregated for people of all ages, and specific data about children's language use are frequently absent (cf. McLeod, 2011a). Martin (2009) reports that there is no updated national database in the United Kingdom related to language use and proficiency. Education, health, and social services are therefore basing their service planning and provision on alternative sources, such as local databases, and these may not necessarily address the diversity of language use.

Finally, it is important to remember that research regarding children's speech and language also is published in languages other than English. For example, the world's largest study of typical monolingual speech acquisition reported data was published in Hungarian and was based on 7602 children (Nagy, 1980; Zajdó, 2007, provides a summary in English). One of the next largest studies was conducted in Japanese reporting data from 1600 children (Sumio, 1978; Ota & Ueda, 2007, provide a summary in English). In contrast, the largest study of speech acquisition in the United States assessed 997 children (Smit et al., 1990). SLPs (especially those who are multilingual) should access journals published in languages other than English to expand their knowledge beyond what is published in English.

In conclusion, the urgent need for developing an international knowledge base concerning multilingualism and speech and language disorders cannot be overstated. Language is a tool that helps us with learning and to understand what goes on around us and therefore is not merely used for communication purposes (Martin, 2009). Research on multilingualism should therefore receive its due attention. As multilingualism becomes more prevalent worldwide, SLPs need to address specific needs of children who speak the world's languages rather than just a few languages. Multilingualism brings with it better solidarity among diverse populations and promotes tolerance of a multicultural society. Multilingualism strengthens social cohesion as citizens participate more in social interaction. It also mitigates the spread of xenophobia and parochialism (Lassagabaster & Huguet, 2007). SLPs have an important role to play within society as they work with children from multilingual backgrounds.

DISCUSSION QUESTIONS

1. Use the four quadrants presented by Genesee and colleagues (2004) to classify the linguistic and cultural heritage of yourself, your family, your friends, and your clients. How do you think speech and language acquisition and proficiency may be different in each of the quadrants?

2. Consider to what extent child language acquisition is influenced by global migration.

3. Prepare a list of questions to ask a multilingual child's parents during the preassessment phase.

4. What advice would you give to a multilingual child's parents about the languages the child and the family should speak? What factors may change your recommendation?

5. Consider how the desire of the parent can influence the language of intervention. What are the best decisions the SLP should make when preparing a child for school when the family does not use the language of the school at home?

6. What resources are available to assist the SLP when she or he does not speak the language of the family?

REFERENCES

American Speech-Language-Hearing Association (2004). *Knowledge and skills needed by speech-language pathologists and audiologists to provide culturally and linguistically appropriate services.* Retrieved January 31, 2011, from www.asha.org/docs/pdf/KS2004-00215.pdf.

American Speech-Language-Hearing Association (2010). Cultural competence in professional service delivery. Retrieved November 1, 2010, from www.asha.org.

Ball, M. J., Müller, N., & Munro, S. (2001). The acquisition of rhotic consonants by Welsh-English bilingual children. *International Journal of Bilingualism, 5,* 71-86.

Ball, M., Müller, N. & Munro, S. (2006). Phonological development and disorder of bilingual children acquiring Welsh and English. In Zhu Hua & B. Dodd (Eds.), *Phonological development and disorders: A multilingual perspective.* Clevedon, UK: Multilingual Matters.

Ballard, E., & Farao, S. (2008). The phonological skills of Samoan speaking 4-year-olds. *International Journal of Speech-Language Pathology, 10,* 379-391.

Bates, E., & MacWhinney, B. (1982). Functionalist approaches to grammar. In E. Wanner & L. R. Gleitmann (Eds.), *Language acquisition: The state of the art.* New York: Cambridge University Press.

Bates, E., & MacWhinney, B. (1987). Competition, variation, and language learning. In *Mechanisms of language acquisition.* Hillsdale, NJ: Erlbaum.

Battle, D. E. (2002). *Communication disorders in multicultural populations* (3rd ed.). Boston: Butterworth-Heinemann.

Bedore, L. M., & Peña, E. D. (2008). Assessment of bilingual children for identification of language impairment: Current findings and implications for practice. *International Journal of Bilingual Education and Bilingualism, 11,* 1-29.

Bedore, L. M., Peña, E. D., Gillam, R. B., & Ho, T.-H. (2010). Language sample measures and language ability in Spanish-English bilingual kindergarteners. *Journal of Communication Disorders, 43(6),* 498-510.

Berman, R. A. (1977). Natural phonological processes at the one-word stage. *Lingua, 43,* 1-21.

Bialystok, E., Luk, G., & Kwan, E. (2005). Bilingualism, biliteracy, and learning to read: Interactions among languages and writing systems. *Scientific Studies of Reading, 9,* 43-61.

Brice, A. E., Carson, C. K., & Dennis O'Brien, J. (2009). Spanish-English articulation and phonology of 4- and 5-year-old preschool children: An initial investigation. *Communication Disorders Quarterly, 31,* 3-14.

Bruner J. S. (1986). *Actual minds, possible worlds.* Cambridge, MA: Harvard University Press.

Bunta, F., & Ingram, D. (2007). The acquisition of speech rhythm by bilingual Spanish- and English-speaking 4- and 5-year-old children. *Journal of Speech, Language, and Hearing Research, 50,* 999-1014.

Bunta, F., Davidovich, I., & Ingram, D. (2006). The relationship between the phonological complexity of a bilingual child's words and those of the target languages. *International Journal of Bilingualism and Bilingual Education, 10,* 71-86.

Bunta, F., Fabiano, L., Ingram, D., & Goldstein, B. (2009). Phonological whole-word measures in three-year-old bilingual children and their monolingual peers. *Clinical Linguistics and Phonetics, 23,* 156-175.

Caesar, L. G., & Kohler, P. D. (2007). The state of school-based bilingual assessment: Actual practice versus recommended guidelines. *Language, Speech, and Hearing Services in Schools, 38,* 190-200.

Cataño, L., Barlow, J. A., & Moyna, M. I. (2009). A retrospective study of phonetic inventory complexity in acquisition of Spanish: Implications for phonological universals. *Clinical Linguistics and Phonetics, 23,* 446-472.

CEC (1995). *Teaching and learning: Towards the learning society.* Luxemburg: European Commission.

Cheng, L., & Butler, K. (1993). *Difficult discourse: Designing connections to deflect language impairment.* Paper presented at the annual meeting of the California Speech-Language Hearing Association, Palm Springs, California.

Cheng, L. (2004). The challenge of hyphenated identity. *Topics in Language Disorders, 24,* 216-224.

Cheng, L. L. (2006). Lessons from the *Da Vinci Code*: Working with bilingual/multicultural children and families. *The ASHA Leader, 26,* 14-15.

Cheng, L., Battle, D., Murdoch, B., & Martin, D. (2001). Educating speech-language pathologists for a multi-cultural world. *Folia Phoniatrica et Logopaedica, 53,* 121-127.

Cheng, L. R., & Butler, K. (1989). Code switching: A natural phenomenon versus language deficiency. *World Englishes, 8,* 293-309.

Child Welfare Information Gateway (2008). *Total adoptions to the United States.* Retrieved February 7, 2011, from: http://adoption.state.gov/news/total_chart.html.

Child Welfare Information Gateway (2010). *2010 Annual report on intercountry adoptions.* Retrieved February 7, 2011, from http://adoption.state.gov/content/pdf/fy2010_annual_report.pdf.

Cleave, P. L., Girolametto, L. E., Chen, X., & Johnson, C. J. (2010). Narrative abilities in monolingual and dual language learning children with specific language impairment. *Journal of Communication Disorders, 43,* 511-522.

Collins, M. F. (2005). ESL preschoolers' English vocabulary acquisition from storybook reading. *Reading Research Quarterly, 40,* 406-408.

Crutchley, A., Conti-Ramsden, G., & Botting, N. (1997). Bilingual children with specific language impairment and standardised assessments: Preliminary findings from a study of children in language units. *International Journal of Bilingualism, 1,* 117-134.

Cruz-Ferreira, M. (1999). Prosodic mixes: Strategies in multilingual language acquisition. *International Journal of Bilingualism, 3,* 1-21.

Cruz-Ferreira, M. (2010). *Multilinguals are . . . ?* London: Battlebridge Publications.

Crystal, D. (1997). *The Cambridge encyclopedia of language* (2nd ed.). Cambridge, UK: Cambridge University Press.

Cummins, J. (2003). Bilingual education: Basic principles. In J. M. Daelewe, A. Housen, & L. Wei (Eds.), *Bilingualism: Beyond basic principles.* Clevedon, UK: Multilingual Matters.

De Houwer, A. (2009). *Bilingual first language acquisition.* Clevedon, UK: Multilingual Matters.

De Houwer, A., Bornstein, M. H., & De Coster, S. (2006). Early understanding of two words for the same thing: A CDI study of lexical comprehension in infant bilinguals. *International Journal of Bilingualism, 10,* 331-347.

Deuchar, M., & Quay, S. (2000). *Bilingual acquisition: Theoretical implications of a case study.* Oxford: Oxford University Press.

Dodd, B., Holm, A., & Li, W. (1997). Speech disorder in preschool children exposed to Cantonese and English. *Clinical Linguistics and Phonetics, 11,* 229-243.

Dodd, B., So, L., & Li, W. (1996). Symptoms of disorder without impairment: The written and spoken errors of bilinguals. In B. Dodd, R. Campbell & L. Worrall (Eds.), *Evaluating theories of language.* London: Whurr.

Dollaghan, C. A. (2007). *The handbook for evidence-based practice in communication disorders.* Baltimore: Paul H. Brookes.

Dollaghan, C. A., & Horner, E. A. (2010, in press). Bilingual language assessment: A meta-analysis of diagnostic accuracy. *Journal of*

Speech, Language, and Hearing Research, DOI 10.1044/1092-4388 (2010/10-0093).

Fabiano, L., & Goldstein, B. (2005). Phonological cross-linguistic influence in sequential Spanish-English bilingual children. *Journal of Multilingual Communication Disorders, 3,* 56-63.

Fabiano-Smith, L., & Barlow, J. A. (2010). Interaction in bilingual phonological acquisition: Evidence from phonetic inventories. *International Journal of Bilingual Education and Bilingualism, 13,* 81-97.

Fabiano-Smith, L., & Goldstein, B. (2010). Phonological acquisition in bilingual Spanish-English speaking children. *Journal of Speech, Language, and Hearing Research, 53,* 160-178.

Fabiano-Smith, L., & Goldstein, B. A. (2010). Early-, middle-, and late-developing sounds in monolingual and bilingual children: An exploratory investigation. *American Journal of Speech-Language Pathology, 19,* 66-77.

Faingold, E. D. (1996). Variation in the application of natural processes: Language-dependent constraints in the phonological acquisition of bilingual children. *Journal of Psycholinguistic Research, 25,* 515-526.

Gadesmann, M., & Miller, N. (2008). Reliability of speech diadochokinetic test measurement. *International Journal of Language and Communication Disorders, 43,* 41-54.

Gatt, D. (2010). *Early expressive lexical development: Evidence from children brought up in Maltese-speaking families.* Unpublished doctoral dissertation. University of Malta, Malta.

Gauthier, K., & Genesee, F. (2011, in press). Language development in internationally-adopted children: A special case of early second language learning. *Child Development.*

Genesee, F., Paradis, J., & Crago, M. B. (2004). *Dual language development and disorders: A handbook on bilingualism and second language learning.* Baltimore: Paul H. Brookes.

Gierut, J. (2004, 11-13 June). *Enhancement of learning for children with phonological disorders* (pp. B164-B172). Sound to Sense Conference. Massachusetts Institute of Technology, Boston, MA.

Gildersleeve, C., Davis, B., & Stubbe, E. (1996, November). When monolingual rules don't apply: Speech development in a bilingual environment. Paper presented at the annual convention of the American Speech-Language-Hearing Association, Seattle, WA.

Gildersleeve-Neumann, C., & Goldstein, B. A. (2011). Intervention for multilingual children with speech sound disorders. In S. McLeod & B. A. Goldstein (Eds.), *Multilingual aspects of speech sound disorders in children.* Bristol, UK: Multilingual Matters.

Gildersleeve-Neumann, C., Kester, E., Davis, B., & Peña, E. (2008). English speech sound development in preschool-aged children from bilingual English-Spanish backgrounds. *Language, Speech, and Hearing Services in Schools, 39,* 314-328.

Gildersleeve-Neumann, C. E., & Wright, K. E. (2010). English phonological acquisition in 3- to 5-year-old children learning Russian and English. *Language, Speech, and Hearing Services in Schools, 41,* 429-444.

Goldstein, B. A. (2000). *Cultural and linguistic diversity resource guide for speech-language pathologists.* San Diego, CA: Singular Thomson Learning.

Goldstein, B., & Bunta, F. (2010, in press). Positive and negative transfer in the phonological systems of bilingual speakers. *International Journal of Bilingualism.*

Goldstein, B., Bunta, F., Lange, J., Burrows, L., Pont, S., & Bennett, J. (2008, November). *Interdependence in the phonological systems of bilingual children with speech sound disorders.* Seminar presented at the convention of the American Speech-Language-Hearing Association, Chicago, IL.

Goldstein, B., Bunta, F., Lange, J., Rodriguez, J., & Burrows, L. (2010). The effects of measures of language experience and language ability on segmental accuracy in bilingual children. *American Journal of Speech-Language Pathology, 19,* 238-247.

Goldstein, B., Fabiano, L., & Washington, P. (2005). Phonological skills in predominantly English, predominantly Spanish, and Spanish-English bilingual children. *Language, Speech, and Hearing Services in Schools, 36,* 201-218.

Goldstein, B. A., & McLeod, S. (2011, in press). Typical and atypical speech acquisition. In S. McLeod & B. A. Goldstein (Eds.). *Multilingual aspects of speech sound disorders in children.* Bristol, UK: Multilingual Matters.

Goldstein, B., & Washington, P. (2001). An initial investigation of phonological patterns in 4-year-old typically developing Spanish-English bilingual children. *Language, Speech, and Hearing Services in Schools, 32,* 153-164.

Gorman, B., Fiestas, C. E., Peña, E. D., & Clark, M. R. (2011). Creative and stylistic devices employed by children during a storybook narrative task: A cross-cultural study. *Language, Speech, and Hearing Services in Schools, 42,* 167-181.

Grech, H. (1998). *Phonological development of normal Maltese speaking children.* Unpublished doctoral dissertation, University of Manchester, UK.

Grech, H., & Cheng, L. (2010). Communication in the migrant community in Malta. *Folia Phoniatrica et Logopaedica, 62,* 246-254.

Grech, H., & Dodd, B. (2007). Assessment of speech and language skills in bilingual children: An holistic approach. *Stem-, Spraak- en Taalpathologie, 15,* 84-92.

Grech, H., & Dodd, B. (2008). Phonological acquisition in Malta: A bilingual learning context. *International Journal of Bilingualism, 12,* 155-171.

Grech, H., Franklin, S., & Dodd, B. (n.d.). *Maltese-English Speech Assessment (MESA).* Unpublished assessment tool.

Gupta, A., & Chandler, H. (1993). Paediatric speech and language therapy referral in Singapore: Implications for multilingual language disabilities. *European Journal of Disorders of Communication, 28,* 309-318.

Gutiérrez-Clellen, V. (2001). Language choice in intervention with bilingual children. *American Journal of Speech-Language Pathology, 8,* 291-302.

Gutiérrez-Clellen, V. F., & Peña, E. (2001). Dynamic assessment of diverse children: A tutorial. *Language, Speech, and Hearing Services in Schools, 32,* 212-224.

Gutiérrez -Clellen, V. F., Simon-Cereijido, G., & Erickson Leone, A. (2009). Code-switching in bilingual children with specific language impairment. *International Journal of Bilingualism, 13,* 91-109.

Ha, S., Johnson, C. J., & Kuehn, D. P. (2009). Characteristics of Korean phonology: Review, tutorial, and case studies of Korean children speaking English. *Journal of Communication Disorders, 42,* 163-179.

Hammer, C. S., Lawrence, F. R., & Miccio, A. W. (2008). The effect of summer vacation on bilingual preschoolers' language development. *Clinical Linguistics and Phonetics, 22,* 686-702.

Hemsley, G., Holm, A., & Dodd, B. (2006). Diverse but not different: The lexical skills of two primary age bilingual groups in comparison to monolingual peers. *International Journal of Bilingualism, 10,* 453-476.

Hemsley, G., Holm, A., & Dodd, B. (2010). Patterns in diversity: Lexical learning in Samoan-English bilingual children. *International Journal of Speech-Language Pathology, 12,* 362-374.

Holm, A., & Dodd, B. (1999a). A longitudinal study of the phonological development of two Cantonese-English bilingual children. *Applied Psycholinguistics, 20,* 349-376.

Holm, A., & Dodd, B. (1999b). Differential diagnosis of phonological disorder in two bilingual children acquiring Italian and English. *Clinical Linguistics and Phonetics, 13,* 113-129.

Holm, A., & Dodd, B. (1999c). An intervention case study of a bilingual child with phonological disorder. *Child Language Teaching and Therapy, 15*(2), 139-158.

Holm, A., & Dodd, B. (2001). Comparison of cross-language generalisation following speech therapy. *Folia Phoniatrica et Logopaedica, 53,* 166-172.

Holm, A., & Dodd, B. (2006). Phonological development and disorder of bilingual children acquiring Cantonese and English. In Z. Hua & B. Dodd (Eds.), *Phonological development and disorders in children: A multilingual perspective* (pp. 286-325). Clevedon, UK: Multilingual Matters.

Holm, A., Dodd, B., Stow, C., & Pert S. (1999). Identification and differential diagnosis of phonological disorder in bilingual children. *Language Testing, 16,* 271-292.

Holm, A., Dodd, B., Stow, C., & Pert, S. (1998). Speech disorder in bilingual children: Four case studies. *Osmania Papers in Linguistics, 22-23,* 46-64.

Holm, A., Ozanne, A., & Dodd, B. (1997). Efficacy of intervention for a bilingual child making articulation and phonological errors. *International Journal of Bilingualism, 1,* 55-69.

Hua, Z., & Dodd, B. (Eds.). (2006). *Phonological development and disorders: A multilingual perspective.* Clevedon, UK: Multilingual Matters.

Huguet, A., & Lasagabater, D. (2007). European bilingual contexts: Some final considerations. In D. Lassagabaster, & A. Huguet, (Eds.), *Multilingualism in European bilingual contexts: Language use and attitudes.* Clevedon, UK: Multilingual Matters.

IALP (2006). Recommendations for working with bilingual children: Prepared by the multilingual affairs committee of IALP. *Folia Phoniatrica Logopaedica, 58,* 456-464.

IALP (2010). The revised education guidelines of the IALP. *Folia Phoniatrica et Logopaedica, Special Issue, 62,* 210-216.

Ingram, D. (2011, in press). Prologue: Cross-linguistic and multilingual aspects of speech sound disorders in children. In S. McLeod & B. A. Goldstein (Eds.), *Multilingual aspects of speech sound disorders in children.* Bristol, UK: Multilingual Matters.

Isaac, K. M. (2007). Working with interpreters In S. McLeod (Ed.), *The international guide to speech acquisition* (pp. 122-126). Clifton Park, NY: Thomson Delmar Learning.

Jacobs, E. L., & Coufal, K. L. (2001). A computerized screening instrument of language learnability. *Communication Disorders Quarterly, 22,* 67-76.

Jakobson, R. (1968). *Child language aphasia and phonological universals.* The Hague: Mouton.

Johnson, C., & Lancaster, P. (1998). The development of more than one phonology: A case-study of a Norwegian-English bilingual child. *International Journal of Bilingualism, 2,* 265-300.

Johnston, J. R., & Wong, M. Y. A. (2002). Cultural differences in beliefs and practices concerning talk to children. *Journal of Speech, Language, and Hearing Research, 45,* 916-926.

Jordaan, H. (2008). Clinical intervention for bilingual children: An international survey. *Folia Phoniatrica et Logopaedica, 60,* 97-105.

Jordaan, H., Shaw-Ridley, G., Serfontein, J., et al. (2001). Cognitive and linguistic profiles of specific language impairment and semantic-pragmatic disorder in bilinguals. *Folia Phoniatrica et Logopaedica, 53,* 153-165.

Kan, P. F. (2010). Measuring word learning ability in sequential bilingual children. *Perspectives on Communication Disorders and Sciences in Culturally and Linguistically Diverse Populations, 17,* 25-32.

Kan, P. F., & Kohnert, K. (2005). Preschoolers learning Hmong and English: Lexical-semantic skills in L1 and L2. *Journal of Speech, Language, and Hearing Research, 48,* 372-383.

Karrebæk, M. S. (2003). Iconicity and structure in codeswitching. *International Journal of Bilingualism, 7,* 407-442.

Kayser, H. (1995). *Bilingual speech-language pathology: An Hispanic focus.* San Diego, CA: Singular Publishing.

Kayser, H. G. (1990). Social communicative behaviors of language-disordered Mexican-American students. *Child Language Teaching and Therapy, 6,* 255-269.

Kehoe, M., Trujillo, C., & Lleó, C. (2001). Bilingual phonological acquisition: An analysis of syllable structure and VOT. In K. F. Cantone & M. O. Hinzelin (Eds.), *Proceedings of the colloquium on structure, acquisition and change of grammars: Phonological and syntactic aspects* (pp. 38-54). Universität Hamburg: Arbeiten zur Mehrsprachigkeit.

Keshavarz, M., & Ingram, D. (2002). The early phonological development of a Farsi English bilingual child. *International Journal of Bilingualism, 6,* 255-269.

Kohnert, K., Kan, P. F., & Conboy, B. T. (2010). Lexical and grammatical associations in sequential bilingual preschoolers. *Journal of Speech, Language, and Hearing Research, 53,* 684-698.

Kohnert, K., Yim, D., Nett, K., et al. (2005). Intervention with linguistically diverse preschool children: A focus on developing home language(s). *Language, Speech, and Hearing Services in Schools, 36,* 251-263.

Kritikos, E. P. (2003). Speech-language pathologists' beliefs about language assessment of bilingual/bicultural individuals. *American Journal of Speech-Language Pathology, 12,* 73-91.

Laing, S. P., & Kamhi, A. (2003). Alternative assessment of language and literacy in culturally and linguistically diverse populations. *Language, Speech, and Hearing Services in Schools, 34,* 44-55.

Lanza, E. (2004). *Language mixing in infant bilingualism: A sociolinguistic perspective.* Oxford: Oxford University Press.

Lassagabaster, D., & Huguet, A. (Eds.) (2007). *Multilingualism in European bilingual contexts: Language use and attitudes.* Clevedon, UK: Multilingual Matters.

Law, N. C. W., & So, L. K. H. (2006). The relationship of phonological development and language dominance in bilingual Cantonese-Putonghua children. *International Journal of Bilingualism, 10,* 405-427.

Lin, L.-C., & Johnson, C. J. (2010). Phonological patterns in Mandarin-English bilingual children. *Clinical Linguistics and Phonetics, 24,* 369-386.

Lleó, C., Kuchenbrandt, I., Kehoe, M., & Trujillo, C. (2003). Syllable final consonants in Spanish and German monolingual and bilingual acquisition. In N. Müller (Ed.), *(In)vulnerable domains in multilingualism* (pp. 191-220). Amsterdam: John Benjamins.

Marchman, V. A., Martínez-Sussmann, C., & Dale, P. S. (2004). The language-specific nature of grammatical development: Evidence from bilingual language learners. *Developmental Science, 7,* 212-224.

Martin, D. (2009). *Language disability in cultural and linguistic diversity.* Clevedon, UK: Multilingual Matters.

Martin, D., Krishnamurthy, R., Bhardwaj, M., & Charles, R. (2003). Language change in young Panjabi/English children: Implications for bilingual language assessment. *Child Language Teaching and Therapy, 1,* 245-265.

Másdóttir, T. (2011, in press). Translation to practice: Typical and atypical multilingual speech acquisition in Iceland. In S. McLeod & B. A. Goldstein (Eds.), *Multilingual aspects of speech sound disorders in children.* Bristol, UK: Multilingual Matters.

McLeod, S. (Ed.). (2007). *The international guide to speech acquisition*. Clifton Park, NY: Thomson Delmar Learning.

McLeod, S. (2010). Laying the foundations for multilingual acquisition: An international overview of speech acquisition. In M. Cruz-Ferreira (Ed.), *Multilingual norms* (pp. 53-71). Frankfurt: Peter Lang Publishing.

McLeod, S. (2011a, in press). Multilingual speech assessment. In S. McLeod & B. A. Goldstein (Eds.), *Multilingual aspects of speech sound disorders in children*. Bristol, UK: Multilingual Matters.

McLeod, S. (2011b, in press). Translation to practice: Creating sampling tools to assess multilingual children's speech. In S. McLeod & B. A. Goldstein (Eds.), *Multilingual aspects of speech sound disorders in children*. Bristol, UK: Multilingual Matters.

Meyerstein, R. (1970). *Functional load: Descriptive limitations, alternatives of assessment and extensions of application*. The Hague: Mouton.

Miller, N., & Abudarham, S. (1984). Management of communication problems in bilingual children. In N. Miller (Ed.), *Bilingualism and language disability* (pp. 177-198). San Diego, CA: College-Hill Press.

Miller, N. (1984). *Bilingualism and language disability: Assessment and remediation*. San Diego, CA: College Hill.

Munro, S., Ball, M. J., Müller, N., Duckworth, M., & Lyddy, F. (2005). The acquisition of Welsh and English phonology in bilingual Welsh-English children. *Journal of Multilingual Communication Disorders, 3*, 24-49.

Murphy, J., & Dodd, B. (2010). A diagnostic challenge: Language difficulties and hearing impairment in a secondary-school student from a non-English speaking background. *Child Language Teaching and Therapy, 26*, 207-220.

Nagy, J. (1980). *5-6 éves gyermekeink iskolakészültsége* [Preparedness for school of five to six year old children] [in Hungarian]. Budapest: Akadémiai Kiadó.

Navarro, A., Pearson, B., Cobo-Lewis, A., & Oller, D. (1995, November). *Early phonological development in young bilinguals: Comparison to monolinguals*. Paper presented to the American Speech, Language and Hearing Association Conference.

Ng, M., Hsueh, G., & Leung, C. S. (2010). Voice pitch characteristics of Cantonese and English produced by Cantonese-English bilingual children. *International Journal of Speech-Language Pathology, 12*, 230-236.

Nicholls, R. J., Eadie, P. A., & Reilly, S. (2011, in press). Monolingual versus multilingual acquisition of English morphology: What can we expect at age 3? *International Journal of Language and Communication Disorders*.

Omark, D. R. (1981). Pragmatics and ethnological techniques for the observational assessment of children's communicative abilities. In J. G. Erikson, & D. R. Omark (Eds.), *Communication assessing bilingual exceptional children: In-service manual*. San Diego, CA: Los Amigos Research.

Ota, M., & Ueda, I. (2007). Japanese speech acquisition In S. McLeod (Ed.), *The international guide to speech acquisition* (pp. 457-471). Clifton Park, NY: Thomson Delmar Learning.

Paradis, J. (2001). Do bilingual two-year-olds have separate phonological systems? *International Journal of Bilingualism, 5*, 19-38.

Paradis, J. (2005). Grammatical morphology in children learning English as a second language. *Language, Speech, and Hearing Services in Schools, 36*, 172-187.

Paradis, J., Crago, M., Genesee, F., & Rice, M. (2003). Bilingual children with specific language impairment. How do they compare with their monolingual peers? *Journal of Speech, Language, and Hearing Research, 46*, 1-15.

Paradis, J., Emmerzael, K., & Duncan, T. S. (2010). Assessment of English Language Learners: Using parent report on first language development. *Journal of Communication Disorders, 43*, 474-497.

Paradis, J., Nicoladis, E., & Genesee, F. (2000). Early emergence of structural constraints on code-mixing: Evidence from French-English bilingual children. *Bilingualism: Language and Cognition, 3*, 245-261.

Patterson, J. L. (1998). Expressive vocabulary development and word combinations of Spanish-English bilingual toddlers. *American Journal of Speech-Language Pathology, 7*, 46-56.

Peña, E. D., Bedore, L. M., & Zlatic-Giunta, R. (2002). Category-generation performance of bilingual children: The influence of condition, category, and language. *Journal of Speech, Language, and Hearing Research, 45*, 938-947.

Peña, E. D., Gutiérrez-Clellen, V. F., Iglesias, A., et al. (n.d.). *Bilingual English Spanish Assessment* (BESA). Unpublished assessment tool.

Perozzi, J. A., & Sanchez, M. L. C. (1992). The effect of instruction in L1 on receptive acquisition of L2 for bilingual children with language delay. *Language, Speech, and Hearing Services in Schools, 23*, 348-352.

Pollock, K. E. (2007). Speech acquisition in second first language learners (Children who were adopted internationally). In S. McLeod (Ed.), *The international guide to speech acquisition* (pp. 107-113). Clifton Park, NY: Thomson Delmar Learning.

Prathanee, B., Thanaviratananich, S., & Pongjanyakul, A. (2003). Oral diadochokinetic rates for normal Thai children. *International Journal of Language and Communication Disorders, 38*, 417-428.

Pray, L. (2005). How well do commonly used language instruments measure English oral-language proficiency? *Bilingual Research Journal, 29*, 387-408.

Preston, J. L., & Seki, A. (2011). Identifying residual speech sound disorders in bilingual children: A Japanese-English case study. *American Journal of Speech-Language Pathology, 20*(2), 73-85.

Quinn, C. (2001). The developmental acquisition of English grammar as an additional language. *International Journal of Language and Communication Disorders, 36*(Suppl.), 309-314.

Raval, A., Hooke, E., Martin, Q. T., & Anderson, S. (1999). *Teaching about bilingualism and linguistic minority in speech and language therapy courses*. London: Royal College of Speech and Language Therapists' National Special Interest Group in Bilingualism.

Ray, J. (2002). Treating phonological disorders in a multilingual child: A case study. *American Journal of Speech-Language Pathology, 11*, 305-315.

Roger, P., & Code, C. (2011). Lost in translation? Issues of content validity in interpreter-mediated aphasia assessments. *International Journal of Speech-Language Pathology, 13*, 61-73.

Roseberry-McKibbin, C. (2002). Principles and strategies in intervention. In A. E. Brice (Ed.), *The Hispanic child: Speech, language, culture and education*. Boston, MA: Allyn & Bacon.

Roseberry-McKibbin, C., & O'Hanlon, L. (2005). Nonbiased assessment of English Language Learners: A tutorial. *Communication Disorders Quarterly, 26*, 178-185.

Royal College of Speech and Language Therapists (RCSLT). (2006). *Communicating quality* (3rd ed.). London: Author.

Sackett, D. L., Rosenberg, W. M. C., Muir Gray, J. A., et al. (1996). Evidence-based medicine: What it is and what it isn't. *British Medical Journal, 312*, 71-72.

Salameh, E., Håkansson, G., & Nettelbladt, U. (2004). Developmental perspectives on bilingual Swedish-Arabic children with and without language impairment: A longitudinal study. *International Journal of Language and Communication Disorders, 39*, 65-91.

Salameh, E.-K., Nettlebladt, U., & Norlin, K. (2003). Assessing phonologies in bilingual Swedish-Arabic children with and without language impairment. *Child Language Teaching and Therapy, 19,* 338-364.

Scott, K. A., Roberts, J. A., & Glennen, S. (2011, in press). How well do children who are internationally adopted acquire language? A meta-analysis. *Journal of Speech, Language and Hearing Research,* DOI 1092-4388_2010_1010-0075.

Shin, H. B., & Kominski, R. A. (2010). *Language use in the United States: 2007.* Washington, DC: U.S. Census Bureau.

Simard, I. (2011, in press). Translation to practice: Intervention for multilingual children with speech sound disorders in Montréal, Québec, Canada. In S. McLeod & B. A. Goldstein (Eds.), *Multilingual aspects of speech sound disorders in children.* Bristol, UK: Multilingual Matters.

Simmons, N., & Johnston, J. (2007). Cross-cultural differences in beliefs and practices that affect the language spoken to children: Mothers with Indian and Western heritage. *International Journal of Language and Communication Disorders, 42,* 445-465.

Skahan, S. M., Watson, M., & Lof, G. L. (2007). Speech-language pathologists' assessment practices for children with suspected speech sound disorders: Results of a national survey. *American Journal of Speech-Language Pathology, 16,* 246-259.

Smit, A. B., Hand, L., Freilinger, J. J., Bernthal, J. E., & Bird, A. (1990). The Iowa articulation norms project and its Nebraska replication. *Journal of Speech and Hearing Disorders, 55,* 779-798.

Snow, C. (1981). Social interaction and language acquisition. In P. Dale & D. Ingram (Eds.), *Child language: An international perspective.* Baltimore: University Park Press.

Sollors, W. (2009). Multilingualism in the United States: A less well-known source of vitality in American culture as an issue of social justice and of historical memory. *Nanzan Review of American Studies, 31,* 59-75.

Steenge, J. (2006). *Bilingual children with specific language impairment: Additionally disadvantaged?* The Netherlands: Radboud University Nijmegen.

Stokes, S., & Surendran, D. (2005). Articulatory complexity, ambient frequency and functional load as predictors of consonant development in children. *Journal of Speech, Language, and Hearing Research, 48,* 577-591.

Stow, C., & Dodd, B. (2003). Providing an equitable service to bilingual children in the UK. *International Journal of Language and Communication Disorders, 38,* 351-378.

Stow, C., & Dodd, B. (2005). A survey of bilingual children referred for investigation of communication disorders: A comparison with monolingual children referred in one area in England. *Journal of Multilingual Communication Disorders, 3,* 1-23.

Stow, C., & Pert, S. (1998). *Rochdale Assessment of Mirpuri Phonology with Punjabi, Urdu and English: A speech and language therapy resource for the phonological assessment of bilingual children.* Rochdale: Pert.

Stow, C., & Pert, S. (2006a). *BiSSS—Bilingual Speech Sound Screen: Pakistani heritage languages.* Milton Keynes, UK: Speechmark.

Stow, C., & Pert, S. (2006b). Phonological acquisition in bilingual Pakistani heritage children in England. In Zhu Hua & B. Dodd (Eds.), *Phonological development and disorders in children: A multilingual perspective.* Clevedon, UK: Multilingual Matters.

Sumio, K. (1978). *Yōjikyōiku sensho Ryōikihen: Gengo.* [in Japanese]. Tokyo: Kawashima Shoten.

Sundara, M., Polka, L., & Genesee, F. (2006). Language-experience facilitates discrimination of /d-_/ in monolingual and bilingual acquisition of English. *Cognition, 100,* 369-388.

Sundara, M., Polka, L., & Molnar, M. (2008). Development of coronal stop perception: Bilingual infants keep pace with their monolingual peers. *Cognition, 108,* 232-242.

Thordardottir, E. (2010). Towards evidence-based practice in language intervention for bilingual children. *Journal of Communication Disorders, 43,* 523-537.

Valdés, G., & Figueroa, R. A. (1994). *Bilingualism and testing: A special case of bias.* Norwood, NJ: Ablex.

Vihman, M. M. (1985). Language differentiation by the bilingual infant. *Journal of Child Language, 12,* 297-324.

Vogel, I. (1975). One system or two: An analysis of a two-year-old Romanian-English bilingual's phonology. *Papers and Reports on Child Language Development, 9,* 43-62.

Wagner, L. (2008). Screemik Version 2. *Screening der Erstsprachefähigkeit bei Migrantenkindern: Russisch-Deutsch. Türkisch-Deutsch* [in German]. Eugen: Wagner Verlag.

Winter, K. (2001). Numbers of bilingual children in speech and language therapy: Theory and practice of measuring their representation. *International Journal of Bilingualism, 5,* 465-495.

Yang, H. Y., & Hua, Z. (2010). The phonological development of a trilingual child: Facts and factors. *International Journal of Bilingualism, 14,* 105-126.

Yavaş, M. (2010). Acquisition of /s/-clusters in Spanish-English bilingual children with phonological disorders. *Clinical Linguistics and Phonetics, 24,* 188-198.

Yavaş, M. & Barlow, J.A., (2006). Acquisition of #sC clusters in Spanish-English bilingual children. *Journal of Multilingual Communication Disorders, 4,* 182-193.

Yavaş, M., & Beaubrun, C. (2006). Acquisition of #sC clusters in Haitian Creole-English bilingual children. *Journal of Multilingual Communication Disorders, 4,* 194-204.

Yavaş, M. & Goldstein, B. (2006). Aspects of bilingual phonology: The case of Spanish-English bilingual children. In Zhu Hua, & B. Dodd. (Eds.), *Phonological development and disorders: A multilingual perspective.* Clevedon, UK: Multilingual Matters.

Yazıcı, Z., İlter, B. G., & Glover, P. (2010). How bilingual is bilingual? Mother-tongue proficiency and learning through a second language. *International Journal of Early Years Education, 18,* 259-268.

Yip, V., & Matthews, S. (2007). Relative clauses in Cantonese-English bilingual children: Typological challenges and processing motivations. *Studies in Second Language Acquisition, 29,* 277-300.

Zajdó, K. (2007). Hungarian speech acquisition In S. McLeod (Ed.), *The international guide to speech acquisition* (pp. 412-436). Clifton Park, NY: Thomson Delmar Learning.

ADDITIONAL RESOURCES

Cruz-Ferreira, M. (2010). *Multilinguals are . . . ?* London: Battlebridge Publications.

Cruz-Ferreira, M. (Ed.) (2010). *Multilingual norms.* Frankfurt: Peter Lang Publishing.

De Houwer, A. (2009). *Bilingual first language acquisition.* Clevedon, UK: Multilingual Matters.

Genesee, F. (2007, January/February). A short guide to raising children bilingually. *Multilingual Living Magazine,* 1-9.

Genesee, F., Paradis, J., & Crago, M. B. (2004). *Dual language development and disorders: A handbook on bilingualism and second language learning.* Baltimore: Paul H. Brookes.

Goldstein, B. A. (2000). *Cultural and linguistic diversity resource guide for speech-language pathologists.* San Diego, CA: Singular Thomson Learning.

Goldstein, B. A. (Ed.) (2004). *Bilingual language development and disorders in Spanish-English speakers.* Baltimore: Paul H. Brookes.

Harding-Esch, E., & Riley, P. (2003). *The bilingual family: A handbook for parents* (2nd ed.). Cambridge, UK: Cambridge University Press.

Hua, Z. & Dodd, B. (Eds) (2006). *Phonological development and disorders: A multilingual perspective.* Clevedon, UK: Multilingual Matters.

Langdon, H. (2008). *Assessment and intervention for communication disorders in culturally and linguistically diverse populations.* Clifton Park, NY: Thomson Delmar Learning.

McLeod, S. (Ed.) (2007). *The international guide to speech acquisition.* Clifton Park, NY: Thomson Delmar Learning.

McLeod, S., & Goldstein, B. A. (Eds.) (2011). *Multilingual aspects of speech sound disorders in children.* Bristol, UK: Multilingual Matters.

Studies of Multilingual Children's Speech and Language Development*

Languages	Country	Study	Age of Children	Total No. of Children (No. of Multilingual Children)†
Arabic-Swedish	Sweden	Salameh, Nettlebladt, & Norlin (2003)	3;10-6;7 years	20 (20)
Cantonese-English	UK	Dodd, So, & Li (1996)	3-5 years	16 (16)
	UK	Dodd, Holm, & Li (1997)	5;2 and 3;7 years	2 (2)
	Australia	Holm & Dodd (1999a)	2;3-3;1 and 2;9-3;5 years (longitudinal)	2 (2)
	Australia and UK	Holm & Dodd (2006)	2-5 years	56 (56)
	Canada	Ng, Hsueh, & Leung (2010)	5-15 years	86 (86)
Cantonese-Putonghua	Hong Kong and Shenzhen, China	Law & So (2006)	2;6-4;11 years	100 (100)
Dutch-French	Belgium	De Houwer, Bornstein, & De Coster (2006)	13 months	31 (31)
Farsi-English	UK and Iran	Keshavarz & Ingram (2002)	8-20 months	1 (1)
French-English	Canada	Paradis (2001)	23-35 months	53 (17)
	Canada and USA	Paradis, Crago, Genesee, & Rice (2000)	About 7;0 to 7;6 years (mean = 83-91 months)	47 (16)
	Canada	Sundara, Polka, & Genesee (2006)	4;0-5;09 years	36 (12) + 12 adults
	Canada	Sundara, Polka, & Molnar (2008)	6-8 months + 10-12 months	96
Haitian-Creole-English	Unknown	Yavaş & Beaubrun (2006)	3;1-4;11	40 (40)
Hebrew-English	Israel	Berman (1977)	18-23.5 months	1 (1)
Hindi-Gujarati-English	USA	Ray (2002)	5 years	1 (1)
Hmong-English	USA	Kan (2010)	Preschoolers	3 (3)
	USA	Kan & Kohnert (2005)	3;4-5;2	19 (19)
	USA	Kohnert, Kan, & Conroy (2010)	2;11-5;2	19
Hungarian-English	USA	Bunta, Davidovich, & Ingram (2006)	2;0	1 (1)
Italian-English	UK	Holm & Dodd (1999b)	4;2, 4;4	2 (2)
Korean-English	USA	Ha, Johnson, & Kuehn (2009)	3;10, 6;0, 11;0	3 (3)
Maltese-English	Malta	Grech & Dodd (2008)	2;0-6;0	241 (93)
Mandarin-English	Taiwan	Lin & Johnson (2010)	Bilingual mean = 5;0; monolingual mean = 5;3	48 (25)
Norwegian-English	Canada	Johnson & Lancaster (1998)	1;2-1;8 (Language) 1;9 (speech)	1 (1)
Pakistani heritage languages (Mirpuri, Punjabi, Urdu)-English; Punjabi-English	UK	Stow & Pert (2006b)	1;4-7;11	246 (246)
	UK	Holm, Dodd, Stow, & Pert (1999)	4;8-7;5	35 (35)
	UK	Holm & Dodd (1999c)	—	1 (1)

*Studies of typically and atypically developing multilingual children published in English were included; however, studies that only included monolingual children were excluded.
†The total number of children may have included both multilingual and monolingual children, so the number in parentheses provides the total number of multilingual children.

Typically Developing Children	Atypically Developing Children	Speech (Articulation and/or Phonology)	Language (Semantics, Morphology, Syntax, and/or Discourse)	Production/ Expressive Language	Perception/ Receptive Language
Typical	Atypical	Speech		Production	
Typical		Speech		Production	
	Atypical	Speech		Production	
Typical		Speech		Production	
Typical		Speech		Production	
Typical		Speech		Production	
Typical		Speech		Production	
Typical			Language		Perception
Typical		Speech		Production	Perception
Typical		Speech		Production	
	Atypical		Language	Production	
Typical		Speech			Perception
Typical		Speech			Perception
Typical		Speech		Production	
Typical		Speech		Production	
	Atypical	Speech		Production	
Typical			Language	Production	
Typical			Language	Production	Perception
Typical			Language	Production	Perception
Typical		Speech		Production	
	Atypical	Speech		Production	
Typical		Speech		Production	
Typical		Speech		Production	
Typical		Speech		Production	
Typical		Speech	Language	Production	
Typical		Speech		Production	
Typical	Atypical	Speech		Production	
	Atypical	Speech		Production	

Languages	Country	Study	Age of Children	Total No. of Children (No. of Multilingual Children)[†]
Portuguese-English	USA	Collins (2005)	Preschoolers	70 (70)
Portuguese-Swedish-English	—	Cruz-Ferreira (1999)	—	3 (3)
Romanian-English	USA	Vogel (1975)	1;6-2;0	1 (1)
Russian-English	USA	Gildersleeve-Neumann & Wright (2010)	3;3-5;7	42 (14)
Samoan-English	New Zealand	Ballard & Farao (2008)	4;0-4;11	20 (20)
	Australia	Hemsley, Holm, & Dodd (2006)	Mean = 11;2	101 (62) (28 = Samoan-English)
	Australia	Hemsley, Holm, & Dodd (2010)	4 to 5 years	18 (9)
Spanish-English	USA	Brice, Carson, & Dennis O'Brien (2009)	4 to 5 years	16 (16)
	USA	Bunta, Fabiano-Smith, Goldstein, & Ingram (2009)	3;0-4;0	24 (8)
	USA	Bunta & Ingram (2007)	3;9-5;2	30 (10)
	USA	Cataño, Barlow, & Moyna (2009)	0;11-5;1	16 (6)
	USA	Fabiano-Smith & Goldstein (2010)	3;0-4;0	24 (8)
	USA	Fabiano-Smith & Barlow (2010)	3;0-4;0	24 (8)
	USA	Fabiano & Goldstein (2005)	5;0, 6;2, and 7;0	3 (3)
	USA	Gildersleeve-Neumann, Kester, Davis, & Peña (2008)	3;1-3;10	33 (23)
	USA	Goldstein & Bunta (2010)	Mean age 5;10-6;0	30 (10)
	USA	Goldstein, Bunta, Lange, Rodriguez, & Burrows (2010)	4;3-7;1	50 (50)
	USA	Goldstein, Fabiano, & Washington (2005)	5;0-5;5	15 (5)
	USA	Goldstein & Washington (2001)	4;0-4;11	12 (12)
	USA	Gorman, Fiestas, Peña, & Clark (2011)	6;6-8;4	60 (20 Latino)
	USA	Gutierrez-Clellen, Simon-Cereijido, & Erickson Leone (2009)	—	58 (58)
	USA	Hammer, Lawrence, & Miccio (2008)	Preschool	83 (83)
	USA	Marchman, Martínez-Sussmann, & Dale (2004)	17-30 months	113 (113)
	USA	Patterson (1998)	21 to 27 months	102 (102)
	USA	Yavaş & Barlow (2006)	2;11-4;5	40 (40)
	USA	Yavaş (2010)	3 to 7 years	30

Typically Developing Children	Atypically Developing Children	Speech (Articulation and/or Phonology)	Language (Semantics, Morphology, Syntax, and/or Discourse)	Production/ Expressive Language	Perception/ Receptive Language
Typical			Language	Production	
Typical		Speech	Language	Production	
Typical		Speech		Production	
Typical		Speech		Production	
Typical		Speech		Production	
Typical			Language	Production	Perception
Typical			Language	Production	Perception
Typical		Speech		Production	
Typical		Speech		Production	
Typical		Speech		Production	
Typical		Speech		Production	
Typical		Speech		Production	
Typical		Speech		Production	
Typical		Speech		Production	
Typical		Speech		Production	
Typical		Speech		Production	
Typical		Speech		Production	
Typical		Speech		Production	
Typical		Speech		Production	
Typical			Language	Production	
	Atypical		Language	Production	
	Atypical		Language		Perception
Typical			Language	Production	
Typical			Language	Production	
Typical		Speech		Production	
	Atypical	Speech		Production	

Continued

Languages	Country	Study	Age of Children	Total No. of Children (No. of Multilingual Children)[†]
Spanish-German	Germany	Lleó, Kuchenbrandt, Kehoe, & Trujillo (2003)	1;0-3;0	11 (5)
Spanish-Mandarin- Taiwanese	Not specified (most likely Paraguay and Taiwan)	Yang & Hua (2010)	1;3-2;0	1 (1)
Spanish-Portuguese-Hebrew	Israel	Faingold (1996)	0;11-1;11	1 (1)
Turkish-German; Turkish-Norwegian	Germany, Austria, Norway, Turkey	Yazıcı, İter, & Glover (2010)	5-6 years	120 (90)
Vietnamese-English	Australia	Hemsley, Holm, & Dodd (2006)	Mean = 11;5	101 (62) (34 = Vietnamese-English)
Welsh-English	Wales	Munro, Ball, Müller, Duckworth, & Lyddy (2005)	2;6-5;0	83 (83)
	Wales	Ball, Müller, & Munro (2001)	2;6-5;0	83 (83)

Typically Developing Children	Atypically Developing Children	Speech (Articulation and/or Phonology)	Language (Semantics, Morphology, Syntax, and/or Discourse)	Production/ Expressive Language	Perception/ Receptive Language
Typical		Speech		Production	
Typical		Speech		Production	
Typical		Speech		Production	
Typical			Language		Perception
Typical			Language	Production	Perception
Typical		Speech		Production	
Typical		Speech		Production	

Neurogenic Disorders of Speech, Language, Cognition-Communication, and Swallowing

Constance Dean Qualls

Globalization has compelled ways of thinking that express a model for inclusion in its highest and purest form. As such, notwithstanding cultural peculiarities (Geertz, 1983), people around the world can no longer overlook the universality of many aspects of the human existence, including its nature, behavior, and environment. For instance, demographers of aging show global trends that reflect significant increases in the numbers of individuals, both within the United States and internationally, who are living longer and living longer with disabilities. The hallmark of this global demographic shift is the explosion in the growth of nonwhite populations. It is therefore imperative that a multicultural worldview be embraced, cultivated, and promoted when working with individuals with neurogenic communication and swallowing disorders. The World Health Organization (WHO) responded to the call for integral inclusion of personal and cultural factors related to health and disability, including communication disorders, when developing the International Classification of Functioning, Disability and Health (ICF, 2001). Further, evidence-based practice (EBP) for communication disorders integrates within its framework clinician's expertise, current best evidence, and client values and preferences. According to the American Speech-Language-Hearing Association (2010), the goal of EBP is "... to provide high quality services that reflect the interests, values, needs, and choices of the individuals we serve." Threats (2010) contends that both the ICF model and EBP are client-based approaches; therefore, integration of the tenets of both will ensure culturally relevant rehabilitation outcomes.

WHO ICF MODEL AND NEUROGENIC COMMUNICATION DISORDERS

The WHO developed the ICF (2001) model as a system for classifying health and health-related domains. Domains of the ICF are body structure and function, activity, participation,

and environmental factors. The ICF recognizes the concepts of health and disability as universals within the human experience and allows for a common metric that can be used globally to capture the essence of health and disability for all humans. Importantly, ICF takes into account the social aspects of disability (contextual factors) to account for the impact of the environment on human functioning. In this regard, one's cultural beliefs, practices, and preferences are integrated within the clinical enterprise.

In recent years, the WHO has focused greater attention on health and disability associated with chronic diseases such as stroke and Alzheimer's disease (AD). As the number of older individuals grows, so will the incidence and prevalence of stroke and AD. Clinical management of individuals with neurogenic communication and swallowing disorders can be based on the ICF model. In this regard, body structure and function deal with impairments of the brain and its functions; activity deals with a person's ability to speak, listen, and understand language, and to read and write; and participation deals with a person's ability to effectively communicate needs, wants, and ideas when participating in everyday life activities such as working, shopping, and dining. Unlike the traditional approach of focusing largely on assessment and treatment of language modalities (i.e., activity), the ICF framework amplifies rehabilitation of functional communication abilities (i.e., the ability to interact effectively in home, work, and social settings). The fourth aspect of the ICF model deals with environmental or contextual factors; that is, cultural milieu must be integrated within the clinical process to achieve the best outcome.

Evidence-Based Practice

EBP can be defined as the clinician's "conscientious, explicit, and judicious use of current best evidence in making decisions about the care of individual patients" (Sackett et al.,

1996, p. 71). For communication sciences and disorders, EBP is a process in which the clinician systematically gathers and integrates information from a variety of resources, including scientific evidence, prior knowledge, and client preferences, to arrive at a decision (Justice, 2008). To this definition, the context in which services are delivered has been added. Therefore, EBP is grounded in the following four types of evidence: external evidence, clinical expertise, client values and preferences, and service delivery context.

External evidence includes both scientific research and objective performance measures (i.e., test results, direct patient observation, and ancillary reports from other health professionals) used by clinicians to evaluate and monitor progress. Clinical expertise is acquired through experience, continuing education, and consensus building among professionals and allows us to provide services in areas in which scientific evidence is absent, incomplete, or equivocal. Client values and preferences enable us to serve individuals appropriately by taking into account personal and individual factors (i.e., beliefs, communication style, language choice). Incorporating client values and preferences throughout the clinical management process ensures the delivery of culturally competent professional services. The service delivery context includes the pressures, policies, and practices of employment facilities, government agencies, and other regulatory bodies that have an unavoidable and profound effect on practice patterns (American Speech-Language-Hearing Association [ASHA], 2010; Gottfred, 2008).

Cultural Competence

Culture and communication are integrally related. Individuals express held cultural views, values, beliefs, and preferences by means of verbal and nonverbal communication as well as in behaviors and actions. Cultural anthropologist Clifford Geertz (1983) asserted that "culture is always local." If one espouses to this way of thinking about culture, it is clear to see how egocentricity (self-interest) too often prevails over altruism (selflessness). Examination of egocentricity is essential in communication disorders. Paul and Elder (2009) state that:

Egocentric thinking results from the unfortunate fact that humans do not naturally consider the rights and needs of others. We do not naturally appreciate the point of view of others or the limitations in our point of view. We become explicitly aware of our egocentric thinking only if trained to do so. We do not naturally recognize our egocentric assumptions, the egocentric way we use information, the egocentric way we interpret data, the source of egocentric concepts and ideas, the implications of our egocentric thought. We do not naturally recognize our self-serving perspective. (p. 21)

Embodied within this statement are two important points. First, broad, global ways of thinking can be taught and learned. Second, if one accepts that there are individual,

culture-driven differences in basic assumptions in ways of collecting, using, and interpreting information and data, and in the source of concepts and ideas, then one fully understands what it means to be culturally competent.

Cultural competence deals with attitudes and behaviors that dictate a person's actions. Accordingly, it " . . . is a set of cultural behaviors and attitudes integrated into the practice methods of a system, agency, or its professionals, that enable them to work effectively in cross cultural situations" (Administration on Aging [AoA], 2010). In this view, there are two dimensions to cultural competence: surface structure and deep structure (AoA, 2010; Myers, 1987). Surface structure deals with understanding the people, including the beliefs and values they hold and the language, traditions, music, food, and clothing familiar to and preferred by them. Deep structure involves understanding sociodemographic and racial/ethnic population similarities and differences, and the influences of ethnic, social, cultural, historical, and environmental factors on behaviors. Specific to communication disorders, Battle (2002) characterizes the essence of cultural competence as follows:

Cultural competence involves far more than an understanding of language form and dialectical considerations. It involves understanding all dimensions of culture and communication and how they impact on the individual. Because culture permeates every dimension of communication, the culturally competent clinician understands that most, if not all, truths are merely perceptions of truth viewed through the prism of culture. (p. xviii)

Of import in Battle's characterization are (1) the impact of culture for effective and efficient communication, and (2) that all individuals view and interpret the world from the perspective of their own cultural lens (see Klein, 2004). There are some basic tenets of cultural competence for clinicians providing services to individuals from multicultural and international populations who have neurogenic communication and swallowing disorders. First, one must understand the demographics of normal and pathologic aging. This is particularly important because persistent and significant health disparities exist among U.S. populations as well as non-U.S. populations, and because of the specific diseases and disorders that lead to neurogenic communication and swallowing disorders. Second, there are some identified differences in the neuropathophysiologic changes and neural recovery patterns that are driven by race and ethnicity. Complete understanding of the impact of the differences in brain structure and function will effectively inform patient-based clinical management. Third, evidence-based clinical practice accommodates for the cultural competence of the health professional within its framework; this tenet assumes reflection on and integration of the sociodemographic and sociocultural values and preferences of the patient throughout the clinic decision-making process (see Threats, 2010).

Clinicians who fully understand the influence of cultural and linguistic diversity in research and practice appreciate the significance of adopting a culturally competent, evidence-based approach to their clinical and professional pursuits. It is possible that providers of culturally competent services will see improved patient participation, increased compliance, and improved follow-up. A systematic, qualitative review of the literature showed excellent evidence that cultural competence training can (1) favorably affect knowledge of attitudes of health care providers, and (2) improve their attitudes and skills when working with individuals from various racial/ethnic backgrounds (Levine et al., 2004). Similarly, good data suggest that cultural competence training will improve patient satisfaction, although it is yet unclear what the impact is on patient adherence (Agency for Health Care Research and Quality, 2004).

There is an undeniable "sea change" evolving in the United States and throughout the world: people are living longer and living longer with disability. The combination of shifting demographics, technology, medical advancements, and changes in education level (e.g., more college-educated individuals) and lifestyle (e.g., less cigarette smoking, healthy eating, and exercise) has increased the average life span. On the other hand, given that advancing age increases significantly the risk factors that can lead to cardiovascular diseases such as heart attack and stroke and degenerative brain disorders such as AD and Parkinson's disease, it is reasonable to expect that greater numbers of older adults will be living with neurologic impairments, and many of these individuals will need services to address cognitive-linguistic, communicative, or swallowing difficulties.

The remainder of this chapter focuses on multicultural and international considerations for the management of individuals with acquired communication and swallowing disorders as a result of brain damage. The research cited reflects the findings of researchers from the United States and around the globe. The topics of interest in this writing fall into two broad categories: situational factors and clinical management issues. Situational factors are those factors that have the potential to increase significantly the risk for medical conditions such as stroke that often lead to neurogenic communication and swallowing disorders. The situational factors discussed in this chapter are global aging, the epidemiology of cardiovascular and related diseases among populations, and the incidence and prevalence of acquired neurogenic communication and swallowing disorders.

The second broad topic to be discussed is clinical management issues. Included in this section is an overview of neurogenic communication and swallowing disorders followed by discussion of the cultural, linguistic, communication, and clinical issues that warrant attention when working with individuals with these disorders. The organizational structure of the remaining discussions in this section includes implications for assessment and treatment for the following categories of neurologic disorders: language, speech, cognitive-communicative, and swallowing disorders.

Demographics of Normal and Pathologic Aging

Worldwide, population aging is unprecedented, pervasive, and enduring and has profound implications (World Population Ageing, 2010). At the beginning of the 21st century, approximately 600 million people worldwide were aged 60 years and older; by 2050; this population is expected to number more than 1 billion. Globally, the older adult population is growing by 2% per year, with expected future growth of 2.8% per year between 2025 and 2030. Women make up the overwhelming majority of the older population. In the United States, the number of individuals who are 65 years and older is growing exponentially, reflecting the "graying of America." The AoA (2009) highlights the most recent demographics of aging and disability. The number of individuals 65 years and older reached 38.9 million in 2008 (12.8% of the U.S. population), a 13% increase over 1998, and that number is expected to increase by 31% by 2020. Further, persons who reach age 65 years have a projected life expectancy of an additional 18.6 years (19.8 years for females and 17.1 years for males); thus, the older population itself is aging, with the most significant increase among the oldest-old, those aged 80 to 85 years and older.

This trend is also seen among individuals from culturally and linguistically diverse groups. In 2008, 19.6% of persons 65 years and older were from racial or ethnic minority groups. Approximately 8.3% were African Americans. Persons of Hispanic origin (who may be of any race) represented 6.8% of the older population. About 3.4% were Asian or Pacific Islander, and less than 1% were American Indian or Native Alaskan. In addition, 0.6% of persons 65 years and older identified themselves as being of two or more races. Growing faster than majority populations of elderly people, elderly people from racial/ethnic minority groups increased from 5.7 million (16.3% of the elderly population) in 2000 to 8.0 million (20.1% of the elderly population) in 2010 and are projected to increase to 12.9 million (23.6% of the elderly population) by 2020. The growing numbers of adults who are living longer, and the ever-increasing cultural diversity within older adult populations, both in the United States and around the world, have major implications for the health and well-being of individuals in these groups.

Epidemiology of Neurogenic Communication and Swallowing Disorders

Epidemiologic data on neurogenic communication and swallowing disorders are severely limited. Epidemiology is the study of the distribution and determinants of health-related states or events in a specified population, taking into account factors (e.g., inequalities, community, family, work) and risks (e.g., habits, genetics, lifestyle) that influence patterns of health and disease for the purpose of understanding how to control and prevent health problems (Enderby & Pickstone, 2005). Increased attention to prevention in the current health care climate makes it imperative for speech-language pathologists to understand the principles of epidemiology and how epidemiologic data can inform clinical practice (Enderby & Pickstone, 2005; Lubker, 1997). This is particularly salient for clinicians who work with older individuals. Three factors are critical to understanding issues in working with older persons. First, there is a high prevalence of diseases and disorders of the brain in this population. Second, there is a significant increase in individual and group differences due to unique life experiences or circumstances. Third, there are increasing numbers of aging individuals who do not speak American English (e.g., recent immigrants), who do not speak English well, who speak English as a second language, or who speak more than one language.

Given the growing numbers of older adults and the significant increase in the diversity of the older adult population, one can expect a significant increase in disabilities, including communication and swallowing disorders, in culturally and linguistically diverse individuals. An estimated 6.2 million Americans from culturally and linguistically diverse backgrounds have a communication disorder (ASHA, 2010). More than 2.3 million Hispanics/Latinos need speech, language, and hearing services. Approximately 69% are adults older than 18 years of age. Approximately 21 in every 1000 African Americans between the ages of 45 and 65 years are living with a communication disorder. In general, the burden of neurogenic communication disorders is greater in these populations because of the high prevalence of chronic diseases that adversely affect the cardiovascular system, namely heart disease, hypertension, and diabetes. Between 2005 and 2007, hypertension was the number one chronic condition in African Americans (84% prevalence rate compared with 71% for all older persons), and in 2008, there was a higher incidence of diabetes in African Americans (10.9%) and Hispanics/Latinos (10.7%) compared with non-Hispanic whites (6.9%) (AoA, 2009).

Neuropathophysiologic Diversity

Research has provided limited but compelling evidence for cultural variability (race and gender) in the distribution of neurologic lesions in stroke (see Table 8-1; Gorelick, 1998; Li, Lam, & Wong, 2002). Notably, African Americans, Japanese, and women tend to show a prevalence of intracranial (within the skull/cranium; see Markus et al., 2007) lesions affecting small arteries such as those located in the subcortical and midbrain regions. White males, on the other hand, show an overwhelming prevalence of extracranial

TABLE 8-1 Incidence (%) of Stroke by Type and Race-Ethnicity

Type	White	Hispanic	Native American
	(N = 1085)	(N = 220)	(N = 70)
Hemorrhage	37	48	27
Lacunar	16	15	30
Cardioembolic	16	9	14
Atherothrombotic	14	10	11
Unknown	11	9	14
Other	6	9	4

From Frey, J. L., Jahnka, H. K., Bulfinch, E. W. (1998). Differences in stroke between White, Hispanic and Native American Patients. *Stroke, 29,* 29-33.

(outside of the cranium) lesions that affect the large carotid arteries. Frey and colleagues (1998) reported lesion distribution data for Hispanics/Latinos, Native Americans, and whites. They found few significant differences between the races for type of stroke. As shown in Table 8-1, Native Americans (30%) had a greater prevalence of stroke related to lacunes than either whites (16%) or Hispanics (15%). Whites (16%) had a greater incidence of stroke related to cardioembolism than Hispanics (9%). There was no difference in the strokes related to hemorrhagic, atherothrombotic, or other types of stroke. Although these trends appear to be stable, additional research is needed to determine the implications of these racial and ethnic and gender differences. It is possible that, in addition to other prognostic factors such as size and site of lesion, age of onset, premorbid education level and social functioning, and family support, the distribution of the lesion may have implications for differences in neurobehavioral expectations (i.e., the particular deficits or skill sets of an individual after stroke) and assessment and treatment outcomes. The latest research shows that combination *or* tandem intracranial and extracranial arterial occlusions are found in a unique group of patients (Malik et al., 2011). These patients generally show a poor prognosis and, to date, race-ethnicity has yet to be identified as a distinct feature in this group of patients.

Neurogenic Communication and Swallowing Disorders

Neurologic disorders of communication and swallowing result from a variety of diseases of the brain and nervous system, including demyelinating, degenerative, inflammatory, systemic, cardiovascular, extrapyramidal, episodic and paroxysmal, nerve, nerve root and plexus, polyneuropathies and other disorders of the peripheral nervous system, myoneural junction and muscle, cerebral palsy and other paralytic syndromes, as well as other disorders of the nervous system (ICD, 2010). Adult (acquired) neurogenic language disorders include aphasia, alexia, agraphia, and cognitive-communicative disorders secondary to stroke, dementia, mild cognitive impairment (MCI), traumatic brain injury (TBI), and right hemisphere damage (RHD). Acquired neurogenic speech disorders include apraxia of speech (AOS) and the dysarthrias. Approximately 24% of individuals who experience stroke have primary speech impairments following brain damage (see Byles, 2005). Acquired neurogenic swallowing disorders (also referred to as dysphagia) range from oral to oropharyngeal to pharyngeal to esophageal dysphagia. Dysphagia is highly prevalent among stroke patients; 45% to 65% of these patients will experience swallowing difficulties within 6 months after the onset of stroke (Schindler & Keller, 2002). It is impossible to cover, with any depth, the vast collection of research and clinical practice information on acquired neurogenic communication and swallowing disorders in this chapter. Payne (1997) and Wallace (1997) have focused specifically on adult neurogenics in multicultural populations. Others have focused on communication disorders in multicultural populations over the life span that included adult neurogenics (e.g., Battle, 2002). The following section presents a brief overview of major acquired language disorders of aphasia and cognitive-communicative impairments secondary to dementia, TBI, and RHD. Included in the discussion is the available research on incidence and prevalence of each of the disorders in multicultural and international populations.

Aphasia

Aphasia is a disruption in one or more language modalities, including comprehension of language, speech production, reading, writing, and gesturing, that can significantly impair one's ability to communicate her or his needs, wants, feelings, and ideas and, therefore, adversely affects the person's quality of life. Only a very small number of stroke patients completely recover from aphasia. It is widely held that, in most people, language is lateralized to the left hemisphere (also referred to as the language-dominant hemisphere), although new research suggests that there is no one-to-one correlation between where the lesion occurs in the brain and the type of aphasia (e.g., nonfluent, fluent, Broca's, Wernicke's, global) (Dronkers et al., 2004).

Stroke and Neurogenic Disorders of Communication and Swallowing

Stroke is the second leading cause of death and a leading cause of disability in older adults throughout the world. It is the principal cause of older adult communication and swallowing disabilities, including aphasia, motor speech disorders (apraxia of speech and dysarthria), and dysphagia. Incidence of stroke varies markedly in different world

populations. The WHO (2005) estimates that, worldwide, 15 million persons have a stroke annually, resulting in 5.7 million deaths and 5 million persons with long-term disability. Stroke accounts for 9.9% of all deaths, affecting 8.6% of males and 11.0% of females worldwide. The WHO estimates that, in Europe, there are 650,000 deaths from stroke annually. Eighty-five percent of the persons having a stroke live in low- and middle-income countries, and one third are younger than 70 years of age. In developing countries, the number of strokes is declining owing to control of high blood pressure and reduction in the use of tobacco; however, the aging population has an effect on the overall rate.

Recent data show that stroke or brain attack is the fourth most common cause of death in the United States (Centers for Disease Control and Prevention [CDC], 2010). The general rate of stroke in the United States is 2.6% of the population; however, according to the CDC (Neyer et al., 2005), the prevalence of stroke varies by education level, race and ethnicity, and geographic region. Risk factors related to education level include poverty and lack of economic opportunity, social isolation, and cultural norms for diet and exercise. They report that the prevalence of stroke varies across racial/ethnic groups in the United States is as follows: American Indians/Alaskan Natives (6.0%), multiracial (4.6%), African Americans/blacks (4.0%), Hispanics (2.6%), whites (2.3%), and Asians and Pacific Islanders (1.6%). According to the CDC data, African Americans/blacks, Hispanics, Asians and Pacific Islanders, and American Indians/Alaskan Natives die from a stroke at younger ages than whites. The report suggests that the higher prevalence of stroke in certain racial/ethnic groups may be related to higher incidence of chronic health conditions such as high blood pressure, heart disease, high cholesterol, diabetes, tobacco and alcohol use, inactivity, and obesity. Further, these data indicate that individuals who are at greater risk for stroke are also at greater risk for communication and swallowing disorders.

African Americans

The frequency of stroke and stroke-associated mortality is approximately twice as high for African American males and females as it is in among whites (Gorelick, 1998). This disparity is most pronounced at younger ages. For example, African American men aged 45 to 59 years are about four times more likely to die of stroke than white men of the same age. By age 75 years or older, however, this ratio falls to about 1.26. In the United States, the disparity in the ratio of African American to Hispanic mortality is greatest for stroke.

Several of the known risk factors for stroke, such as hypertension, diabetes, and obesity, are more common in blacks than whites, and sickle cell disease and HIV infection are stroke risk factors with particular relevance to Africans (Imam, 2002). Wertz and associates (1997) reported that there are several differences between strokes experienced by African Americans and those experienced by whites. African American women are more likely to have a stroke than African American males; among whites, there are minimal gender differences in the incidence of stroke. Among African Americans, the lesion leading to the stroke is more often located within the cranium (skull), whereas among whites, it is more often located outside the cranium. Among African Americans, after a stroke, physical and functional impairment is more severe, and functional improvement occurs at a slower rate than among whites. African Americans are particularly prone to aphasia owing to a higher incidence of stroke and stroke-related diseases such as diabetes and hypertension.

Pratt and colleagues (2003) reported that, as a group, African Americans have less knowledge about stroke, its risk factors, and prevention than whites. Those who have a history of diabetes, hypertension, or heart disease and who had a history of stroke in their family had more knowledge about strokes than those who did not have this history. Younger and college-educated African Americans had more knowledge about stroke and stroke prevention than those with less education, regardless of age.

A small group of researchers have investigated one aspect of aphasia (narratives) in African Americans. The results were mixed. Ulatowska and colleagues (2000, 2003) observed narrative style in African Americans with stroke. They reported that when blacks communicate with each other or tell stories, they have the tendency to repeat themselves or have other people repeat what they say. An example is that African American ministers encourage the congregation to repeat what they say in a call-and-response pattern during the sermon. Some African Americans with aphasia involuntarily repeat all or part of the utterances of speech partners, even when no one is talking about that subject anymore. In severe cases, the person may experience stereotypic self-repetition of single recurrent syllables, words, or phrases (Ulatowska, et al., 2000). On the other hand, Olness and associates (2010) recently reported no differences between African American and white persons with aphasia in assigning prominence to information in narratives.

Hispanics/Latinos

An American Heart Association study conducted in the late 1990s reported that Hispanics between the ages of 45 and 59 years have more than three times the risk for suffering a stroke than non-Hispanic whites. Stroke is the fourth highest killer of Hispanics. Nearly 25% of all deaths in Hispanic men are due to stroke, and the number rises to 33% for Hispanic women (Gillum, 1995).

Frey and colleagues (1998) reported on differences in stroke types (see Table 8-1) and risk factors such as hypertension, diabetes, cardiac disease, and smoking in 1700 white, Hispanic, and Native American stroke patients admitted to a hospital in Arizona. Mean age at stroke onset was significantly lower in Native Americans (56 years) than Hispanics (61 years) and whites (69 years). The mean age of onset of stroke for Hispanics was significantly lower than for whites. They report that hypertension was significantly more prevalent in Hispanics (72%) and Native Americans (71%) than whites (66%). Diabetes was significantly more prevalent in Native Americans (62%) than both Hispanics (36%) and whites (17%). Cigarette smoking was significantly more common in whites (61%) than either Hispanics (46%) or Native Americans (41%). Cardiac disease was significantly more prevalent in whites (34%) than Hispanics (24%). History of hypercholesterolemia was not significantly different between the races. Heavy alcohol intake was significantly more prevalent in Native Americans than Hispanics and whites and significantly more prevalent in Hispanics than whites.

Asians and Pacific Islanders

Although racial and ethnic disparities in the incidence of stroke and aphasia within the United States have been a recent interest, most studies have focused on African Americans and Hispanics, and few reports describe stroke in Asians and Pacific Islanders. However, stroke is a major concern in Asia. The stroke incidence rates in China and Japan are among the higher ones in the world. Reported incidence rates vary dramatically but are generally higher than those of the United States. For example, compared with incidence in the United States, reported rates for overall stroke are 39% greater in Japan, 23% greater in Taiwan, and 81% greater in Northern China. Stroke is the second leading cause of death in China, Korea, and Taiwan; third in Japan and Singapore; sixth in the Philippines; and tenth in Thailand. In 2005, there were a reported 1.4 million fatal strokes in China, including an annual 3000 in Hong Kong alone (Ng, 2007).

The variation in the proportion of stroke subtypes among Chinese populations could be as large as or larger than that between Chinese and Western populations. Zhang and colleagues (2003a, 2003b) reported that ischemic stroke is more frequent in Chinese than in Western populations. Overall, Asian and Pacific Islander adults are less likely than white adults to die from a stroke; they have lower rates of being overweight or obese, lower rates of hypertension, and are less likely to have hypertension, be obese, and be current cigarette smokers.

Bilinguals and Aphasia

Given the increase in the bilingual population in the United States, it is expected that there will be as many as 45,000 persons with cognitive impairment, including aphasia, reported in bilinguals each year (Paradis, 2001). Although much attention has been given to the development of language in bilingual speakers, little attention has been given to recovery of language in bilinguals with aphasia. Until recently, no data existed to determine whether there are differences in the manifestations and recovery from aphasia among bilinguals, trilinguals, and multilinguals. Research has primarily focused on describing symptoms, language localization, and recovery patterns (Roberts & Kiran, 2007). In the past decade, there has been a virtual explosion in published research dedicated to assessing and treating the speech and language abilities of bilingual individuals with aphasia, with much of the emphasis on Spanish-English or English-Spanish speakers. Ardila and Ramos (2007) report on research on generative naming tasks on bilingual aphasics in several countries and languages, including French, Greek, Russian, and Italian. In an extensive review of the literature, Lorenzen and Murray (2008) state that there are differences among bilinguals in impairment patterns in both output or expression and translation or comprehension abilities among bilingual aphasics, making the study of bilingual aphasia complicated. They provide information on differences in recovery of language skills for bilinguals as reported by Fabbro (2001). For example, parallel recovery is when recovery of language parallels the patients premorbid abilities (i.e., one language is stronger than the other), differential recovery occurs when one language is recovered much better than the other compared with premorbid abilities, and blending is when there is uncontrollable mixing of words and grammatical constructions of two or more languages even when attempting to speak in only one language (not to be confused with code switching) (Fabbro, 2001; Paradis, 2004, as cited in Lorenzen & Murray, 2008). Similarly, bilingual and multilingual persons with aphasia demonstrate different patterns of impairment and recovery of translation skills: they may no longer have the ability to translate from one language to another, they may be able to translate but without comprehension, they may be able to translate in one language and not in the other, or they may continuously and spontaneously translate (see Lorenzen & Murray, 2008). A number of variables have been cited as predictors of recovery patterns and often include age of the speaker, proficiency in each language, when and where each language was learned, premorbid language status, lesion site, environmental and social situations where the languages were used, and aphasia type. However, there is no confirmation of the importance of any one of these variables as a predictor of recovery; rather, it is more likely a combination of the variables with the importance of each dependent on the individual speaker (Fabbro, 2001).

Understanding of these recovery patterns cannot be overstated because traditional linguistic and cognitive treatments may require modification or revision to meet the needs of the bilingual patient. Few studies have targeted treatment for bilingual and multilingual speakers with aphasia, and the findings from these studies are largely mixed. Further, existing studies concentrated heavily on the lexical (e.g., word naming) and semantic (e.g., explaining the use of an item; categorizing) aspects of language, with virtually no research on writing, reading, or using gestures. Lorenzen and Murray (2008) caution the use of augmentative and alternative communication (AAC) with bilingual and multilingual speakers because these devices likely present cultural barriers (e.g., non-English background, cultural traditions, values or preferences).

Faroqi-Shah and associates (2010) worked with the National Center for Evidence-based Practice in Communication Disorders of the American Speech-Language-Hearing Association to conduct a systematic review of the language used in the treatment of bilingual aphasics. Based on their review of 14 studies involving 45 patients, they concluded that treatment in L2 yields positive results in recovery of the receptive and expressive language abilities of bilinguals with aphasia. The age of acquisition of L2 had little differential effect on the outcomes, and finally, there was cross-language transfer in at least half of the studies reviewed, especially when L1 was used in treatment. The evidence supported the belief that, because bilinguals possess an intermixed lexical and morphosyntactic organization with shared neural networks in both languages, treatment in L2 transfer to L1 resulted in cross-language transfer (Kohnert, 2009).

Lorenzen and Murray (2008) concluded there are continuing controversies regarding " . . . how best to quantify and qualify bilingualism and other linguistic concepts (e.g., cognate status) unique to bilingual speakers" (p. 213) and how particular linguistic (e.g., lexical) and cognitive (e.g., inhibition) factors affect recovery patterns. They further point out that many studies on bilingual aphasia use weak study designs (e.g., case studies, small descriptive studies) with poor controls and that the development and testing of assessment of treatment protocols for bilingual aphasia have been severely limited. Essentially, more and better studies are needed to provide the necessary information to effectively and efficiently treat persons with aphasia who are bilingual.

Assessment of Bilingual Aphasia

Roberts and Kiran (2007) have provided a rather comprehensive review of the available assessment tools for bilingual aphasia. They report that many of the tests used for English speakers are available in other languages. For example, the Boston Naming Test (BNT; Kaplan et al., 1983, 2001) is available in French, Spanish, Chinese, Greek, Swedish, Norwegian, Dutch, Finnish, and Korean. However, because of the psychometric properties, the tests may have limited value in the assessment of aphasic bilinguals. For example, there are differences in the names given to objects in different countries. In addition, because the tests may be translations without concern for the cultural and linguistic differences between languages, the difficulty level of the items may differ across languages.

The Boston Diagnostic Aphasia Examination (BDAE) (Goodglass & Kaplan, 1983), The Aachen Aphasia Test

(German), and the Multilingual Aphasia Examination English and Spanish) (Benton et al., 1994) are also available; however, a recent review by the Agency for Health Care Research and Quality (Biddle et al., 2002) concluded that the BDAE (second edition) did not meet the recognized standard for either reliability or validity when used with bilingual aphasics. Several databases are being developed to assist with assessment of language naming in various languages that may be helpful in assessment of bilingual aphasic. Kremin and colleagues (2003) developed a set of 269 pictures with normative data for 90 to 130 participants who were native speakers of Dutch, English, German, French, Italian, Russian, Spanish, and Swedish. The International Picture-Naming Project (Bates et al., 2003) provides data on more than 520 black-and-white drawings of common object names and 275 verbs in English, German, Mexican Spanish, Italian, Bulgarian, Hungarian, and a Taiwanese dialect of Mandarin. Although these tests are not without limitation, they may provide useful information in the assessment of individuals with aphasia who are bilingual.

Dementia

Dementia is an acquired, progressive deterioration in communicative functioning, personality traits, and intellectual functioning (e.g., Froelich, Bogardus, & Inouye, 2001). There is a range of dementia types, with AD constituting 50% to 80% and vascular dementia constituting 20% to 30% of all of the dementias (Alzheimer's Association, 2010). Unlike the insidious onset and largely focal nature of aphasia, dementia results from widespread, progressive neurophysiologic changes that will eventually affect one's activities of daily living (e.g., eating, self-care, socialization). As a progressive disorder, dementia is classified in stages, and, depending on the stage, language and communication deficits are manifest in naming, reading, writing, and auditory comprehension (Bhatnagar, 2008). Since the mid-1990s, published research has documented effective interventions for persons with dementia, and therefore the belief that cognitive deficits limit learning is being reexamined. For example, some people with dementia have demonstrated new learning from direct training (i.e., recognizing and using cues) that is maintained over time and generalized to other contexts (Brookshire, 2007). Spaced retrieval and errorless learning are two specific direct interventions that are gaining increasing attention from researchers in communication sciences and disorders. The implications of these findings will support reimbursement for direct interventions for persons with dementia that will increase significantly the quality of life for these individuals and their families.

There are global differences in the incidence and prevalence of dementia. Arai and colleagues (2004) reported on the incidence of dementia in Japan. They found a prevalence rate of slightly more than 2.8 per 1000 Japanese adults aged 70 to 74 years who presented with dementia, with a slightly higher rate for men than women, but a significantly higher prevalence among individuals 85 years and older (75.5 per 1000). Raina and coworkers (2008) reported a low incidence of dementia in Kashmiri (India) migrants of 5.34 per 1000 individuals aged 60 years and older. In Australia, along with the growing numbers of aging individuals, the prevalence of dementia without prevention methods is projected to increase from 172,000 individuals in 2000 to 588,000 in 2050 (Jorm et al., 2005). Similarly, the incidence and prevalence of dementia in Beijing, China is rising along with the increasing numbers of individuals 60 years and over; AD is the most common type of dementia seen in this population (Li et al., 2007). In Japan, vascular dementia has a higher prevalence than AD; this may be due to the differential distribution of lesions as cited by Gorelick (1998) or to other factors such as environment or genetics (Fratiglioni et al., 1999). One study compared elderly African Americans living in Indianapolis, Indiana, and Yoruba living in Ibadan, Nigeria (Hendrie et al., 2001). The authors found that African Americans were more than twice as likely to develop AD than Yoruba; that African Americans are at greater risk for development of AD, likely owing to a higher prevalence of hypertension; and that the presence of APOE-4 exerted some influence for African Americans, but not for Yoruba. From a global perspective, these numbers compel international leaders and professionals in health care to work together to (1) gain complete understanding of dementia and its socioeconomic impact (2) adequately identify, assess, and treat individuals with dementia; and (3) identify and train health care professionals to provide highly skilled services to these individuals and their families.

In the United States, there is some evidence that, neurophysiologically, dementia may look different between African Americans and whites (Froelich et al., 2001; Lichtenberg, 2009). First, it appears that vascular dementia accounts for a larger proportion of cases in African Americans than in whites; this is similar to the results found in Japan. Second, genetic etiologies of dementia of the AD type may also differ. For example, it appears that, although the presence of dementia is proportionally higher in African Americans (Froelich et al., 2001), the presence of the APOE-4 allele (associated with the development of AD) is greater in whites (Hendrie et al., 2004; Tang et al., 2001). Lichtenberg (2009) pointed out that, as the older population becomes increasingly diverse, it is important to understand the factors that affect diagnosis and treatment. Froelich and colleagues (2001) suggested that differences in etiology would have implications for customizing clinical services according to racial/ethnic group.

Incidence and prevalence studies indicate that African Americans and Hispanics aged 71 and older are more likely to have AD than older whites (i.e., 21.3% of African Americans versus 11.2% for whites). The high incidence of AD among African Americans and Hispanics may be related to the higher incidence of high blood pressure and diabetes in these groups, which are risk factors for AD (Alzheimer's Association, 2010).

Traumatic Brain Injury

The International Brain Injury Association (IBIA, 2010), and the North American Brain Injury Society (NABRS, 2010) have both cited brain injury as the leading cause of death and disability worldwide (2010), and the CDC states that "Traumatic brain injury is a significant public health problem in the United States." At least 1.7 million people sustain a TBI each year: of these, about 52,000 die, 275,000 are hospitalized, and 1.365 million are treated and released from an emergency department (CDC, 2010). According to the CDC, in the United States and the European Union, falls constitute the major cause of brain injury in adults 65 years and older; adults aged 75 years and older have the highest rates of TBI-related hospitalization and death.

There are several reported disparities in the treatment of TBI along racial/ethnic lines. In their comprehensive review of racial/ethnic differences in postinjury outcomes following TBI, Gary and colleagues (2009) found that "African Americans and Latinos have worse functional outcomes and community integration and are less likely to receive treatment and be employed than whites post-TBI" (p. 775). They further highlight the need for additional research to determine the efficacy or effectiveness of rehabilitation after TBI, citing only two studies that examined racial/ethnic information. This is also the case for mild TBI.

Bazarian and associates (2008) studied racial, ethnic, and gender disparities in the emergency department care of mild TBI at the National Hospital Ambulatory Medical Care Survey for the years 1998 through 2000. Cases of mild TBI were identified, and care variables related to imaging, procedures, treatments, and disposition were analyzed along racial, ethnic, and gender categories. The relationship among race, ethnicity, and selected care variables was analyzed using multivariate logistic regression with control for associated injuries, geographic region, and insurance type. The incidence of mild TBI was highest among men (590 per 100,000), Native Americans/Alaska Natives (1026.2 per 100,000), and non-Hispanics (391.1 per 100,000). After controlling for important confounders, Hispanics were more likely than non-Hispanics to receive a nasogastric tube; nonwhites were more likely to receive care by a resident and less likely to be sent back to the referring physician after discharge. Men and women received equivalent care.

Motor Speech Disorders

Motor speech disorders are impairments in the systems and mechanisms that control the movements necessary for the production of speech. They are a group of disorders resulting from disturbances in muscular control, weakness, slowness, or incoordination of the speech mechanism due to damage to the central nervous system. The term encompasses coexisting neurogenic disorders of several or all the underlying processes of speech: respiration, phonation, resonance, articulation, and prosody.

Dysarthria is a group of disorders that result from brain damage, largely stroke, and that impair speech intelligibility. Characterized by weakness, slowness, incoordination, and imprecise movements of the muscles of speech, dysarthria is classified as either progressive or nonprogressive. Progressive dysarthrias can be seen in patients with Parkinson's disease, Huntington's disease, multiple sclerosis, motor neuron disease, and so forth. Although the decline can be delayed in some cases, patients with progressive dysarthria show progressively declining function in the muscles over time. In contrast, patients with nonprogressive dysarthrias resulting from stroke and TBI can improve muscle function with treatment. Apraxia of speech is a motor speech disorder in which motor function is intact, but the neurologic mechanisms for planning and programming the motor speech sequences are impaired. Stroke is the primary cause of motor speech disorders in adults, and there is a high incidence and prevalence of stroke in nonmainstream cultural groups. Yet, until recently, literature on the impact of cultural and linguistic variability for assessment and treatment of acquired motor speech disorders has been extremely limited. Researchers have examined the affects of dysarthria on speech tone and prosody in some non-U.S. populations, including Bengali and Chinese Cantonese and Mandarin. For example, Chakraborty and colleagues (2008) studied dysarthric speech in Bengali adults and found that imprecise consonants were the most universal feature in the speech across five types of dysarthria studied. Other speech problems present included phonatory deficiency, strained voice, vocal tremor, monoloudness, and prosodic difficulties such as reduced stress, slow rate, and irregular articulatory breaks and hyperventilation. Many findings for Chinese speakers with dysarthria support earlier findings for English speakers, thus affirming the language-universal aspect of dysarthria. However, certain differences, which can be attributed to the distinct phonologies of Cantonese and Mandarin, highlight the language-specific aspects of the condition in speakers of Cantonese and Mandarin-Chinese who had Parkinson's disease and cerebral palsy. Because Chinese languages are highly tonal, dysarthria affects not only the segmental features of the languages but also the suprasegmental features, highlighting the interplay between the neurophysiologic features of dysarthria and the language-specific phonotactic aspects of different languages. In the United States, a prevailing question deals with the influence of dialect relative to dysarthric speech, particularly in African Americans who use African American Vernacular English (AAVE). This question warrants empirical study.

Neurogenic Dysphagia

Dysphagia is a condition of difficulty in swallowing owing to problems with nerve or muscle control. Dysphagia compromises nutrition and overall health and may lead to aspiration pneumonia and hydration. Acquired neurogenic dysphagia can result from a variety of etiologies, the most common of which is stroke. Although prevalence rates vary widely (Reilly & Ward, 2005), each year, between 300,000 and 600,000 people in the United States develop dysphagia as a result of stroke (ECRI, 1999). Approximately 51,000 of those individuals will develop dysphagia as a result of other neurologic conditions, including degenerative diseases such as AD, Parkinson's disease, and amyotrophic lateral sclerosis. Patients with head and neck cancers suffer with dysphagia, not to mention some medications for older adults will compromise the ability to swallow. Regardless of the etiology, dysphagia can lead to other, potentially life-threatening medical conditions in this population, including aspiration pneumonia and malnutrition (ECRI, 1999). Speech-language pathologists focus most of their attention on oropharyngeal dysphagia, although more and more, clinicians are being requested to work with patients who exhibit esophageal dysphagia.

In 2003, Code and Heron published the findings of their survey of speech and language therapists in the United Kingdom, showing that, between 1990 and 2000, there was an increase in the numbers of individuals with neurogenic disorders of communication and swallowing. However, they found that speech and language therapists primarily work with individuals with swallowing disorders and that the amount of time spent in aphasia therapy falls significantly below what is recommended in the literature. Although the response rate from the survey was low (33%), these findings give some indication of the variable treatment of the communication and swallowing disorders among the speech and language therapists in the United Kingdom.

Dysphagia receives considerable attention among speech-language pathologists; however, little attention has been given to the cultural issues involved in dysphagia treatment or in the prevalence of dysphagia across racial/ethnic groups. In a recent study, Gonzales-Fernandez, Kuhlemeier, and Palmer (2008) investigated racial disparities among a group of white, black, and Asian patients with stroke, Parkinson's disease, and oral cancer in California and New York. No significant differences were found among the patients with Parkinson's disease or oral cancer; however, Asians were more likely to have dysphagia after a stroke than members of the other two groups. The association was statistically significant after adjusting for age, sex, stroke severity, comorbidities, and stroke type.

McFarland (2008) reminds speech-language pathologists that there is a relationship between culture and food and feeding practices across cultures. The beliefs of the patient and the patient's family regarding nutrition and health play an important part in the evaluation and treatment of dysphagia. Issues, including religious practices regarding what to eat and what not to eat, the importance of food and feeding to the family, and language barriers

in providing dysphagia assessment and intervention, are important variables to consider.

Management of Neurogenic Communication and Swallowing Disorders

Racial and ethnic disparities in the occurrence and impact of neurogenic communication and swallowing disorders increase the need for culturally competent management of these disorders. African Americans and Hispanics experience poorer quality of health care and medical outcomes in the context of general medical care and in rehabilitation (Balcazar et al., 2010). It is therefore critical that management of neurogenic communication and swallowing disorders be delivered in a culturally competent manner.

Individuals with acquired neurogenic communication and swallowing disorders require the collaborative efforts of a multidisciplinary team of health care professionals who will be involved in the assessment, treatment, and discharge planning of the individual. The speech-language pathologist orchestrates the work of the team in conjunction with the primary medical physician.

Implications for Assessment

Providing culturally appropriate services to multicultural populations is a special challenge for speech-language pathologists. The challenges go beyond the language or languages used by the client and the family to many issues related to the culture of the client. Comprehensive assessment of communication and swallowing disorders entails four major areas: (1) patient staffing, (2) the clinical interview, (3) formal testing, and (4) feedback, planning, and follow-up (Brookshire, 2007). Each of these areas presents the opportunity to provide culturally competent, evidence-based services. For example, chart review allows the clinician to gain an understanding of the patient as a "whole person" prior to seeing the patient. Using the ICF model, information related to the patient's medical or health condition and demographic, educational, occupational, and sociocultural background provides insight about the aspects of communication or swallowing that are affected (based on the impairment; body structure and function), the severity of the disorder (the patient's level of activity and participation), the language and communication needs of the patient (e.g., if they are nonnative speakers of American English), and the level of family or friend support (personal and environmental factors). The goal of the assessment is to understand the client's experience of disability in relation to impairments and in relation to interaction with environmental and personal factors. It is the responsibility of the clinician to assess how the client functions in their unique environment and how they are able to participate in the activities important to themselves and their family according to their culture.

Functional assessment considers evaluating the natural course of client functioning and her or his potential to change. Equally important is determining what is important to the client and her or his family relative to functioning in their environment.

The clinical interview, importantly, confirms or disconfirms some or all of the clinician's impressions and, in most cases, adds greatly to the clinician's understanding of the individual's communication or swallowing difficulties. The clinical interview provides the initial opportunity for direct observation and assessment of the patient's strengths and weaknesses (activity) that will allow the clinician to make decisions about the next step in the clinical process (e.g., comprehensive speech and language assessment, bedside swallow examination or videofluoroscopic swallow examination, no services warranted at this time due to medical or health status). Even more important, during the clinical interview, the clinician establishes rapport, and helps to allay fears and apprehension about what has happened to the patient, and informs the patient as to what will happen next. As an alternative to the traditional interview, Westby (2009) suggested using ethnographic techniques with culturally and linguistically diverse individuals. For example, start by having a friendly conversation with the patient, family, and friends and then gradually introduce open-ended questions to facilitate sharing of experiences. Many individuals from nonmainstream populations have little appreciation for rapid-fire questioning because this can feel like formal interrogations that will quickly evaporate rapport (Westby, 2009). Ask the right questions. For example, ask questions that reveal information not in the chart review, shared by other health care professionals, or directly observed, such as "What do you hope to get out of therapy?" or "How can I help you communicate better with your wife/husband?" or "Do you have any questions?" Also, clinicians can ask questions to clarify what was written or said or to get more information that will be useful in planning the patient's program. When working with interpreters or family members who interpret, clinicians should maintain the same level of conversational tone and use appropriate body language (e.g., eye contact, gestures) as if they were speaking directly to the patient or family member (ASHA, 2004). If the individual does not have a family member present (e.g., the client is Hindi or Iranian and does not have family in the United States), it may be necessary to ask someone in their language community to serve as an interpreter, cultural broker, and advocate. The key to gathering good data through the clinical interview involves three characteristics: respect, reciprocity, and responsiveness (see Westby, 2009 for a full description of each). Briefly, respect refers to the acknowledgement and acceptance of the boundaries that exist among persons; reciprocity refers to the recognition that each person in the interaction has something valuable to contribute; and responsiveness refers to the willingness to listen without making judgments, to fully understand another's perspective, and to defer any and all stereotypes based on known racial, cultural, or ethnic information.

Changes in health care practice have led to the need for a paradigm shift in assessment practices to the extent that assessment tools should (1) assess a range of cognitive abilities, (2) quantify the impact of impairments on everyday activities, (3) allow for rapid test administration, and (4) meet psychometric standards. Depending on a number of factors, including the health care facility, the patient's medical condition, the patient's ability to pay, and so forth, the speech-language pathologist may have shorter periods in which to assess and treat patients. A study by Appeleros (2007) of hospitals in Sweden reported the mean length of stay as 12 days for stroke patients in acute-care hospitals, 30 days when the person was in a stroke unit, and longer stays (56 and 83 days) when the person is being seen in a rehabilitation unit and long-term-care facility, respectively. The challenge is to use the assessment to prioritize the salient aspects of the patient's speech, language, cognitive-communication, and swallowing abilities so that the patient will get the maximum benefit from the time spent with the speech-language pathologist.

Another challenge has to do with the particular assessments used to determine the patient's speech, language, communication, and swallowing abilities. The BDAE (Goodglass et al., 2000), the Western Aphasia Battery (WAB) (Shewan & Kertesz, 1980), and the Aachen Aphasia Test (Huber et al., 1984) are the most commonly used aphasia tests in the world. The Agency for Health Care Research and Quality (Biddle, 2002) noted that, despite the existence of a large number of tests and assessments for speech and language disorders, there continues to be only a few that reliably and validly assess the speech and language of individuals from culturally and linguistically diverse populations. For adult language assessments, the WAB met their relaxed standards for reliability and validity. For adult swallowing disorders, the evidence-based report by the Agency for Health Care Research and Quality concluded that full bedside examination sensitivities were nearly 80% accurate, suggesting that clinicians are capable of detecting most aspiration, even when it is silent.

Cross-language translations must be considered to ensure validity of the tests developed and produced in languages other than English and for cultural differences among client populations. For example, low levels of performance in a group of African Americans was associated with lack of familiarity with some test items on a neuropsychological test battery, resulting in lower performance than their counterparts in tests of cognitive functioning after TBI. The findings suggested that differences in cultural experience may be an important factor in the neuropsychological assessment of African Americans after TBI and provided support for the hypothesis that cultural factors may partially account for the differences among ethnic and cultural groups on neuropsychological tests (Kennepohl et al., 2004). Also, owing to lack of familiarity with some of the items, Cruice and colleagues (2000) found that Australians had lower scores on the BNT compared with North American and European populations. Similarly, a South African study (Mosdell et al., 2010) concluded that the BNT contained language and cultural bias that favored English speakers, even when education level was controlled. Clinicians should avoid using tests that have been simply translated from English because they may not capture the totality of the nonnative speaker's language and culture; rather, Paradis (2004) suggested using tests that evaluate equivalent ability levels, difficulty levels, and so forth. Also, language tests are particularly sensitive to cultural effects and education level, and, therefore, some individuals may show naming deficits where there are none.

Accurate interpretation of performance on communication and swallowing assessments must take into account the patient's cultural milieu. For example, patient preferences: Is the patient not able to swallow because of neurologic impairment or lack of preference for the food? A prevailing multicultural and international issue for clinicians is the ability to differentiate between a speech or language difference and speech or language disorder. According to ASHA (2010), a communication difference is a variation of a symbol system used by a group of individuals that reflects and is determined by shared regional, social, or cultural and ethnic factors. A regional, social, or cultural and ethnic variation of a symbol system should not be considered a disorder of speech or language. The comprehensive assessment should consider the language and speech of the patient before neurologic insult and make appropriate decisions about the patient based on that information. When an interpreter is used, it is imperative that, before testing, the speech-language pathologist assist the interpreter with making distinctions between the person's accent or dialect and a speech error. Examples can be provided and the interpreter can attend a brief training session before seeing the patient (ASHA, 2004).

The last area of assessment has to do with providing feedback, planning, and follow-up. When providing feedback, the speech-language pathologist should employ the same communication strategies as in the clinical interview. Cultural-ethnic background, level of acculturation, and other factors (e.g., time of day) will dictate whether the patient will have a single family member (i.e., a spouse) or additional family and/or non-family members present when communicating the diagnosis. The session provides another opportunity for the speech-language pathologist to observe the patient, keeping in mind that adults with neurogenic disorders display variable behavior over time. Importantly, one must be able to distinguish between those behaviors that result from the neurologic impairment (e.g., a woman who exhibits long silences) and culturally acceptable behaviors (e.g., quiet, deferential, particularly when her husband or a man is present). Planning for treatment should incorporate the patient's specific goals (e.g.,

returning to work); however, for persons with neurologic impairments, this may be difficult. If the person has difficulty speaking, it may be necessary to construct a low-technology augmentative-alternative means of communication such as a "yes-no" communication board to allow the patient to participate actively in the planning session. Use interpreters and cultural brokers as needed and involve the patient's family members. (See Chapter 14 for a further discussion of the issues involved in culturally appropriate assessment of adults with neurogenic disorders.)

Implications for Treatment

Speech-language pathologists are ethically bound to implement "best practices" when assessing and treating multicultural and international individuals who have acquired neurogenic disorders of speech, language, cognitive-communicative, and swallowing disorders. Providing culturally competent speech-language pathology services requires an understanding of (1) the cultural beliefs, values, traditions, and practices of the client; (2) the culturally defined, health-related needs of the client, the family, and the community; (3) the culturally based, health-related knowledge and belief systems that include illness, disease, healing, rehabilitation, and death and dying; and (4) the attitudes toward seeking help from health care providers.

The Academy of Neurologic Communication Disorders and Sciences has published Practice Guidelines that consist of systematic reviews of existing research studies that investigated treatment efficacy and treatment effectiveness for aphasia, apraxia of speech, dementia, dysarthria, and TBI. This rather extensive compilation of reviews of published research consists largely of early-stage studies (pre-efficacy) with small numbers of participants that used both group experimental and single-subject designs. Noticeably missing is research in multicultural populations, as pointed out by Turkstra and coworkers (2005).

For multicultural and international populations with neurogenic disorders, many of the treatment approaches may be appropriate. However, cultural factors can sometimes present barriers for the patient, and thus, they may not fully benefit from the services. Cultural factors can include level of acculturation, dialect, communication style, socioeconomic status, world view, and values and beliefs. Simpson and colleagues (2000) examined cultural variations in the understanding of TBI and rehabilitation with Italian, Lebanese, and Vietnamese individuals in Australia. Individuals in all three groups experienced stigma associated with brain injury and reported feeling socially isolated. They suggested that understanding the concept of "rehabilitation" varied widely among patients and their family members. Connotations of what rehabilitation means can run the gamut from training or retraining to outcomes to an "ongoing process" (p. 132). Depending on the patient's cognitive status, clinicians should have a frank conversation with the patient and family members at the beginning of the patient's treatment or rehabilitation. It is likely that when the patient and family members understand what they will be participating in, why, and what they hope to gain from therapy, the patient will stay with and complete the prescribed treatment. Still, some patients may be apprehensive about the process.

When treating persons with neurogenic disorders of communication and swallowing, culturally competent speech-language pathologists will:

- Be knowledgeable about possible cultural differences (relative to their own culture) that may impede the therapeutic process, and respond appropriately
- Gain a clear understanding of how patients feel about their communication or swallowing status
- Understand how to communicate effectively with patients and family members, including using friendly, nonverbal communication
- Treat the patient as an individual and provide support and reassurance without stereotyping
- Work closely with interpreters and cultural brokers and assist them in understanding the process before working with the patient
- Make treatment decisions using critical thinking and problem-solving abilities (clinical judgment) and incorporate within those decisions the most up-to-date and best available evidence (empirical research, consensus, expert opinion)
- Educate patients (and family members) about their brain and the injury they suffered, including how it functions and how they can live with their new communication and swallowing status, but also how to prevent further damage
- Adequately observe the patient to determine whether her/his communication or swallowing behavior is typical or atypical for their ethnic-cultural background (when in doubt, ask)

SUMMARY AND FUTURE RESEARCH

This chapter discussed acquired neurogenic disorders of speech, language, cognition-communication, and swallowing, with particular emphasis on the salient considerations important to multicultural and international populations. Discussions centered on providing culturally competent, evidence-based clinical practice in the context of an international framework using the most up-to-date research. Researchers in the communication sciences and disorders continue to investigate the efficacy and effectiveness of treatments for aphasia, apraxia of speech, dysarthria, dysphagia, and cognitive-communicative impairments secondary to stroke or brain attack, dementia, right hemisphere damage, and TBI in all individuals. However, very little research has examined the impact of racial, ethnic, and cultural variables on assessment and treatment of neurologic communication and swallowing disorders. Future research is needed to (1) provide an accurate picture of the epidemiology of neurogenic disorders in individuals from culturally and linguistically diverse backgrounds; (2) determine the impact of neurophysiologic differences in lesion distribution and its impact on treatment of neurologic communication and swallowing disorders; (3) assess the fairness and accuracy of standardized speech and language assessments; (4) determine the variable impacts of socioeconomic status and race and ethnicity to illuminate "true" cultural effects; (5) investigate neurologic communication disorders using stronger research designs (e.g., in bilingual persons with aphasia); (6) replicate findings of published studies to better understand treatment effects; and (7) come to consensus about the role of the speech-language pathologist for some of the relatively new classifications of neurogenic language disorders, including mild cognitive impairment and primary progressive aphasia (not covered in this writing).

DISCUSSION QUESTIONS

1. Discuss the ways in which dialect could interact with acquired motor speech disorders and the implications for assessment and treatment.
2. What are the implications for considering racial, ethnic, and gender differences in the neurophysiology of brain damage?
3. Using the WHO ICF framework, provide an example of an assessment or treatment plan with a multicultural or international individual who presents with a neurogenic communication or swallowing disorder.
4. Understanding the complexity of closed head injury, how might one disentangle cultural behaviors from those of brain injury? Include in your discussion specific examples of cognitive-communicative impairment (e.g., divergent versus convergent thinking), as well as some tools, tests, or tasks, that will assist with differentiating a cultural difference from a disorder.
5. Persons with dementia show a range of behaviors attributable to the disorder. What psychological construct appears to be intact for people with dementia? Discuss this construct and how it may provide a means for speech-language pathologists to treat some aspects of communicative decline in some persons with dementia.

REFERENCES

Administration on Aging (2010). Profile on older Americans. Retrieved from www.aoa.gov/aoaroot/aging_statistics/Profile/index.aspx.

Alzheimer's Association (2010). *Alzheimer's disease facts and figures* (vol. 6). Special Report: Race, Ethnicity and Alzheimer's Disease. Chicago: Author

American Speech-Language-Hearing Association (2010). Evidence-based practice link, retrieved December 19, 2010: http://www.asha.org/members/ebp/.

Arai, A., Katsumata, Y, Konno, K., & Tamashiro, H. (2004). Sociodemographic factors associated with incidence of dementia among senior citizens of a small town in Japan. *Care Management Journals, 5(3)*, 159-165.

Ardila, A., & Ramos, E. (2007). *Speech and language disorders in bilinguals.* New York: Nova Science Publishers.

Appeleros, P. (2007). Prediction of length of stay for stroke patients. *Acta Neurologica Scandinavica, 116*, 15-19.

Balacazar, F., Suarez-Balacazar, Y., Taylor-Ritzler, T., & Keys, C. (2010). *Race, culture and disability: Rehabilitation science and practice.* Boston: Jones & Bartlett.

Bates, E., D'Amico, S., Jacobsen, T., et al. (2003). Timed picture naming in seven languages. *Psychonomic Bulletin & Review, 10*, 344-380.

Battle, D. E. (2002). *Communication disorders in multicultural populations* (3rd ed). Boston: Butterworth Heinemann.

Bazarian, J., Pope, C., McClung, J., et al. (2008). Ethnic and racial disparities in emergency department care for mild traumatic brain injury. *Academic Emergency Medicine, 10*, 1209-1217.

Benton, A., Hamsher, K., & Sivan, A. *Multilingual aphasia examination* (3rd. ed.) (1994). Lutz, FL: Psychological Assessment Resources.

Bhatnagar, S. C. (2008). *Neuroscience for the student of communicative disorders* (3rd ed). Philadelphia: Lippincott Williams & Wilkins.

Biddle, A., Watson, L., Hopper, C., et al. (2002). *Criteria for determining disability in speech and language disorders.* Summary. Evidence Report/Technology. #52. AHRO Publication 02-E009. Rockville, MD: Agency for Health Care Research and Quality. Retrieved from http://archive.ahrq.gov/clinic/tp/spdistp.htm.

Brookshire, R. H. (2007). *Introduction to neurogenic communication disorders* (7th ed). St. Louis: Mosby Elsevier.

Byles, J. (2005). The epidemiology of communication and swallowing disorders. *Advances in Speech-Language Pathology, 7*, 1-7.

Centers for Disease Control and Prevention (2010). *Deaths: Preliminary data for 2008.* National Vital Statistics Reports, 59(2). Washington, DC: Author. (CDC). Retrieved February 24, 2011, from www.cdc.gov/nchs/data/nvsr/nvsr59/nvsr59_02.pdf.

Centers for Disease Control and Prevention (2010). *Traumatic brain injury.* Washington, DC: Author. Retrieved February 24, 2011, from www.cdc.gov/traumaticbraininjury/.

Chakraborty, N., Roy, T., Hazra, A., et al. (2008). Dysarthria in Bengali speech: A neurolinguistic study. *Postgraduate Medical Journal, 54*, 268-272.

Code, C., & Heron, C. (2009). Services for aphasia, other acquired adult neurogenic communication and swallowing disorders in the United Kingdom, 2000. *Disability and Rehabilitation, 25*, 1231-1237.

Cruice, M., Worrall, L., & Hickson, L. (2011). Psychological well-being of older adults in chronic aphasia in the context of unaffected peers. *Disability and Rehabilitation, 33*, 219-228.

Dronkers, N. F., Wilkins, D. P., Van Valin, R. D., et al. (2004). Lesion analysis of the brain areas involved in language comprehension. *Cognition, 92*, 145-177.

ECRI Health Technology Assessment Group (1999). Diagnosis and treatment of swallowing disorders (dysphagia) in acute-care stroke patients. Rockville, MD: Agency for Healthcare Research and Quality. Retrieved September 30, 2010, from http://archive.ahrq.gov/clinic/epcsums/dysphsum.htm.

Enderby, P., & Pickstone, C. (2005). How many people have communication disorders and why does it matter? *Advances in Speech-Language Pathology, 7*, 8-13.

Fabbro, F. (2001). The bilingual brain: bilingual aphasia. *Brain and Language, 79*, 201-210.

Faroqi-Shah, Y., Frymark, I., Mullen, R., & Wang, B. (2010). Effect of bilingual individuals with aphasia: A systematic review of the evidence. *Journal of Neurolinguistics, 23*, 319-341.

Fratiglioni, L., De Ronchi, D., & Torres, H. (1999). Worldwide prevalence and incidence of dementia. *Drugs, 15*, 365-375.

Frey, J. L., Jahnka, H. K., Bulfinch, E. W. (1998). Difference in stroke between white, Hispanic and Native American patients. *Stroke, 29*, 29-33.

Froehlich, T. E., Bogardus, S. T., & Inouye, S. K. (2001). Dementia and race: Are there differences between African Americans and Caucasians? *J Am Geriatr Soc, 49*, 477-484.

Gary, K. W., Arango-Laspilla, J. C., & Stevens, L. F. (2009). Do racial/ethnic difference exist in post-injury outcomes after TBI? A comprehensive review of the literature. *Brain Injury*, 23, 775-789.

Geertz, C. (1983). *Local knowledge: Further essays in interpretive anthropology.* New York: Basic Books.

Gillum, R. F. (1995). Epidemiology of stroke in Hispanic Americans. *Stroke, 26*, 1701-1712.

Gonzalez-Fernandez M., Kuhlemeier, K., Palmer J. (2008). Racial disparities in the development of dysphagia after stroke: Analysis of the California and New York inpatient databases. *Archives of Physical Medicine and Rehabilitation, 89*, 1358-1365.

Goodglass, H., & Kaplan, E. (1983). *Boston Diagnostic Examination of Aphasia.* San Antonio: Psychological Corporation.

Goodglass, H., & Kaplan, E. & Barresi, B. (2000). *Boston Diagnostic Examination of Aphasia* (3rd ed). San Antonio: Pearson Assessments.

Gorelick, P. B. (1998). Cardiovascular disease in African Americans. *Stroke, 29*, 2656-2664.

Gottfred, K. (2008, November 25). Scientifically based professional practice. *The ASHA Leader.*

Hendrie, H. D., Hall, K. S., Ogunniyi, A., & Gao, S. (2001). Incidence of dementia and Alzheimer's disease in 2 communities. *Journal of the American Medical Association, 285*, 739-747.

Hendrie, H., Ogunniyi, A., Hall, K., et al. (2004). Alzheimer's disease, genes, and environment: The value of international studies. *Canadian Journal of Psychiatry, 49*, 92-89.

Huber, W., Poeck, K., & Willmes, K. (1984). The Aechen Aphasia Test (AAT). *Advances in Neurology, 42*, 291-303.

Imam, I. (2002). Stroke: A review with an African perspective. *Annals of Tropical Medicine and Parasitology, 96*, 435-445.

International Brain Injury Association (2010). Retrieved from www.internationalbrain.org/?q=Brain-Injury-Facts.

International Classification of Functioning, Disability and Health (ICF). Retrieved December 19, 2010, from www.who.int/classifications/icf/en/.

Jorm, A., Dear, K., & Burgess, N. (2005). Projections of future numbers of dementia cases in Australia with and without prevention. *Australian and New Zealand Journal of Psychiatry, 39*, 959-964.

Justice, L. (2008). Evidence-based terminology. *American Journal of Speech-Language Pathology, 17*, 324-325.

Kaplan, E., Goodglass, H., & Weintraub, S. (1983). *The Boston Naming Test.* Philadelphia: Lea & Febiger.

Kaplan, E., Goodglass, H., & Weintraub, S. (2001). *The Boston Naming Test.* Baltimore: Lippincott Williams & Wilkins.

Kennepohl, S., Shore, D., Nabors, E., & Hanks, R. (2004). African American acculturation and neuropsychological test performance following traumatic brain injury. *Journal of International Neuropsychological Society, 101*, 566-577.

Klein, H. A. (2004). Cognition in natural settings: The cultural lens model. In M. Kaplan (Ed.), *Cultural ergonomics: Advances in human performance and cognitive engineering research* (vol. 4) (pp 249-280). Philadelphia: Elsevier.

Kremin, H., Akhatino, T., Basso, A., et al. (2003). A crosslinguistic data base for oral picture naming in Dutch, English, German, French, Italian, Russian, Spanish, Swedish (PEDI). *Brain & Cognition, 53,* 243-246.

Kohnert, K. (2009). Cross-language generalization following treatment in bilingual speakers with aphasia: A review. *Seminars in Speech and Language, 30,* 174-186.

Levine, C., Fahrbach, K., Siderowf, A., et al. (2004). *Diagnosis and treatment of Parkinson's disease: A systematic review of the literature. Evidence Report/Technology Assessments No.* 57, 1-4. Rockville, MD: Agency for Healthcare Research and Quality.

Li, H., Lam, W. W. M., & Wong, K. S. (2002). Distribution of intracranial vascular lesions in the posterior circulation among Chinese stroke patients. *Neurology Journal of Southeast Asia, 7,* 65-69.

Li, S., Yan, F., Li, G., et al. (2007). Is the dementia rate increasing in Beijing? Prevalence and incidence of dementia 10 years later in an urban elderly population. *Acta Psychiatrica Scandinavica, 115,* 73-79.

Lichtenberg, P. A. (2009). Disparities in dementia in later life among African Americans. *Annual Review of Gerontology and Geriatrics, 29,* 115-130.

Lorenzen, B., & Murray, L. L. (2008). Bilingual aphasia: A theoretical and clinical review. *American Journal of Speech-Language Pathology, 17,* 299-317.

Lubker, B. B. (1997). Epidemiology: An essential science for speech-language pathology and audiology. *Journal of Communication Disorders, 30,* 251-268.

Markus, H. S., Khan, U., Birns, J., et al. (2007). Differences in stroke subtypes between black and white patients with stroke: the South London Ethnicity and Stroke Study. *Circulation, 116*(19), 2157-2164.

Malik, A. M., Vora, N. A., et al. (2011). Endovascular treatment of tandem extracranial/intracranial anterior circulation occlusions: preliminary single-center experience. *Stroke, 42*(6), 1653-1657.

McFarland, E. (2008). Family and cultural issues in a school swallowing and feeding program. *Language, Speech, and Hearing Services in Schools, 39,* 119-213.

Mosdell, J., Balchin, R., & Ameen, O. (2010). Adaptation of aphasia tests for neurocognitive screening in South Africa. *South African Journal of Psychology, 40,* 250-261.

Myers, L. J. (1987). The deep structure of culture: Relevance of traditional African culture in contemporary life. *Journal of Black Studies, 18,* 72-85.

Neyer, J. R., Greenland, K. J., Denny, C. H., et al. (2005, May 18). Prevalence of stroke in the U.S.—2005. National Center for Chronic Disease and Health Promotion, Centers for Disease Control and Prevention. *Morbidity and Mortality Weekly Report, 56,* 469-474.

Ng, P. W. (2007). The stroke epidemic. *Hong Kong Medical Journal, 13,* 92-94.

North American Brain Injury Society (2010). Retrieved from http://www.nabis.org/, 2010).

Olness, G. S., Matteson, S. E., & Stewart, C. T. (2010). "Let me tell you the point": How speakers with aphasia assign prominence to information in narratives, *Aphasiology, 24,* 697-708.

Paradis, M. (2001). The need for awareness of aphasia symptoms in different languages. *Journal of Neurolinguistics, 14,* 85-94.

Paradis, M. (2004). *A neurolinguistic theory of bilingualism.* Amsterdam: John Benjamins.

Paul, R., & Elder, L. (2009). Miniature guide to critical thinking: concepts and tools. Foundation for Critical Thinking. Available at: www.criticalthinking.org.

Payne, J. C. (1997). *Adult neurogenic language disorders: Assessment and treatment—a comprehensive ethnobiological approach.* San Diego: Singular Publishing.

Pratt, C. A., Ha, L., Levine, S. R., & Pratt, C. B. (2003, July-August). Stroke knowledge and barriers to stroke prevention among African Americans: Implications for health communication. *Journal of Health Communication, 8,* 369-381.

Raina, S., Razdan, S., Pandita, K., & Raina, S. (2008). Prevalence of dementia among Kashmiri migrants. *Annals of Indian Academy of Neurology, 11,* 106-108.

Reilly, S., & Ward, E. (2005). The epidemiology of dysphagia. Describing the problem—are we too late? *Advances in Speech-Language Pathology, 7,* 14-23.

Roberts, P., & Kiran, S. (2007). Assessment and treatment in bilingual aphasia and bilingual anomia. In A. Ardila & E. Ramos (Eds.), *Speech and language disorders in bilinguals* (pp. 109-130). New York: Nova Science.

Sackett, D. L., Rosenberg, W. M. C., Gray, J. A. M., et al. (1996). Evidence based medicine: What it is and what it isn't. *British Medical Journal, 312,* 71.

Schindler, J. S., & Kelly, J. H. (2002). Swallowing disorders in the elderly. *Laryngoscope, 112,* 589-602.

Shewan, C., & Kertesz, A. (1980). Reliability and Validity of the Western Aphasia Battery. *Journal and Speech and Hearing Disorders, 45,* 208-324.

Simpson, G., Mohr, R., & Redman, A. (2000). Cultural variations in the understanding of traumatic brain injury and brain injury rehabilitation. *Brain Injury, 14,* 125-140.

Tang, M., Cross, P., Andrews, H., et al. (2001). Incidence of AD in African Americans, Caribbean Hispanics and Caucasians in northern Manhattan. *Neurology, 56,* 49-56.

Threats, T. T. (2010). The complexity of social/cultural dimension in communication disorders. *Folia Phoniatr Logop, 62,* 158-165.

Turkstra, L., Ylvisaker, M., Coelho, C., et al. (2005). Practice guidelines for standardized assessment for persons with traumatic brain injury. *Journal of Medical Speech-Language Pathology, 13,* ix-xxviii.

Ulatowska, H. K., Olness, G., Hill, C., et al. (2000). Repetition in narratives of African Americans: The effects of aphasia. *Discourse Processes, 30,* 265-283.

Ulatowska, H. K., & Olness, G. (2003, May). Relationship between discourse and Western Aphasia Battery performance in African Americans with aphasia. *Aphasiology, 17,* 511-521.

Wallace, G. (1997). *Multicultural neurogenics: A resource for speech-language pathologists providing services to neurologically-impaired adults from culturally and linguistically diverse backgrounds.* San Antonio: Psychological Corporation.

Westby, C. (2009). Considerations in working successfully with culturally/linguistically diverse families in assessment and intervention of communication disorders. *Seminars in Speech and Language, 30,* 279-289.

Wertz, R. T., Auther, L. L., & Ross, K. B. (1997). Aphasia in African Americans and Caucasians: Severity, improvement and rate of improvement. *Aphasiology, 11.*

United Nations Department of Economic and Social Affairs (2010). World Population Ageing: 1920-1950. Retrieved December 19, 2010, from www.un.org/esa/population/publications/worldageing19502050/.

Zhang, L. F., Yang, J., Hong, Z., et al. (2003a). Proportion of different subtypes of stroke in China. *Stroke, 34,* 2091-2096.

Zhang, L., Yang, J., Wu, Y., et al. (2003b). Incidence of ischemic and hemorrhagic stroke in Chinese populations. *Zhonghua Nei Ke Zazhi 42,* 94-97.

ADDITIONAL RESOURCES

Academy of Neurologic Communication Disorders and Sciences. Available at: www.ancds.org.

Promotes high-quality services to persons with neurologic communication disorders by developing standards of clinical practice, developing evidence-based practice guidelines, certifying clinical specialists in this area of practice, and providing continuing education programs.

Alzheimer's Association. Available at: www.alz.org/index.asp.

This nonprofit organization is the leading organization in the world for Alzheimer's disease care and support. The primary mission is to enhance care and support for people affected by Alzheimer's disease and related dementias. They do this by running over 4500 support groups, connecting people across the globe; delivering 20,000 education programs annually in 17 languages; funding research; hosting a comprehensive library; providing safety services; and hosting a 24/7 Help Line as well as other services.

American Speech-Language-Hearing Association. Available at: http://www.asha.org.

The professional, scientific, and credentialing association for 145,000 members and affiliates who are speech-language pathologists, audiologists, and speech, language, and hearing scientists in the United States and internationally. The organization provides educational programs and resources that support the work of its members who provide clinical services and conduct research with individuals with speech, language, voice, swallowing, hearing, and balance disorders. ASHA advocates on behalf of persons with communication and swallowing disorders, advances the science of communication and its disorders, and promotes effective human communication in all persons.

American Speech-Language-Hearing Association (2004). Knowledge and Skills Needed by Speech-Language Pathologists and Audiologists to Provide Culturally and Linguistically Appropriate Services [Knowledge and Skills]. Available at: www.asha.org/policy.

American Speech-Language-Hearing Association (2005). Cultural Competence [Issues in Ethics]. Available at: www.asha.org/policy.

International Association of Logopedics and Phoniatrica. Available at: www.ialp.info.

To improve the quality of life of individuals with disorders of voice, speech, language, swallowing, and hearing. The organization has members in 55 countries around the world and has 13 committees, including aphasia, motor speech disorders, and dysphagia, that study, report, and hold conferences on the issues related to international perspectives.

International Brain Injury Association. Available at: www.internationalbrain.org/.

Established to encourage international exchange of information, to support research, to provide training especially in developing countries and to advocate for brain injury.

National Aphasia Association. Available at: www.aphasia.org/.

A nonprofit organization that promotes public education, research, rehabilitation, and support services to assist people with aphasia and their families. The association is a network of 440 support groups for persons with aphasia in the United States and international locations. Its members include bilingual clinicians who work to enhance the understanding and management of aphasia and its consequences in different linguistic and sociocultural environments, including Spanish, Hindi, German, French, Russian, Chinese, Korean, Urdu and other languages.

WHO World Report on Disability. Availiable at: www.who.int/disabilities/world_report/2011/report/en.

The first ever WHO/World Bank World report on disability reviews evidence about the situation of people with disabilities around the world.

Chapter 9

Cultural Diversity and Fluency Disorders

Tommie L. Robinson, Jr.

The relevance of cultural and international factors in the assessment and treatment of communication disorders has been discussed in the literature (Battle, 1997; Guitar, 2006; Taylor, 1986; Terrell & Hale, 1992; Proctor et al., 2008). Essentially, the relevance is, in order for assessment to be accurate and meaningful and for treatment to be maximally effective, both should be conducted with regard to the client's cultural identity, cultural assimilation, cultural environment, and cultural system (Crowe et al., 2000; Robinson & Crowe, 1998). Clinicians and researchers have attempted to address this issue by providing models for service delivery in various clinical settings and with various cultures (Robinson & Crowe, 1994; Robinson & Crowe, 1998; Seymour, 1986; Seymour & Seymour, 1977; Taylor, 1986; Taylor & Payne, 1983; Taylor & Samara, 1985; Van Kleeck, 1994; Vaughn-Cooke, 1983, 1986). These models, for the most part, have been discussed relative to nonbiased assessment of speech articulation disorders, with little reference to the treatment process.

Attention has been given to the influence of cultural factors on the evaluation and treatment of stuttering (Bullen, 1945; Cooper & Cooper, 1993; Crowe et al., 2000; Robinson & Crowe, 2000, Watson & Kayser, 1994). Consideration of cultural variables should begin when clients or their families first contact clinical centers to schedule evaluations or merely to obtain information. Clinical intervention for treatment of stuttering should be structured within the context of each client's *cultural system* and *cultural environment*. After determining the client's *cultural identity* and *degree of assimilation* into the culture, in order for therapy to be maximally effective and also for therapy to be efficient in regard to time spent setting and achieving goals. Clinicians' attention to these cultural dimensions of the therapy relationship also will increase the probability that counseling for the prevention of stuttering will be effective (Crowe, 1995).

Cultural system pertains to all that composes the belief systems of clients. This includes values, attitudes, perceptions, myths, and so on, and to a large extent these culture-based factors determine the perceived reality in which clients operate. The client's perceptions of reality may or may not match the clinician's; if their perceptions do not match, there is likelihood that intervention, and especially counseling, will not be maximally effective. Of course, cultural variables account for only one of the reasons that a client and clinician's phenomenal field may not match, but different cultural systems is a frequent reason why they do not. Phenomenal field in this context refers to the comprehensive experiences and belief systems of individuals.

Cultural environment is also important to take into consideration when structuring a plan for counseling in fluency intervention. This includes all aspects of the client's environment: his or her phenomenal field; access to experience; semantic environment; relationships with significant others; and language environment. In the case of child clients, it is important for clinicians to remember that parents are the chief architects of their child's environment and should be counseled to be active in designing an environmental gestalt for their child that is conducive to speech fluency and to normal personality development (Crowe, 1994). The environment of the child with disfluencies should be conducive to him or her developing the use of ego functions that might in turn help prevent the development of defensive reactions to speech disfluency and to speech therapy.

A general model for inclusion of these cultural factors in assessment and therapy planning for individuals who stutter is discussed later in this chapter. Also discussed later are techniques for identifying aspects of the client's cultural identity, cultural assimilation, cultural environment, and cultural system as well as the influence of culture on beliefs and behavior related to stuttering.

UNIVERSALITY OF FLUENCY DISORDERS

Like most disorders that affect the human condition, fluency disorders, in specific stuttering, are not restrained by geographic demarcations. Stuttering appears on every continent, in every country, in every corner of the globe. The evidence for the universality of stuttering is summarized effectively by Van Riper (1982), Bloodstein (1995), and Bloodstein and Bernstein Ratner (2008).

The universality of stuttering pertains to cultures as well as continents and countries. There is strong evidence that stuttering appears in all cultures, or to put it more conservatively, there is no compelling evidence for any culture that indicates stuttering does exist within it.

Cultural groups that have been studied include Native Americans (Clifford et al., 1965; Johnson, 1944a, 1944b; Lemert, 1953; Snidecor, 1947; Stewart, 1960; Zimmerman et al., 1983), African Americans (Anderson, 1981; Brutten & Miller, 1988; Conrad, 1985; Ford, 1986; Goldman, 1967; Leith & Mims, 1975; Nathanson, 1969; Proctor et al., 2008; Robinson, 1992; Robinson & Crowe, 1987, 1998; Robinson et al., 2000), Asians (Lemert, 1962; Toyoda, 1959; Wakaba, 1983), Hispanics (Bernstein-Ratner & Benitez, 1985; Dale, 1977; Jayaram, 1983; Nwokah, 1988; Travis et al., 1981), West Indies (Ralston, 1981); and African (Aron, 1962; Goodall & Brobby, 1982; Kirk, 1977; Morgenstern, 1953, 1956; Nwokah, 1988). Results of these studies generally suggest that cultural differences influence speech fluency and that there are differences in perceptions, beliefs, values, and norms about speech fluency and fluency disorders among various cultural groups. One possible significance of these suggestions is that cultural factors might appreciably affect the outcomes of clinical intervention with fluency disorders.

There has been disputation about the universality of stuttering with argument that it is not universal based on sparse, largely anecdotal data that for the most part were later refuted. The best known case of this was the assertion by Johnson (1944) and two of his students, Snidecor (1947) and Stewart (1960), that stuttering did not exist in the Utes, Bannock, and Shoshone American Indian tribes. This idea was on the researchers' findings that no stuttering was reported in interviews with numbers of the tribes, social pressures on communication appeared to be minimal within the tribes, and no word in the tribal languages could be found for stuttering. Evidence was later presented (Zimmerman, 1983) that stuttering does exist in these American Indian tribes.

PREVALENCE OF STUTTERING AMONG CULTURES

Although the idea that in some cultures stuttering may not exist is given little credence today. The thought associated with it that social demand on communication and stuttering might be positively correlated may be one possible explanation for varying prevalence among cultures. Cooper and Cooper (1998) stated that "universally accepted definitions do not exist regarding what constitutes the fluency disorders that the English terms *stuttering* and *stammering* and their equivalents in other languages have come to encompass and symbolize" (pp. 252-253). They also pointed to a great deal of variability in the data collection process across cultures. Van Riper (1982) and Bloodstein (1995) indicated that the prevalence of stuttering in the general population is about 0.8%, whereas the incidence of stuttering in some cultural groups is between 5% and 10%. Tables 9-1 through 9-5 depict prevalence research in various cultural groups.

Factors that Influence Stuttering in Cultural Groups

Researchers have reported a number of factors that may influence all aspects of speech and language. Some of these factors have been discussed earlier in this text and have been highlighted over the years by researchers and scholars as having great impact on the service delivery to clients and their families. Specific to the area of stuttering, such influences have been linked to attitudes, myths and beliefs, religion, nonverbal behaviors, and events in the life cycle.

Attitudes

An attitude is a state of mind, feeling, orientation, or disposition (American Heritage Dictionary, 1996). For years, researchers and clinicians have examined the relationship between stuttering and attitude. It has been determined that attitude plays a major role in both the diagnostic and treatment processes. The feelings that accompany stuttering are a major component of the stuttering syndrome. Starkweather (1980) indicated that treating one aspect and ignoring the other dooms any therapeutic approach to failure.

From a cultural prospective, the attitude toward communication disorders and, more specifically, stuttering changes from cultural group to cultural group. Harris (1986) indicated that attitudes evolve from individuals' value systems

TABLE 9-1 African American Populations

Study	No. of Subjects	Findings
Waddle (1934)	1582	1.7:1 Ratio in children
Carson & Kanter (1945)	NA	60% Higher than white children
Neely (1960)	NA	No differences
Pritchett (1966)	NA	1.3:1.0 Ratio of African American to white children
Goldman (1967)	694	2.4:1.0 Ratio of African American male to female children
Gillespie & Cooper (1973)	5054	2.8%
Conrad (1980)	1271	2.7% African American adults (2:1 ratio male to female)
Proctor et al. (2008)	2223	2.60%

TABLE 9-2 African Populations

Study	No. of Subjects	Findings
Morgenstern (1953, 1956)	5618	2.67% Ibo schoolchildren
Aron (1962)	6581	1.26% Bantu schoolchildren
Kirk (1977)	NA	High incidence of disfluent speech (non-pathologic) among children from Ghana
Goodall & Brobby (1982)	NA	5.5% Prevalence in Dakar schoolchildren 3.5% Prevalence in Accra district
Nwokah (1988)	NA	Incidence in Nigerians and West Africans may be the highest in the world

TABLE 9-3 Caribbean Populations

Study	No. of Subjects	Findings
*McCartney (1971)	NA	1.07-4.46% Prevalence among Bahamians
Ralston (1981)	1999	4.7% Prevalence in Caribbean children
Leith & Gibson (1991)	1217	3.6% Prevalence in children in Nassau

Cited in Leith and Gibson (1991).

TABLE 9-4 Hispanic Populations

Study	No. of Subjects	Findings
Leavitt (1974)	10,455	0.84% Prevalence in New York City Puerto Ricans
Leavitt (1974)	10,499	1.50% Prevalence in Puerto Ricans in San Juan
Ardila et al. (1994)	1879	2% Prevalence among Spanish-speaking university students from Bogota, Colombia

TABLE 9-5 Asian Populations

Study	No. of Subjects	Findings
Toyoda (1959)	140,000	0.82% Prevalence in Japanese schoolchildren
Ozawa (1960)	7600	0.90% Prevalence in Japanese school children
Lemert (1962)	NA	More stuttering among Japanese than among Polynesians

disabilities, the elements necessary for a difference in the value of rehabilitation, and the differences between their own belief systems and those of their clients (p. 229).

Myths and Beliefs

It is important for clinicians to be familiar with the myths and beliefs of the culture group relative to the etiologic factors and approaches to intervention for stuttering. It is also important to note that some myths and beliefs are rooted in the fact that in some cultures, families do not see the value in speech-language services. Clinicians must take these myths very seriously because they represent the parents' honest understanding of stuttering. Robinson and Crowe (1998) provided the following examples of African American myths about stuttering.

Stuttering is caused by:
- The mother eating improper foods when breastfeeding the infant
- Allowing an infant to look in the mirror
- Tickling the child too much
- Cutting the child's hair before he or she says his or her first words
- The mother seeing a snake during pregnancy
- The mother dropping the baby
- The child being bitten by a dog
- The work of the devil

Stuttering can be treated by:
- Stuttering can be controlled by the child.
- Stuttering can be controlled by telling the child not to move his or her feet when talking.
- Stuttering can be cured by hitting the child in the mouth with a dish towel.
- Stuttering can be cured by having the child hold nutmeg under his or her tongue.

Religion

Some cultural groups are deeply rooted in religious practice. Clinicians should be mindful that, sometimes, religious practices might greatly influence family's acceptance

and culture. She further indicated that these value systems are often so ingrained in a person's mind that his or her values become truth, usually not only for that particular person but for all humans. Practitioners must acknowledge the potential for differences in perception of the causes and meaning of of the stuttering intervention process. For example, in some cultural interactions, clinicians may find that the group views stuttering as a curse from God. Yet in another group, seeking the service in general may be against religious practices.

Nonverbal Behaviors

During their interactions with children and adults, clinicians should be mindful of nonverbal behaviors such as silence, eye contact, and physical activity levels (e.g., excessive gross motor behavior, constant body movements, out-of-seat behavior, extraneous hand movements). These are often misconstrued as secondary mannerism or avoidance behaviors when they are in fact cultural differences in nonverbal behaviors.

Events in the Life Cycle

Stuttering has been linked with a number of holidays, family activities, and events in the lives of clients. Clinicians find themselves developing clinical strategies to address the stressors that may develop from these events. Further, clinicians also see correlation with the degree of stuttering with regard to these events. It is important to know the events that individuals find stressful in various cultural groups. For example, a Jewish person who stutters might find it stressful to read from the Torah during synagogue or Bar Mitzvah service, whereas in a Central American family, a young lady who stutters might have exceptional difficulty with her speech at the time of her *quincianera* (celebration of the 15th birthday symbolizing womanhood).

A CULTURE-BASED MODEL

Robinson and Crowe (1998) presented a decision model for inclusion of multicultural variables in stuttering intervention. In this model, six levels are presented: preintervention; intake; evaluation; client counseling; treatment; and carryover or generalization. Decisions are made at each intervention level as to the relevance of cultural variables in the intervention process. At each level, the decision is also made whether to revisit previous levels or to expedite progress through a given level.

Decision level I (preintervention). In this level, the client's cultural identification, age, gender, and communication norms are determined.
Decision level II (intake). This level includes general disorder typing, specific cultural variables relative to stuttering, myths, attitudes, terminology, and beliefs.
Decision level III (evaluation). At this level, the clinician is encouraged to make cultural adjustments for nonverbal behaviors of the client as well as verbal

language and interaction and visual stimuli. The clinician should also look at cognitive learning styles, parental-child interaction, and how the client interacts with the clinician.
Decision level IV (client counseling). This level allows the clinician to look at rules for interaction and how they affect the counseling process. The clinician should also examine the family unit for cultural identity, residential history, generational factors, and the language spoken in the home and its importance.
Decision level V (treatment). At this level, the clinician should build cultural-based experiences, factors, and interactions into the treatment process.
Decision level VI (carryover or generalization). This is when the clinician involves the home, peers, and client to ensure that the skills learned in therapy are taken outside of the treatment room.

This model may be used from an international perspective as well if one thinks of the notion that culture touches everyone and everyone is from a culture. Regardless of one's background, each of the principles in the model affect the individual client as an individual.

CULTURE-RELATED ISSUES IN ASSESSMENT AND TREATMENT

Making assumptions about a client's cultural identity is a mistake. Clinicians must be mindful that cultural identity goes beyond the race of individuals and that just because a culture has been assigned to the client does not mean that the client identifies with that particular culture. Second, after the cultural identity of the client has been determined, his or her age and gender must also be considered before evaluation because, in some cultures, these variables influence the communication norms that are expected by clients or parents of clients. At this point, clinicians will have enough information to make generalizations regarding the culture-based beliefs and values about communication that the clients and their significant others bring to the clinical setting (Watson & Kayser, 1994).

A factor that should be considered when gathering culture background information about a client is his or her degree of cultural assimilation. This is the idea that although clients may identify with a given culture, they may not be fully assimilated into the culture. This degree of assimilation in a particular culture may vary from client to client.

Assessment

Most standardized assessment programs often do not consider cultural information, so clinicians should add this information to the clinical protocol. First of all, clinicians should consider areas such as the cultural identity, cultural assimilation, cultural environment, and cultural system (i.e. attitudes and beliefs). Crowe and colleagues (2000) provide an example of a format that can be used to guide clinicians' discovery in these areas. Their form examines the extent to which the child understands areas like cultural identity, cultural assimilation, cultural environment, and cultural systems and beliefs.

Next, clinicians may find it necessary to modify test items or testing procedures to make them more inclusive of culturally specific visual stimuli. Clinicians should also note that when working with children who stutter, parent-child interaction is an important part of the data-gathering process. Clinicians should consider the differences based on cultural backgrounds. Particular attention should be given to issues such as directive behaviors, child-rearing practices, and verbal expectations, which often influence parent-child interaction (Conrad, 1985; Hartfield et al., 2005). With adults, clinicians must note culture-specific pragmatic and social interaction styles, such as who is allowed to speak and when, what are the rules for interruptions, and how topics are introduced. Finally, commercial programs are often used during the evaluation process. They are often standardized based on normative data or items that were developed with the mainstream population in mind. Clinicians should feel comfort in knowing that modifications to these testing instruments can and should be made with the client's cultural background in mind.

Culture-Specific Test Items

During the evaluation process, clinicians should consider the cultural experiences of the clients. When using commercial programs as a means for evaluating speech fluency, it is important to take these experiences into consideration. For example, a clinician using the Stuttering Prediction Instrument for Young Children with an urban Hispanic child may want to review the suggested "topics to elicit conversation" presented by Riley (1981). In the review, the clinician needs to determine the experiences that the child has had relative to his or her presentation. If a child has never had a traditional birthday party or planted a garden, as suggested in the instrument, it may be difficult to expect a response. By the same token, the story plates used in this instrument depict middle-class white America. Clinicians may want to substitute these story plates with pictures that reflect the child's specific culture and culturally relevant experiences.

Similar test modification can be easily made with adults in mind. Conversational samples should reflect their experiences and their culture rather than the experience and expectations of the clinician. As clinicians gather speech samples, topics should be of interest to the client and include a representative sample of the client's speech fluency behavior. Although a number of procedures may be implemented to address the specific needs of individual clients, clinicians must be responsible to ensure that the integrity of the instrument is not at risk.

Parent-Child Interaction

An important aspect of conducting a speech fluency evaluation on preschool- and early school-aged children is observation of the parent-child interaction. It is crucial that clinicians are aware of the interaction styles that are specific to different cultures. There is nothing more demeaning to parents than being told their child-rearing practices and interaction skills are causing their child to stutter. The clinician can avoid this by selectively seeking to understand the cultural dynamics of the family. During the evaluation process, clinicians should use caution in conveying this information to the parent and also should seek to research and understand the culture's interaction style. Rules that govern when children are allowed to talk, how conversations are initiated with children, who initiates the conversation, emotionality, and nonverbal behaviors within the culture should be examined.

Pragmatic and Social Interaction Style

Social language behavior also plays a major role in speech fluency behavior, especially with adults who stutter. Often during the evaluation process, clinicians tend to observe and evaluate the client's level of interaction as it pertains to verbal behaviors (e.g., interruptions, initiating conversation, turn-taking, vying for the floor) and nonverbal behaviors (e.g., hand, facial, head, and whole-body movements; eye contact). In cases in which there is no understanding of the culture, clinicians can easily diagnose behaviors as abnormal in these areas. In reality, these observations should be evaluated as differences rather than disorders.

Treatment

Commercial Programs

When using a commercial fluency treatment program that involves specific activities and materials, clinicians may have difficulty developing strategies to enhance the cultural sensitivity of the program. However, clinicians may find that the program's concepts can be preserved and used with other activities for cultural enrichment. For example, a component of the Fluency Development System for Young Children (Meyers & Woodford, 1992) can be adjusted by substituting characters that are familiar to the client rather than the "Tortoise and Hare" story as a basis for establishing the cognitive linguistic components of the therapy program. For programs that do not require adherence to specific activities and materials, modification for inclusion of culturally sensitive materials can be made easily. For example, when using the Fluency Rules Therapy Program for Young Children (Runyan & Runyan, 1986) or the Stuttering Therapy for Children (Gregory & Hill, 1980) with a school-aged child who is interested in sports, clinicians can use sport activities and can easily incorporate sports-related narrative discourse activities.

Intervention

Intervention for stuttering and fluency disorders should be based in factors previously discussed such as values, beliefs, attitudes, religion, and interaction styles. Strategies should be developed and incorporated to minimize cultural bias and to ensure clients and families of the value in their beliefs. Here again, clinicians should make an effort to modify stimuli so that they represent the client's cultural background. In addition, clinicians should focus on ways to enhance the clinician-child interaction, clinician-family interaction when necessary, cognitive learning styles with children (Robinson & Crowe, 1998), and social interaction styles of the adults. Some suggestions for each area are presented next.

Clinician-Child Interaction

1. *Use culturally relevant and culturally appropriate topics during discussion.* This will aid the clinician in understanding the client and will make culture an ongoing focus in the treatment process. Selecting the right topic for discussion will make the client feel as if the focus of therapy has his or her interests at heart. This also helps with motivation in adolescents and adults.
2. *Incorporate the physical activity levels of the individuals.* This technique is important when working with children whose physical activity levels are high and whose cognitive learning style is different. Teaching children to maintain speech fluency control during high-energy movements is more feasible than trying to change physical behaviors.
3. *Monitor the client's secondary mannerisms to distinguish them from "normal" behaviors.* During the therapy process, it is important for clinicians to devote time to ongoing assessment of secondary mannerisms. In some cultures, expressive verbal communication may be accompanied by nonverbal movements that may be reflected in facial contortions, extraneous body movements, hand gestures, or eye contact. Clinicians should provide ongoing study of these behaviors to rule out cultural influence. This can be done through observing others in the culture (i.e., parents, significant others, community), interviewing individuals from the culture, and reading information about the specific culture.
4. *Expand the treatment program by using peers and the family unit as a part of remediation.* Including friends and family members as a part of the treatment process will provide the client with a support system to aid in building self-esteem and will encourage carryover. Culturally, some groups are more comfortable with the extended family units, and clinicians will find that the family works better than peers in this regard.

Clinician-Family Interaction

1. *Understand and correct myths.* It is important for clinicians to be familiar with the myths of the culture group relative to etiologic factors and approaches to therapy for stuttering. Clinicians must take these myths very seriously because they represent the parents' and clients' honest understanding of stuttering. Clinicians should be able to offer alternative approaches to the myths or aid the family in understanding the origin of the myths, or both.
2. *Address the learning style of all individuals involved.* Clinicians should consider the learning styles of everyone involved with the well-being and care of the client. In addition to recognizing the low literacy rate of in some cultures, clinicians may also want to incorporate learning styles in the therapy process. For example, with some African American children, physical activity levels, language use, and whole-to-part or relational learning should be given close attention. Hilliard (1976) and Hale-Benson (1987) described relational learning styles in opposition to analytic learning styles. They indicated that analytical cognitive styles may include characteristics such as stimulus centered; parts specific; long attention span; standard English language style; formal and stable rules for language organization; and long concentration span. Aspects of relational cognitive style may include self-centeredness; global; fine descriptive characteristics; fluent spoken language; short attention span; short concentration span; gestalt learning; and language dependent on unique context, interactional characteristics of the communicants, time and place, inflection, muscular movements, and other nonverbal cues. Many, but not all, African American children use relational learning styles. Although this is one example, our clinical encounters lead us to a variety of cultures, and for each, these characteristics should be considered.
3. *Incorporate parents and significant others in the intervention process as culturally appropriate.* Depending on the cultural group, some parents feel more a part of the treatment process if they are "hand-on" participants. Yet with another group, more expectations are placed on the clinicians as the primary change agent. With this in mind, clinicians should take under considerations such characteristics as parental involvement, literacy skills, educational level, and employment when giving assignments and modeling techniques for parents and significant others.

Cognitive Learning Style

1. *Develop functional and hands-on activities.* At this level, clinicians should be mindful of the need to make treatment activities as engaging and exciting as possible. With individuals from diverse backgrounds, clinicians must determine whether their learning style is relational or analytic and develop activities accordingly.

2. *Switch activities frequently.* The learning style of the individual will also determine the frequency of variability activities. From a cultural standpoint, clients with a relational learning style will need engaging speech fluency activities that take into consideration their attention span and concentration span.

3. *Make treatment programs reflective of the cultural experiences of the clients.* This concept has been emphasized throughout this chapter. It is factor that should be applied to each clinical encounter so that individuals from diverse cultures are not penalized for experiences that have not been a part of their lives. It is important for clinicians to conduct extensive interviews, interactions, and observations as well as to keep an open line of communication with all individuals involved in the client's environment. When developing speech fluency goals and activities, the clinician should include specific experiences of the client.

Social Interaction Style

1. *Learn how the individual communicates in his or her culture.* Clinicians should be mindful of attributes such as silence, interruptions, topic maintenance, and verbal expectations in both children and adults. Often, clients and their families are penalized for interaction styles that clinicians judge to be inappropriate. The clients' evidence may in fact be a culturally specific interaction style that has no deleterious effect on speech.

2. *Create mock social interactions.* Clinicians may find use in creating social settings that can be used to prepare the client for actual events. Creating scenarios such as ordering in a restaurant, talking on the telephone, asking someone out on a date, or making a class presentation are pragmatic and functional communication processes. These also prove to be invaluable to meeting the social needs of clients. Using this approach also allows for individuality of goals and objectives and allows the clinician the opportunity to work with the unique culture of the client.

3. *Use verbal conflict as a therapy tool.* For cultural groups that place high regard on being verbal, it is important that clinicians incorporate as much activity in this regard as possible. An effective way to accomplish this is by engaging the client in verbal conflict. This is done by taking an opposing viewpoint on an issue of discussion between the client and the clinician. Using this strategy helps the client prepare to engage in conversation and verbal exchange with peers and family members.

THE ARC OF COUNSELING

Although counseling is an ongoing process, it should definitely begin at the speech fluency evaluation. This is an especially important level in clinical intervention with multicultural clients because it is here that the stage is set for therapy, ideally with the complete comprehension and support of clients and their families. Clinicians should be mindful of the three aspects of counseling. The first aspect is that counseling should begin, when possible, before stuttering develops and definitely before stuttering becomes severe. This becomes a challenge to clinicians, especially because there are cultural myths and beliefs about the necessity of the intervention process. The second aspect of counseling concerns the interpretation of test results to clients, definition of the disorders and its treatment, and explanation of prognosis. Clinicians should remember to observe rules for cultural interaction. This will remove potential sources of miscommunication between clients and clinicians. The third aspect of counseling addresses personal adjustments of the clients and significant others as an ongoing part of the treatment process. Here it is important that the clinician explore the possible significance of cultural identity, residential history, and generational factors.

It is also important that clinicians understand rules about interacting with individuals from diverse backgrounds. Important attributes such as touching, establishing eye contact, and observing levels of emotion are crucial to the counseling session. Clinicians must be able to adjust to cultural differences in order to win the trust of clients and parents so that counseling with them will be maximally effective.

SUMMARY

There remains a dearth of information relative to examining speech fluency and stuttering in populations other than the mainstream. A review of the literature reveals limited research pertaining to cultural groups, and clinical experience indicates that there is a need for future study. Specifically, there is a need for study of cultural influences in the following areas:

Development of Stuttering

There still exists the need to study the development of stuttering in multicultural populations. Limited information is available on the course that stuttering takes in multicultural groups. Perhaps there are developmental differences that might warrant a course of intervention that is quite different from our current offerings. Such studies might examine the development of stuttering in various populations as well as parent-child interaction, family-child interaction, and general characteristics. For example, Einarsdóttir and Ingham's (2005; 2008; 2009; 2010) work focuses on Icelandic clients but has great implications for international studies and what the needs are in those populations. The same holds true for Boey and associates' (2009) work with Dutch-speaking children and the work with populations in the United Kingdom undertaken by Fry and colleagues

(2009), Millard and coworkers (2008; 2009), and Biggart and associates (2006).

Manifestation

There is also the need to explore those attributes that mark speech fluency disorders in multicultural populations. It has been suggested that there are differences in interaction styles, attitudes, secondary mannerisms, disfluency types, and beliefs that related to stuttering. There is now a need to provide empirical data that support these hypotheses and suggestions.

Intervention

The intervention process continues to be the most challenging area for clinicians. Given the rich diversity of the individuals who seek our services, applying the cookie-cutter approach to intervention is not sufficient. There is a need to further explore both the evaluation and therapy processes to maximize service delivery options to multicultural populations. For example, the Lidcombe program (Onslow et al., 2003) can be easily adapted to meet cultural expectations.

LAST WORDS

Finally, as a word of caution, it is important that contemporary research move away from comparing cultural groups in research protocols and begin to examine and explore groups for their own uniqueness. There is no clinical value in comparing individuals from multicultural groups to the mainstream population. However, there is clinical value in understanding how specific populations function in terms of stuttering and what the needs and concerns might be regarding the roles of particular clients and particular cultures in stuttering, thus contributing to evidence-based practice.

REFERENCES

American heritage dictionary of the English language (3rd ed.) (1996). Boston: Houghton Mifflin.

Anderson, B. (1981). An analysis of the relationship of age and sex to type and frequency of disfluencies in lower socioeconomic preschool Black children. Unpublished doctoral dissertation, Northwestern University, Evanston, IL.

Ardila, A., Bateman, J. R., & Nino, C. R. (1994). An epidemiologic study of stuttering. *Journal of Communication Disorders, 27,* 37-48.

Aron, M. (1962). The nature and incidence of stuttering among a Bantu group of school going children. *Journal Speech and Hearing Disorders, 27,* 116-128.

Battle, D. (1997). Multicultural considerations in counseling communicatively disordered persons and their families. In T. A. Crowe (Ed.), *Applications of counseling in speech-language pathology and audiology* (pp. 118-141). Baltimore: Williams & Wilkins.

Bernstein-Ratner, N., & Benitez, M. (1985). Linguistic analysis of the bilingual stutterer. *Journal of Fluency Disorders, 10,* 211-219.

Biggart, A., Cook, F., & Fry, J. (2006). The role of parents in stuttering treatment from a cognitive behavioural therapy perspective. Proceedings of the Fifth World Congress on Fluency Disorders, Dublin, Ireland, July 25-28.

Bloodstein, O. (1995). *A handbook on stuttering* (5th ed.). San Diego: Singular.

Bloodstein, O., & Bernstein Ratner, N. (2008). *A handbook on stuttering* (6th ed) Scarborough, Ontario: Thompson Delmar Learning.

Boey, R, Wuyts, F, Van de Heyning, P, et al. (2009). Stressors associated with the onset of stuttering in native Dutch-speaking children. *Journal of Stuttering Advocacy and Research, 3,* 71-87.

Brutten, G., & Miller, R. (1988). The disfluencies of normally fluent Black first graders. *Journal of Fluency Disorders, 13,* 291-299.

Bullen, A. K. (1945). A cross-cultural approach to the problem of stuttering. *Child Development, 16,* 1-88.

Carson, C., & Kanter, E. (1945). Incidence of stuttering among white and colored children. *Southern Speech Journal, 10,* 57-59.

Clifford, S., Twitchell, M., & Hull, R. (1965). Stuttering in South Dakota Indians. *Central States Speech Journal, 16,* 59-60.

Conrad, C. (1980). An incidence study of stuttering among black adults. Unpublished research project, Northwestern University.

Conrad, C. (1985). A conversational act analysis of black mother-child dyads including stuttering and nonstuttering children. Unpublished doctoral dissertation, Northwestern University, Evanston, IL.

Cooper, E. B., & Cooper, C. S. (1993). Fluency disorders. In D. Battle (Ed.), *Communication disorders in multicultural populations* (pp. 189-211). Boston: Andover Medical.

Cooper, E. B. & Cooper, C. S. (1998). Fluency disorders. In D. Battle (Ed.), *Communication disorders in multicultural populations* (pp. 189-211). Boston: Andover Medical Pulishers.

Crowe, T. (1994). Preventative counseling with parents at risk. In. C. W. Starkweather, & H. F. M. Peters (Eds.), *Proceedings of the First World Congress on Fluency Disorders* (pp. 232-235). Nijmegen, The Netherlands: University Press.

Crowe, T. A. (1995, December). Counseling for fluency disorders: Rationale, strategy and technique. Paper presented as part of a short course (with W. Manning and G. W. Blood) at the American Speech-Language-Hearing Association Convention, Orlando, FL.

Crowe, T. A., Di Lollo, A., & Crowe, B. (2000). *Crowe's protocols: A comprehensive guide to stuttering assessment.* San Antonio, TX: Psychological Corporation.

Dale, P. (1977). Factors related to dysfluent speech in bilingual Cuban-American adolescents. *Journal of Fluency Disorders, 2,* 311-314.

Einarsdóttir, J., & Ingham, R. (2005). Have disfluency type measures contributed to the understanding and treatment of developmental stuttering? *American Journal of Speech-Language Pathology, 14,* 260-273.

Einarsdóttir, J., & Ingham, R. (2008). The effect of the Stuttering Measurement and Assessment Training (SMAAT-child) on preschool teachers' ability to identify stuttering. *Journal of Fluency Disorders, 33,* 167-179.

Einarsdóttir, J., & Ingham, R. (2009). Does language influence the accuracy of judgments of stuttering in children? *Journal of Speech, Language and Hearing Research, 52,* 766-780.

Einarsdóttir, J., & Ingham, R. (2009). Accuracy of parent identification of stuttering occurrence. *International Journal of Language and Communication Disorders, 44,* 847-863.

Ford, S. (1986). Pragmatic abilities in black disfluent preschoolers. Unpublished master's thesis, Howard University, Washington, DC.

Fry, J., Botterill, W., & Pring T. (2009). The effect of an intensive group therapy programme for young adults who stutter: A single subject study. *International Journal of Speech-Language Pathology, 11,* 12-19.

Gillespie, S., & Cooper, E. (1973). Prevalence of speech problems in junior and senior high schools. *Journal of Speech and Hearing Research, 16,* 739-743.

Goldman, R. (1967). Cultural influences on the sex ratio in the incidence of stuttering. *American Anthropology, 69,* 78-81.

Goodall, H. B & Brobby, G. W. (1982). Stuttering, sickling and cerebral malaria: A possible organic basis for stuttering, *Lancet, 824,* 1279-1281.

Gregory, H., & Hill, D. (1980). Stuttering therapy for children. *Seminars in Speech, Language and Hearing, 1,* 351-363.

Guitar, B. (2006). Stuttering: An integrated approach to its nature and treatment. (3rd Ed.) Philadelphia, PA: Lippincott Williams & Wilkins.

Hale-Benson, J. E. (1987). *Black children: Their roots, culture, and learning styles.* Baltimore, MD: The Johns Hopkins University Press.

Harris, L. (1986). Barriers to the delivery of speech, language, and hearing services in Native Americans. In O. L. Taylor (Ed.), *Nature of communication disorders in culturally and linguistically diverse populations* (pp. 219-236). San Diego: College Hill.

Hartfield, K., Payne, K., Robinson, T. L. Jr., & Conture, E. (2005). Parent-based treatment of childhood stuttering: Two case studies. *E-Journal for Black and Other Ethnic Group Research and Practices in Communication Sciences and Disorders, 1* (2).

Hilliard, A. (1976). *Alternative to IQ testing: An approach to the identification of gifted minority children (final report).* Sacramento: California State Department of Education.

Jayaram, M. (1983). Phonetic influences on stuttering in monolingual and bilingual stutterers. *Journal of Communication Disorders, 16,* 287-297.

Johnson, W. (1944a). The Indians have no word for it: I. Stuttering in children. *Quarterly Journal of Speech, 30,* 330-337.

Johnson, W. (1944b). The Indians have no word for it: II. Stuttering in adults. *Quarterly Journal of Speech, 30,* 456-465.

Kirk, L. (1977). Stuttering and quasi-stuttering. *Georgia Journal of Communication Disorders, 10,* 109-126

Leavitt, R. R. (1974). *The Puerto Ricans: Cultural change and language deviance.* Tucson, AZ: University of Arizona Press.

Leith, W. R., & Gibson, A. (1991). The prevalence of stuttering among school children in Nassau, the Bahamas. Unpublished manuscript, Wayne State University.

Leith, W. R., & Mims, H. A. (1975). Cultural influences in the development and treatment of stuttering: A preliminary report on the Black stutterer. *Journal of Speech and Hearing Disorders, 40,* 459-466.

Lemert, E. M. (1953). Some Indians who stutter. *Journal of Speech and Hearing Disorders, 18,* 168-174.

Lemert, E. M. (1962). Stuttering and social structure in two Pacific societies. *Journal of Speech and Hearing Disorders, 27,* 3-10.

Millard, S., Edwards, S., & Cook, F. (2009). Parent-child interaction therapy: Adding to the evidence. *International Journal of Speech-Language Pathology, 11,* 61-76.

Mallard, S., Nicholas, A. , & Cook, F. (2008). Is parent-child interaction therapy effective in reducing stuttering? *Journal of Speech, Language and Hearing Research, 51,* 636-650.

McCartney, T. O. (1971). *Neurosis in the sun.* Nassau, Bahamas: Executive Ideas of the Bahamas Publisher

Meyers, S. C., & Woodford, L. L. (1992). *The fluency development system for young children.* Buffalo, NY: United Educational Services.

Morgenstern, J. J. (1953). Psychological and social factors in children's stammering. Unpublished doctoral dissertation, University of Edinburgh.

Morgenstern, J. J. (1956). Socioeconomic factors in stuttering. *Journal of Speech and Hearing Disorders, 21,* 25-53.

Nathanson, S. (1969). A study of the influence of race, socioeconomic status and sex on the speech fluency of 200 nonstuttering fifth graders. Unpublished doctoral dissertation, Northwestern University, Evanston, IL

Neely, M. (1960). An investigation of the incidence of stuttering among elementary school children in the parochial schools of Orleans parish. Unpublished master's thesis, Tulane University, New Orleans, LA.

Nwokah, E. (1988). The imbalance of stuttering behavior in bilingual speakers. *Journal of Fluency Disorders, 13,* 357-373.

Onslow, M., Packman, A., & Harrison, E. (2003). *The Lidcombe program of early stuttering intervention: A clinician's guide.* Austin, TX: Pro-Ed.

Ozawa, Y. (1960). Studies of misarticulation in Wakayama District. *Journal of Medicine, University of Osaka, 5,* 319.

Pritchett, M. (1966). The role of the East St. Louis Schools: A study of the effectiveness of the multi-approach in stuttering therapy. Proceedings of the annual meeting of the Illinois Speech Association, Chicago.

Proctor, A. Yairi, E, Duff, M., & Zhang, J. (2008). Prevalence of stuttering in African American preschoolers. *Journal of Speech, Language and Hearing Research, 51,* 1465-1479.

Ralston, L (1981). Stammering: A stress index in Caribbean classrooms. *Journal of Fluency Disorders, 6,* 119-133.

Riley, G. D. (1981). *Stuttering prediction instrument.* Austin, TX: Pro-Ed.

Robinson, T. L. Jr. (1992). An investigation of speech fluency skills in African American preschool children during narrative discourse. Unpublished dissertation, Howard University, Washington, DC.

Robinson, T. L. Jr., & Crowe, T. A. (1994, November). A model for inclusion of multicultural variables in fluency intervention programming. Paper presented at the American Speech-Language-Hearing Association Annual Convention, New Orleans, LA.

Robinson, T. L. Jr., & Crowe, T. A. (1987). A comparative study of speech disfluencies in nonstuttering black and white college athletes. *Journal of Fluency Disorders, 12,* 147-156.

Robinson, T. L. Jr., & Crowe, T. A. (1998). Culture-based considerations in programming or stuttering intervention with African American clients and their families. *Language Speech and Hearing Services in the Schools, 29,* 172-179.

Robinson, T. L. Jr., & Crowe, T. A. (2000). Multicultural issues in speech fluency. In T. Coleman (Ed.), *Clinical management of communication disorders in culturally diverse children* (pp. 251-269). Boston: Allyn and Bacon.

Robinson, T. L. Jr., Davis, J. G., & Crowe, T. A. (2000). Disfluency in nonstuttering African-American preschoolers during conversation and narrative discourse. *Contemporary Issues in Communication Science and Disorders, 27,* 64-171.

Runyan, C. M., & Runyan, S. E. (1986). A fluency rules therapy program for young children in the public schools. *Language, Speech and Hearing Services in Schools, 17,* 276-284.

Seymour, H. N. (1986). Clinical principles for language intervention. In O. L. Taylor (Ed.), *Nature of communication disorders in culturally and linguistically diverse populations* (pp.115-133). Austin, TX: Pro-Ed.

Seymour, H. N., & Seymour, C. M. (1977). A therapeutic model for communication disorders among children who speak black English vernacular. *Journal of Speech and Hearing Disorders, 42,* 247-256.

Snidecor, J. C. (1947). Why the Indian does not stutter. *Quarterly Journal of Speech, 33,* 493-495.

Starkweather, C. W. (1980). A multiprocess behavioral approach to stuttering therapy. *Seminars in Speech, Language and Hearing, 1,* 327-337.

Stewart, J. L. (1960). The problem of stuttering in certain North American Indian societies. *Journal of Speech and Hearing Disorders (Monograph Supplement 6), 87.*

Taylor, O. L. (1986). Historical perspectives and conceptual framework. In O. L. Taylor (Ed.), *Nature of communication disorders in culturally and linguistically diverse populations* (pp. 1-17). Austin, TX: Pro-Ed.

Taylor, O. L., & Payne, K. T. (1983). Culturally valid testing: A proactive approach. *Topics in Language Disorders, 3,* 8-20.

Taylor, O. L., & Samara, R. (1985). Communication disorders in underserved populations: Developing nations. Paper presented at the National Colloquium on Underserved Populations, American Speech-Language-Hearing Association, Washington, DC.

Terrell, B. Y., & Hale, J. E. (1992). Serving a multicultural population: Different learning styles. *American Journal of Speech-Language Pathology, 1,* 5-8.

Toyoda, B. (1959). A statistical report. *Clinical Paediatrica, 12,* 788.

Travis, L. E., Johnson, W., & Shover, J. (1981). The relationship of bilingualism to stuttering. *Journal of Speech Disorders, 2,* 185-189.

Van Kleeck, A. (1994). Potential cultural bias in training parents as conversational partners with their children who have delays in language development. *American Journal of Speech-Language Pathology, 3,* 67-78.

Van Riper, C. (1982). *The nature of stuttering* (2nd ed). Englewood Cliffs, NJ: Prentice-Hall.

Vaughn-Cooke, F. B. (1983). Improving language assessment in minority children. *ASHA, 25,* 29-34.

Vaughn-Cooke, F. B. (1986). The challenge of assessing the language of non-mainstream speakers. In O. L. Taylor (Ed.), *Treatment of communication disorders in culturally and linguistically diverse populations* (pp. 23-48). Austin, TX: Pro-Ed.

Waddle, E. (1934). A comparison of speech defects in colored and white children. Unpublished master's thesis, University of Iowa.

Wakaba, Y. (1983). Group therapy for Japanese children who stutter. *Journal of Fluency Disorders, 8,* 93-118.

Watson, J. B., & Kayser, H. (1994). Assessment of bilingual/bicultural children and adults who stutter. *Seminars in Speech and Language, 15,* 149-164.

Zimmerman, G., Liljeblad, S., Frank, A., & Cleeland, C. (1983). The Indians have many terms for it: Stuttering among the Bannock-Shoshone. *Journal of Speech and Hearing Research, 26,* 315-318.

ADDITIONAL RESOURCES

American Speech Language Hearing Association Division 4: Fluency and Fluency Disorders. A nationally recognized authority providing education, research, and support to help speech-language pathologists achieve excellence in treating people who stutter. The Division provides speech-language pathologists with resources and education that (a) facilitate understanding of fluency disorders and (b) promote effective treatment of people with fluency disorders; supports new and ongoing research on the nature, diagnosis, and treatment of fluency disorders; and improves the quality of life for people with fluency disorders through advocacy and public education. Available at: http://www.asha.org/Members/divs/div_4.htm.

Canadian Stuttering Association (CSA). A national not-for-profit organization that is committed to offering an impartial forum for sharing information, to speak as advocates for Canadians who stutter, and to promote greater acceptance of people who stutter by educating the public about the condition of stuttering. Available at: http://www.stutter.ca.

European Clinical Specialization in Fluency Disorders (ECSF). A one-year program developed by eight different universities and colleges in five European countries for speech-language therapists wanting to become European Fluency Specialists. Available at: http://www.ecsf.eu.

European League of Stuttering Associations (ELSA). A nonprofit transnational, cross-cultural organization of 12 countries was founded in 1995 as a worldwide network of people who stutter, to promote a greater knowledge and understanding of stuttering. Available at: http://www.stutterisa.org/What_Why_ISA.html.

International Fluency Association (IFA). A not-for-profit, international, interdisciplinary organization devoted to the understanding and management of fluency disorders, and to the improvement in the quality of life for persons with fluency disorders. Available at: http://theifa.org.

Chapter 10

International and Intercultural Aspects of Voice and Voice Disorders

Mara Behlau and Thomas Murry

BACKGROUND

About 20 years ago, we met at the annual meeting of the Voice Foundation. Since that time, we have become professional colleagues and personal friends. During those past 20 years, we have been privileged to speak at more than 300 conferences on voice and voice disorders in more than 100 countries. In many of those early meetings and workshops, we arrived with our talks well prepared and our slides in perfect order only to learn that care of the voice in those countries is much different from what goes on in our respective countries. Since those first years, we have learned that the voices of carnival singers are much different from those of the Broadway singers and that the chanting prayers of Tibetan monks are not at all like the chanting prayers of Jewish cantors. We also learned that school teachers in Austria do not have the same voice problems as the teachers in Greece. Cultures, environments, education level, and personal health all play a role in defining the types of voices and the types of voice problems that we have encountered on our individual professional journeys.

Our training, teaching, and travels to many countries of the world have taught us that the voice is a dynamic instrument of communication. We have learned that the voice is used to communicate. It tells us something about the people and the environment in which they live. Without voice, communication is possible, but it is neither efficient nor timely. A normal voice can be convincing, motivating, and stimulating to any conversation, whether it be a casual conversation between two individuals or from the front of the lecture hall to the very last row. Even with country, regional, or local speech dialects, a clear and pleasant voice draws the listener and maintains attention. From the government halls of the United Nations to the middle of the Sahara desert, a clear voice delivering an important speech commands much more attention when it comes from a person with a pleasant resonant voice. But, what is a pleasing and resonant voice? How can we improve the voice to be more resonant? How can we protect the clear voice, and how can we rehabilitate the injured voice? Those questions

may never be answered entirely because the voice varies with culture, with need, and with emotion. Of importance, when a speaker develops voice problems, the treatment must be addressed within the framework of the patient's need, culture, emotion, and personality.

During the period of July to December 2009, 60 questionnaires were electronically sent out to voice specialists all over the world to survey voice assessment and diagnosis, voice education and training, and voice clinic practice profiles. The rate of return was 76.6% sampled over 26 countries. The goal was to obtain data on the variety of approaches to the training of voice therapists and the manner in which they offer assessment and treatment of voice disorders. The questionnaire and results are given in Appendix 10-1 at the end this chapter. The information from the survey is used throughout this chapter to show the international and cultural issues in understanding voice and its disorders.

BEGINNING OF AN INTERCULTURAL RELATIONSHIP

The information in this chapter evolved through multiple streams. One stream, the visual stream, was initiated by Moore and Von Leden, who sought to understand the diagnosis of voice problems in more detail and to identify methods that may be used to treat the problems (Cooper & Von Leden, 1996; Moore, 1998). Their work in the 1940s and 1950s remains a guide to the importance of a team approach.

As speech pathologists, we have traditionally used the auditory sense to provide treatment. We have learned the importance of listening because the visual information is not always present and was rarely present when the field of speech pathology was in its infancy. Moreover, voice therapy involves a strong auditory-perceptual basis for changing vocal behavior. As listeners, we have learned to pay attention initially to the articulation, accent, or speed of a talker rather than his or her voice. Only when the voice falls out of the range that we consider normal do we focus on the vocal characteristics of the speaker. For that reason, the early work of Shipp and associates must be acknowledged. They began to examine the characteristics of normal voices in the late 1960s (Shipp & Hollien, 1969). They were interested in identifying the healthy voice and in how healthy voices vary with age. They found that listeners had little difficulty categorizing age simply by listening to a sample of the voice. Later, they pointed out the importance of the fundamental frequency as an indicator of age (Hollien & Shipp, 1972), with a gap of 5 years of certainty. Thus, the voice gives us much more information than simply a message. The message is steeped with information about the speaker as well as the context of the message. We are well aware of the need to understand the normal voice and its multiple messages. Germinal work, such as the studies by Hollien and Shipp, has propelled clinicians and scientists all over the world to search for a better understanding of vocal fold vibration, of the characteristics of the normal voice, and of the degree to which the voice can be developed, trained, and improved.

The second stream of knowledge independently evolved from the work of individuals such as Black and Tosi, which has culminated in a seminal work on voice identification (Tosi, 1979). Their interests, along with determining how to assess normal from abnormal, were focused on how the ear perceives severity and what instruments besides the ear can best measure the changes in severity of the pathologic voice. Thus, the two areas of laryngeal visualization and psychoacoustics have brought together the modern voice specialist's approach to voice disorders. This chapter updates the degree to which those two streams of evidence have evolved over the years and throughout many countries.

DIMENSIONS OF VOICE PRODUCTION

Traditional Definition of the Normal Voice

In the narrowest sense, a normal voice is the result of an air stream driving the vocal folds into vibration through a series of resonance chambers. Conversely, in a broader sense, voice is one of the most important expressions of a human being and his or her culture. It is very difficult to draw a definite boundary to classify normal and abnormal samples because voice is not a descriptive category (like male and female). Instead, it is a series of measures (like weight and height) that can vary from more to less, depending on the subject characteristics, spoken language, occupational demands, and environmental factors. A voice is usually considered normal when it properly represents a person; corresponds to the expectations of the person's gender, age, group, occupation, society, and community; and does not call attention to itself. An abnormal voice is one that impairs communication or reduces voice-related quality of life (Schwartz et al., 2009). Therefore, the social and professional aspects of someone's life may be vocally at risk because of the way he or she sounds or the effort needed to produce sound.

Range of Abnormal or Dysphonic Voice

A voice can be considered *dysphonic* when an alteration in its production impairs social and professional communication (Schwartz et al., 2009). Some patients can have complaints of vocal quality (hoarseness, breathiness, or tension), some others can have pitch deviations (too high, too low, or monotone voice), whereas some others do not have clear auditory deviations but a sense of effortful phonation, which can clearly limit communication performance. A diagnostic assessment is performed, preferably with information from the physician and speech-language pathologist (SLP). Therefore, this label of abnormal or dysphonic should only be used after a proper medical evaluation.

Individuals with unhealthy voices usually experience vocal complaints despite an occasional normal-sounding voice. However, there are several situations during the life span that can be characterized by a particular vocal quality that may be considered dysphonic or abnormal. For instance, the typical physiologic manifestations of infanthood (baby cries) and childhood (breathy and mild roughness phonation) and the instabilities during puberty and senescence are expected vocal qualities. However, temporary changes may ultimately turn into dysphonias.

The *adapted voice* is a term employed in cases of specific vocal demands, such as the use for commercial voiceover recordings and acting roles. These voices are sometimes called supranormal voices, owing to their specific controlled vocal quality. Voice after therapy does not always reach an optimal level, and we can use the term *rehabilitated voice* to express this condition, which may still include aspects of dysphonia.

A final concept is the *preferred voice* that may be used to express the set of parameters that represent a specific professional category, such as newscaster or auctioneer. These individuals must be watched carefully; their voice use may lead to dysphonias because their preferred voice is usually not their voice in daily conversation.

The disordered voice may be an exclusive result of vocal behavior or a partial result of that behavior. If vocal behavior is abusive, overly driven, or combined with injuries to other systems (pulmonary, neurologic, digestive), lesions, usually benign in nature, may result. In some situations, the relationship between the use of voice and the voice disorder is evident both to the clinician and to the patient. In other circumstances, this relationship is not very straightforward. The patient and the clinician must understand the importance of the vocal behavior as a contributor to the genesis of the dysphonia. Designing a therapeutic program to define the intervention options and also to reestablish an acceptable voice is an educational and therapeutic contract between the clinician and the patient. Stress related to communication in different cultural settings can play a major role in the development of a vocal problem; thus, the reduction of stress may help in rehabilitation of the voice problem.

The Preferred Voice

The *preferred voice* is the result of a coordinated set of parameters that include breathing, phonatory mode, resonance, articulation, psychodynamics, and behavioral parameters. A preferred voice for a specific occupation can be the result of training, imitation, or both. As an example, the modern jazz or rock singer usually starts a career with limited training and makes several attempts to approximate his or her voice to a successful singer of his or her preference. For the classical singer, the training aspect is more intense, but some imitation or fashion preferences can also play a role. It is important to understand that preferred traits undergo continuous changes.

Some professions have healthier preferences than others: examples include voiceover speakers with a low pitch and loudness compared with rock singers with a high-pitched voice, occasional growling, and laryngeal tension; and news announcers with habitual use of microphones compared with teachers who project their voices in classrooms with poor acoustics.

Some cultures have their own preferences that can be identified using objective procedures (e.g., a nasal tone in French or a pharyngeal resonance in Arabic). The preferred voice in one culture may be viewed as having a negative impact on another culture; as an example, Japanese women usually prefer using a high pitch and low volume to indicate politeness, which can be interpreted in the Unites States as a sign of lack of power or immaturity.

The Artistic Voice

Singing is one of the best expressions of a culture. The *artistic voice* serves both to represent a culture and to convey the singer's personality. Some cultural expressions may amplify certain vocal traits. For example, Hamdan and colleagues (2008) studied 78 Middle Eastern singers and concluded that this specific and very admired singing style, with a rich musical mode (Maqam system), is characterized by moderate tension, hypernasality, and thoracic breathing. This combination of features is different from Western singing, which is characterized by balanced tension, oral resonance, and abdominal breathing, particularly for the operatic singers. So, even if the Arabic singing voices are somehow displaced toward the region of deviated voices, it does not reflect pathology but rather expresses different vocal characteristics valued differently in the culture.

Voice as a Cultural Construct

Voice is a *cultural construct*. Vocal expression has been the mirror of cultural differences throughout mankind. There is a relationship among voice, linguistic code, and cultural behavior. The study of the cultural aspect of voice has not been a major focus of the SLP. Nonetheless, when cultural modifications lead to qualitative changes in the voice, a voice disorder must be considered.

The long drone of the Tibetan chant is much different than the pulsatile and rhythmic prayers of Chilean Indian tribes. Rock music sung in English, German, Japanese, or Brazilian Portuguese may sound extremely similar. The same happens with the music from a Broadway show sung in English, French, Italian, Brazilian Portuguese, or Spanish. There is an expectation of what a rock tune or a Broadway show must sound like, regardless the listeners' linguistic code. For example, American actors may be required to use a British accent in a play. The level of awareness and training to master accent requirements is higher. So, the use of the accent will require extra tension from phonatory and articulatory muscles. It is interesting to note that several SLPs have informally reported an increase of voice problems during the first months of a Broadway show performed outside of the United States, which may reflect the effort to accommodate a specific sound (the voice of musical theater) to a different one from the original. Even if a Broadway play is sung in Spanish, the audience wants to hear the typical Broadway sound. Although there is a worldwide trend toward globalization, voice clinicians who serve clients from cultural backgrounds with which they are not familiar may find it difficult to assess the culturally different vocal patterns, particularly with actors or singers. Moreover, it may be a challenge to offer them a directed course for healthy voice use based only on the standards of the clinician's country.

Only recently, specific books produced by SLPs have addressed the issue of voice as a contributor to reduce accent in English and produce a better interaction between articulation and phonation (Menon, 2007). Although this work often goes undocumented, there are many anecdotal reports of the changes in voice following singing in the Russian opera literature, singing in the Indian movie industry (Bollywood), and acting in roles requiring the use of Asian cultural intonation. Not only are these cultural differences important in the acting world, they also reflect how the average listener perceives normal and dysphonic voices of various cultures.

PREVALENCE OF VOICE DISORDERS
General Findings

Prevalence data on voice disorders are difficult to obtain. Demographic variation is largely due to country (even regions), age, gender, ethnicity, and occupation. Even where prevalence data are available, comparisons among studies are difficult owing to different sampling techniques, tools for assessment, and statistical power. Many issues are related to this difficulty. Normal voice is a negotiable concept, and there is no clear indication to establish what is a voice problem. Moreover, vocal style and vocal behavior may vary, largely owing to cultural expression, and this can interfere with a vocal screening program. Above all, well-designed prevalence studies are still limited in our specialty. The belief is that prevalence of voice disorders appears to vary widely across the spectrum of countries. Several studies have reported the prevalence of voice disorders in various countries and cultures, but most of the data come from evaluation of school-aged children.

According to two recent epidemiologic studies done in the United States, nearly one third of the population may experience impaired voice production at some point in their lives (Roy, 2004a; Roy et al., 2005). Data from the United Kingdom obtained during the past 20 years (Carding & Hillman, 2001) indicate prevalence ranging from 28 per 100,000 population in 1986 (Enderby & Phillipp, 1986), to 89 per 100,000 population in 1995 (Enderby & Emerson, 1995), to 121 per 100,000 population in 2001 (Mathieson, 2001). Although this trend suggests an increase of voice disorders during the past 25 years, it may simply represent more accurate sampling and reporting from a broader-based network.

In the United States, the general prevalence of a vocal problem has been estimated to be about 6.6% in adults (Roy et al., 2005), with a high lifetime prevalence of voice complaints of 28.8% in the general population (Roy et al., 2004a). Some professionals worldwide, such as teachers, are recognized as having the highest prevalence rates of vocal problems, reaching up to 57% and 3.87 new cases per year per 1000 teachers (Preciado-Lopez et al., 2007). Telemarketers, aerobic instructors, sport coaches, military personnel, and ministers generally have the highest prevalence of voice disorders after teachers. In addition, older adults are also at particular risk, with a prevalence of 29% (Roy et al., 2007), and a lifetime incidence of up to 47% (Roy et al., 2007) was found in groups of patients older than 55 years.

Women are more frequently affected by voice disorders than men, with a 6:4 female-to-male ratio (Coyle et al., 2001; Roy et al., 2005; Titze et al., 1997). Among children, prevalence rates vary from 3.9% to 23.4% (Duff et al., 2004; Silverman & Zimmer 1975), with the most affected age range being 8 to 14 years (Angelillo et al., 2008). This large range may be due to the screening protocol, to the type of testing used for the analysis (perceptual analysis only, visual inspection of the larynx, patient complaints), and to the threshold level set for failing. Data show that African American and European American students present similar rates of dysphonia (Duff et al., 2004).

One cultural finding in the data, which may be unique to American female adolescents, is the specific task-attributed dysphonia, "cheerleading." There is nothing similar to American cheerleading in the rest of the world.

Carnival in Brazil is known to produce a peak of acute dysphonia in the people that attend the parties, dancing and singing for many hours. The carnival celebrations in Brazil are noisy owing to the high level of amplification and intense use of percussion instruments accompanying the long-term singing. Specific strategies and vocal emergency programs have been developed in the country to assist the carnival singers, who make a substantial portion of their income during those few days of the year. There is no information on voice problems during Mardi Gras in New Orleans or other national celebrations such as Bastille day.

Specific Findings

Children with Voice Disorders

The prevalence of voice disorders in children has been estimated to be between 6% and 9% during the past 25 years. Results of studies vary, but in children up to the age of 14 years, the prevalence is about 6 in 100, or 6% (Leske, 1981). This apparently decreases during adulthood, ages 15 to 44 years, when the incidence is reported to be as low as 1% of the population, and then increases to 6.5% in those 45 to 70 years old. Although these numbers may be low, they reflect reporting in medical settings, and one should consider that many voice disorders, such as mild hoarseness or breathiness, go untreated or even unnoticed for years. This is especially true in countries where the health care is limited to serious, life-threatening illnesses.

Senturia and Wilson (1968) reported that 6% of school-aged children in a Midwest city in the United States had a voice disorder. Others have reported the prevalence to be more in the range of 6% to 9%, with one study (Silverman & Zimmer, 1975) reporting 4% of school-aged children with a voice disorder. Duff and colleagues (2004), in a study of 2445 African American and European American preschool children (1246 males and 1199 females, aged 2 to 6 years), found that only 3.9% of African American and European American preschoolers interviewed by SLPs had a voice disorder. Statistical analysis revealed no significant differences for age, gender, or race.

Adults with Voice Disorders

Prevalence of voice disorders in the adult population appears to vary based on the presence of other diseases. According to a study by Verdolini and Ramig, about 30% of working adults will experience a voice disorder during some time in their lives (Verdolini & Ramig, 2001).

The most common group of individuals who experience voice disorders consists of teachers (Roy et al., 2005). Roy reported that more than 3 million teachers in the United States use their voice as a primary tool of trade and are thought to be at higher risk for occupation-related voice disorders than the general population. However, estimates regarding the prevalence of voice disorders in teachers and the general population vary considerably. Roy and associates (2004b) found that the prevalence of teachers reporting a current voice problem was significantly greater compared with nonteachers. In their study, 11% of the teachers had a current voice problem, and 57% of the teachers indicated that they had a voice problem at some time in their lives. That is compared with only 28% of nonteachers reporting a voice problem at some time in their lives. Compared with men, women not only had a higher lifetime prevalence of voice disorders (46.3% vs. 36.9%) but also had a higher prevalence of chronic voice disorders (>4 weeks in duration), compared with acute voice disorders (20.9% vs. 13.3%). The same Roy study was replicated in Brazil (Behlau et al., 2011), in which data from 26 Brazilian states were gathered and analyzed including 3265 individuals consisting of 1651 teachers and 1614 nonteachers. Several similarities were found, despite deep economic, social, and cultural differences between the two countries. The Brazilian teachers reported a higher number of current (3.7) and past (3.6) voice symptoms when compared with nonteachers (1.7 present, 2.3 past) and attributed these to their occupation ($P < .001$). Sixty-three percent of teachers (1041) and 35.3% of nonteachers (569) reported having suffered a voice problem at some time in their life. Teachers missed more work days than nonteachers (4.9 days for voice problems). Teachers indicated the possibility of changing their occupation in the future because of their voice more than nonteachers (276, or 16.7%, and 14, or 0.9%; $P < .001$). Regional characteristics were not significantly different, with the two exceptions of more symptoms in dry regions than in humid areas and more access to medical and rehabilitative services in rich states than in poor regions. This disturbing panorama was consistent all over Brazil and similar to the United States, which reveals the strength and uniformity of data.

These results support the notion that teaching is a high-risk occupation for voice disorders, regardless the country, even if there are important variables in this profession related to the country.

One would expect teachers who work in countries with higher class sizes and who teach in classrooms less protected from noise and in the countries where there is a higher incidence of smoking would have the same or higher prevalence of voice disorders than in the United States.

Laryngeal Cancer: A Special Case

Although few prevalence data exist for specific voice problems, the best available data are on the incidence of laryngeal cancer. In 2009, the American Cancer Society reported 12,290 new cases of laryngeal cancer, 3660 deaths from laryngeal cancer, and 2850 new cases of hypopharyngeal cancer (American Cancer Society, 2010). The agency indicated that these numbers are decreasing in the United States owing to the reduction in smoking. Conversely, it suggests these numbers are increasing in countries where smoking is stable or increasing, such as Russia, China, and Greece.

The International Agency of Research on Cancer (Parkin, 2004) recently reported an estimated 161,000 new cases of laryngeal cancer per year, which can lead to a severe vocal limitation, particularly when diagnosis is delayed and treatment requires total ablation of the larynx (including the vocal folds). Laryngeal cancer is a predominantly male cancer, and it represents 2.7% of all cancer cases. The sex ratio (more than 7:1 male-to-female ratio) is greater than for any other site. For men, the high-risk world areas are Europe (East, South, and West), South America, and Western Asia. In Western Asia, larynx cancer accounts for more than 5% of cancers in men. Tobacco smoking is estimated to cause two thirds of all cancer cases in men. The risk for cancer development is the combined results of the relative contributions of "environment" and "genetics," which can at least partially explain some prevalence peaks in certain countries or areas of the globe, such as India and Brazil. The variation in exposure to carcinogens, pollution in the external environment, and lifestyle choices (tobacco and alcohol consumption) are the three factors contributing to cancer in the head and neck areas. This so-called triangular hypothesis plays a major role in countries where tobacco restriction laws are not reinforced. The Brazilian Academy of Laryngology and Voice (http://www.ablv.com.br) states that Brazil (São Paulo city) occupies the second worldwide position on laryngeal cancer, after India (Mumbai), and reinforces the need to consider hoarseness as a threatening symptom. The World Voice Day, an initiative that started in Brazil in 1999 and has quickly spread internationally, has one of its main goals to reduce this alarming trend (Švec & Behlau, 2007).

The outcome of laryngeal cancer is loss of normal voice. After total removal of the larynx because of cancer, communication is accomplished through tracheoesophageal prosthesis or classical esophageal speech (more used in underdeveloped countries). This is an alternative form of communicating that has severe limitations, such as restriction in pitch and loudness range for social communication, singing, or acting. The frequency, intensity range, and rate of speaking impair vocal projection and use of the voice for many professional voice situations. If the cancer is caught early, conservative procedures may be used to treat the disease, and voice communication remains, albeit with restrictions in voice quality and voice clarity.

Laryngeal cancer is not the only form of cancer that impairs normal voice communication. Oral cavity cancer accounted for 267,000 cases in 2000 in the United States (Parkin, 2004). Almost two thirds of those cases were in men. The geographic area with the highest incidence is Melanesia (36.3 per 105 in men and 23.6 per 105 in women). Similar to laryngeal cancer, rates of oral cancer in men are higher than in women in most regions, such as Western (12.5 per 105) and Southern Europe (9.2 per 105), South Asia (13.0 per 105), Southern Africa (12.4 per 105), and Australia and New Zealand (12.1 per 105). However, in females, the incidence is relatively high in Southern Asia (8.6 per 105).

The specific risk factors that can explain this difference in prevalence are tobacco and alcohol in Western and Southern Europe and Southern Africa, and the chewing of *betel quid* (a combination of betel leaf, areca nut, and slaked lime) in South Central Asia and Melanesia. The high rate of oral cancer in Australia is due to lip cancer (related to solar irradiation). It is difficult to identify all related factors involved in specific areas of high prevalence because protocols used for screening do not follow the same criteria of administration and assessment.

Prevalence Summary

The issue of prevalence is highly variable across cultures. To some extent, it is based on the manner in which prevalence is identified. Several studies have focused on voice qualities and how they affect the presence or absence of a voice disorder. The incidence of voice disorders increases when one considers the effects of conditions such as cerebral vascular accidents, Parkinson's disease, and other neurologic and neuromuscular diseases, primarily in aging adults, that often bring on changes in the voice that affect one's ability to communicate. The most studied and treated neuromuscular disorder with vocal impairment is surely Parkinson's disease (Sapir et al., 2009), affecting an estimated 8 million individuals in the world; of these, 80% to 90% are likely to develop speech disorders (dysarthria), in which reduced voice loudness and monotone are the primary voice characteristics.

It is clear that voice disorders affect children and adults to various degrees depending on how one defines a voice disorder and how a culture perceives the voice quality. Behavior-based dysphonias and their diagnosis can be influenced by the culture and language of the speaker.

The contribution of the environmental aspects in the development of dysphonias has been studied only recently. Because the vocal output is often greatly determined by the environment in which the individual lives or works, environment may be a significant underlying cause of a voice disorder. In general, the environment sets the loudness, the amount of use, and the speech rate. The environment introduces physical and psychological reactions revealed by the voice production. Thus, the voice that the patient displays in the clinic is not always the one he or she uses during his or her professional or social activity. In professional voice users, it is important to understand and to characterize the preferred voice for the specific professional category.

The world has shrunk and has become more similar. Cosmopolitan cities share similar problems and challenges, and their inhabitants develop a similar attitude as an answer to the stress factors of their environment.

ASSESSMENT OF VOICE DISORDERS

Self-Assessment Tools

The World Health Organization Quality-of-Life (WHO QOL) assessment group proposed that the perceptions and interpretations of an individual's QOL are rooted in that person's culture (Skevington, 2002). The cultural background of an individual may influence the manner in which a person experiences a voice disorder (Krischke et al., 2005). These cultural constraints, coupled with limited social interactions, can produce different strategies in interpreting and coping with a voice problem.

Traditionally, assessment of voice disorders has focused on attempts to measure the vocal output. This assessment strategy remains prominent to this day. In the early 1980s and 1990s, the main efforts for assessment of the voice-related outcomes were directed to the development and improvement of computerized objective analysis of acoustic and aerodynamic measures. However, these objective measures did not consider the patient's perspective regarding his or her vocal function. Similarly, improved and magnified endoscopic images of the larynx, including stroboscopic images, have been used to diagnose and assess vocal function in diseased and post-treatment states (Woo, 1996). However, neither objective voice measures nor video endoscopic measures have been shown to be useful in assessing the patient's feelings about the severity of either their voice problem or their satisfaction with the outcomes of their treatments (Jacobson et al., 1997).

Voice Handicap Index

Several self-evaluation protocols have been developed and disseminated worldwide for understanding the patient's perception of the impairment, disability, and handicap. In 1997, a group from the Henry Ford Hospital in Detroit developed an assessment tool to focus on the patient's perception of the severity of his or her voice: the Voice Handicap Index (VHI; Jacobson et al., 1997). The VHI is a patient self-administered assessment of voice handicap. It has been shown to be a valid and reliable instrument for assessing patients' self-perceived voice handicap. A handicap, as described by the WHO, is a social, economic, or environmental disadvantage (WHO, 1980). This is the result of an impairment or disability that limits or prevents the fulfillment of one or several roles regarded as normal, depending on age, sex, and social and cultural factors (Barbotte et al., 2001). The term *disability* refers to a restriction or lack of ability to perform a daily task. Therefore, the handicap associated with a voice disorder cannot be fully assessed by either objective voice measurements or videoendoscopic measurements. Rather, the measurement of a patient's handicap due to a voice disorder must take into account social and cultural factors, such as whether a teacher can teach all day and throughout the week or whether a factory foreman can talk loudly enough to be heard over the noise of factory machines.

The VHI consists of 30 items. These items are equally distributed over three domains: functional, physical, and emotional aspects of voice disorders. The functional domain includes statements that describe the "impact of a person's voice disorders on his or her daily activities." The emotional domain indicates the patient's "affective responses to a voice disorder." Items making up the physical domain are statements representing self-perceptions of laryngeal discomfort and voice output characteristics.

The VHI was acknowledged by the Agency of Healthcare Research and Quality (2002) as a reliable and valid diagnostic tool. Since then, the VHI has been translated and adapted to many different languages. Table 10-1 lists current references to the adapted and validated VHI.

It is interesting to note that there are only five comments on validation particularities. The Brazilian group mentions that the VHI presented a higher linguistic challenge because of similarities in some of the sentences (Behlau et al., 2009). In European Portuguese, one word did not achieve direct translation and had to be adapted (Guimarães & Aberton, 2004). The French version was appointed as deserving a review in translation (Woisard et al., 2004). The German modification may not represent all statements equally (Günther et al., 2005); and the Polish version has suffered modifications as well (Pruszewicz et al., 2004).

Despite its wide clinical and research application, the reliability of the VHI was questioned when being correlated with objective voice laboratory measurements (Hsiung et al., 2002). Hsiung and coworkers (2002) reported a large discrepancy between the results of VHI and voice laboratory measurements testing. Accordingly, they concluded that no objective parameter can yet be regarded as a definitive prognostic factor in a subjective evaluation of dysphonic patients.

A recent study showing the strength of the VHI was published by Verdonck-de Leeuw and colleagues (2008) using confirmatory factor analysis to assess equivalence of the American version and several translations, including Dutch, Flemish Dutch (Belgium), Great Britain English, French, German, Italian, Portuguese, and Swedish. VHI questionnaires were gathered from a cohort of 1052 patients from eight countries. They found that the internal consistency of the VHI proved to be good. Confirmatory factor analysis across countries revealed that a three-factor fixed-measurement model was the best fit for the data. The three subscales appeared to be highly intercorrelated, especially in the American data. The underlying structure of the

TABLE 10-1 Countries where the Voice Handicap Index Is Used as a Valid and Reliable Tool for Self-Assessment of the Severity of the Voice Disorder

Country	Study Authors, Year
United States	Jacobson, Johnson, Grywalsky, Silbergleit, Jacobson, Benninger, Newman, 1997
Germany	Nawka, Wiesmann, Gonnermann, 2003
Taiwan	Hsiung, Lu, Kang, Wang, 2003
Portugal	Guimarães, Aberton, 2004
France	Woisard, Bodin, Puech, 2004
Poland	Pruszewicz, Obrebowski, Wiskirska-Woznica, Wojnowski, 2004
United Kingdom	Franic, Bramlett, Bothe, 2005
Germany	Günther, Rasch, Klotz, Hoppe, Eysholdt, Rosanowski, 2005
The Netherlands	Hakkesteegt, Wieringa, Gerritsma, Feenstra, 2006
Israel	Amir, Ashkenazi, Leibovitzh, Michael, Tavor, Wolf, 2006
Scotland	Webb AL, Carding PN, Deary IJ, MacKenzie K, Steen IN, Wilson, 2007
Spain	Núñez-Batalla, Corte-Santos, Señaris-González, Llorente-Pendás, Górriz-Gil, Suárez-Nieto, 2007
Turkey	Kiliç, Okur, Yildirim, Oğüt, Denizoğlu, Kizilay, Oğuz, Kandoğan, Doğan, Akdoğan, Bekiroğlu, Oztarakçi, 2008
Sweden	Ohlsson, Dotevall 2009
Italy	Schindler, Ottaviani, Mozzanica, Bachmann, Favero, Schettino, Ruoppolo, 2010
Greece	Helidoni, Murry, Moschandreas, Lionis, Printza, Velegrakis, 2010
Saudi Arabia	Malki, Mesallam, Farahat, Bukhari, Murry, 2010
Brazil	Behlau, Alves dos Santos, Oliveira, 2011

VHI was also equivalent regarding various voice lesions. Distinct groups were recognized according to the severity of the VHI scores, indicating that various voice lesions lead to a diversity of voice problems in daily life. Verdonck-de Leeuw and colleagues concluded that the American Voice Handicap Index and the translations studied appeared to be equivalent. This would suggest that results from studies from the various countries included can be compared.

Although the VHI may be the only reliable and valid assessment tool used worldwide, investigators have found some discrepancies in the country-to-country data. Thus, whereas the internal consistency appears to be high from country to country, terminology across certain questions may reflect some of the difficulties that persist when trying to validate any test across countries and cultures. Cultural variations exist in every language and in the interpretation of specific words. For example, the terms *handicap* and *creaky* proved difficult to translate into the Greek version of the VHI (Helidoni et al., 2010). The Arabic version from Saudi Arabia went through an exhaustive review before publication because many Arabic countries use some modification of the Arabic language of Saudi Arabia (Malki et al., 2010). Nonetheless, the Arabic VHI has been shown to be highly reliable and related to the original VHI for the Saudi Arabian population.

One problem that may arise with the use of the VHI is due to its length. In routine diagnostics, voice patients may need to undergo several measurements. Therefore, the 30 items of the VHI might require too much time (about 10 to 15 minutes). For this reason, two shortened versions of the VHI have been proposed: the VHI-10 (Lam et al. 2006; Rosen et al., 2004) and the VHI-12 (Nawka et al., 2009). The VHI-10 has been constructed by selecting those items that have the largest differences between patients and a control group as well as between pretreatment and post-treatment (Rosen et al., 2000; 2004). The VHI-12 is based on factors with test-retest validation. Both scales have already been applied in numerous clinical studies around the world. However, each of these short scales was only constructed on the basis of data from the United States and using American English. The VHI-12 was from a subject sample from Germany using the German language.

To address the population of professional singers, VHI adaptations for assessing singing voice were proposed (Cohen et al., 2007; Morsomme et al., 2007), including a short version, the SVHI-10 (Cohen et al., 2009). An Italian phoniatrician, Franco Fussi, proposed two versions after analyzing more than 400 singers, called the Modern Singing Handicap Index (MSHI) for popular singers and the Classical Singing Handicap Index (CSHI) for classical singers (Fussi, 2005). Fussi showed that singers do respond to specific questions related to their vocal health and work status. These protocols have been used in the United States (Cohen et al., 2007), Belgium (Morsomme et al., 2007), Italy (Fussi, 2005), Spain (García-López et al., 2010), and Brazil (Moreti et al., 2010), with benefits to both the singer and the SLP. Results are comparable among the cultures, despite different singing styles. The Fussi modern and classical singing versions have been translated and adapted in Brazil (Moreti et al., 2010) after analyzing data from 229 singers (170 popular and 59 classical). Classical singers with voice complaint had higher scores than the popular singers. Classical singers with voice complaint seem to perceive a higher impact on quality of life due to their problem, reflecting a greater sensitivity to the dysphonic condition. The organic aspects showed the greatest deviations for the popular singers. The classical singers with and without vocal complaint had greater deviations than the popular singers on both the organic and functional aspects. Both protocols proved to be a useful tool for helping SLPs, singing teachers, and conductors to map voice problems of popular and classical singers. These data suggest that modern and classical singers deserve to be evaluated with specific protocols. Although there are currently no data to compare singers from all over the world, one might hypothesize that differences between classical and modern seem to follow a general trend and are not culturally bound.

Recently, the VHI-10 was adapted to the professional singer (Murry et al., 2009). Data from singers and nonsingers were analyzed in terms of overall subject self-rating of voice handicap and then rank-ordered from least to most important. The overall difference between the mean VHI-10s for the singers and nonsingers was not statistically significant, thus supporting the validity of the VHI-10. However, the 10 statements were ranked differently in terms of their importance by both groups. In addition, when three statements related specifically to the singing voice were substituted in the original VHI-10, the singers judged their voice problem to be more severe than when using the original VHI-10. Thus, the type of statements used to assess self-perception of voice handicap may be related to the subject population. Singers with voice problems do not rate their voices to be more handicapped than nonsingers unless statements related specifically to singing are included.

Other Assessment Tools

Other self-assessment tools have been developed recently. Most of these came from the initial American efforts in trying to quantify vocal handicap or quality of life, such as the specific Italian protocols to assess modern and classical singers (MSHI and CSHI; Fussi, 2005), and some others are country based, such as the Hong Kong protocol to assess voice activity and participation (VAPP; Ma & Yiu 2001). Others focus on specific aspects, such as the British protocol to evaluate vocal performance (VPQ; Carding et al., 1999) and the British coping questionnaire to assess the strategies used to deal with a voice problem (VDCQ; Epstein et al., 2009). Table 10-2 summarizes the major instruments to address self-perceived voice handicap and voice-related quality of life.

Most of the tools in Table 10-2 are less widely used than the VHI. The V-RQOL measure is a 10-item, disease-specific outcome instrument for voice disorders. All items are straightforward and easily translated and were validated in Brazilian Portuguese (Gasparini et al., 2009). The V-RQOL has a physical functioning domain, a social-emotional domain, and a total score. The VAPP (Ma & Yiu, 2001), originally written in English with data from a Hong Kong population, is a 28-item assessment tool that evaluates the perception of a voice problem, activity limitation, and participation restriction based on the International Classification of Functioning concept of WHO. It consists of five

TABLE 10-2 Major Voice-Disordered Quality of Life Instruments

Name of Instrument	Acronym	Study Country; Authors, Year	Characteristics
Vocal Performance Questionnaire	VPQ	United Kingdom; Carding, Horsley, Docherty, 1999	12-Item questionnaire: single score, questions on the sound of the voice, physical discomfort, effort to talk, voice usage, comments from the others Scaling: 5-point Likert scale to assign the severity of vocal performance Score range: 12 to 60 Population addressed: adult patients with voice disorder, to assess the physical symptoms and socioeconomic impact of the voice disorder
Voice-Related Quality of Life	V-RQOL	United States; Hogikyan, Sethuraman, 1999	10-Item questionnaire: total score, physical functioning domain and social-emotional domain Scaling: 4-point Likert scale—none, small amount, moderate amount, a lot and problem "as bad as it can be" Score range: 0 to 100 Population addressed: adult patients with any voice disorder
Voice Outcome Survey	VOS	United States; Gliklich, Glovsky, Montgomery, 1999	5-Item questionnaire: single score, questions on speaking voice, limitation to be understood over noise, interference in social activities or work, swallowing difficulties and effort to talk Scaling: 3 or 5 options according to the question Score range: 0 to 100 Population addressed: unilateral vocal fold paralysis
Voice Activity and Participation Profile	VAPP	China (Hong-Kong); Ma, Yiu, 2001	28-Item questionnaire, 5 aspects: total score and scores on self-perceived severity of voice problem, effect on job, effect on daily communication, effect on social communication, and effect on emotion. Two extra scores for activity and participation Scaling: visual analog scale of 10 cm (100-point range) Score range: 0 to 280; activity and participation scores from 0 to 40 Population addressed: active adult patients with dysphonia (working individuals)
Pediatric Voice Outcomes Survey	PVOS	United States; Hartnick, 2002	5-Item questionnaire: single score, information on the child's speaking voice, limitation to be understood over noise, interference in social activities or school, swallowing difficulties and effort to talk Scaling: 3 or 5 options according to the question Score range: 0 to 100 Population addressed: parental proxy; parents of children with tracheotomy or surgical decannulation
Voice Symptom Scale	VoiSS	United Kingdom; Deary, Wilson, Carding, MacKenzie, 2003	30-Item questionnaire: total score, impairment subscale, emotional subscale and physical subscale. Scaling: 5-point Likert scale—never, occasionally, some of the time, most of the time and always Score range: 0 to 120 Population addressed: adult patients with any voice disorder
Classical Singing Handicap Index	CSHI	Italy; Fussi, 2005	30-Item questionnaire: total score and organic, emotional and functional subscales Scaling: 4-point Likert scale—never, sometimes, almost always, and always Score range: 0 to 90 Population addressed: classical singers with specific singing voice complaints

TABLE 10-2 Major Voice-Disordered Quality of Life Instruments—cont'd

Name of Instrument	Acronym	Study Country; Authors, Year	Characteristics
Modern Singing Handicap Index	MSHI	Italy; Fussi, 2005	30-Item questionnaire: total score and organic, emotional and functional subscales Scaling: 4-point Likert scale—never, sometimes, almost always, and always Score range: 0 to 90 Population addressed: modern singers from any style, with specific singing voice complaints
Pediatric Voice-Related Quality of Life	PV-RQOL	United States; Boseley, Cunningham, Volk, Hartnick, 2006	10-Item questionnaire: total score, social-emotional and physical-functional subscales Scaling: 5-point Likert scale—none, small amount, moderate amount, a lot, and problem "as bad as it can be" Score range: 0 to 100 Population addressed: parental proxy; parents of children with all types of dysphonia
Pediatric Voice Handicap Index	pVHI	United States; Zur, Cotton, Kelchner, Bake, Weinrich, Leel, 2007	23-Item questionnaire: total score, functional, physical and emotional subscales plus rating the child talkativeness (7-point from quiet listener to extremely talkative) Scaling: 5-point Likert scale—never, almost never, sometimes, almost always, always Score range: 0 to 92 Population addressed: parental proxy; parents of children with dysphonia following surgical, medical, and behavioral interventions
Voice Handicap Index—Partner	VHI-P	United States; Zraick, Risner, Smith-Olinde, Gregg, Johnson, McWeeny, 2007	30-Item questionnaire: total score, physical, functional, and emotional subscales Scaling: 5-point Likert scale—never, almost never, sometimes, almost always, and always Score range: 0 to 120 Population addressed: proxy instrument, general dysphonic patients, close relatives
Voice Handicap Index Adapted to the Singing Voice	VHIC	Belgium; Morsomme, Gaspar, Jamart, Remacle, Verduyckt, 2007	30-Item questionnaire: total score, physical, functional, and emotional subscales Scaling: 5-point Likert scale—never, almost never, sometimes, almost always, and always Score range: 0 to 120 Population addressed: classical singers with specific singing voice complaints
Singing Voice Handicap Index	SVHI	United States; Cohen, Jacobson, Garrett, Noordzij, Stewart, Attia, Ossoff, Cleveland, 2007	36-Item questionnaire: single score, questions on physical, emotional, social, and economic impact of singing voice problems Scaling: 5-point Likert scale—never, almost never, sometimes, almost always, and always Score range: 0 to 144 Population addressed: singers with voice complaints, from any style, classical or modern
Voice Disability Coping Questionnaire	VDCQ	United Kingdom; Epstein, Hirani, Stygall, Newman, 2009	15-Item questionnaire: four coping subscales—social support, passive coping, avoidance, and information seeking Scaling: 5-point Likert scale—never, almost never, quite often, very often, and always Score range: 0 to 75 Population addressed: adult dysphonic patients

Continued

TABLE 10-2 Major Voice-Disordered Quality of Life Instruments—cont'd

Name of Instrument	Acronym	Study Country; Authors, Year	Characteristics
Voice Handicap Index for Singers	VHI-10 S	United States; Murry, Zschommler, Prokop, 2009	10-Item questionnaire: single score, questions similar to the VHI-10 plus singing voice causes client to lose income, client strains to produce singing voice, and clarity of singing voice is unpredictable Scaling: 5-point Likert scale—never, almost never, sometimes, almost always, and always Score range: 0 to 40 Population addressed: singers with voice complaints, from any style, classical or modern
Singing Voice Handicap Index-10	SVHI-10	United States; Cohen, Statham, Rosen, Zullo, 2009	10-Item questionnaire: single score, questions on singing voice Scaling: 5-point Likert scale—never, almost never, sometimes, almost always, and always Score range: 0 to 40 Population addressed: singers with voice complaints, from any style, classical or modern

sections: self-perceived severity of voice problem, effect on job, effect on daily communication, effect on social communication, and effect on emotion. The VAAP is a valid tool available in Finnish (Sukanen et al., 2007) and Brazilian Portuguese (Behlau et al., 2009). Because of this specific configuration, the VAPP helps to obtain a map on the scenario where the voice problem interferes the most (on the job, daily communication, social communication, and effect on emotion).

Each protocol to assess the impact of a voice problem in the individual's life has its peculiarities, advantages, and limitations. The many validation processes undertaken by several clinicians and researchers all over the world occurred in a quasi-steady fashion. Nonetheless, minimum adaptations were needed, and not a single item had to be withdrawn owing to lack of cultural representation. Recently, an Indian study has proposed a self-assessment protocol to be used in India (Konnai et al., 2010). This tool considers some prominent aspects of the environment and culture, such as noise and dust pollution, lack of acoustic amplification, lifestyle (spicy foods, excessive consumption of coffee, tea, and carbonated soft drinks), the tropical climate, and excessive voice use. The Voice-DOP is the only culture-specific QOL assessment tool developed for individuals with voice disorders and was created for the Kannada-speaking population in India. There are 21 different languages and many dialects spoken in India, suggesting that assessment tools may have to be developed for different languages despite occurrence in the same country (Konnai et al., 2010).

Specific cultural examples appropriate to India have been highlighted in the literature. For example, a street merchant selling food in a public railway station has to increase his vocal intensity above the noise of the loud trains and the congested crowd, in the dusty environment for long hours. A full-time teacher is likely to teach an average of about 30 classes per week, the duration of each class being about 40 minutes (Prakash, 2008). Moreover, in India most women have no paid employment, so questions related to the need for changing jobs because of a voice problem or to risk earning less money because of vocal difficulties may not be not applicable to females. Undoubtedly, other countries also retain certain cultural situations that are not readily addressed by the VHI or any self-assessment tool.

Auditory Perceptual Assessment of Voice

Perceptual Assessment and Tools

The SLP's clinical tradition is to describe numerous vocal parameters related to vocal quality, such as type of voice, glottal attack, resonance, pitch, loudness, respiratory dynamics, and vocal registers. It is known that the type of voice assessment protocol has a direct relation to the vocal physiology and an indirect relation to the acoustic analysis. It is well known that poor breath control and pulmonary pathologies may contribute to dysphonia; thus, it is necessary to develop a good respiratory pattern and coordination when treating dysphonia. It is also known that resonance, pitch, and loudness are more likely the genesis of a voice problem, which produces a negative psychodynamic impact. However, voice endurance to continuous speech, a central and vital use of voice-related aspect particularly for professional voice users, has been clinically underevaluated. Recent studies have superficially understood the impact of either the intensive voice use or the use of voice in adverse environmental conditions. There is not a screening or evaluation test that can be used in the clinic to characterize such parameters that is a frequent complaint of the dysphonic patient. Except for singers and actors, who represent the vocal elite, a voice produced with effort and fatigue should be more carefully considered than vocal quality deviations such as hoarseness and breathiness.

The worldwide basis of the clinical evaluation of the voice is still the auditory perceptual analysis that is performed by means of standardized protocols. Such an option allows information exchange between different centers. However, as the voice is multidimensional, its variables are numerous and they usually represent a specific center, country, and professional category profile. There are a wide range of perceptual protocols available, from which we can highlight: the Grade,

Roughness, Breathiness, Asthenia, Strain (GRBAS) scale (Hirano, 1981), Voice Profile Analysis (VPA) (Laver, 1980), Stockholm Voice Evaluation Approach (SVEA) (Hammarberg & Gauffin, 1995), Sound Judgment (SJ) (Oates & Russell, 2003), and Consensus Auditory Perceptual Evaluation of Voice (CAPE-V) (Kempster et al., 2009). The CAPE-V was designed to analyze a minimum set of perceptual parameters that specialists agreed on, and also to have the possibility of including additional parameters in the analysis. The CAPE-V seems to offer an interesting solution that can be internationally employed; however, particular aspects of clinical needs must be considered. The main information in these five protocols is organized in Table 10-3.

TABLE 10-3 Major Protocols for Perceptual Voice Analysis

Name of Protocol	Study Country; Authors, Year	Main Characteristics of Protocol	Scaling Properties
GRBAS (Grade, Roughness, Breathiness, Asthenia, Strain)	Japan; Hirano, 1981	Five parameters: G, degree of deviation; R, roughness; B, breathiness; A, asthenicity; S, strain Speech material: 5 vowels and reading passage suggested for the analysis Laryngeal focused scale, too superficial for clinical purpose No training material	Four-point Likert scale: absent, mild, moderate, and severe

Voice Profile Analysis (VPA)	United Kingdom; Laver, 1980	Voice described according to deviation of the neutral settings in four main dimensions:
		  I. Vocal quality features: A. Supralaryngeal features: 1. labial, 2. mandibular, 3. lingual (tip/blade), 4. lingual body, 5. velopharyngeal, 6. pharyngeal, and 7. supralaryngeal tension; B. Laryngeal features: 8. laryngeal tension, 9. larynx position, 10. phonation type
		  II. Prosodic features: 1. pitch, 2. consistency, 3. loudness
		  III. Temporal organization features: 1. continuity, 2. rate
		  IV. Comments: breaths support and rhythmicality
		Speech material: reading standard passage suggested for the analysis
		Phonetic description of vocal quality
		Too long and laborious for clinical purpose
		Training material available
			First pass: neutral X non-neutral; second pass for non-neutral: normal or abnormal; with 3-point scalar degree (1, 2, 3 for normal and 4, 5, 6 for abnormal)

Stockholm Voice Evaluation Approach (SVEA)	Sweden; Hammarberg, Gauffin, 1995	Eleven aspects of vocal quality: aphonic/intermittent aphonic; breathy, hyperfunctional/tense, hypofunctional/lax, vocal fry/creaky, with glottal attacks, rough, grating/scrapy, unstable voice quality/pitch, register/pitch breaks, diplophonia. Additional marks for register (modal, falsetto, or undetermined) and pitch (high versus low) Speech material: no specific task for the analysis Clinically developed Some items difficult to translate into English No loudness option to recording condition No training material	Two options of scaling: 5-point Likert scale, equal interval (0 = absent to 4 = high degree of presence); or a 10-cm visual analog scale (100 points)

Continued

TABLE 10-3 Major Protocols for Perceptual Voice Analysis—cont'd

Name of Protocol	Study Country; Authors, Year	Main Characteristics of Protocol	Scaling Properties
Sound Judgment (SJ)	Australia; Oates, Russell, 2003	Three main aspects: pitch (high, low, and monotone), loudness (loud, soft, and mono-loud) and quality (breathy, strained, rough, glottal fry, pitch breaks, phonation breaks, voice arrests, falsetto, tremor and diplophonia) Speech material: no specific task for the analysis Perceptual voice profile clinically oriented No information on overall degree of dysphonia Training material available (DVD with several clinical voice samples)	Six-point Likert scale for degree of impairment: normal, slight, mild, moderate, moderate-severe, severe
Consensus Auditory Perceptual Evaluation of Voice (CAPE-V)	United States; Kempster, Gerrat, Verdolini-Abott, Barkmeier-Kraemer, Hillman, 2009	Six parameters under consensus: overall severity, roughness, breathiness, strain, pitch, and loudness. Two extra lines are provided for additional features. Consistent or intermittent presence of each feature can be marked. Comments on resonance can be included at the end of the protocol. Speech material: three tasks for the analysis: vowels, selected sentences, and spontaneous speech Parameters listed are the result of a consensus meeting with specialists Force of recommendation by ASHA Training material will be available	Visual analog scale of 100 mm length, which corresponds to 100 possibilities of marking Anchor abbreviation of words along the line: DI for discrete, MO for moderate, and SE for severe deviation

The scale most widely used worldwide for perceptual auditory analysis is the GRBAS system, developed by the Japanese Committee of Phonatory Functions (Hirano, 1981). This system is composed by five parameters (G, overall deviation; R, degree of roughness; B, degree of breathiness; A, degree of asthenicity; and S, degree of strain) evaluated by a four-point Likert scale (0, absent; 1, mild; 2, moderate; and 3, severe). Despite lack of clear definition of parameters and training material, this scale was disseminated all over the world. Some evident problems such as concentration on laryngeal contribution of the vocal quality and the fact that asthenicity and strain are the opposite of each other (therefore, one single parameter), the system appears in international publications in numerous countries. Recently, the CAPE-V protocol, proposed by the American Speech-Language and Hearing Association Special Interest Group 3 (Kepmster et al., 2009) has produced a change in the paradigm of vocal analysis. The strength of the consensus protocol relates to a clear definition of six vocal parameters (overall severity, roughness, breathiness, tension, pitch, and loudness) and the fact that it was designed after a task force project to understand trends in psychoacoustic analysis and after considering all available protocols (such as GRBAS, John Laver, and SVEA protocols). The protocol is short, is specific to voice, and offers the possibility of marking two extra parameters, if

needed, plus the use of resonance. Moreover, this protocol is assessed by means of a visual analog scale with 100 points, which offers a more precise and detailed analysis.

The perceptual threshold for considering a voice normal is an interesting question for research. The worldwide singing expression is a live example of vocal variety, in which some cultures and musical styles clearly present certain preferences. For example, an opera singer must present a clear tone, with powerful projection, without any sign of roughness or breathiness. The rock singer's production can be characterized by roughness and strain and still be acceptable. Another interesting example is the degree of breathiness welcomed in bossa nova singing, a traditional Brazilian music now embraced worldwide. The difficult task is to differentiate a personal and culturally accepted vocal style from the expression of a voice problem. A clear cutoff point for separating normal variation of vocal quality and abnormal vocal quality through auditory perceptual analysis was suggested by a Finnish group (Simberg et al., 2000) as 34 mm (on a total scale of 100 mm), using the G parameter from the GRBAS scale (overall deviation). This criterion was chosen based on a pilot study and tested on the analysis of 226 students. The results indicate that this specific point can be used as a screening criterion. A similar cutoff limit was defined by two Brazilian studies analyzing 211 voice samples (plus 10% of repetition for reliability analysis) from adults with and without vocal complaints (Yamasaki et al., 2010). Two evaluation analyses were performed, the first one by using a visual analog scale with 100 units and the second a four-point numerical scale (NS). The results provided a reference system for perceptual analysis, with four ranges: 0 to 35.5 units for normal variation of voice quality or mild dysphonia (0 to 1 NS); 35.6 to 50.5 units for mild to moderate deviation (1 to 2 NS); 50.6 to 90.5 units for moderate deviation (2 NS) and 90.6 to 100 for severe deviation (3 NS). The limit of 35.5 units, close to the Finnish study, is suggested as a screening level for perceptual auditory analysis. These results provide some evidence to support the claim that cultural and language backgrounds of the listeners would affect perception for some voice quality types. Thus, the cultural and language backgrounds of judges should be taken into consideration in clinical voice evaluation. Despite these discrepancies, the GRBAS scale may be an excellent tool for perceptual evaluation of voice quality by linguistically diverse groups.

The major change from the 1980s is to focus only on three vocal types that can be consistently identify regardless the culture (roughness, breathiness, and strain) instead of trying to detail any peculiarity of the voice type (Oates, 2009). Although clinicians also make judgments about other factors, such as strain in the client with spasmodic dysphonia and rate of speaking in the client with Parkinson's disease, these parameters are usually less reliable when judged by groups of listeners or even the same listener repeatedly. Even though voice strain is a behavioral parameter that can be discretely rated in some cultures and languages, it may not be universally translated to others with the same degree of consistency and reliability as roughness and breathiness. Thus, roughness and breathiness, which have a more consistent construct across languages and cultures, are the most studied cross-cultural voice qualities (Yiu et al., 2008).

Linguistics, Voice, and Perception

Literature presents evidence that voice quality varies across languages and can even vary when an individual speaks two languages, as shown by Bruyninckx and associates (1994), when comparing voices produced by Catalan-Spanish bilinguals. The influence of language, particularly considering the way in which the phonetic properties may affect the manifestation of a voice problem, has not been studied properly. However, it seems plausible that certain vocal gestures regarding a specific linguistic code may introduce some adjustments that can interfere in the voice production of nonhealthy speakers. Lorch and Whurr (2003) reported that characterization of abductor spasmodic dysphonia in French speakers differs from that of English speakers in that the French did not show evidence of pitch breaks, only phonatory breaks, harshness, and breathiness. The frequency of occurrence of phonemes in French and English

is different and may have been one of the factors regarding the expression of some of the vocal features.

Nguyen and colleagues (2009) studied female primary school teachers with muscle tension dysphonia (MTD) who use Vietnamese, a tonal language, to determine whether professional voice users of a tonal language presented with the same symptoms of speakers of a nontonal language. The results showed that MTD was associated with a larger number of vocal symptoms than previously reported. They found that the Vietnamese teachers did not have the same vocal symptoms as those reported in English-speaking teachers. For example, hard glottal attack, pitch breaks, unusual speech rate, and glottal fry were rare in the Vietnamese speakers. The authors highlight the potential contribution of linguistic-specific factors besides the teaching-related aspects to the presentation of this voice disorder.

Cross-linguistic variables, such as those reported by Lorch and Whurr (2003) and by Nguyen and colleagues (2009) and Nguyen and Kenny (2009a), may interfere in the diagnostic criteria of specific dysphonias and may interfere with the clinician's ability to propose a clear diagnosis in speakers who use languages different from his or her native one. In the international arena, an understanding of speech-related effects on the voice provides the clinician with additional information when approaching the goals of treatment. Moreover, with the world population moving more and more toward large diverse metropolitan areas, there is more need to understand cultural variations. The current authors live in cities where the populations are higher than 5 million, and it is clear that cultural variations within the language play a major role in treatment planning and acceptance of the treatment outcome.

Few studies have investigated the cross-language perception of the voice in specific pathologies. To investigate this issue, Hartelius and coworkers (2003) compared the perceptual assessments of dysarthric samples by 10 Australian and 10 Swedish speakers with multiple sclerosis (MS) analyzed by 2 Australian and 2 Swedish clinically experienced judges. The consensus ratings from both judges were high for both the Australian and the Swedish speakers. They concluded that perceptual assessments of speech characteristics in individuals with MS are informative and can be achieved with high interjudge reliability irrespective of the judge's knowledge of the speaker's language. Thus, the universality of the voice parameters contributed to the perception of the disorder, regardless the language spoken.

Because voice quality is the expression of behavioral and cultural characteristics, different linguistic backgrounds may affect the evaluation of certain voice parameters. Few studies have explored these questions: Yamaguchi and associates (2003) studied the way in which Japanese and American clinicians (both SLPs and MDs) rated 35 Japanese voice samples using the GRBAS scale. There was no significant difference between the Japanese and American listeners in the use of the grade, roughness, and breathiness (G, R, B) scales. However, the asthenicity (A) and strain (S) scales, which reflect a more behavioral continuum, were judged differently between the two groups of listeners. The same vowel samples were judged by 74 Brazilian listeners (Behlau et al., 2001), and once again asthenicity and strain were judged differently from the Japanese listeners. The G factor achieved highest intercultural agreement, followed by roughness and breathiness. Thus, asthenicity and strain may be considered as discrete by the Japanese listeners but not by the American or Brazilian listeners.

Speakers identify voices from their own culture more accurately than voices from other cultures. Doty (1998) and Anders and associates (1988), in separate studies, demonstrated that accuracy in perceptual judgments was higher when judges identified speakers from their own country than speakers from other countries. In the Anders study, American listeners rated German symphonic voices with less severe dysphonias compared with German and Finnish listeners. The authors suggested that the lack of familiarity with the German language may have produced a more conservative evaluation.

The cultural and language backgrounds of judges interfere in the assessment of the vocal quality, even when using controlled synthesized signals and when listeners are from two different cultural and language backgrounds (Yiu and coworkers found significant differences between Australian and Hong Kong SLPs) when judging synthesized samples of various voice qualities (Yiu et al., 2008).

Acoustic Analysis of Voice

Acoustic Basis of Assessment

Measurement of the acoustic signal is currently a substantial portion of voice assessment. During the past 30 to 40 years, acoustic analysis of the voice has been refined, in large part owing to the hardware and software that have become available. The perceptual analysis of the voice by an experienced clinician may never be replaced in some cultures; however, it is unquestionable that acoustic analysis has added a new dimension to the voice evaluation.

Acoustic analysis allows the clinician to have a quantifiable baseline for treatment follow-up. There are two basic options: extraction of measures (fundamental frequency, frequency perturbation, and noise measurement) and spectrographic analysis, which requires a specific training for reading the spectrographic wave. The options for computerized programs vary from free to elaborated, complex, and expensive systems. The clinicians must identify their needs and choose the most available alternative because voice evaluation and treatment rely on both perceptual and acoustic analysis.

The literature indicates that, particularly, perturbation measure thresholds can be culturally influenced; however, not all voices can be reliably classified according to perturbation

measures. Voice is a quasi-periodic signal, and when that signal becomes buried in sufficient noise (hoarseness or roughness or breathiness), there is not enough quasi-periodic information to obtain a reliable analysis. The work of Titze and his colleagues (1995) suggests that, of the three types of signals usually produced by the voice, only two types will produce valid measures consistently (Titze, 1995). Clinicians often overlook this important information in attempting to obtain "objective" data. Highly dysphonic samples may be better studied with other types of analysis, such as chaos analysis (Baken, 1990).

When appropriate, acoustic analysis of a voice sample offers a clear benefit in understanding the voice production using objectivity. This analysis can lead to a better understanding of the parameters of the vocal output that are distorted, allow for better documentation for the client database, help to monitor treatment, and provide professional voice development follow-up and reliable outcome measures.

For acoustic analysis, the voice signal must be properly recorded and stored. This is one of the key issues of the evaluation because recording conditions can deeply interfere with the ultimate outcome of the signal analysis. Acoustic characteristics are highly influenced by the recording conditions, type of microphone, system and software of analysis, speech tasks, algorithms involved, and human interaction with the vocal laboratory. Therefore, information gathered from different software and systems can be difficult to compare. Acoustic analysis can offer two main options for the average SLP, shown in Table 10-4.

Measurements in the voices of adults are usually stable between 20 and 50 years of age (Dehqan et al., 2010), but variations can be found in the voices of children and elderly people, which need to be interpreted with caution.

Voice, when combined with speech, is culturally determined to a large extent, as we have previously discussed. Just as the cultural aspects of voice influence how a speaker

TABLE 10-4 Two Categories for the Acoustic Analysis of the Voice Signal

Parameter Extraction	Spectrographic Analysis
Fundamental frequency	Spectrographic trace reading
Jitter	Formant structure
Shimmer	Singing formant
Tremor	Harmonic components
Vibrato	Noise components
Signal-to-noise ratio or similar measurements (harmonic-to-noise ratio, glottal noise excitation)	Signal durations (VOT)
	Articulatory precision
	Prosodic elements
Voice range profile	
Speech range profile	

is perceived, culture and language may also have an influence on the acoustic properties of the voice. Fundamental frequency is a cultural mark and can be deeply associated with physical characteristics. For example, the low-pitched voice from the typical bass Russian singer is usually found in Russia and hardly ever in other countries, owing to a combination of general body, anatomic characteristics, cultural inheritance, and environmental reinforcement. It is known that ethnicity, gender, and spoken language affect the fundamental frequency and other acoustic measures (O'Neil et al., 1997). However, the degree of this influence is difficult to access because of the need for a large collection of data to derive strong conclusions and specifically well-designed and controlled studies of various cultures simultaneously.

The information available in the literature offers opportunity for reflection and helps the clinician to develop a proper attitude when evaluating or treating a patient with a cultural identity different from his or her own. For example, Malki and associates (2009) found significant differences for fundamental frequency in adult males and females from Saudi Arabia compared with North American data from a normative database. In the male group, 10 of 15 perturbation parameters and 12 of 15 parameters in the female group were found to be significantly different from the KayPentax database that is based on U.S. adults with English as their first language. The authors hypothesized that the differences may reflect ethnic anatomic and tissue differences. Similar results were found by Xue and Fucci (2000) and by Sapienza (1997), who studied African Americans and compared their voice data to the KayPentax database. Although the actual numbers vary considerably, it is clear that the incidence of voice disorders from an international perspective varies considerably depending on the age, the occupation, and culturally accepted norms from the perceptual and acoustical domains. More recently, Xue and colleagues (2006) reported that volumetric differences in the vocal tract of white American, African American, and Chinese speakers would contribute to the acoustic characteristics of these individuals and could be at least partially responsible for the formant frequency differences in a vowel sound void of specific language and dialectal impacts.

Walton and Orlikoff (1994) have shown that measures of amplitude and frequency perturbation in African American adult males higher than those of white adult males. Also, Sapienza (1997) analyzed the vowel /a/ in a group of 20 African Americans and 20 European Americans. She found that African American males and females had higher mean fundamental frequencies and lower sound pressure levels for the voice samples, but the differences were not significant. She did find significant differences for both males and females between the African American group and the European American group for maximum flow declination rate. This difference was partially attributed to the

larger ratio of membranous to cartilaginous portion of the vocal folds and increased thickness, a finding previously reported by Boshoff (1945).

Differences in acoustic parameters are usually small, and gender differences are quite consistent. For example, female Iranian speakers have aslightly higher harmonic-to-noise ratio (Dehqan et al., 2010) than Brazilian Portuguese (Felippe et al., 2006) and English speakers (Ferrand, 2000).

A variety of acoustic software programs are used by clinicians in the different cultures. The differences are mostly price, options in parameters settings, and output protocols. The availability of freeware or shareware software for acoustic analysis has definitely brought the acoustic laboratory to the clinical setting in a wide variety of countries and cultures where it was previously too expensive to obtain. The average SLP anywhere in the world with a low-cost computer can have a clinical voice laboratory to record the patient's voice and document the treatment outcome acoustically. Two examples are PRAAT (Paul Boersma and David Weenink) and GRAM (Visualization Software LLC, Richard Horne) software. Low-cost systems have been developed for specific purposes. For example, Brazil invested in developing low-cost software as Voxmetria, Fonoview, and Vocalgrama (CTS Informatica, Brazil), three programs for voice evaluation that offer different possibilities of acoustic measures, such as spectrography, phonatory deviation diagrams, voice and speech range profiles, perturbation measures such as jitter, shimmer, and noise-to-glottal rate.

Acoustic analysis of voice is not without its problems. For example, children's voices are more unstable than adults' voices. Therefore, the available normative databases usually derived from adult voices are not reliable for comparison. Acoustic measurements for children have been defined for English-speaking children (Bennett, 1983; Campisi et al., 2002; Hollien & Maclik 1962; Wheat & Hudson 1988), for English-speaking African American and European American children (Hollien & Maclik, 1962; Steinsapir et al.,1986; Wheat & Hudson 1988), for Arabic-speaking children (O'Neil et al., 1997) and for Jordanian Arabic–speaking children (Natour & Wingate, 2003). Although the acoustic normative values vary from one language to another, this variation has been found to be rather subtle for most children's voices studied.

Voice Acoustics and Cultural Influences

Some studies show that even in different cultures, some prosodic aspects of the vocal output are nearly universal. Across languages and cultures certain signaling functions of the frequency of voice are remarkably similar (Ohala, 1983; 1984; Stoel-Gamon et al., 1994). These include the following:

1. High or rising frequency to mark questions, low or falling frequency to mark nonquestions

2. High frequency to signal politeness, low tones to signal assertiveness

3. In "sound symbolic" vocabulary, high tone used with words connoting smallness or diminutive, low tone with words connoting largeness

Human vocal communication exploits the "frequency code," a cross-species association of high-pitched vocalizations with smallness and lack of threat of the speaker, and of low-pitched vocalizations with the speaker's largeness and threatening intent.

Most of the acoustic information on speakers from different languages deals with phonatory traits, such as voice onset time (VOT), in stop phonemes across the languages (Henton et al., 1992; Hoonhorst et al., 2009; Schmidt & Flege 1996; Williams & Buder, 1994). Some studies have shown differences in vowel formants in different languages (Andrianopoulos et al., 2001) and also with bilingual individuals (Morris, 1997; Rinker et al., 2010). This subject is beyond the focus of this chapter but may be an important concern when assessing a patient with a vocal problem outside of the clinician's normal culture and language.

Normative cultural data must be collected to properly access patients with voice disorders, and international standardization of assessment protocols can clearly indicate some trends in the acoustic analysis of voice. However, this requires an international workforce under the guidance of an international body, such as the International Association of Logopedics and Phoniatrics (IALP) or the World Voice Consortium (WVC), an organization of world leaders devoted to upgrading the standards for management of voice disorders and disseminating those standards through meetings around the world.

Aerodynamic Analysis of the Voice

It is understood that in any culture, the power of the voice comes from the pulmonary system. Aerodynamic studies have shown that aerodynamic measures provide information regarding the competency of the voice valving system. The dynamic breath stream of the power system, coupled with the complex channeling of the air stream through the glottis (mass, tension, and glottic configuration) and out through the mouth and nose, allows the human to generate a multitude of intensities regardless of his or her size. Early studies by Isshiki (1965) found increased flow rate with increased intensity. Regardless of the cultural limitations placed on loud or quiet voice, as the aerodynamic system of lungs, vocal folds, and supraglottic cavities becomes tuned, the voice becomes an efficient transmitter of emotion and information.

VOICE, EMOTIONS, AND CULTURE

Scherer (2000) elaborated on the hypothesis of the universality of the emotional effects on vocal production (versus language variability). There has been considerable research into perceptual correlates of emotional state of the voice, but a very limited amount of the literature examines the voice and emotions with regard to the cultural influences. We are subconsciously competent to understand the main emotional information that is constantly offered by a speaker, regardless of the language spoken and the comprehension of what is really being said.

There are more than 400 recognized emotions; however, a certain number of emotions are more basic than others and share similar vocal expressions among different cultures and languages. The six basic emotions according to Ekman (1992) include fear, anger, happiness, sadness, surprise, and disgust. Such a classification is based on the hypothesis that these emotions reflect survival-related patterns of responses to events in the constantly changing environment. It is assumed that these emotions are universal as a result of the human evolutionary history. Therefore, some of the vocal manifestations are collective, and others are defined by cultural constraints, in a similar fashion to what is observed in gesture communication (universal body language versus specific cultural gestures).

Identifying the emotion of a speaker from a different culture is not an easy task. If the listeners have access to facial expression (visual information), greater information is provided to help to identify emotion, as reported by Shigeno (2009), who studied Japanese and American speakers and listeners. However, the overall tendency to identify emotions from the voice is similar in cultures as different as Hebrew and Japanese, as seen in the study that analyzed the perception of Japanese voices by Hebrew speakers (Teshigawara et al., 2009). They found that speakers exhibiting laryngeal constriction were rated unfavorably for positive traits (laryngeal constriction was associated with the "bad guy"). The general correlation patterns between phonetic measures and trait items (physical characteristics such as tall and short, and personality such as good and evil) were similar across the two cultures, suggesting underlying perceptual similarities. Their findings also suggested that there may be fine differences in vocal pitch patterns between the two cultures. Low-pitched male voices might be more favored by Hebrew listeners, whereas a high-pitched female voice might be more favored by Japanese listeners.

The voice parameters affected by emotion are found to be of three main types: voice quality, utterance timing, and utterance pitch contour. The voice fundamental frequency (pitch) is the central parameter of the vocal expression of emotion, on both perceptual and expressive perspective; however, energy (intensity), duration, and speaking rate are also relevant. Vocal effects are associated with five basic emotions, specified in Table 10-5.

Happiness and anger have high energy owing to the high level of physiologic activation. Conversely, sadness and disgust are subdued because of reduced physiologic activation. Anger is characterized by a loud and harsh voice implemented by an attenuation of the low to middle frequency.

TABLE 10-5 Vocal Effects Associated with Basic Emotions

Vocal Effects	Basic Emotions				
	Fear	*Anger*	*Sadness*	*Happiness*	*Disgust*
Speech rate	Much faster	Slightly faster	Slightly slower	Faster or slower	Very much slower
Articulation	Precise	Tense	Slurring	Normal	Normal
Pitch average	Very much higher	Very much higher	Slightly lower	Much higher	Very much lower
Pitch range	Much wider	Much wider	Slightly narrower	Much wider	Slightly wider
Pitch changes	Normal	Abrupt on stressed syllables	Downward inflections	Smooth upward inflections	Wide downward terminal inflections
Intensity	Normal	Higher	Lower	Higher	Lower
Vocal quality	Irregular voicing Tremulous and breathy	Breathy chest tone Loud and harsh	Resonant breathy blaring Breathy	Grumbled Loud and breathy	Chest tone Harsh

Data reported by Cosi and Drioli (2009) regarding vocal quality; all other data from Murray and Arnot (1993).

Fear voice quality is tremulous and breathy. Joy and surprise are usually loud and breathy. Disgust has a harsh voice quality, and sadness is manifested by a breathy vocal quality (Cosi & Drioli, 2009). This has been overemphasized by actors and also in research with simulated emotions or machine-produced affects (Cahn, 1990).

Experiments on the automatic discrimination of emotions from voice have concentrated primarily on the English language. Nonetheless, the importance of voice and emotions is already playing out in business, as evidenced by the work of Toivanen and colleagues (2009).

Research using speech and voice recognition has also shown that voice may play a role in the cultural basis of recognizing emotions (González & Ramos, 2009). The authors developed a bilingual computerized speech recognition program for screening depression through voice and concluded that the vocal response latency is usually larger for depressive than for normal people and is even larger for Latinos. Moreover, utterances from depressive individuals are shorter (straight answers) and with a low level of energy. Thus, the possibility of using automatic detection software may contribute to the diagnosis of depression and direct proper attention to this population.

Another important challenge regarding voice and emotions is to identify emotions through voice in the tonal languages because pitch is used as part of speech to change the meaning of a word, such as happens in Chinese, Thai, and Vietnamese. In these languages, the larynx is used as an articulator, with additional features that add meaning to words. Kitayama and Ishii (2002) found Stroop-like perceptual interference due to vocal emotional tone when Japanese and American listeners are drawn to word content, and vice versa. The drawing away of attention from the word items can be interpreted as a mandatory reallocation of attentional resources to process this particular property

of the utterance. The amount of interference was greater for word content for Americans and greater for vocal tone for Japanese, reflecting differences in the importance of tone across the languages. Patients with voice problems in tonal languages may exhibit larger difficulty in communicating emotions and meaning because of the specific characteristic of their languages (Nguyen et al., 2009).

Even if the expression of at least the basic emotions is universal, languages may differ in the way they encode vocally transmitted emotions. For example, in Spanish (Montero et al., 1998) sadness and surprise are expressed with prosodic elements (pitch, loudness, and duration), whereas happiness and cold anger are represented by segmental features (spectrum and energy). On the contrary, in Japanese, the elements of anger, surprise, and sorrow are prosodic; those of joy and fear are segmental (Moriyama & Ozawa, 1999).

Learning a second language and mastering the expression of emotions by means of voice requires at least a good level of fluency and may vary depending on the speaker's native language. Steinberg (2009a) notes that native speakers of East Asian lexical tonal languages are often extraordinarily sensitive to intonation and, when learning American English, are generally adept at mastering intonation paradigms for various syntactic patterns and emotional expressions in casual conversation. Yet it is often difficult for native English speakers to listen to East Asian speakers who are presenting academic papers in English, quite possibly because the speakers are concentrating on articulating smaller units of speech and have never been trained in how native English speakers use vocal intonation across phrases. Second language speakers may become more competent by learning to use the voice in the same way native speakers of a certain culture do in order to express affect.

Heroes and enemies in cartoons easily express recognizable vocal manifestations. Exaggerated pitch slides and extremely high (and glottalized) registers characterize baby talk, "motherese" and expressions of sympathy, as well as the speech of cartoon villains (whose villainy is identified by the incongruent association between body language and voice). On the contrary, the simple, conversational speech of trusted American heroes contains less variety but offers correspondingly less reason for listeners to suspect the speaker of disguising his voice or speaking falsely (Steinberg, 2009b). Steinberg (2009b) states that the acoustic and articulatory characteristics of a caricatured voice of a villain may be culturally universal, but an insincere-sounding voice may be less sensitive to context and culture than an honest-sounding one.

Laryngeal constriction, often thought of as an underlying feature of dysphonia, plays a major role in vocal emotions. The degree of laryngeal constriction appears to be negatively correlated with ratings of favorable traits in Japanese. In other words, the presence of vocal constriction has an important role in differentiating heroic and villainous voices in the perceptual analysis with the constriction state associated to the villain (Teshigawara, 2009; Teshigawara et al., 2009).

Listeners attribute less favorable physical traits, personality traits, emotional states, and vocal characteristics to speakers who exhibit non-neutral supraglottic states. It appears that there is at least some universality with respect to emotional speech and that universal characteristics of emotional speech have some relevance to vocal stereotypes of good and bad characters (because villains in English are also associated with vocal constriction). However, it is important to determine whether these findings can be extended to other cultures.

The history of colonization can teach us many important lessons on merging cultures and transforming the expression of a language. Filipinos have embodied the Hispanic open expressiveness of emotions in their speech, adding expressiveness to their childlike playfulness which has produced the most effusive way of speaking among all Asians (Seneriches, 2009). Several American words have been introduced and successfully incorporated into the Filipino language. However, the typical American frankness has not replaced the Filipino polite characteristic profile of using a roundabout way of speaking, with lots of joking around, laughter, and use of familiarization (Seneriches, 2009).

Burkhardt et al. (2006) specifically addressed the question of whether parameters from emotional speech are universal in a diphone synthesis context. They compared the effects of parameter variations taken from the literature on French, German, Greek, and Turkish listeners. They found that general trends were quite consistent across language groups but that there were nevertheless differences that may have been caused by cultural differences.

Although automatic voice recognition systems may be developed to monitor and identify the basic human emotions as reported earlier, they may not be completely adaptable to the fine changes found within cultures to express all existing emotions. The universality of the voice to express emotion may be useful in marketing of speech technology products because little customization is necessary for basic emotional expression. However, special adaptations for specific languages or countries may be required to interpret the unique characteristics associated with Asian, Latin, and various English emotional content (Sidorova et al., 2009).

COPING WITH VOICE DISORDERS ACROSS CULTURES

The previous section discussed voice and emotions as they relate to the normal voice. However, when the voice is disordered, confusion may lead to a misinterpretation of the emotions expressed by the speaker. An interesting aspect recently explored for voice patients is how a dysphonic individual copes with a voice problem. That is, how does one get the message intended and the emotional intent across to a listener? Coping is defined as the cognitive and behavioral efforts directed to the management of either external or internal demands of a specific stressful encounter that may be exceeding an individual's adaptation resources (Folkman, 1984; Folkman & Lazarus, 1985, Folkman et al., 1986a, 1986b; Lazarus 1993, 1998; Lazarus & Folkman, 1984). It is seen as a process, not a goal, and the general aim of coping actions is to reduce the imbalances between demand by stressors and capacities of the individual. A reference point in this area is the cognitive theory of stress and coping of Lazarus and Folkman (1984). According to this model, coping is viewed as a response to specific stressful situations, in which cognitive appraisals of potential threat function as a mediating link between life stressors and the individual's coping response. This theory classifies the strategies as problem focused, which are the efforts directed to modify the stress source, and emotion focused, which are the attempts to regulate the emotional stress caused by a stressor.

The literature reviewing coping with voice disorders primarily focused on the impact of emotion on voice instead of on the effect of a voice problem on emotional aspects and on the role of coping (Aronson, 1990; Brodnitz, 1976; Moses 1948, 1956). The pioneer research on coping with dysphonia by Epstein (1998) investigated coping strategies used by individuals with spasmodic dysphonia and with muscle tension dysphonia. The findings of this research were used for the development of a self-reporting questionnaire that assesses coping in voice disorders, the Voice Disability Coping Questionnaire (VDCQ; Epstein et al., 2009). Many investigators undertook research on this issue with the hope that the concept of coping might help explain why some individuals fare better than others when encountering stress in their lives (Folkman & Moskowitz

2004). Many other concepts, such as culture, developmental history, or personality, can also help explain these individual differences (Folkman & Moskowitz, 2004).

Culture is one of the main aspects of society that permeates the whole process of stress and coping (Chun et al., 2006). The parameters that define a culture are complex and undergo continuous modification. They are learned within the culture, shared, transmitted, and changed from one generation to the other. Cultural parameters have inherent normal values based on the beliefs of the general population. These normal values shape the human behavior that may bring on stress when a voice problem develops. It is apparent that the manner of coping with the stress of a voice problem may be highly culturally bound (Chun et al., 2006; Oyserma et al., 2002; Screen & Anderson, 1994). Voice is the universal common means of communication, but the coping strategies to deal with a voice problem are significantly different from culture to culture. Therefore, it is expected that the way a Spanish individual copes with a voice problem may be different from the way a British person does, even though they are experiencing the same health problem (Screen & Anderson, 1994).

An important perspective of the analysis of the cultural influence on human behavior relates to the concepts of individualism and collectivism, which have been extensively studied for the past 20 years (Oyserman et al., 2002). In the so-called collectivist cultures, it is more likely to have a lifestyle centered in the society. On the other hand, in the individualist cultures, the emphasis is on the individual. Bearing in mind this concept, it seems reasonable that an individual who lives in a collectivist country is more likely to seek for social help to deal with a stressful event such as a voice disorder.

Two studies applied a specific voice-related coping questionnaire, the original British study by Epstein and colleagues (2009) and the Brazilian version of the research protocol by Oliveira and associates (2011). The results clearly indicated that there are cultural preferences in coming up with specific types of strategies for facing a voice problem. The challenge to the clinician is to identify maladaptive vocal strategies that may interfere with the rehabilitation outcome.

THE CHALLENGES OF VOICE TREATMENT AROUND THE WORLD

From a historical perspective, voice therapy requires the clinician to have a unique combination of personal characteristics and specific scientific knowledge. Treatment of dysphonia was historically an art-based approach, using the singing pedagogy or drama training to help patients with voice problems. The possibility of assessing the phonatory mechanisms with clinical instruments has brought physiologic data to change this scenario to a more scientific procedure. There are many challenges that voice specialists face to assess and treat clients with an optimal practice attitude, which is even more defying when considering cultural aspects.

From the clinical perspective, broad diagnostic diversity presents as a major problem. Even though the voice area has evolved from a more abstract and artistic nature to a more structured scientific standpoint, there is still a lag to routinely used practice-based evidence interventions. Clinicians face the challenge of applying the best available evidence to each patient. The decision to administer programmatic or custom therapy, the selection of approaches to treatment, and the dismissal and follow-up procedures remain to be assessed at a more basic level of evidence.

Modern Developments

Currently, there is positive evidence that voice rehabilitation is effective and efficacious. The recent panel of specialists that produced an important document that has been spread all over the world (Schwartz et al. 2009), popularly known as the "hoarseness guideline," has made the strong recommendation that "the clinician should advocate for voice therapy for patients diagnosed with hoarseness that reduces voice-related quality of life." The strong recommendation status was made by SLPs after systematic reviews and randomized trials that indicated a preponderance of benefit over harm.

In the past, the format of therapy was usually a long-term commitment to treatment, including classical approaches such as relaxation and breathing techniques. The current research on treatment outcomes has changed this picture. Currently, there are three main options in treating patients with behavioral dysphonia:

1. Hygienic approach (elimination of negative behaviors and habits harmful to the vocal mechanism)
2. Symptomatic approach (direct modification of altered vocal characteristics)
3. Physiologic approach (holistic treatment with retraining and rebalancing breathing, phonation, and resonance subsystems)

All three are easily identified in clinical references throughout the world. A systematic review of the efficacy literature by Thomas and Stemple (2007) revealed various levels of support for the three approaches.

Symptomatic approaches usually produce good immediate changes, but there is a need for well-designed studies to understand its applicability, particularly when combined on a programmatic approach.

Vocal hygiene is a component of several programs, used all over the world, but the real contribution is inconclusive. Even the observance of some rules may produce small positive changes (Behlau & Oliveira, 2009). The basics of vocal care are shared among many countries, with some particularities regarding the detriment of using cold drinks or air conditioning.

Of the three methods, the strongest evidence of change has been found for the physiologic approach known as the Lee Silverman Voice Treatment (LSVT), a therapy regimen based on improving vocal fold closure. This method, developed almost 20 years ago by Ramig and colleagues (Fox et al., 2006; Ramig et al., 1995, 1996, 2001, 2008; Sapir et al., 2002, 2003), was initially suggested and applied to patients with Parkinson's disease. It is a specific voice therapy that has generated a global interest among clinicians and researchers because of its powerful effects on various aspects of voice and speech in individuals with Parkinson's disease as well as with various neurologic disorders. According to the authors, this method is delivered in an intensive regimen and in a manner consistent with theories of motor learning and skill acquisition, as well as with principles of neural plasticity. It is a high-effort healthy, loud phonation method to encourage maximum phonatory efficiency and coactivation and coordination of speech subsystems. This may be the most international of all modern approaches in treating a specific voice disorder.

The programmatic approaches, such as LSVT, Vocal Function Exercises (VFE), and the Accent Method have produced a broad range of evidence, but even if the results from these approaches are widely known, it is clear from a survey of clinicians from 26 countries as reported in Appendix 10-1 that all clinicians use custom-based approaches, when needed.

Aside for the LSVT, other physiologic approaches have evolved with various levels of evidence to support their efficacy. This is due particularly to the simultaneous emergency of these methods and instrumentation to assess the vocal production that favored gathering data. Four methods have strong evidence data (Thomas & Stemple, 2007). These methods include the following: Accent Method, Vocal Function Exercises, Resonant Voice Therapy, and Manual Laryngeal Musculoskeletal Reduction Technique.

The *Accent Method* was originally developed in Scandinavia (Smith & Thyme 1976) and mostly used in Egypt (Bassiouny, 1998; Kotby et al., 1991) and Japan (Kotby et al., 1993). The basis of this method is to associate an abdominal diaphragmatic breathing with accentuated vowels in syllable, sentences, and texts. The goal is to optimize respiratory-phonatory connection and improve vocal fold closure.

VFE were developed in the United States (Roy et al., 2001; Stemple et al., 1994) and are mostly used in Brazil, Australia, and European countries and also with a tonal language (Nguyen & Kenny, 2009b). This is a simple method, with four well-structured exercises aimed at restoring proper balance among the speech subsystems of respiration, phonation, and resonance.

The *Resonant Voice Therapy*, based on theater tradition and mostly used in the United States (Roy, 2003; Verdolini-Marston et al., 1995), is recognized worldwide (Barrichelo-Lindstrom & Behlau, 2009a, 2009b; Chen et al., 2003).

This method uses auditory and tactile cues to obtain optimum resonance in the midportion of the face.

The *Manual Laryngeal Musculoskeletal Reduction Technique* is a technique to manipulate and massage the extrinsic laryngeal musculature in order to reduce tension. It was originally described by Aronson (1969) in the United States and later popularized by others (Roy et al., 1993, 1997). It appears with variations, as in Belgium (Van Lierde et al., 2004), with a more structured strategy in the United Kingdom (Mathieson et al., 2009) or other manual approaches, such as in Finland (Leppänen et al., 2009).

Specific Cultural Issues Related to Voice Treatment

There may be some personal preferences in the way a patient wants to be treated, but some general trends are clear. A Muslim woman may prefer using a melodic approach and not laryngeal massage. A business man may feel more comfortable being treated with VFE rather than body exercises. Universal techniques, such as the use of resonance exercises (e.g., humming, nasal sounds, nasal sounds with vowels, nasal sequences) are seen in most traditional textbooks for voice treatment all over the world, with large variations in the way the exercises are presented and monitored. The clinician's expertise and preferred approaches may also determine the therapy format. Popular techniques in one country, even with acceptable evidence, may not be frequently used in other countries. For example, the French Tearing Out Technique (Arnoux-Sindt, 1991) for granuloma amputation through intense aggressive vocal maneuvers and specific body postures and exercises is administered mostly by Italian clinicians (Bergamini et al., 1995) and in some cases in Brazil (Behlau & Pontes, 2001). It is hardly used anywhere else in the world. The Accent Method, originally from Scandinavia (Smith & Thyme 1976), despite the body of evidence, is frequently used in Japan and Egypt and less frequently in other parts of the world.

The multidisciplinary treatment for dysphonia may also require the contributions from singing teachers, acting coaches, and specialists whose scope of practice may vary around the world (such as those who teach specific materials to specific individuals, e.g., synagogue cantors).

THE CHALLENGES OF MULTICULTURAL POPULATIONS WITH VOICE DISORDERS

A New World of Information Interchange

The world has shrunk as a result of the ease in traveling, international job opportunities, and democratic Internet communication. A person does not have to travel to face the challenges of communicating with someone abroad. Cellular telephone networks, cable television, and the Internet have brought the world to almost everybody's living room. Multicultural populations can be seen in large cities, in small villages, and in refugee camps. Multicultural populations face challenges not only because of language proficiency but also because of the use of certain vocal parameters that do not match the preferred voice of the primary local culture. Mature adults are particularly concerned owing to embodied accents and deviated vocal parameters from the expected ones that can reduce their opportunity for employment and impede their opportunity for promotion and advancement.

Elderly individuals may prefer to live inside the communities protected by their cultural group, reducing chances of integration. Moreover, the current culture would surely benefit from the richness of multiple perspectives and cross-cultural experiences. The more we are touched by international and true multicultural scenarios, the more tolerant, understanding, and accepting we become and the freer we can be from single-culture bandages. The use of the voice embodies these principles.

Multicultural Approach to a Preferred Voice

The international world can knock at anyone's door. The multiplicity of cultural presentations is large. It would be a challenging task for the SLP to treat a patient from a culture other than his or her original culture. Besides any cultural preference, there are also social specificities and certain occupational demands that may require the clinician's attention. The clinician must not feel reluctant to seek information in order to provide a competent cultural service. Bearing this in mind, we would like to present a set of useful questions to guide the clinical attitude, to create value in the case history for the clinician and client, and to establish a basis for a culture-related context leading to a successful voice intervention program. We have highlighted the main concerns a clinician must be aware of before managing the case.

Proposed Guide to a Multicultural Approach to Assessment in the Voice Clinic

In this chapter, we have demonstrated that there are both similarities and differences in the normal voices and disordered voices of clients from countries and within cultures around the world. The survey reported in Appendix 10-1, although not scientific in the strictest sense, opens the door to expose significant differences and the limitations in the manner of assessment and treatment of voice disorders used around the world. Based on that survey, the literature reviewed in this chapter, and our experiences of 20 years of interaction with clinicians around the world, we have proposed an approach to assessment that includes cultural aspects of the voice that should be addressed. These are presented in a question format.

Do you think you have a voice problem, or does someone think you have a problem? Certain vocal style characteristics of a culture can be seen as deviations of the habitual pattern in another society. For example, speaking with a soft voice is a sign of education and respect in Japan and can be seen as a lack of assertiveness and timidity in the United States or Brazil. A more projected voice may be a requirement for a teacher from Japan to be respected in a classroom in the Western world.

Is your voice considered a problem in your country or community? As mentioned earlier, voice is a cultural construct that is influenced by the spoken language and can mirror a specific social or cultural group. Therefore, a so-called problem can reflect a particular interpretation of someone's vocal pattern. In order to be a competent speaker in a second language, besides mastering the vocabulary and prosody, some persons need to work specifically in certain vocal acoustic parameters, such as resonance, pitch, and loudness.

Does anyone make comments (humorous or not) about your voice? Comments are usually made in a negative perspective. When someone masters a second language, people generally have more patience with beginners (or avoid communication totally) and less patience with proficient speakers. Some accents can be the motivation for jokes and can produce a profound impact on the speaker. Vocal deviations can be seen as lack of intelligence or may be used to misjudge one's ability to learn. It is important to identify any comments (negative or not) in order to verify whether they can be used as feedback toward improvement. Moreover, the patient may need to receive some coaching on how to properly react to these difficulties.

Do you suffer any limitation due to your voice in the community where you live, work, and socialize? It is important to know whether the patient crosses cultural communities in his or her typical daily life. In some contexts, social and familial lives are mostly limited to the original culture, and the work setting presents a multicultural scenario. Some religious and Latin groups may prefer to maintain their cultural traditions in their personal life but do not make efforts to adapt to a competitive multicultural or international environment.

How long have you been aware of these limitations? The longer a person lives with a limitation without searching for help, the bigger the inner belief that little can be done to change the current situation. Coping strategies to deal with a problem can be generally divided into emotional and problem-focused strategies. Some cultures are more collectivist, such as the Latino culture, and the familial and social networking will play a major role in dealing with stressful situations. Individualistic societies may easily use problem-focused strategies, and they may even consider that this is the appropriate way to solve an issue, misjudging any other type of procedure. The clinician must be aware of the different strategies to use when dealing with a voice problem depending on the culture of the client. A specific protocol can be used to address these questions (e.g., Epstein et al., 2009).

Have you experienced any setbacks in your work or social life because of your voice? A voice problem can impair professional performance. Most of the modern professions require the use of the voice as the main tool in their work. Depending on the vocal demands, these individuals may experience frequent abnormal dysphonias related to their work. Teachers, lawyers, call center operators, health professionals, and salespersons do not need a special voice, like those of actors and singers, but the fact is that any vocal deviation that draws listeners' attention may misplace the focus of the communication and impair the message. The simple fact of asking someone to repeat what was just said may raise the stress level during communication.

Can you describe the ideal voice for you? Is there anyone's voice that you would like to have or sound similar to? Who and why? An ideal voice can largely vary according to someone's fantasy about what is a good voice. By describing the ideal voice, an abstract problem can be brought to a concrete level in order to be addressed during therapy. Usually, successful television or movie stars are seen as model voices. Voices do not come on menus, but to explore what specifically attracts someone to another speaker's voice may help to guide the therapy and to make the whole process more concrete (e.g., female teachers may want to have a lower pitch to be more authoritarian). This can be an opportunity to explore the knowledge that every human being has a specific vocal tract and a unique vocal identity. Moreover, if a person understands that his or her voice was wired on a specific cultural context during childhood, an extra effort can be made to create new connections toward a desired or required pattern.

How distant from the ideal voice are you now? The treatment process includes giving proper information on how behavior can be changed. The individual needs to understand that there is a highway to travel and that any behavior can be implemented under the general laws of learning. Behavioral information reduces anxiety and helps the individual to proceed and understand the active role he or she will have to play in the rehabilitation process.

How different is your voice from your original community? If the person's voice is already different from the peers in the community, the issue is more related to a health problem (dysphonia itself) instead of a cultural matter. On the contrary, two options should be addressed: the person may have developed a health-related voice problem owing to the efforts in communicating in a second language in a different culture, or the vocal style does not fit the new perspective and now requires adjustment.

How different is your voice from your peer group? Some persons have a clear understanding of the differences (too soft, too loud, excess nasal tone, or too high or low pitch), they present when compared with their peer group.

Some others do not have a clear auditory perception of the differences. In such cases, an auditory training program is required. In some cases, the main reason of not addressing these aspects is an inner belief that vocal styles and accent cannot be changed.

Do you strain your voice to talk or sing in your first language? Does it change when you are using a second language? Straining the voice is one of the main causes of a voice disorder. Lack of confidence in speaking a second language or trying too hard to communicate can generate more tension on the vocal apparatus. Some cultures have original lax general patterns, such as French, compared with others in which a tense vocal system is the default, such as Arabic. Strain can be a linguistic trait or an acquired state and must be clarified.

Is a loud voice a positive or negative aspect in your culture? A loud voice can be interpreted in some cultures (particularly in the Western world) as a sign of power, leadership, and confidence. On the other hand, it can also be interpreted as lack of education, lack of politeness, hostility, and aggressiveness. In some cultures (particularly in the Eastern or Asian world), a loud voice can be seen as abrasive and a sign of low income and poor breeding. There is no general rule, and this has to be asked in order to be adjusted. Moreover, personality features have to be taken into consideration because extroverted individuals tend to speak louder than introverted ones.

Is a high-pitched voice a positive or negative aspect in your culture? Pitch is an important gender maker, and it is directly related to the fundamental frequency (number of vocal fold vibration cycles per second). Females have higher pitch than males, regardless the culture. Even if fundamental frequency derives from the anatomic configuration, there is a range of possibilities of setting up the average pitch: culture and personality play major roles. High-pitched voices in Japanese women and some Indian men are a sign of proper education; however, in Brazilian women, they can indicate dependence and immaturity.

Is a low-pitched voice a positive or negative aspect in your culture? Similar to the previous question, this has to be addressed.

Is a fast speech rate a positive or negative aspect in your culture? Speech rate is related both to inner and society timing. People tend to speak faster when under stress or anxious, because of lack of time, or when they do not receive proper attention from the listener. Conversely, speaking at a slower rate transfers politeness, education, self-control, and concerns toward the listener. A too slow rate can risk losing the listener's attention and must be avoided.

CONCLUSION

The knowledge, enthusiasm, and appreciation of the normal voice and voice disorders have become a worldwide interest, as evidenced by the diverse current literature on the topic. Regardless of the cultural limitations placed on language and the interpretation of the language, the sound of the voice can send a message across cultural barriers. The recent explosion of the translation of the VHI is but one example of the need to communicate issues of normal and pathologic voice descriptions to colleagues around the world. Three other factors have fueled this interest. The first is the concept of a voice team that began with G. Paul Moore and Hans von Leden more than 50 years ago (Moore & von Leden, 1958). Since then, leaders in laryngology and speech-language pathology have worked to emphasize the team concept of voice research and patient management. Second, the availability of conferences and workshops that bring SLPs and laryngologists together has opened a dialogue around the world for interested professionals in both disciplines to share their specific expertise about the understanding of voice production in the normal and disordered voice. Third, the specific use and knowledge of clinical instruments to refine the diagnostic and treatment plan has contributed to a broad focus in the patient rather than a strictly "listen" approach that has fragmented treatment in the past.

In this chapter, we have emphasized the importance of SLPs' role in the assessment and treatment of voice disorders and their contributions to the database of knowledge about the normal voice. As these aspects of team management, conference opportunities, and instrumentation continue to improve around the world, there is no doubt that knowledge of normal voice production and voice disorders will also improve the study of this exciting discipline.

Although the contributions of language and culture may increase the complexity of interpreting specific voice tools in various countries, the questionnaire that formed the basis of this chapter suggests that voice transcends many of those barriers. To further understand the multicultural contributions to voice production, perceptual studies across cultures that combine the constraints of the language are needed.

Treatment of voice in the future may rely additionally on such developments as the use of handheld monitors to validate therapeutic exercise regimens, interactive devices to offer telemedicine treatment that will be approved by insurance companies, development of international standards to assess outcomes in addition to the VHI, and cultural standards for objective measures that reflect the basic parameters of the voice, namely frequency, amplitude, voice spectrum, and intonation.

We have shown that the SLP plays a shared role in the patient's voice problem, the assessment of the problem, and most importantly the outcome of the treatments extended to the patient for his or her problem. We have also shown that the study of voice is a cultural expedition that includes attention to the variables of voice use across the world. Although voice can be changed, modified, and adapted to specific cultures and situations through accent reduction, acting, training, disguise, and imitation, the consequences of those changes must be within the normal range of voice production for each individual. To be aware of the vocal implications and the flexibility of the voice across cultures is one of the main challenges of the modern SLP.

DISCUSSION QUESTIONS

1. Discuss the differences between a bilingual child with a voice problem diagnosed as hoarseness with vocal nodules and a bilingual adult with the same diagnosis. What concerns would you expect of each? Would you alter their treatment simply because of their age or voice needs?

2. The Chinese population is growing rapidly, and large groups of Chinese and other Asians are located in many parts of South America. What advice can you give Asian teachers and Asian business people for the use of their voice in their chosen professions? Do you think the Asian teacher or Asian business person would have the same voiced problem if he or she lived in São Paulo, Brazil or Montevideo, Uruguay? Why or why not?

3. Most acoustic data on voice are based on American men and women. What are the needs, if any, to identify additional acoustic data on diverse populations such as Chinese, African, or Indian individuals who live in their mother country and those who now live in adopted countries?

4. When there is a need to curb noise, what role does the SLP play? How does the SLP counsel clients and their families to manage noise in their work situations, in their home, and in their social life?

REFERENCES

Agency for Healthcare Research and Quality. Criteria for determining disability in speech-language disorders. *Evidence Report/Technology Assessment,* 2002.

American Cancer Society: What are the key statistics about laryngeal and hypopharyngeal cancers. ACS Report 8/16/2010.

Amir, O., Ashkenazi, O., Leibovitzh, T., et al. (2006). Applying the voice handicap index (VHI) to dysphonic and nondysphonic Hebrew speakers. *Journal of Voice, 20,* 318-324.

Anders, L. C., Hollien, H., Hurme, P., et al. (1988). Perception of hoarseness by several classes of listeners. *Folia Phoniatrica et Logopedica, 40,* 91-100.

Andrianopoulos, A. V., Darrow, K. N., Chen, J. (2001). Multimodal standardization of voice among four multicultural populations: Fundamental frequency and spectral characteristics. *Journal of Voice, 15,* 194-219.

Angelillo, N., Di Costanzo, B., Angelillo, M., et al. (2008). Epidemiological study on vocal disorders in paediatric age. *Journal of Preventive Medicine and Hygiene, 49,* 1-5.

Arnoux-Sindt, B. P. (1991). A propos de la technique rééductative des granulomas larynges. *Cahiers D'ORL, 26,* 13-15.

Aronson, A. E. (1969). Speech pathology and symptom therapy in the interdisciplinary treatment of psychogenic aphonia. *Journal of Speech and Hearing Disorders, 34,* 321-341.

Aronson, A. E. (1990). *Clinical voice disorders* (3rd ed). Stuttgart, New York: Georg Thieme Verlag.

Baken, R. J. (1990). Irregularity of vocal period and amplitude: A first approach to the fractal analysis of voice. *Journal of Voice, 4,* 185-197.

Barbotte, E., Guillemin, F., Chau, N., for the Lorhandicap Group (2001). Prevalence of impairments, disabilities, handicaps and quality of life in the general population: A review of recent literature. *Bulletin of the World Health Organization, 79,* 1047-1055.

Barrichelo-Lindstrom, V., Behlau, M. (2009a). Resonant voice in acting students: Perceptual and acoustic correlates of the trained Y-Buzz by Lessac. *Journal of Voice, 23,* 603-609.

Barrichelo-Lindstrom, V., Behlau, M. (2009b). The contribution of Lessac's Y-buzz from two Brazilian voice therapists' perspectives. In M. Munro, S. Turner, A. Munro, K. Campbell (Eds.), *Collective writings on the Lessac voice and body work: A festschrift* (pp. 351-361). Coral Springs, FL: Ilumina.

Bassiouny, S. (1998). Efficacy of the Accent Method of voice therapy. *Folia Phoniatrica et Logopedica, 50,* 146-164.

Behlau M, Alves Dos Santos L de M, Oliveira G. (2011). Cross-cultural adaptation and validation of the voice handicap index into Brazilian Portuguese. *Journal of Voice, 2011, 25,* 354-359.

Behlau, M., Oliveira, G., Santos, L. M. A., Ricarte, A. (2009). Validation in Brazil of self-assessment protocols for dysphonia impact (original title: Validação no Brasil de protocolos de auto-avaliação do impacto de uma disfonia). *Pró-Fono Revista, 21,* 326-332.

Behlau, M., Oliveira, G. (2009). Vocal hygiene for the voice professional. *Current Opinion in Otolaryngology and Head and Neck Surgery, 17,* 149-154.

Behlau, M., Pontes, P. (2001). Eliminação de granuloma pós-cordectomia por técnica vocal de arrancamento. In M. Behlau (Ed.), *O melhor que vi e ouvi III: Atualização em laringe e voz* (pp 334-343). Rio de Janeiro, Revinter.

Behlau, M., Yamaguchi, H., Andrews, M. (2001). Escala GRBAS em três diferentes culturas. In: Proceedings of the 9th Brazilian Congress of Speech Language Pathology and Audiology (p. 586). Guarapari, ES, Brazil.

Behlau, M., Zambon, F., Guerrieri, A. C., Roy, N. (2010, June). Voice disorders in teachers and general population in Brazil. Paper presented at the 39th Voice Foundation Symposium: Care of Professional Voice, Philadelphia.

Bennett, S. (1983). A 3-year longitudinal study of school aged children's fundamental frequencies. *Journal of Speech and Hearing Research, 26,* 137-142.

Bergamini, G., Luppi, M. P., Dallari, D., et al. (1995). La rieducazione logopedica dei granulomi laringei. *Acta Otorhinolaringolica Italica, 15,* 375-382.

Boseley, M. E., Cunningham, M. J., Volk, M. S., Hartnick, C. J. (2006). Validation of the pediatric voice-related quality-of-life survey. Archives of Otolaryngology—Head and Neck Surgery, *132,* 717-720.

Boshoff, P. H. (1945). The anatomy of the south African Negro larynx. *South African Journal of Medical Sciences, 10,* 113-119.

Brodnitz, F. S. (1976). Spastic dysphonia. *Annals of Otolaryngology, 85,* 210-214.

Bruyninckx, M., Harmegnies, B., Llisterri, J., Pocholive, D. (1994). Language-induced voice quality variability in bilinguals. *Journal of Phonetics, 22,* 19-31.

Burkhardt, F., Audibert, N., Malatesta, L., et al. (2006). Emotional prosody: Does culture make a difference? In R. Hoffmann and H. Mixdorff (Eds.), *CD-ROM proceedings of the Third International Conference on Speech Prosody Conference.* Dresden, Germany: TUDpress Verlag der Wissenschaften.

Cahn, J. E. (1990). The generation of affect in synthesized speech. *Journal of the American Voice I/O Society,* 1-19.

Campisi, P., Tewfik, T. L., Manoukian, J., et al. (2002). Computer-assisted voice analysis: Establishing a pediatric database. *Archives of Otolaryngology—Head and Neck Surgery, 128,* 156-160.

Carding, P. N., Horsley, I. A., Docherty, G. J. (1999). A study of the effectiveness of voice therapy in the treatment of 45 patients with nonorganic dysphonia. *Journal of Voice, 13,* 172-104.

Carding, P. N., Hillman, R. (2001). More randomised controlled studies in speech and language therapy. *British Medial Journal, 323,* 645-646.

Chen, S. H., Huang, J. L., Chang, W. S. (2003). The efficacy of resonance method to hyperfunctional dysphonia from physiological, acoustic and aerodynamic aspects: the preliminary study. *Asia Pacific Journal of Speech, Language, and Hearing, 8,* 200-203.

Chun, C., Moos, R. H., Cronkite, R. C. (2006). Culture: A fundamental context for the stress and coping paradigm. In: Wong, P. T. P., & Wong, L. C. J. (Eds.), *Handbook of multicultural perspectives on stress and coping* (p. 31). New York: Springer.

Cohen, S. M., Jacobson, B. H., Garrett, C. G., et al. (2007). Creation and validation of the Singing Voice Handicap Index. *Annals of Otology, Rhinology, and Laryngology, 116,* 402-406.

Cohen, S. M., Statham, M., Rosen, C. A., Zullo, T. (2009). Development and validation of the Singing Voice Handicap-10. *Laryngoscope, 119,* 1864-1869.

Cooper, D., Von Leden, H. (1996). The discipline of voice: An historical perspective. In W. S. Brown, B. P. Vinson, M. A. Crary (Eds.), *Organic voice disorders: assessment and treatment* (pp. 1-22). San Diego: Singular.

Cosi, P., Drioli, C. (2009). LUCIA, a new emotive/expressive Italian talking head. In K. Izdebski (Ed.), *Emotions in the human voice: Culture and perception* (Vol. III) (pp. 153-176). San Diego: Plural.

Coyle, S. M., Weinrich, B. D., Stemple, J. C. (2001). Shifts in relative prevalence of laryngeal pathology in a treatment-seeking population. *Journal of Voice, 15,* 424-440.

Deary, I. J., Wilson, J. A., Carding, P. N., MacKenzie, K. (2003). VoiSS: A patient-derived Voice Symptom Scale. *Journal of Psychosomatic Research, 54,* 483-489.

Dehqan, A., Ansari, H., Bakhtiar, M. (2010). Objective voice analysis of Iranian speakers with normal voices. *Journal of Voice, 24,* 161-167.

Doty, N. D. (1998). The influence of nationality on the accuracy of face and voice recognition. *American Journal of Psychology, 111,* 191-214.

Duff, M. C., Proctor, A., Yairi, E. (2004). Prevalence of voice disorders in African American and European American preschoolers. *Journal of Voice, 18,* 348-353.

Ekman, P. (1992). An argument for basic emotions. In: N. L. Stein, & K. Oatley (Eds.). *Basic emotions* (pp. 169-200). Hove, UK: Lawrence Erlbaum.

Enderby, P., Emerson, J. (1995). *Does speech and language therapy work?* London: Whurr.

Enderby, P., Phillipp, R. (1986). Speech and language handicap towards knowing the size of the problem. *British Journal of Disorders of Communication, 21,* 151-165.

Epstein, R., Hirani, S. P., Stygall, J., Newman, S. P. (2009). How do individuals cope with voice disorders? Introducing the Voice Disability Coping Questionnaire. *Journal of Voice, 23,* 209-217.

Epstein, R. (1998). *The impact of botulinum toxin injections in adductor spasmodic dysphonia: A cross sectional and longitudinal study* [tese]. Londres: University College and Middlesex School of Medicine.

Felippe, A. C. N., Grillo, M. H. M. M., Grechi, T. H. (2006). Standardization of acoustic measures for normal voice patterns. *Revista Brasileira de Otorrinolaringologia, 72,* 659-664.

Ferrand, C. T. (2000). Harmonics-to-noise ratio in normally speaking prepubescent girls and boys. *Journal of Voice, 14,* 17-21.

Folkman, S. (1984). Personal control and stress and coping processes: A theoretical analysis. *Journal of Personality and Social Psychology, 46,* 839-852.

Folkman, S., Lazarus, R. S., Dunkel-Schetter, C., et al. (1986a). Dynamics of a stressful encounter: Cognitive appraisal, coping, and encounter outcomes. *Journal of Personality and Social Psychology, 50,* 992-1003.

Folkman, S., Lazarus, R. S., Gruen, R. J., DeLongis, A. (1986b). Appraisal, coping, health status, and psychological symptoms. *Journal of Personality and Social Psychology, 50,* 571-579.

Folkman, S., Lazarus, R. S. (1985). If it changes it must be a process: Study of Emotion and Coping During Three Stages of a College Examination. *Journal of Personality and Social Psychology, 48,* 150-170.

Folkman, S., Moskowitz, J. T. (2004). Coping: Pitfalls and promise. *Annual Review of Psychology, 55,* 745-774.

Fox, C. M., Ramig, L. O., Ciucci, M. R., et al. (2006). The science and practice of LSVT/LOUD: neural plasticity-principled approach to treating individuals with Parkinson disease and other neurological disorders. *Seminars in Speech and Language, 27,* 283-299.

Franic, D. M., Bramlett, R. E., Bothe, A. C. (2005). Psychometric evaluation of disease specific quality of life instruments in voice disorders. *Journal of Voice, 19,* 300-315

Fussi, F. (2005). *La voce del cantante* (Vol. 3). Florence, Italy: Omega.

García-López, I., Núñez-Batalla, F., Gavilán Bouzas, J., Górriz-Gil, C. (2010). Validation of the Spanish version of the voice handicap index for vocal singing (SVHI) [in Spanish]. *Acta Otorrinolaringologica Española, 61,* 247-254.

Gasparini, G., Behlau, M. (2009). Quality of life: Validation of the Brazilian version of the voice-related quality of life (V-RQOL) measure. *Journal of Voice, 23,* 76-81.

Gliklich, R. E., Glovsky, R. M., Montgomery, W. W. (1999). Validation of a voice outcome survey for unilateral vocal cord paralysis. *Otolaryngology—Head and Neck Surgery, 120,* 153-158.

González, G. M., Ramos, A. L. (2009). Assessing voice characteristics of depression among English- and Spanish-speaking populations. In K. Izdebski (Ed.), *Emotions in the human voice: Culture and perception* (Vol. III) (pp. 49-65). San Diego: Plural.

Guimarães, I., Abberton, E. (2004). An investigation of the Voice Handicap Index with speakers of Portuguese: Preliminary data. *Journal of Voice, 18,* 71-82.

Günther, S., Rasch, T., Klotz, M., et al. (2005). Bestimmung der subjektiven Beeinträchtigung durch Dysphonien. Ein Methodenvergleich. *HNO, 53,* 895-904.

Hakkesteegt, M. M., Wieringa, M. H., Gerritsma, E. J., Feenstra, L. (2006). Reproducibility of the Dutch version of the Voice Handicap Index. *Folia Phoniatrica et Logopedica, 58,* 132-138.

Hamdan, A. L., Deeb, R., Tohme, R. A., et al. (2008). Vocal technique in a group of Middle Eastern singers. *Folia Phoniatrica et Logopedica, 60,* 217-221.

Hammarberg, B., Gauffin, J. (1995). Perceptual and acoustic correlates of quality differences in pathological voices as related to physiological aspects. In O. Fujimura, M. Hirano (Eds.), *Vocal fold physiology: Voice quality control* (pp. 283-303). San Diego: Singular.

Hartelius, L., Theodoros, D., Cahill, L., Lillvik, M. (2003). Comparability of perceptual analysis of speech characteristics in Australian and Swedish speakers with multiple sclerosis. *Folia Phoniatrica et Logopedica, 55,* 177-188.

Hartnick, C. J. (2002). Validation of a pediatric voice quality-of-life instrument: The pediatric voice outcome survey. *Archives of Otolaryngology—Head and Neck Surgery, 128,* 919-922.

Helidoni, M. E., Murry, T., Moschandreas, J., et al. (2010). Cross-cultural adaptation and validation of the Voice Handicap Index into Greek. *Journal of Voice, 24,* 221-227.

Henton, C., Ladefoged, P., Maddieson, I. (1992). Stops in the world's languages. *Phonetica, 49,* 65-101.

Hirano, M. (1981). *Clinical examination of voice.* Vienna, Austria: Springer-Verlag.

Hogikyan, N. D., Sethuraman, G. (1999). Validation of an instrument to measure voice-related quality of life (V-RQOL). *Journal of Voice, 13,* 557-569.

Hollien, H., Maclik, E. (1962). Adolescent voice change in Southern Negro males. *Speech Monographs, 29,* 53-58.

Hollien, H., Shipp, T. (1972). Speaking fundamental frequency and chronological age in males. *Journal of Speech and Hearing Research, 15,* 155-159.

Hoonhorst, I., Colin, C., Markessis, E., et al. (2009). French native speakers in the making: from Language-general to language-specific voicing boundaries. *Journal of Experimental Child Psychology, 104,* 353-366.

Hsiung, M. W., Lu, P., Kang, B. H., Wang, H. W. (2003). Measurement and validation of the voice handicap index in voice-disordered patients in Taiwan. *Journal of Laryngology and Otology, 117,* 478-481.

Hsiung, M. W., Pai, L., Wang, H. W. (2002). Correlation between voice handicap index and voice laboratory measurements in dysphonic patients. *European Archives of Otorhinolaryngology, 259,* 97-99.

Isshiki, N. (1965). Vocal intensity and air flow rate. *Folia Phoniatrica et Logopedica, 17,* 92-104.

Jacobson, B. H., Johnson, A., Grywalsky, C., et al. (1997). The Voice Handicap Index (VHI): Development and validation. *American Journal of Speech and Language Pathology, 6,* 66-70.

Kempster, G. B., Gerrat, B. R., Verdolini-Abbott, K., et al. (2009). Consensus auditory-perceptual evaluation of voice: Development of a standardized clinical protocol. *American Journal of Speech and Language Pathology, 18,* 124-132.

Kiliç, M. A., Okur, E., Yildirim, I., et al. (2008). Reliability and validity of the Turkish version of the Voice Handicap Index. *Kulak Burun Bogaz Ihtisas Dergisi, 18,* 139-147.

Kitayama, S., Ishii, K. (2002). Word and voice: Spontaneous attention to emotional utterances in two languages. *Cognition and Emotion, 16,* 29-59.

Konnai, R. M., Jayaram, M., Scherer, R. C. (2010). Development and validation of a voice disorder outcome profile for an Indian population. *Journal of Voice, 24,* 206-220.

Kotby, M. N., Shiromoto, H. M. (1993). The Accent Method of voice therapy: Effects of accentuation on F0, SLP, and airflow. *Journal of Voice, 7,* 319-325.

Kotby, M. N., El-Sady, S., Abou-Rass, Y., Regazi, M. (1991). Efficacy of the Accent Method of voice therapy. *Journal of Voice, 5,* 316-320.

Krischke, S., Weigelt, S., Hoppe, U., et al. (2005). Quality of life in dysphonic patients. *Journal of Voice, 19,* 132-137.

Lam, P. K., Chan, K. M., Ho, W. K., et al. (2006). Cross-cultural adaptation and validation of the Chinese Voice Handicap Index-10. *Laryngoscope, 116,* 1192-1198.

Laver, J. (1980). *The phonetic description of voice quality* (pp. 184-208). London, Cambridge University Press.

Lazarus. R. S. (1993). Coping theory and research: Past, present, and future. *Psychosomatic Medicine, 55,* 234-47.

Lazarus, R. S. (1998). *Fifty years of the research and theory of RS Lazarus: An analysis of historical and perennial issues*. Mahwah, NJ: Lawrence Erlbaum, 1998.

Lazarus, R. S., Folkman, S. (1984). *Stress: Appraisal and coping*. New York: Springer.

Leppänen, K., Laukkanen, A. M., Ilomäki, I., Vilkman, E. (2009). A comparison of the effects of voice massage and voice hygiene: Lecture on self-reported vocal well-being and acoustic and perceptual speech parameters in female teachers. *Folia Phoniatrica et Logopedica, 61,* 227-238.

Leske, M. C. (1981). Prevalence estimates of communicative disorders in the U.S. Speech disorders. *ASHA, 23,* 217-225.

Lorch, M., Whurr, R. (2003). A cross-linguistic study of vocal pathology: Perceptual features of spasmodic dysphonia in French-speaking subjects. *Journal of Multilingual Communication Disorders, 1,* 35-52.

Ma, E. P. M., Yiu, E. M. L. (2001). Voice activity and participation profile: Assessing the impact of voice disorders on daily activities. *Journal of Speech, Language, and Hearing Research, 44,* 511-524.

Malki, K. H., Al-Habib, S. F., Hagr, A. A., Farahat, M. M. (2009). Acoustic analysis of normal Saudi adult voices. *Saudi Medical Journal, 30,* 1081-1086.

Malki, K. H., Mesallam, T. A., Farahat, M., et al. (2010). Validation and cultural modification of Arabic voice handicap index. *European Archives of Otorhinolaryngology, 267,* 1743-1751.

Mathieson, L., Hirani, S. P., Epstein, R., et al. (2009). Laryngeal manual therapy: A preliminary study to examine its treatment effects in the management of muscle tension dysphonia. *Journal of Voice, 23,* 353-366.

Mathieson, L. (2001). *The voice and its disorders* (6th ed) (pp. 139-140). London: Whurr.

Menon, M. S. (2007). *Foreign accent management*. San Diego: Plural.

Montero, J. M., Gutirrez-Arriola, J., Cordoba, R., et al. (1998). Spanish emotional speech: Towards concatenative synthesis. In E. Keller, G. Bailly, A. Monaghan, J. Terken, M. Huckvale (Eds.), *Improvements in speech synthesis. Cost 258: The naturalness of synthetic speech* (pp. 246-251). Chichester, UK: John Wiley and Sons.

Moore, G. P., Von Leden, H. (1958). Dynamic variations of the vibratory pattern in the normal larynx. *Folia Phoniatrica et Logopedica, 10,* 205-238.

Moore, G. P. (1998). A sketch of the partnership between speech-pathology and laryngology. In R. T. Sataloff (Ed.), *Voice perspectives* (pp. 1-14). San Diego: Singular.

Moreti, F., Ávila, M. E. B., Rocha, C., et al. (2010). Self-assessment protocols for modern and classical singing voice: Brazilian versions of MSHI and CSHI. Proceedings of the 28th World Congress of the International Association of Logopedics and Phoniatrics, Athens, Greece.

Moriyama, T., Ozawa, S. (1999). Emotion recognition and synthesis system on speech. *ICMCS, 1,* 840-844.

Morris, R. (1997). Speaking fundamental frequency characteristics of 8- through 10-year-old white- and African-American boys. *Journal of Communication Disorders, 30,* 101-114; quiz, 115-116.

Morsomme, D., Gaspar, M., Jamart, J., et al. (2007). Voice handicap index adapted to the singing voice [in French]. *Revue de Laryngologie-Otologie-Rhinologie, 128*(5), 305-314.

Moses, P. J. (1948). Vocal analysis. *Archives of Otolaryngology, 48,* 171-186.

Moses, P. J. (1956). *The voice of neurosis*. New York: Grune & Stratton.

Murray, I. R., Arnot, J. L. (1993). Towards the simulation of emotion in synthetic speech: A review of the literature on human vocal emotion. *Journal of the Acoustic Society of America, 2,* 1097-1108.

Murry, T., Zschommler, A., Prokop, J. (2009). Voice handicap in singers. *Journal of Voice, 23,* 275-279.

Natour, Y. S., Wingate, J. M. (2003). Fundamental frequency characteristics of Jordanian Arabic speakers. *Journal of Voice, 23,* 560-566.

Nawka, T., Verdonck-de-Leeuw, I., De Bodt, M., et al. (2009). Item reduction of the Voice Handicap Index based on the original version and on European translations. *Folia Phoniatrica et Logopedica, 61,* 37-48.

Nawka, T., Wiesmann, U., Gonnermann, U. (2003). Validierung des Voice Handicap Index (VHI) in der deutschen Fassung [Validation of the German version of the Voice Handicap Index]. *HNO, 51,* 921-930.

Nguyen, D. D., Kenny, D. T., Tran, N. D., Livesey, J. R. (2009). Muscle tension dysphonia in Vietnamese female teachers. *Journal of Voice, 23,* 195-208.

Nguyen, D. D., Kenny, D. T. (2009a). Impact of muscle tension dysphonia on tonal pitch target implementation in Vietnamese female teachers. *Journal of Voice, 23,* 690-698.

Nguyen, D. D., Kenny, D. T. (2009b). Randomized controlled trial of vocal function exercises on muscle tension dysphonia in Vietnamese female teachers. *Journal of Otolaryngology: Head and Neck Surgery, 38,* 261-278.

Núñez-Batalla, F., Corte-Santos, P., Señaris-González, B., et al. (2007). Adaptation and validation to the Spanish of the Voice Handicap Index (VHI-30) and its shortened version (VHI-10). *Acta Otorrinolaringologica Española, 58,* 386-392.

Oates, J. (2009). Auditory-perceptual evaluation of disordered vocal quality: Pros, cons and future directions. *Folia Phoniatrica et Logopedica, 61,* 49-56.

Oates, J., Russell, A. (2003). *A sound judgement*. La Trobe University, COMET.

Ohala, J. J. (1983). Cross-language use of pitch: an ethological view. *Phonetica, 40,* 1-18.

Ohala, J. J. (1984). An ethological perspective on common cross-language utilization of F0 of voice. *Phonetica, 41,* 1-16.

Ohlsson, A. C, Dotevall, H. (2009). Voice handicap index in Swedish. *Logopedics, Phoniatrics, Vocology, 34,* 60-66.

Oliveira, G., Hirani S. P., Epstein, R., Yazigi, L., Behlau, M. (2011). Coping Strategies in Voice Disorders of a Brazilian Population. *Journal of Voice* [in press].

O'Neil. E. N., Jones, G., Chad, N. (1997). Acoustic characteristics of children who speak Arabic. *International Journal of Pediatric Otorhinolaryngology, 42,* 117-124.

Oyserman, D., Coon, H. M., Kemmelmeier, M. (2004). Rethinking individualism and collectivism: Evaluation of theoretical assumptions and meta-analyses. *Psychological Bulletin, 128,* 3-45.

Parkin, D. M. (2004). International variation. *Oncogene, 23,* 6329-6340.

Prakash, B. (2008). Voice analysis: Care of professional voice users. In Proceedings of the National Workshop on Voice: Assessment and management. AIISH Publications.

Preciado-Lopez, J., Perez-Fernandez, C., Calzada-Uriondo, M., Preciado-Ruiz, P. (2007). Epidemiological study of voice disorders among teaching professional of La Rioja, Spain. *Journal of Voice, 22,* 489-508.

Pruszewicz, A., Obrebowski, A., Wiskirska-Woznica, B., Wojnowski, W. (2004). Complex voice assessment: Polish version of the Voice Handicap Index (VHI). *Otolaryngology (Poland), 58,* 547-549.

Ramig, L. O., Countryman, S., Thompson, L., Horii, Y. (1995). Comparison of two forms of intensive speech treatment for Parkinson disease. *Journal of Speech, Language, and Hearing Research, 38,* 1232-1251.

Ramig, L. O., Dromey, C. (1996). Aerodynamic mechanisms underlying treatment-related changes in vocal intensity in patients with Parkinson disease. *Journal of Speech and Hearing Research, 39,* 798-807.

Ramig, L. O., Fox, C., Sapir, S. (2008). Speech treatment for Parkinson's disease. *Expert Review of Neurotherapeutics, 8,* 297-309.

Ramig, L. O., Sapir, S., Fox, C., Countryman, S. (2001). Changes in vocal loudness following intensive voice treatment (LSVT) in individuals with Parkinson's disease: a comparison with untreated patients and normal age-matched controls. *Movement Disorders, 16,* 79-83

Rinker, T., Alku, P., Brosch, S., Kiefer, M. (2010). Discrimination of native and non-native vowel contrasts in bilingual Turkish-German and monolingual German children: Insight from the Mismatch Negativity ERP component. *Brain and Language, 113,* 90-95.

Rosen, C. A., Murry, T., Zinn, A., et al. (2000). Voice handicap index change following treatment of voice disorders. *Journal of Voice, 14,* 619-623.

Rosen, C. A., Lee, A. S., Osborne, J., et al. (2004). Development and validation of the Voice Handicap Index-10. *Laryngoscope, 114,* 1549-1556.

Roy N. (2003). Functional dysphonia. *Current Opinion in Otolaryngology and Head and Neck Surgery, 11,* 144-148.

Roy, N., Merrill, R. M., Thibeault, S., et al. (2004a). Voice disorders in teachers and the general population: effects on work performance, attendance, and future career choices. *Journal of Speech, Language, and Hearing Research, 47,* 542-551.

Roy, N., Merrill, R. M., Thibeault, S., et al. (2004b). Prevalence of voice disorders in teachers in the general population. *Journal of Speech, Language, and Hearing Research, 47,* 281-293.

Roy, N., Gray, S. D., Simon, M., et al. (2001). An evaluation of the effects of two treatment approaches for teachers with voice disorders: a prospective randomized clinical trial. *Journal of Speech, Language, and Hearing Research, 44,* 286-296.

Roy, N., Merril, R. N., Gray, S. D., Smith, E. M. (2005). Voice disorders in the general population: Prevalence, risk factors and occupational impact. *Laryngoscope, 115,* 1988-1995.

Roy, N., Stemple, J., Merrill, R. M., Thomas, L. (2007). Epidemiology of voice disorders in the elderly: preliminary findings. *Laryngoscope, 117,* 628-633.

Roy, N., Leeper, H. A. (1993). Effects of the manual laryngeal musculoskeletal tension reduction technique as a treatment for functional voice disorders: Perceptual and acoustic measures. *Journal of Voice, 7,* 242-249.

Roy, N., Bless, D. M., Heisey, D., Ford, C. N. (1997). Manual circumlaryngeal therapy for functional dysphonia: An evaluation of short- and long-term treatment outcomes. *Journal of Voice, 11,* 321-331.

Sapienza, C. M. (1997). Aerodynamic and acoustic characteristics of the adult African American voice. *Journal of Voice, 11,* 410-416.

Sapir, S., Ramig, L., Fox, C. (2009). Speech therapy in the treatment of Parkinson's disease. In A. Blitzer, M. Brin, L. Ramig (Eds.), *Neurologic voice disorders.* New York: Thieme Medical.

Sapir, S., Ramig, L. O., Hoyt, P., et al. (2002). Speech loudness and quality 12 months after intensive voice treatment (LSVT) for Parkinson's disease: A comparison with an alternative speech treatment. *Folia Phoniatrica et Logopedica, 54,* 296-303

Sapir, S., Spielman, J., Ramig, L. O., et al. (2003). Effects of intensive voice treatment (the Lee Silverman Voice Treatment [LSVT]) on ataxic dysarthria: A case study. *American Journal of Speech and Language Pathology, 12,* 387-399.

Scherer, K. (2000). A cross-cultural investigation of emotion interferences from voice and speech: implications for speech technology. In: Proceedings of the Sixth International Conference on Spoken Language Processing (Vol. 2) (pp. 379-382).

Schindler, A., Ottaviani, F., Mozzanica, F., et al. (2010). Cross-cultural adaptation and validation of the Voice Handicap Index into Italian. *Journal of Voice, 24,* 708-714.

Schmidt, A. M., Flege, J. E. (1996). Speaking rate effects on stops produced by Spanish and English monolinguals and Spanish/English bilinguals. *Phonetica, 53,* 162-179.

Schwartz, S. R., Cohen, S. M., Dailey, S. H., et al. (2009). Clinical practice guideline: Hoarseness (dysphonia). *Otolaryngology—Head and Neck Surgery, 141,* S1-S31.

Screen, R. M., Anderson, N. B. (1994). An understanding of the professions. In R. M. Screen, N. B. Anderson (Eds.), *Multicultural perspectives in communication disorders* (pp. 14-15). San Diego: Singular.

Seneriches, J. S. (2009). Voice and emotions in the Philippine culture. In K. Izdebski (Ed.), *Emotions in the human voice: Culture and perception* (Vol. III) (pp. 289-295). San Diego: Plural.

Senturia, B. H., Wilson, F. M. (1968). Otorhinolaryngologic findings in children with voice deviations. *Annals of Otology, Rhinology, and Laryngology, 77,* 1027-1042.

Shigeno, S. (2009). Recognition of vocal and facial emotions: Comparison between Japanese and North Americans. In K. Izdebski (Ed.), *Emotions in the human voice: Culture and perception* (Vol. III) (pp. 187-204). San Diego: Plural.

Shipp, T., Hollien, H. (1969). Perception of the aging male voice. *Journal of Speech and Hearing Research, 12,* 704-710.

Sidorova, J., McDonough, J., Badia, T. (2009). Automatic recognition of emotive voice and speech. In K. Izdebski (Ed.), *Emotions in the human voice: Culture and perception* (Vol. III) (pp. 205-230). San Diego: Plural.

Silverman, E. M., Zimmer, C. H. (1975). Incidence of chronic hoarseness among school age children. *Journal of Speech and Hearing Disorders, 40,* 211-215.

Simberg, S., Laine, A., Sala, E., Rönnemaa, A. M. (2000). Prevalence of voice disorders among future teachers. *Journal of Voice, 14,* 231-235.

Skevington, S. M. (2002). Advancing cross-cultural research on quality of life: Observations drawn from the WHOQOL development. *Quality of Life Research, 11,* 135-144.

Smith, S., Thyme, K. (1976). Statistic research on changes in speech due to pedagogic treatment (the Accent Method). *Folia Phoniatrica et Logopedica, 28,* 98-103.

Steinberg, C. (2009a). Dazed and confused: Possible processing constraints on emotional response to information-dense motivational speech. In K. Izdebski (Ed.), *Emotions in the human voice: Culture and perception* (Vol. III) (pp. 79-103). San Diego: Plural.

Steinberg, C. (2009b). Tokin tuf: True grit in the voice virility. In K. Izdebski (Ed.), *Emotions in the human voice: Culture and perception* (Vol. III) (pp. 239-262). San Diego: Plural.

Steinsapir, C. D., Forner, L. L., Stemple, J. C. (1986). Voice characteristics among black and white children: Do differences exist? ASHA Convention, Detroit.

Stemple, J. C., Lee, L., D'Amico, B., Pickup, B. (1994). Efficacy of vocal function exercises as a method of improving voice production. *Journal of Voice, 8,* 271-289.

Stoel-Gammon, C., Williams, K., Buder, E. (1994). Cross-language differences in phonological acquisition: Swedish and American /t/. *Phonetica, 51,* 146-158.

Sukanen, O., Sihvo, M., Rorarius, E., et al. (2007). Voice Activity and Participation Profile (VAPP) in assessing the effects of voice disorders on patients' quality of life: Validity and reliability of the Finnish version of VAPP. *Logopedics, Phoniatrics, Vocology, 32,* 3-8.

Švec, J. G., Behlau, M. (2007). April 16th: The World Voice Day. *Folia Phoniatrica et Logopedica, 59,* 53-54.

Teshigawara, M., Amir, N., Amir, O., et al. (2009). Perceptions of Japanese anime voices by Hebrew speakers. In K. Izdebski (Ed.), *Emotions in the human voice: Culture and perception* (Vol. III) (pp. 177-186). San Diego: Plural.

Teshigawara, M. (2009). Vocal expressions of emotions and personalities in Japanese anime. In K. Izdebski (Ed.), *Emotions in the human voice: Culture and perception* (Vol. III) (pp. 275-287). San Diego: Plural.

Thomas, L. B., Stemple, J. C. (2007). Voice therapy: Does science support the art? *Communicative Disorders Review, 1,* 49-77.

Titze, I. (1995). *Workshop on acoustic voice analysis: Summary statement.* Denver, Colorado, National Center for Voice and Speech.

Titze, I. R., Lemke, J., Montequin, D. (1997). Population in the U.S. workforce who rely on voice as a primary tool of trade: a preliminary report. *Journal of Voice, 11,* 254-259.

Toivanen, J., Seppänen, T., Väyrynen, E. (2009). Automatic discrimination of emotion from voice: A review of research paradigms. In K. Izdebski (Ed.), *Emotions in the human voice: Culture and perception* (Vol. III) (pp. 67-77). San Diego: Plural.

Tosi, O. (1979). *Voice identification: Theory and legal applications.* Baltimore: University Park Press.

Van Lierde, K. M., De Ley, S., Clement, G., et al. (2004). Outcome of laryngeal manual therapy in four Dutch adults with persistent moderate-to-severe vocal hyperfunction: A pilot study. *Journal of Voice, 18,* 467-474.

Verdolini, K., Ramig, L. O. (2001). Review: Occupational risks for voice problems. *Logopedics, Phoniatrics, Vocology, 26,* 37-46.

Verdolini-Marston, K., Burke, M. K., Lessac, A., et al. (1995). Preliminary study of two methods of treatment for laryngeal nodules. *Journal of Voice, 9,* 74-85.

Verdonck-de Leeuw, I. M., Kuik, D. J., De Bodt, M., et al. (2008). Validation of the voice handicap index by assessing equivalence of European translations. *Folia Phoniatrica et Logopedica, 60,* 173-178.

Walton, J. H., Orlikoff, R. F. (1994). Speaker race identification from acoustic cues in the vocal signal. *Journal of Speech and Hearing Research, 37,* 738-774.

Webb, A. L., Carding, P. N., Deary, I. J., et al. (2007). Optimising outcome assessment of voice interventions, I: Reliability and validity of three self-reported scales. *Journal of Laryngology and Otology, 121,* 763-767.

Wheat, M. C., Hudson, A. I. (1988). Spontaneous speaking fundamental frequency of 6 year old Black children. *Journal of Speech and Hearing Research, 31,* 723-725.

Woisard, V., Bodin, S., Puech, M. (2004). The Voice Handicap Index: Impact of the translation in French on the validation. *Revue de Laryngologie—Otologie—Rhinologie, 125,* 307-312.

Woo, P. (1996). Quantification of videostrobolaryngoscopic findings: Measurements of the normal glottal cycle. *Laryngoscope, 106,* 1-27.

World Health Organization. (1980). *International classification of impairments, disabilities and handicaps: A manual of classification relating to the consequences of disease* (pp. 25-43). Geneva: World Health Organization.

Xue, S. A., Fucci, D. (2000). Effects of race and sex on acoustic features of voice analysis. *Perceptual and Motor Skills, 91,* 951-958.

Xue, S. A., Hao, G. J., Mayo, R. (2006). Volumetric measurements of vocal tracts for male speakers form different races. *Clinics in Linguistic Phonetics, 20,* 691-702.

Yamaguchi, H., Shrivastav, R., Andrews, M. L., Niimi, S. (2003). A comparison of voice quality ratings made by Japanese and American listeners using the GRBAS scale. *Folia Phoniatrica et Logopedica, 55,* 147-157.

Yamasaki, R., Leão, S., Madazio, G., et al. (2010). Overall severity of dysphonia rated in two different scales: Visual analog and numerical. Paper presented at the Voice Foundation's 39th Annual Symposium: Care of the Professional Voice, June 2-6, 2010, Philadelphia.

Yiu, E. M. L., Murdoch, B., Hird, K., Lau, P. (2008). Perception of synthesized dysphonic qualities: A cross-language comparison. *Folia Phoniatrica et Logopedica, 60,* 107-119.

Zraick, R. I., Risner, B. Y., Smith-Olinde, L., et al. (2007). Patient versus partner perception of voice handicap. *Journal of Voice, 21,* 485-494.

Zur, K. B., Cotton, S., Kelchner, L., et al. (2007). Pediatric Voice Handicap Index (pVHI): A new tool for evaluating pediatric dysphonia. *International Journal of Pediatric Otorhinolaryngology, 71,* 77-82.

ADDITIONAL RESOURCES

Throughout the chapter and in specific tables, we have listed resources for the voice diagnostician. Tables 10-2, 10-3, and 10-4 outline assessment resources in voice and their value. In view of the fact that assessment a treatment may be guided by financial constraints rather than by "state of the art" machines, we feel that the clinician will search out the best tools for his or her needs based on the available resources in each clinic. One of the best resources for seeking help in assessment and treatment is the list of exhibitors at the most recent American Speech Language and Hearing Association Meeting (www.asha.org.) We offer this outlet without bias.

Additionally, many websites offer information about the voice. The Voice Foundation (www.voicefoundation.org), now in existence for 40 years, remains the centerpiece for unbiased information, for recent advances in diagnosis and treatment, and as a guide to existing faculty around the world available to discuss specific voice problems. The Voice Foundation is also responsible for the website www.voiceproblem.org, a major effort that counted with the participation of more than 40 colleagues, physicians, speech-language pathologists, and voice teachers, with some international collaboration. You may also visit The Voice Problem Website (www.voiceproblem.org), an important resource for both patients and clinicians on voice problems. This website was made via a consortium of international colleagues and has received the collaboration of 5 editors and 21 contributors and reviewers.

Fully illustrated, helps individuals to understand the complexity of a voice problem and its treatment.

Speech-Language Pathology World Voice Survey

Appendix Table 10-1 shows the countries and the number of participants from each country who responded to the survey. Appendix Table 10-2 classifies the questions according to the six areas surveyed. The complete survey questionnaire with results follows.

The survey revealed that voice disorders as a discipline is offered at the undergraduate and graduate levels. According to the respondents, it is more frequently a course suited for graduate content. Understanding voice production and voice disorders is easily applicable in different cultural scenarios, which facilitates and inspires colleagues to travel and attend conferences in many countries. This may not be the case for other communicative problems because communication aspects of articulation and language disorders may not be easily transferred in other cultures.

Assessment and treatment of voice disorders have cultural differences but commonalities are also seen in the types of voice disorders and their treatment. Differences appear to be in the way assessments are made.

In some countries, assessment is highly dependent on instrumental measurement, whereas in others, it is not. Treatment patterns are also country dependent in that many respondents reported an eclectic approach to treatment whereas others reported programmed treatments such as the Lee Silverman Voice Treatment (LSVT) and the Vocal Function Exercises (VFE). In the United States, referral is almost always through an otolaryngologist or neurologist, but in other countries, referral patterns may come from general practitioners or from self-referrals. One important finding that appeared in almost all questionnaires is that former patients usually refer new patients. That may be interpreted as an aspect of treatment satisfaction. A significant diagnostic advancement toward international voice communication is the validation of self-assessment protocols. Now more than 20 countries have translated and validated the Voice Handicap Index (VHI) and use it as a patient self-assessment of voice severity.

In our questionnaire, which may be considered as a sampling of attitudes about voice and voice care, colleagues responded to issues of treatment with a variety of differences based on location of service delivery, style of treatment, and types of patients seen. We are fully aware that this questionnaire and the results do not represent a randomized sample, yet they reflect worldwide opinions about the management of voice disorders. Despite the lack of involvement in the medical assessment process in many countries, team attitude was seen as a basic element of the speech-language pathologist's (SLP's) approach to treatment. In addition, a general trend indicated that SLPs are likely to seek continuing education from various medical and SLP associations if they are maintaining a significant part of their clinical practice treating voice disorders.

APPENDIX TABLE 10-1 Countries and the Number of Speech-Language Pathologists from Each of the 25 Countries that Responded to the 27-Item Survey on Voice Assessment and Diagnosis, Voice Education and Training, and Voice Practice Profiles

Country	No. of Respondents
United States	7
Brazil	5
Australia	2
Argentina	3
Canada	1
Japan	1
Sweden	3
United Kingdom	3
Hong Kong	2
Finland	1
Austria	1
Belgium	3
Chile	1
Egypt	1
Spain	1
France	1
Germany	1
Greece	1
Italy	1
Malta	1
New Zealand	1
South Africa	1
The Netherlands	1
Uruguay	1
India	1
Colombia	1
Total	**41**

QUESTIONS FOR INTERNATIONAL PRACTICES IN CLINICAL VOICE DISORDERS

1. From where do you get your referrals? Rank: 1 = most to 5 = least
   (41) Medical doctors
   (27) School nurses
   (30) Parents
   (24) Other health professionals
   (31) Former patients

APPENDIX TABLE 10-2 Breakdown of the Number of Questions and Reference to the Questions from the International Practices in Clinical Voice Disorders

Category	No. of Questions (Items)
Training	3 (4, 14, 19)
Licensing	2 (12, 13)
Assessment and treatment	12 (3, 7, 9, 10, 11, 15, 17, 18, 21, 22, 23, 24, 25)
Insurance	3 (5, 6, 7)
Referral patterns	4 (1, 2, 20, 26)
Research	1 (16)

2. What percentage from each? Mark with an X the appropriate range

	<25%	25%-50%	50%-75%	>75%
Medical doctors (39)	1	6	15	23
School (32)	30	1	1	0
Parents (34)	29	5	0	0
Other health professionals (34)	22	11	5	1
Former patients (33)	22	11	3	2

3. How many sessions are usually given for voice therapy? (Three people answered more than one alternative.)
   (16) Less than 6
   (16) 7-10
   (11) 11-20
   (06) More than 20

4. Do the universities in your country offer a course primarily devoted to voice disorders? What percentage of SLPs take this course?

	<25%	25%-50%	50%-75%	>75%
At undergraduate level (37)	16	3	3	15
At graduate level (38)	11	8	3	16

5. Does medical insurance pay for voice therapy? (One person marked both alternatives.)
   (40) Yes
   (07) No

6. How many sessions does public insurance usually pay? Some people said it depends on the fund, but the rough average is 27 sessions (5 to 50).

7. How many sessions does private insurance usually pay? (Some people said it depends on the insurance, about 10 sessions (0-30).)

8. Do SLPs participate in the interpretation of stroboscopic results? (Four did not answer this question.)
   (32) Yes
   (12) No

9. Where is voice therapy carried out in your country? Rank: 1= most to 4= least
   (45) Hospital

1 = 28	2 = 8	3 = 6	4 = 2

   (41) Physician's office

1 = 4	2 = 9	3 = 15	4 = 13

   (43) Private practice

1 = 19	2 =16	3 = 4	4 = 4

   (41) Home care

1 = 2	2 = 3	3 = 10	4 = 26

10. Do you do group voice therapy for children
    (09) Yes
    (24) No
    (12) I do not do voice therapy with children

11. Do you do group therapy for adults?
    (13) Yes
    (30) No
    (01) I do not do voice therapy with adults

12. Are SLPs licensed in your country?
    (39) Yes; colleagues from 19 countries
    (06) No

13. Is there an official recognition for voice specialists (SLPs)?
    (16) Yes; colleagues from 5 countries
    (29) No

14. Are SLPs required to take continuing education courses in your country?
    (15) Specific topics
    (23) General courses
    No = 6

15. What percentage of voice patients are:

	<25%	25%-50%	50%-75%	>75%
Adults (37)	0	2	10	31
Children and adolescents (36)	27	14	0	0

16. Do your patients participate in research? If positive, what percentage?
    (08) No
    (36) Yes
    (11) <25%
    (10) 25%-50%
    (11) 50%-75%
    (4) >75%

17. Do SLPs treat singers with voice disorders?
    (44) Yes
    (00) No

18. What are the limiting factors in treating voice disorders in your country?

	<25%	25%-50%	50%-75%	>75%
Patient compliance (37)	20	14	6	2
Cost/insurance (36)	15	13	9	4
Lack of voice education among speech-language pathologists (34)	19	7	9	4
Others (24)	19	6	0	0

19. How many voice conferences have you been to during the last 5 years?
    In your country: ____

1-10 = 31	11-20 = 7	21-30 = 3	>30 = 2

    In other countries: ____

1-10 = 32		11-20 = 2	

20. What are the most common types of patients seen for voice therapy in your country?

	<25%	25%-50%	50%-75%	>75%
Home-based mothers (32)	33	4	0	0
Business women (37)	24	12	6	1
Business men (35)	21	11	8	0
Female teachers (37)	3	16	16	8
Male teachers (33)	24	10	3	1
Clergy (32)	27	8	0	1
Children (32)	24	10	2	1
Singers/actors (36)	9	21	9	3
Factory workers (29)	28	5	0	1
Others (48)	21	3	1	25

21. Do you assess patients in their professional setting (e.g., school, theater, performances)?
(20) Yes
(25) No

22. Do you use custom-made approaches for voice rehabilitation? If positive, what percentage?
(10) No
(31) Yes
    (4) <25%
    (8) 25%-50%
    (8) 50%-75%
    (11) >75%

23. What tests of voice do you use in your center? (Check all that apply)

(37) VHI/V-RQOL/VAPP	(18) Air Flow
(40) Acoustic Measures	(13) Vital Capacity
(14) Air Pressure	(28) MPT
(25) Spectrogram	(30) Voice Range Profile
(30) GRBAS	(17) CAPE-V
(20) Other	

24. Are there normative values for voice assessment in your country? (Check all that apply)
(24) Perceptual
(30) Acoustic, from 15 countries
(23) Validated self-assessment of vocal problem
(09) Special protocols developed in your country. Please, name it _____

25. Do you use programmatic therapy?

	<25%	25%-50%	50%-75%	>75%
Lee Silverman Voice Treatment (LSVT): 25	23	6	1	0
Vocal Function Exercises (VFE): 30	13	10	8	5
Accent Method: 20	16	4	3	1
Other: 19	8	6	3	7

26. Are there any cultural/ethnic issues you take into consideration when assessing these populations? Please, indicate with a brief statement.

List of issues provided by the respondents: Chinese patients; Orthodox Muslim patients; Afrikaans; language influence; diet and lifestyle; social values; accent; education and vocal hygiene habits, use of confidential voice; religious issues and beliefs; children's expected behavior; variations in prosodic features; age, gender, profession, role in the family, role in the society; customs; language; multilanguage use; loudness; body language; specific articulatory behaviors; teachers; Japanese teachers; attitudes related to self-monitoring; tropical climates; elite families; loudness of the conversational voice; and adult male members of certain groups who associate high-pitched voice with authority (in India). The situation in

India is unique. Multicultural issues certainly call for a focus group and discussion of the international voice community.

ACKNOWLEDGMENT

The authors acknowledge the speech-language pathologists from around the world who contributed their time and information to the survey taken in 2009. Their responses provided the impetus to the authors to seek further information related to the issue explored. The authors also acknowledge the assistants of the Centro de Estudos da Voz (Center for Voice Studies) and also the students of the Graduate Program in Human Communicative Disorders at Universidade Federal de São Paulo (Federal University of São Paulo), Brazil, who helped locate important references for the discussion and formatting the text.

Chapter 11

Multicultural Aspects of Hearing Loss

Zenobia Bagli

The population of the United States is becoming increasingly diverse, and it has been projected that by 2050, minority groups will make up 50% of the U.S. population. Gradually there has also been a shift in the way multiculturalism is perceived and organized in the United States. Blending into the melting pot is no longer mentioned; individuals no longer relinquish their ethnic and cultural values to adopt those of the American culture. Today, minority groups retain their ethnic and cultural values *and* participate fully in society as it exists in the country; that is, they participate fully in ethnic and cultural pluralism. Clinicians who plan to work in this montage of cultures must be prepared to meet the challenge; they must have the boldness, attitude, eagerness, willingness, knowledge, and skills to effectively and efficiently manage multiculturalism.

In this century, some of the greatest changes and challenges facing health care professionals will be related to ethnic diversity. Speech-language pathologists and audiologists will be providing services to persons from a variety of racial and ethnic backgrounds, and culture will influence the way they operate. Professionals will have to become more conscious and knowledgeable of the cultures of the persons they serve because culture may affect the way a family accepts a diagnosis of hearing loss or deafness, copes with the emotional impact of having a deaf child, interacts with the professional, implements treatment, allows the clinician to participate with the family in early intervention, and tolerates what may be perceived as intrusion from the clinician. To achieve successful outcomes, professionals will have to become more culture conscious, develop cultural competence, and design, develop, and implement assessment and treatment protocols that reflect the diversity of the individuals they serve.

In a culturally diverse nation and world such as ours, it is imperative that clinicians show cultural sensitivity, respect for differences, and flexibility. There are likely to be differences in languages, accent, perspective, customs, beliefs, attitudes, experiences, and values. Clinicians must become culturally competent, that is, recognize and respect the beliefs, behaviors, and attitudes of the patient and family, and avoid stereotyping individuals at all costs.

A hearing impairment may be caused by genetic factors or nongenetic factors, such as infections and ototoxic drugs. In a young child, hearing loss can impede normal development of language and speech and, subsequently, affect education. In the adult, it may result in vocational and economic difficulties and lead to social isolation and stigmatization. The increased life expectancy and the growing world population suggest that, in the future, there will be greater numbers of persons with hearing impairment unless decisive public health action is taken to reduce and eventually eliminate preventable hearing impairment and disability by implementing appropriate preventive measures (World Health Organization [WHO], 2001).

Although deafness can occur in persons of all races, genders, and ages, there are differences among ethnic groups depending on the etiological factor under review. For instance, the leading cause of deafness in the Hispanic community is maternal rubella, but in the African American community, it is meningitis (Schildroth & Hotto, 1995). To some extent, health differences and this disparity appear to be related to socioeconomic status. On average, white Americans have better access to the social and economic resources necessary for a healthy environment and lifestyle and better access to preventive medical services than minorities.

The WHO's Global Burden of Disease (GBD) provides a comprehensive and comparable avenue to assess the impact of an illness or injury. The computation takes into account the incidence, average duration of an illness, and the relative risk of mortality. The causes of the global burden of disease are assessed according to the percentage of total disability adjusted life years (DALYs) in the world attributable to each etiological factor. Thus DALYs are a measure of the years of healthy life lost (YLL) and the years lived with disability (YLD). The data used to estimate YLD are incidence of disability, duration of disability, and a weight factor that reflects the severity of the disease. Since 2001, the WHO has included adult-onset hearing loss in the tables of the global burden of disease in the World Health Report. Adult-onset hearing impairment ranks third among contributors to YLD. YLL for hearing loss is zero; therefore, the DALY burden comes from YLD. GBD was first put into use in 1990, and last revised in 2004. DALY estimates will be revised again after the release of the Global Burden of Disease 2010 study (WHO, 2000; Smith, 2008).

It has been estimated that the lifetime costs of severe to profound hearing loss in the United States are about $297,000 per year; 21% of these costs are incurred in the provision of special education services (Mohr et al., 2000). It has been further estimated that with reduced work productivity, hearing health care, and special education, lifetime costs for those with severe to profound hearing loss acquired prelingually are about $1,000,000 (McPherson, 2008).

INCIDENCE OF HEARING IMPAIRMENT IN THE WORLD

Hearing loss is a disability that is widespread throughout the globe. It negatively affects communication and the quality of life and imposes a tremendous social and economic burden on society. The WHO (2006) estimated that in 2005 there were 278 million persons in the world, who had a disabling hearing impairment (i.e., hearing loss of 41 dB HL or greater in the better ear for adults, and 31 dB HL or greater for children up to 15 years of age). Further, it was estimated that for 68 million people, hearing loss began in childhood, and for 210 million during adulthood. An additional 364 million persons were estimated to have a mild hearing loss. According to the WHO, developing countries bear the greater burden (about two thirds) of hearing loss.

Epidemiology of Hearing Loss and Deafness in the United States

In the United States the incidence of permanent hearing impairment resulting from diseases such as mumps, measles, meningitis, and maternal rubella has substantially declined because of rigorous immunization programs. However, the overall incidence of permanent hearing impairment has *not* declined. Fifty percent of hearing loss is caused by mutations in the deoxyribonucleic acid (DNA) sequence of genes. In addition, there is an increase in the incidence of hearing loss due to cytomegalovirus (CMV) and a growing number of babies are born with very low birth weight. When the gestational period is reduced and the baby is born with low birth weight, health and survival are compromised. These babies often have permanent hearing loss and other neurological involvement. According to the Centers for Disease Control and Prevention (CDC), approximately 25% of newborns who are deaf or hard of hearing have another neurodevelopmental condition, such as learning disability, cerebral palsy, mental retardation, attention deficit disorders, and visual problems (CDC, 2011).

The number of adult Americans with hearing loss has increased drastically, possibly because of an aging population

and increased exposure to noise. Agrawal and colleagues (2008) administered a national cross-sectional survey to 5742 adults aged 20 to 69 years, who participated in the audiometric component of the National Health and Nutrition Examination Survey. They reported that in 2003-2004, 16.1% of American adults, or approximately 29 million, had hearing loss in the speech frequencies, whereas in the youngest age group that they tested (20 to 29 years), 8.5% demonstrated hearing loss. Further, they observed that the odds of having a hearing loss were 5.5 times greater in men than in women and 70% greater in whites than in blacks participating in the survey. Also, according to the survey, smoking, noise exposure, and cardiovascular risk increased the prevalence of hearing loss.

Age, Gender, and Race

The U.S. Department of Health and Human Services (2010) reported the results of the National Health Interview Survey, 2009. Overall, 15% of adults, who were 18 years and older, reported having difficulty with hearing (without a hearing aid), and men were more likely to have this problem than women. Age was positively correlated with hearing difficulties; that is, as age increased, so did the percentage of adults with this problem. There was a higher incidence of trouble in hearing in non-Hispanic white adults (16%) than in non-Hispanic black (10%) and Hispanic (10%) adults. Persons who were younger than 65 years and those covered by Medicaid were more likely to have hearing problems.

Mitchell (2006) provided an independent analysis of the federal government's Survey of Income and Program Participation (SIPP) data files for 2001 and reported that across all age groups, approximately 1,000,000 people (0.38% of the population) were "functionally deaf,"and 10,000,000 persons were hard of hearing. Of these, more than half were 65 years or older, and less than 4% were younger than 18 years. However, these findings included only those who reported having difficulty in hearing normal conversation with or without the use of a hearing aid, and excluded those persons with hearing loss whose hearing was affected "outside the range and circumstances of normal conversation."

Similarly, Schoenborn and Heyman (2009) used data from the 2004-2007 National Health Interview Survey and reported on selected health characteristics of four groups of older adults (55 to 85 years or older). They found that health disparities existed across subgroups of older adults and that these appeared to vary with age. For instance, the prevalence of hearing impairment increased with age. Approximately 31.6% of persons 55 years and older, 23% of persons aged 55 to 64 years, and 62.1% of those 85 years and older demonstrated some degree of hearing impairment. Schoenborn and Heyman also reported gender differences; in the 55- to 64-year age group, men (32.2%) were twice as likely as women (16.4%) to have hearing impairment, whereas in the 75- to 84-year age group, men (53.5%) were 1.5 times more likely than women (37.0%) to have hearing impairment. Finally, in the 85 years and older group, there was a smaller difference between the prevalence of hearing loss in men (69.0%) and women (58.5%).

Based on data from the Family Core and the Sample Core components of the 2004-2006 National Interview Surveys conducted by the CDC's National Center for Health Statistics, it was estimated that non-Hispanics, American Indians, and Alaska Natives were two to four times more likely to have a lot of trouble hearing or to be deaf than white, Hispanic, black, or Asian adults (Barnes et al., 2008). Schoenborn and Heyman (2009) also reported racial differences; among those 65 years and older, 4 out of 10 white adults (41.6%) had hearing impairment, compared with 2 out of 10 non-Hispanic black adults (23.6%), and three out of 10 non-Hispanic Asian (30.1%) and Hispanic (28.2%) adults.

Pratt and associates (2009) also examined the impact of age and race on the prevalence and severity of hearing loss in elder adults (72 to 96 years). They concluded that hearing loss was greater in the eighth than seventh decade of life, and that race and gender influenced the decline. These findings are consistent with those of Helzner and colleagues (2005) and Dillon and associates (2010). Helzner and colleagues reported a prevalence of hearing loss of 59.9% and prevalence of high-frequency hearing loss of 76.9% in 2052 adults aged 73 to 84 years. The incidence was higher in white males and females than in black males and females. Older age, race, diabetes mellitus, cerebrovascular disease, smoking, poor cognitive status, exposure to occupational noise, and ear surgery were associated with hearing loss. Race- and gender-specific risk factors included hypertension and occupational noise exposure in white men, poor cognitive factors and smoking in black women, low total hip bone mineral density in black men. Similarly, Dillon and associates reported (1) sensory impairment increased with age; (2) one out of four persons older than 70 years reported hearing loss; (3) older men were more likely to have hearing impairment than older women; (4) non-Hispanic white and Mexican American persons were more likely to have hearing loss than non-Hispanic black persons, and (5) approximately 70% of older Americans with hearing loss in at least one ear potentially could benefit from using a hearing aid but did not use amplification.

Hearing Loss and Deafness in Children and Youth

Hearing loss in the pediatric population has a deleterious effect on communication skills, social skills, and educational achievement. Shargorodsky and coworkers (2010) examined the current prevalence of hearing loss in U.S. adolescents and examined the change in incidence over time. They examined data from the Third National Health and Nutrition Examination Survey (1988-1994) and from the 2005-2006 survey. They reported that the prevalence of hearing loss in 12- to 19-year-olds had increased significantly from 14.9% in 1988-1994 to 19.5% in 2005-2006. Unilateral hearing loss was more prevalent in 2005-2006 (14%) than in 1988-1994 (11.1%). Further, the high frequencies were more involved in 2005-2006 (16.4%) than in 1988-1994 (12.8%). Also, it was reported that children from families below the federal poverty threshold (23.6%) were more likely to have hearing loss than children from above the poverty threshold (18.4%).

To establish an epidemiologic baseline, Mehra and colleagues (2009) compiled data from published studies. The average incidence of neonatal hearing loss in the United States was 1.1 per 1000 infants, with variation across states. Hispanic Americans demonstrated a higher prevalence of hearing impairment than children from other ethnic backgrounds. Although childhood and adolescent prevalence rates were variable, based on the average of comparable audiometric screening studies the prevalence of mild (>20 dB HL) hearing impairment or worse was 3.1%, whereas self-reporting prevalence was 1.9%. Low-income households demonstrated a higher prevalence of hearing loss compared with those with higher incomes. The prevalence of genetic hearing loss was reported to be 23%.

Based on questions from the Family Core and Sample Child Core questionnaires of the 2001-2007 National Health Interview Survey (NHIS), Pastor and coworkers (2009) reported estimates of functional difficulties related to "sensory difficulties" (vision and hearing) in school-aged children (5 to 17 years). They reported that 3% of children had sensory difficulty, of whom 11% had difficulty only in hearing, 88% only in seeing, and 1% in both hearing and seeing. Although a child's age, gender, race/ethnicity had negligible or insignificant impact on the prevalence of sensory deficits, certain other trends were observed. For instance, poor children (5%) were more likely to have sensory difficulty than children who were from middle- and upper-income families. Children who had public health insurance (4%) or who were uninsured (4%) were more likely to have sensory deficits than children with private insurance (3%). Also children in "mother-only" families (4%) were more likely to have sensory deficits than children from two-parent (3%) families.

In its *29th Annual Report to Congress on the Implementation of the Individuals with Disabilities Education Act (IDEA), 2007,* the U.S. Department of Education (2010) reported that in 2005, 0.1% of students who were 3 to 5 years or 18 to 21 years of age, and 0.5% of students who were 6 to 17 years of age, who had hearing impairment, were served under IDEA, Part B. Risk ratios compare the proportion of a particular racial/ethnic group served under Part B to the proportion served among other racial/ethnic groups combined. In 2005, the risk ratios for children 6 to

21 years of age served under IDEA, Part B, for hearing impairment, differentiated by ethnicity, were as follows: American Indian/Alaska Native (1.34), Hispanic (1.28), Asian/Pacific Islander (1.20), black not Hispanic (1.10), and white not Hispanic (0.77). That is, American Indian/Alaska Native students were 1.34 times more likely to be served under IDEA, Part B, for hearing impairment. Further, it was reported that in 2005, only 13.5% of students were educated in separate environments (e.g., Schools for the Deaf), whereas 48.3% students with hearing impairments spent most of the school day in regular classrooms (<21% of the day outside the regular classroom). The percentage of students with hearing impairment graduating with a regular high school diploma showed some improvement between 1995-1996 (58.8%) and 2004-2005 (69.6%). Students with hearing impairment had one of the lowest dropout rates of all disabilities. Twenty percent of students with hearing impairment participated in their state accountability testing without accommodations or modifications, 63% participated with accommodations or modifications, 16% participated in alternate assessments, and only 1% did not participate in standardized tests or alternate assessments. The mean standard scores for assessments in 2001-2002 and 2003-2004 showed that secondary school students with hearing impairment exhibited stronger mathematics calculation skills (mean standard score = 91.5) than knowledge/skills in applied problems (83.9), social studies (80.5), science (75.4), passage comprehension (75.6), and synonyms/antonyms (84.1).

Since 1968, Gallaudet University's Research Institute (GRI) has been administering its Annual Survey of Deaf and Hard of Hearing Children and Youth to collect demographic, audiologic, and other educationally relevant information on children with impaired hearing. GRI samples the population that receives services specified in IDEA, summarizes data for national use, and posts the data on the World Wide Web. The GRI does not representatively sample the geographic distribution of persons who are deaf or those who are hard of hearing. However, it continues to be very effective at obtaining responses from schools and programs that serve large numbers of children and youth who are hearing impaired and provides valuable demographic data and information regarding the services received by this population.

Data from the GRI Annual Survey between 2003 and 2008 demonstrated that the gender ratio of males to females has remained fairly stable; on an average, males make up 54.2% of this population and females 45.8%. Data on the geographic region where the students were located, consistently (for each of the 5 years) showed the highest number of hearing-impaired students (average of 5 years = 14,048.8) residing in the South, whereas the lowest number (average of 5 years = 5672.6) resided in the Northeast. Table 11-1 provides the national counts of deaf and hard-of-hearing children by age. The total number of children younger than 3 years show definite increases each year from 2003-2004 through 2006-2007. On the other hand, fewer students 18 years and older appear to have enrolled after 2003-2004; there was a significant reduction in the number of students in 2004-2005, and the lower count appears to have been maintained in subsequent years.

Table 11-2 summarizes the instructional setting of the students for the years 2003-2004, 2004-2005, 2005-2006, 2006-2007, and 2007-2008. For each of these years, consistent with IDEA, the highest percentage of students were reported to be studying in a regular school setting with hearing students, and this number shows a gradual increment for each of the years. On the other hand, there is a steady decrease in the number of students being taught in self-contained classrooms.

TABLE 11-1 Number of Children and Youth by Age Who Were Deaf or Hard of Hearing during the 2003 to 2008 School Years

Age (yrs)	2003-2004	2004-2005	2005-2006	2006-2007	2007-2008
<3	566	1244	1316	1330	1280
3-5	2490	3419	3611	3448	3431
6-9	7283	7898	8320	7825	7755
10-13	10,634	10,348	10,829	10,198	9712
14-17	11,036	10,230	10,754	10,121	10,000
18 years or older	5897	3520	3839	3712	3899
Info. not reported	748	841	833	718	633
TOTAL	38,744	37,500	39,502	37,352	36,710

From Gallaudet Research Institute (January 2005, December 2005, December 2006, December 2007, November 2008). Regional and National Summary Report of Data from the 2003-04, 2004-05, 2005-06, 2006-07, 2007-08 Annual Survey of Deaf and Hard of Hearing Children and Youth. Washington, DC: GRI, Gallaudet University.

TABLE 11-2 Percentage of Children and Youth with Hearing Impairment in Types of Instructional Settings during the 2003 to 2008 School Years*

Type of Setting	2003-2004	2004-2005	2005-2006	2006-2007	2007-2008
Special school/center	27.1	28.1	26.5	26.0	24.3
Self-contained classroom	31.1	29.9	27.3	20.4	17.4
Resource room	13.9	14.1	14.6	12.1	9.6
Regular educational setting	46.0	47.0	49.6	55.4	59.9
Home	3.0	2.6	2.7	2.4	2.1
Other	4.5	6.6	7.0	3.0	3.1

From Gallaudet Research Institute (January 2005, December 2005, December 2006, December 2007, November 2008). Regional and National Summary Report of Data from the 2003-04, 2004-05, 2005-06, 2006-07, 2007-08 Annual Survey of Deaf and Hard of Hearing Children and Youth. Washington, DC: GRI, Gallaudet University.
*Percentage may total more than 100 because multiple responses were allowed.

The racial/ethnic breakdown of the population in the GRI Survey is provided in Table 11-3. Except for a small increase in the Hispanic/Latino students and a slight decrease in the number of white students, the percentage representation of the other racial/ethnic groups in this population has remained relatively stable. Upon examining the total counts (all race/ethnic groups included) in Table 11-3, it appears that there is a small decrease in the total number of students from 38,744 (2003-2004) to 36,710 (2007-2008), with a peak in 2005-2006 with 39,502 students.

The GRI Annual Survey provided information regarding the children's home environment. For each of the 5 years, data indicated that the majority of students had "hearing" parents. On an average, the mother's hearing status was reported to be hearing for 91.08% of the students, deaf for 4.4% of the students, and hard of hearing for 2.2% of the students. The father was reported to be hearing on an average for 85.18% of the students, deaf for 4.66% of the students, and hard of hearing for 2% of the students. Both parents were reported to be hearing for 82.14% students, and deaf or hard of hearing for 3.94% of the students. When asked about the use of sign language in the home, it was reported that a majority (70.3%) of family members did not regularly use sign language at home. Only an average of 25.34% of family members signed at home. Data on

TABLE 11-3 Number and Percentage of Students with Hearing Impairments by Race/Ethnicity during the 2003 to 2008 School Years*

Race/Ethnicity	2003-2004	2004-2005	2005-2006	2006-2007	2007-2008
White	19,640 (51.5%)	18,712 (50.7%)	19,120 (49.2%)	17,430 (47.4%)	17,782 (48.7%)
Black or African American	5880 (15.4%)	5647 (15.3%)	5846 (15%)	5566 (15.1%)	5789 (15.9%)
Hispanic or Latino	9226 (24.2%)	9226 (25.0%)	10,417 (26.8%)	10,397 (28.3%)	10,975 (30.1%)
American Indian or Alaska Native	329 (0.9%)	307 (0.8%)	314 (0.8%)	272 (0.7%)	334 (0.9%)
Asian or Pacific Islander	1567 (4.1%)	1512 (4.1%)	1547 (4%)	1542 (4.2%)	1565 (4.3%)
Other	688 (1.8%)	708 (1.9%)	770 (2%)	695 (1.9%)	754 (2.1%)
Multiethnic background	819 (2.1%)	805 (2.2%)	871 (2.2%)	879 (2.4%)	868 (2.4%)
Unknown	595 (1.5%)	583 (1.6%)	617 (1.6%)	571 (1.5%)	189 (0.5%)
Total	38,744	37,500	39,502	37,352	36,710

From Gallaudet Research Institute (January 2005, December 2005, December 2006, December 2007, November 2008). Regional and National Summary Report of Data from the 2003-04, 2004-05, 2005-06, 2006-07, 2007-08 Annual Survey of Deaf and Hard of Hearing Children and Youth. Washington, DC: GRI, Gallaudet University.
*Percent may total more than 100 because multiple responses were allowed.

the languages spoken at home were available only for years 2006-2007 and 2007-2008. The vast majority (average = 82.85%) used English to communicate at home, whereas a much smaller number (average = 21.5%) reported that they spoke Spanish at home. Numerous other languages were reported to be used at home, but those figures were miniscule.

Epidemiology of Hearing Loss and Deafness in Other Countries in the World

Southeast Asia

The WHO (2007) estimated that there were more than 100 million persons with deafness or hearing impairment in Southeast Asia. The WHO (2006) estimated that every year about 38,000 deaf children were born in Southeast Asia. Hearing loss accounted for 2.3% of all DALYs in the Southeast Asia region, giving this region a disproportionately high burden of deafness among all the WHO regions. The prevalence rates of hearing loss by countries in the region were as follows: Indonesia (4.2%), India (6%), Maldives (6%), Myanmar (8%), Bangladesh (9%), Sri Lanka (9%), Thailand (13.3%), and Nepal (16.6%).

Childhood deafness yields higher YLD, although adult-onset hearing loss has a significantly higher prevalence. The WHO (2007) reported that there is a high incidence of presbycusis in Southeast Asia. For example, more than 10% of the population in India and 4.1% of the population in Indonesia have presbycusis. Chronic suppurative otitis media, noise-induced hearing loss, and ototoxicity are the other etiologic factors causing adult-onset hearing loss in the region. According to the WHO (2006), the proportion of older persons in this region has increased during the recent past from 6% to 8%, and it is estimated that by 2050, the proportion of older persons in the less developed countries will rise to 19%, whereas the proportion of children will decline to 22%, so that the less developed countries will have an age structure similar to that of more developed countries. After reviewing the etiology, the WHO believes that half of hearing impairments in the region are preventable, but about 30% are not; however, these could be treated or managed with assistive devices. Thus 80% of all hearing impairments are avoidable, which strongly indicates "the need to strengthen ear care services."

Schmitz and colleagues (2010) conducted a study to assess the prevalence and severity of hearing loss and "middle ear dysfunction" in a group of 15- to 23-year-olds in a rural area of Southern Nepal. They reported that 6.1% of the subjects had hearing loss. Further, they reported that persons who were hearing impaired were six to eight times more likely to report problems in hearing sounds of daily living and in communicating with others.

China

Wong and McPherson (2008) reported that the incidence of hearing loss in China is probably higher than the 21 million reported by the National Bureau of Statistics. More than 14 million persons in China, who are older than 60 years, have hearing loss. If only those older than 65 years are considered, the incidence is higher and growing at a rate of 3% to 4% annually. Sun and associates (2008) examined data from the Second China National Sample Survey on Disability and reported that 27.80 million persons were diagnosed with hearing loss, which was an overall prevalence rate of 2.11%, although the incidence was higher (11.04%) among elderly persons. The prevalence was higher among males than females and higher in rural areas compared with urban areas. Fu and coworkers (2010) investigated the prevalence of hearing loss in students enrolled in primary and middle schools in the Hubei province of China. During their 2-year study, 504,348 students were tested; 813 were deaf of whom 232 children were diagnosed with congenital deafness, and 560 had acquired deafness. Of the latter, 276 had aminoglycoside antibiotic–induced deafness. The severity of deafness in 804 other students was distributed as follows: profound (402), severe (363), moderate (21), and mild (18). The age of onset for most children was under 3 years of age. The prevalence rates of congenital and acquired deafness were 0.046% and 0.111%, respectively. Liu and associates (2001) conducted a large-scale epidemiological survey of 126,876 persons (63,741 male, 63,135 female) in Sichuan, China. They reported an overall prevalence of 3.28% for hearing loss, which increased to 12.8% at 60 years of age; 73.03% of all cases had sensorineural hearing loss, whereas 20.39% had conductive, and the remaining 6% had mixed hearing loss. They also reported that 74.5% of the cases had bilateral hearing loss, Further, 63.79% of cases had mild to moderate hearing loss (<55 dB HL), and 5.67% had profound hearing loss (>90 db HL). In children younger than 15 years, the prevalence of hearing loss was 0.67%; 57.7% of the cases had conductive hearing loss, and 38.8 had sensorineural hearing loss. They reported that persons who lived in the flatlands appeared to have a higher prevalence of hearing loss than those who lived in the hills. Further, they reported that several ethnic groups, namely, Tibetans, the Yi, and the Lisu, had a higher prevalence of hearing loss.

The Middle East

Attias and associates (2006) ascertained the prevalence of congenital and early-onset hearing loss in infants in Jordan and Israel using Distortion Product Otoacoustic Emissions (DPOAE) for screening hearing, with follow-up using Auditory Brainstem Response (ABR) when needed. They found that the prevalence of hearing loss in infants in

Jordan (1.37%) was significantly higher than in the infants in Israel (0.48%). Further, the prevalence of bilateral sensorineural hearing loss was seven times higher in the infants in Jordan than in the infants in Israel. Also, in the Israeli sample, the prevalence of hearing loss in the no-risk infants was 0.19%, compared with 8% (42 times greater) in the high-risk infants. In the Jordanian sample, the prevalence was 0.51% in the no-risk infants and 10% (19 times greater) in the high-risk infants. The overall prevalence of hearing loss in the Jordanian sample was remarkably higher (about 2.8 times) than that in the Israeli sample. Risk factors, such as family history, hyperbilirubinemia, bacterial meningitis, and associated syndromes, were more prevalent in infants in Jordan.

Al Khabori and Khandekar (2004) used pure tone audiometry to screen the hearing of 12,400 persons of all ages in Oman. Children younger than 4 years were tested by subjective methods, involving a set of questions and observations. The prevalence of bilateral hearing loss in Oman was 55 per 1000 persons. The prevalence of bilateral hearing loss was highest in persons who were 60 years or older (325 per 1000), and lower (17 per 1000) in children younger than 10 years.

Abdel-Hamid and coworkers (2007) used DPOAE and impedance audiometry to screen 4000 individuals for hearing loss from six randomly selected governorates in Egypt. The prevalence of hearing loss was 16%, but there were differences between age groups and governorates. Marsa Matrrough, a governorate, had the highest prevalence of hearing loss (25.7%), whereas North Sinai had the lowest percentage (13.5%). Persons who were 65 years and older had the highest prevalence (49.3%), followed by children 0 to 4 years of age (22.4%).

Australia

Currently, one in six persons in Australia has a hearing loss, but it is estimated that this figure will rise to one in four by 2050 as the population ages. Approximately 9 to 12 children per 10,000 live births in Australia are born with a bilateral moderate or greater hearing loss, whereas an additional 23 children per 10,000 acquire a hearing impairment by age 17 years that necessitates the use of hearing aids. By the age of 60 to 70 years, more than 50% of Australians have a hearing loss; this figure increases to 70% or more among those who are older than 70 years and to more than 80% for persons older than 80 years. Men have a higher incidence of hearing loss than women, primarily related to exposure to occupational noise, which is the primary cause of hearing loss in adults in Australia. For instance, more than 50% of farmers have hearing loss because of exposure to noise from agricultural machinery. Hearing loss costs Australia approximately $12 billion annually (Australian Hearing, n.d.; Williams, 2010).

Quinn and Rance (2009) investigated the hearing of 109 indigenous prisoners at five prison locations in Victoria, Australia. Primarily the prisoners had mild sensorineural hearing loss. The rate of conductive hearing loss was consistent with that found in an age-matched adult general population in the United Kingdom. Twelve percent of prisoners had a hearing loss of 25 dB or greater in at least one ear, compared with the incidence of 5% in the general adult Australian population. Thirty-six percent of the inmates had unilateral or bilateral high frequency sensorineural hearing loss; 58% reported having hearing problems some of the time, and 4% reported having a lot of trouble in hearing. Ninety-two percent of inmates reported having had exposure to loud noise; 72% reported having tinnitus.

Russ and colleagues (2003) investigated the incidence and clinical characteristics of congenital hearing loss that was sufficient to necessitate fitting hearing aids during the first 6 years of life in children born in 1993 in Victoria, Australia. Only 2.09 per 1000 children had been fitted with hearing aids. Of these, 54 children (40%) had mild hearing loss (20 to 40 dB HL). The researchers reported that the prevalence of moderate or greater loss (>40 dB HL) was 1.12 per 1000 children, that of severe or greater loss (>60 dB HL) was 0.48 per 1000 children, and that of profound hearing loss (>90 dB HL) was 0.17 per 1000 children.

Denmark and The Netherlands

Dammeyer (2010) reported the prevalence of "deaf blindness" in Denmark to be 1:29,000. Meuwese-Jongejeugd and associates (2006) reported on the prevalence of hearing loss in 1598 adults with an intellectual disability (ID) in the Netherlands. The researchers reported a prevalence ranging from 7.5% in a subgroup aged 18 to 30 years, who did not have Down syndrome but did present an ID, to a prevalence of 100% in adults older than 60 years with Down syndrome. The researchers concluded that in persons with Down syndrome, age-related hearing loss occurs approximately three decades earlier than in the general population. Similarly, in persons who have an ID due to causes other than Down syndrome, hearing loss occurs approximately one decade earlier than in the general population.

Canada

The Participation and Activity Limitation Survey (PALS) is a post-censal national survey funded by Human Resources and Social Development Canada (HRSDC) and conducted by Statistics Canada (2009). It is designed to collect information on adults and children who have an activity limitation because of a health problem. Statistics Canada (2001) reported that 23,750 children aged 0 to 14 years had hearing loss, of whom 14,230 were males and 9520 were females. Of the 23,750 children, 3160 children were 0 to 4 years of age, 10,800 were 5 to 9 years of age, and 9790 were 10 to 14 years of age. Brennan and coworkers (2006) reported that 1,266,120 Canadians aged 15 years and older reported having a hearing limitation on the 2006 PALS. The majority (60.8%) of persons with hearing difficulty reported having some hearing loss. More than 8 of 10 (83.2%) hearing limitations were mild in nature, and 16.8% were classified as severe.

Millar (2005) reported the results of the 2003 Canadian Community Health Survey (CCHS), which is a general survey used to collect information on persons 12 years and older; it precludes those on Indian reservations, Canadian forces bases, and some remote areas. Three percent of the Canadian population aged 12 years and older had some difficulty with their hearing. The incidence increased with age. Accordingly, although seniors made up only 14% of the 12 years or older population, they represented 55% of persons with hearing problems. Of those who were 65 years or older, approximately 11% had a hearing problem. Of those who were 65 to 69 years old, 5% had a hearing problem, and among those who were 80 years and older, 23% had a hearing problem. The percentage of persons reporting a hearing problem by province from the lowest incidence to the highest are as follows: Québec (7%), Ontario (10%), Manitoba (11%), Alberta(13%), Nova Scotia (14%), Prince Edward Island, Newfoundland, New Brunswick, British Columbia (15% each), and Saskatchewan (16%).

Costa Rica

Mencher and Madriz (2000) reported on a four-phase study conducted to determine the incidence and prevalence of sensorineural hearing loss in children in Costa Rica. The four phases involved screening the hearing of more than 12,500 children in the public schools, examining children enrolled in programs for the hearing impaired, searching the community for children not enrolled in schools or special programs, and administration of a questionnaire to obtain pertinent information. There were 1174 to 1274 children with hearing impairment in Costa Rica; that is, the prevalence of hearing impairment was 1.5 to 1.63 per 1000 live births.

EARLY IDENTIFICATION OF HEARING LOSS

Early Identification of Hearing Loss in the United States

Undetected permanent bilateral hearing loss in children can lead to significant delays in the development of language, cognition, speech, and literacy, which in turn affects education and increases the burden on society. For instance, the CDC (2004) estimated that the lifetime costs for all people with hearing loss in the United States, who were born in 2000, would total $2.1 billion. During the

1999-2000 school year, the total cost for special education programs for children who were deaf or hard of hearing in the United States was $652 million, or $11,006 per child (Chambers, Shkolnik, & Perez, 2003). The lifetime educational cost of hearing loss of more than 40 dB HL was estimated to be approximately $115,600 per child (Grosse, 2007).

Interest in infant hearing screening dates back to the mid-1940s when behavioral responses to auditory stimuli were observed. Continued interest in infant hearing screening led to the formation of the Joint Committee on Infant Hearing (JCIH). *Healthy People, 2000* included the goal to reduce the average age at which children with significant hearing loss were identified to no more than 12 months of age (U.S. Department of Health and Human Services, 1990). Dramatic advances in technology in the 1990s led to the invention of more sophisticated audiology equipment and automatic hearing screeners. An expert panel convened by the National Institutes on Deafness and Other Communication Disorders (NIDCD) in 1993 concluded that all infants admitted to NICUs should be screened before discharge, and universal hearing screening should be implemented for all infants within the first 3 months of life. The JCIH (2000) endorsed the development of a system for detection and intervention that was family centered and community based and emphasized the need to identify children with permanent sensory or conductive hearing loss averaging 30 to 40 dB HL or more in the frequency region that is important for speech recognition (i.e., 500 to 4000 Hz).

Goal 28-11 of *Healthy People 2010* (U.S. Department of Health and Human Services, 2001) required an increase in the proportion of newborns screened for hearing loss by 1 month of age, required audiologic evaluation by 3 months, and required provision of appropriate intervention services by 6 months of age. The number of infants screened for hearing loss in the United States increased dramatically from 46.5% in 1996 to 97% in 2007. Further, in 2007, 83% of babies with diagnosed hearing loss were referred to Part C Early Identification Services. To identify babies with hearing loss, all states and territories of the United States have established early hearing detection and intervention (EHDI) programs, which ensure that all newborns and infants are screened and receive recommended follow-up through data collection and outreach to hospitals, providers, and families. Although the high percentage of infants lost to follow-up or lost to documentation continues to be a major challenge for EHDI programs, substantial progress has been made toward achieving benchmarks for screening, evaluation, and intervention (CDC, 2010d; 2011). In 2009, 97% of newborns were screened for hearing loss. Of these, 1.6% did not pass the final or most recent screening. Of those who did not pass the screening 67.9% were diagnosed as having or not having a hearing loss by 3 months of age. The current prevalence rate of newborns with hearing loss is approximately 1.4 per 1000 babies (CDC, 2011).

Early Identification of Hearing Loss in Other Countries in the World

Newborn hearing screening has been a focus of the international community. In 1995, the WHO passed a resolution urging member countries to develop plans for early detection of hearing loss in babies. In November 2009, the WHO held an "informal consultation meeting" to develop guiding principles for early detection and intervention of hearing impairment, and thus facilitate the development and conduct of newborn or infant hearing screening programs around the world. Developed countries such as Australia, Canada, and the Netherlands have been conducting newborn hearing screening for many years. During the past decade, many other developing and developed countries have initiated early identification and intervention programs.

The Netherlands

Unlike many European countries and the United States, in the Netherlands, approximately 35% of babies are born at home, and about 85% of those born in hospitals leave within 24 hours of birth. Sixty-five percent of home-based and hospital deliveries are attended by midwives. The Netherlands has had nationwide screening for hearing loss since the 1960s, but was using distraction testing. Although 96% of babies were tested during the first year of life, over the years, there was growing dissatisfaction with the program because of the high and increasing false-positive rate primarily due to conductive hearing loss. The 5% referral rate in the early 1980s grew to 7% within a few years. Additionally, there was concern because children were diagnosed with permanent hearing loss at about 18 months of age or later. Several studies were conducted to ascertain whether universal neonatal hearing screening could be integrated in the youth health care program in the Netherlands, which provides services that include vaccinations; monitoring of cognitive, motor, and language development; and screening for metabolic disorders, visual and hearing problems to children from birth through 19 years. In one such study, the screening was performed by nurses of well-baby clinics on 3114 newborns. Three-stage transient otoacoustic screening was administered in three different screening settings; in one setting parents visited well-baby clinics, and in two other settings the screening was done at home. The researchers determined that the most efficient and effective setting for universal hearing screening was where hearing screening was integrated with screening for metabolic disorders. The participation rate was the highest (89.9%) and the overall referral rate the lowest (1.4%) in this setting. The results of this study formed the basis for nationwide implementation of universal hearing screening in that country (Uilenburg et al., 2009).

Between 2002 and 2006, all 65 regions in the Netherlands replaced distraction hearing screening with newborn hearing screening. During the transition, some regions switched to newborn hearing screening first, whereas other regions continued to use distraction hearing screening. To ascertain whether this change affected developmental outcomes in children with permanent childhood hearing loss, Korver and coworkers (2010) compared the effect of newborn hearing screening and distraction hearing screening conducted at 9 months of age on development, spoken communication, and quality of life in children. All children born in the Netherlands from 2003 to 2005 were included in the study; thus, 335,560 children in newborn hearing screening regions and 234,826 children born in distraction hearing screening regions participated in the study. At follow-up, 263 (0.78 per 1000) children in newborn hearing screening regions and 171 (0.73 per 1000) in the distraction hearing screening regions had been diagnosed with permanent childhood hearing impairment. All children with permanent hearing impairment were identified by 3 to 5 years of age. Of these, 301 (69.4%) children participated in the analysis of the general performance measures. The two groups did not differ in terms of the primary mode of communication or type of education. However, children in the newborn hearing screening regions had higher overall scores for social development, gross motor development, and quality of life measures than children in the distraction hearing screening regions.

Germany

In 2007, the German Society for Phoniatrics and Pediatric Audiology developed a quality assurance program for universal newborn hearing screening (Neumann et al., 2009). The recommendations included the procedures for screening and subsequent follow-up as well as criteria and definitions of levels of hearing loss.

Rohlfs and associates (2010) described a regional interdisciplinary universal hearing screening program started in Hamburg, Germany, in 2002. Reportedly, this was the first time that a comprehensive protocol that included screening, follow-up procedures, tracking, and early intervention was implemented in Germany. Of 65,466 births registered between 2002 and 2006, 63,459 (93%) newborns were screened; 3.3% failed screening, and 31.3% were lost to follow-up. A total of 118 children were diagnosed with hearing loss at a median age of 3.5 months. Seventy-four children were fitted with hearing aids, of whom 6 were subsequently implanted. Rohlfs and associates reported that their biggest challenge was the high percentage of children lost to follow-up.

Italy

Italy has shown considerable growth in implementing universal new born hearing screening (UNHS). Bubbico and colleagues (2008) reported on the degree of coverage of UNHS in Italy. The number of infants screened for hearing loss increased from 156,048 (29.3%) in 2003 to 262,103

(48.4%) in 2006. The researchers reported that the majority of UNHS programs have been implemented in the most economically developed areas; 108,200 (79.5%) of newborns were screened in the northwest, and 92,133 (57.2%) newborns were screened in the northeast. However, because there are fewer UNHS programs in the Italian islands, including Sardinia and Sicily, only 7158 (11.3%) of newborns were screened in the islands.

Canada

Durieux-Smith and coworkers (2008) reported on the ages of diagnosis and hearing aid fitting of 709 Canadian children with congenital or early-onset permanent hearing loss who were identified between 1980 and 2003 through neonatal hearing screening programs or through medical referrals. Analysis showed that children who were screened were diagnosed earlier, at a mean age of 6.3 months, compared with children who were referred and diagnosed at a mean age of 39.5 months. The researchers reported that over the years, the age at which referred children, were diagnosed and fitted with hearing aids improved but still remained unacceptably high. Further, it was observed that children with lesser degrees of hearing loss were diagnosed at older ages than those with severe to profound hearing loss. The results of this study lend strong support to the benefits of implementing a newborn hearing screening program, diagnosis at an early age and possibly early hearing aid fitting, which greatly facilitates the development of language, speech, cognitive and literacy skills.

Developing Countries

In developing countries, hearing loss remains a silent epidemic. Although developed countries, such as the United States and United Kingdom, have legislated the implementation of universal hearing screening programs, unfortunately, such programs for early detection of hearing loss are not well established or not established at all in the developing countries where the incidence of hearing loss is extremely high and the human and financial resources are meager at best (Olusanya, 2006, 2008; Theunissen & Swanepoel, 2008). Although universal hearing screening has been hospital based in most developed countries, it may not be a feasible option in many developing countries where a majority of births occur at home or in birthing facilities.

Olusanya and associates (2008) indicated that hospital-based universal hearing screening programs were unlikely to be effective in Lagos, Nigeria because the majority of births did not occur in hospitals. On the other hand, routine childhood immunization programs often provided an effective community-based avenue for attracting babies born outside of hospitals. To ascertain the effectiveness of such an arrangement, they set up a screening during bacilli Calmette-Guérin (BCG) immunization (first vaccination given typically within the first month of life to Nigerian babies) in an inner-city area at four health care centers that accounted for 75% of BCG vaccinations. They used a two-stage screening protocol; transient evoked otoacoustic emissions (TEOAE) was administered initially, followed by ABR. They observed an overall prevalence rate of 30.7 per 1000, whereas 19.2 per 1000 had moderate to severe hearing loss. Significantly more males than females were found to have hearing loss. The researchers concluded that permanent hearing loss was a highly prevalent disability in Nigeria; it could be detected early, and community health workers at primary care centers could be effectively used for universal hearing screening.

In Benin City, Nigeria, Okhakhu and coworkers (2010) screened 400 neonates using an OAE screener. Ninety neonates (22.5%) failed the screening and were referred for further testing. Of the 90 neonates, 26 (6.5%) were found to have bilateral hearing loss, and 64 (16%) were found to have unilateral hearing loss. Okhakhu and coworkers concluded that neonatal screening was necessary in all developing countries. Similarly, Swanepoel and colleagues (2007) reported on an infant hearing screening program that was developed using immunization clinics in South Africa as part of the primary, secondary, and tertiary levels of health care.

Lin and associates (2002) assessed the feasibility and cost-effectiveness of implementing universal newborn hearing screening in Taiwan. They screened 6765 newborns before discharge from a hospital using TEOAE. The overall pass rate was 93.6%; 6.4% of newborns were referred for diagnostic audiological assessments. Nine newborns were diagnosed to have permanent bilateral hearing impairment, and 26 newborns were identified to have permanent unilateral hearing loss. The newborns with bilateral hearing loss were referred for hearing aids. The researchers concluded that in Taiwan, universal newborn hearing screening using TEOAE was practicable and cost-effective.

Taiwan's health insurance system apparently does not facilitate newborn hearing screening. From March 2000 through December 2002, Lin and associates (2004) piloted a community-based pay-for-test (parents paid for the TEOAE test) newborn hearing screening program in two hospitals and four obstetric clinics. A total of 5938 healthy newborns were tested in newborn nurseries before discharge using TEOAE. Of these, 5403 (91%) newborns passed the screening, whereas 535 (9%) failed it. One hundred and forty babies were lost to 1-month follow-up. However, 395 (73.8%) infants underwent a second test at the outpatient clinic, of whom 91 failed and were referred for ABR testing. Ultimately, 9 babies were diagnosed with sensorineural hearing loss. The researchers concluded that a pay-for-test model was feasible in Taiwan, was well accepted by parents, and could be implemented without financial support from the government.

Bevilacqua and colleagues (2010) developed a newborn hearing screening program in a public hospital in Brazil.

11,466 newborns were screened using TEOAE and a 2-stage approach. The researchers reported that the prevalence rate of sensorineural hearing loss was 0.96 per 1000 newborns. Eight of 11 children were fitted with hearing aids and 4 children were implanted.

Universal newborn hearing screening programs appear to be the most efficient and cost-effective way of identifying hearing loss early so that intervention can begin within the first few months if not weeks of life. Any one particular model of a newborn hearing screening program, for instance, hospital-based screening, may not be appropriate for every community and every country. The setting is not as important as adequate training of primary staff, test criteria and test conditions, proper data collection, rigorous follow-up, and early initiation of intervention.

In 2006, WHO enabled a new collaboration *WWHearing— World Wide Hearing Care for Developing Countries,* to bring together key stakeholders, such as policy makers, service providers, donors, and representatives of hearing aids industries from developing countries. The mission of this partnership was to encourage large-scale provision of affordable hearing aids and services and to eradicate barriers to the provision of needed ear and hearing care in developing countries. The WHO (2010a) also facilitated the formation of a forum for prevention and control of deafness and hearing impairment in the Southeast Asia region. This new initiative, *Sound Hearing 2030,* will include activities that will link it to *WWHearing—World Wide Hearing Care for Developing Countries.*

One of the challenges is the lack of epidemiological data on hearing loss in developing countries (Mencher, 2000). The WHO's (April, 2010b) efforts toward assisting countries to address hearing impairment have focused on prevention, developing a global database on deafness and hearing impairment, developing training materials *(WHO Primary Ear and Hearing Training Resources)* and training primary and secondary health care workers regarding ear and hearing care, developing and disseminating guidelines on preventable etiological factors, building partnerships to make hearing aids accessible and affordable, raising awareness of the costs of hearing impairment and opportunities for prevention, and encouraging countries to establish national prevention programs. Further, the WHO (2010c) started a journal, *Community Ear and Hearing Health,* which focuses on needs in developing countries and provides information on prevention, management, and rehabilitation of ear and hearing disorders. The journal is for distribution to primary and other health care workers with the goal of increasing awareness, knowledge, and skills.

ETIOLOGY

Deafness or hearing loss at birth or in early childhood can have a devastating effect on a child's language, speech, and cognitive development, which in turn negatively affects the child's emotional and educational experiences. As the child grows older, there are social, vocational, and economic consequences that reduce the quality of life. Advances in genetic technology have greatly facilitated identification of the etiology of hearing loss in many cases, which in turn may facilitate management and may provide the information parents want. Harrison and Roush (2002) asked parents what information they wanted to receive pertaining to their child's hearing loss at the time of the initial diagnosis. Parents reported that they wanted to know the cause of their child's hearing loss. Some even reported that the uncertainty of not knowing the cause made it difficult for them to focus on intervention issues.

Morzaria and colleagues (2004) ascertained the frequency of etiologies of moderate to profound bilateral sensorineural hearing loss in children. They found that the most common causes of bilateral sensorineural hearing loss are unknown (37.7%), genetic nonsyndromic (29.2%), prenatal (12%), perinatal (9.6%), postnatal (8.2%), and genetic syndromes (3.2%). Wormald and associates (2010) examined the etiology of sensorineural hearing loss in children presenting at a medical center in Ireland. They reported that 66% of children had hereditary hearing loss, 8% had acquired hearing loss, and the etiology was unknown in 26% of children. Data from the Gallaudet Research Center's Annual Survey of Deaf and Hard of Hearing Children and Youth for the years 2003-2006 indicated that excluding otitis media, the most prevalent etiological factors consistently reported each year on the survey are genetic/hereditary/familial, prematurity, complications of pregnancy, other postbirth causes, and CMV.

Although risk factors associated with deafness have been known for decades, with advances in medicine, genetics, and technology, the focus of research has shifted from diseases, such as maternal rubella, which has been controlled through immunization, to genetics and other diseases, such as CMV. A detailed discussion of every risk factor is beyond the scope of this chapter. Some etiological factors with implications for multicultural and international populations have been selected for discussion.

Low Birth Weight

Birth weight and gestational period are two very important predictors of health and survival of neonates. Infants born too small or too soon have a greater risk for death, as well as short-term and long-term disabilities, than those who are born at term and who weigh 2500 grams or more. Low birth weight and prolonged use of ventilation appear to be the main risk factors associated with sensorineural hearing loss in infants. In 2006, the U.S. infant mortality rate was 6.68 infant deaths per 1000 live births.

Some races and ethnic groups are disproportionately affected by the high infant mortality rate for low-birth-weight infants. Matthews and MacDorman (2010) reported rates that ranged from 4.52 per 1000 live births for Central and South American mothers to 13.35% for non-Hispanic black mothers. Other factors associated with low birth weight in neonates include maternal age (e.g., teenage pregnancies), delayed or no prenatal care, mother's disadvantaged background, maternal education, maternal use of tobacco, and so forth. According to the JCIH (2000), infants weighing less than 1500 grams are at risk for hearing impairment or deafness. Therefore, it may be inferred that more African American babies are at risk for hearing impairment or deafness than other ethnic groups.

Neonatal intensive care units (NICUs) are known to reduce mortality among infants with low birth weight. Barfield and coworkers (2010) analyzed birth data from 19 states to ascertain the prevalence of admission of infants with very low birth weight (VLBW) to NICUs. The rate of admission varied by race and ethnicity among states: a smaller percentage (71.8%) of infants with VLBW born to Hispanic mothers were admitted to NICUs, compared with infants born to non-Hispanic black mothers (79.5%) and infants born to non-Hispanic white mothers (80.5%). The researchers reported that greater prevalence of admission of infants with VLBW to NICUs was associated with three factors: preterm delivery, multiple births, and cesarean delivery.

Coenraad and colleagues (2010) evaluated etiological factors associated with sensorineural hearing loss in infants who were admitted to NICUs in the Netherlands. Normal hearing controls were used for comparison. Of the 3316 infants screened, 58 infants (26 girls, 32 boys) were diagnosed with sensorineural hearing loss. Although numerous risk factors were examined, the incidence of dysmorphic features, low Apgar score (1 minute), sepsis, meningitis, cerebral bleeding, and cerebral infarction were significantly increased in infants with sensorineural hearing loss compared with the normal hearing controls.

After conducting a 30-year longitudinal study in Canada, Robertson and associates (2009) reported that permanent hearing loss is an adverse outcome of extreme prematurity. This hearing loss may have a delayed onset and may be progressive. Their subjects had a gestational age of 28 weeks or less and birth weight of less than 1250 grams. They reported that prolonged supplemental oxygen use was a marker for predicting permanent hearing loss. Tomasik (2008) also examined risk factors for hearing impairment in 218 prematurely born Polish infants with birth weights of 520 to 3000 grams and gestational age of 22 to 36 weeks. Tomasik concluded that the following factors put premature infants at risk for hearing loss: low gestational age or associated with it prolonged mechanical ventilation, hyperbilirubinemia, severe general condition, hypoglycemia, and prolonged treatment with amikacin.

Xoinis and coworkers (2007) conducted a retrospective study on NICU graduates to establish a prevalence rate for auditory neuropathy. They reported a prevalence of

sensorineural hearing loss in 16.7 per 1000 NICU infants and a prevalence of auditory neuropathy in 5.6 per 1000 infants. They reported that compared with infants with sensorineural hearing loss, infants with auditory neuropathy had younger gestational ages and lower birth weights. In fact, two thirds of infants with auditory neuropathy were infants with extremely low birth weight and had significantly longer hospital stays compared with infants with sensorineural hearing loss.

To examine the impact of birth weight on risk for sensorineural hearing loss in Norwegian children, Engdahl and Eskild (2007) compared children with sensorineural hearing loss with those in a control group. They observed that the risk for hearing loss decreased with increasing birth weights. They concluded that the risk for both mild to moderate and severe to profound sensorineural hearing losses were influenced by birth weight. Martinez-Cruz and colleagues (2008) investigated risk factors associated with sensorineural hearing loss in infants in a tertiary level NICU and a control group in Mexico City. They reported that low birth weight, longer stay in a NICU under mechanical ventilation, higher serum bilirubin levels, blood transfusion, intraventricular hemorrhage, and meningitis were the main risk factors associated with sensorineural hearing loss.

Olusanya (2011) studied undernourished infants in sub-Saharan Africa to determine risk factors for early-onset permanent hearing loss. Of 2254 infants, 39 (1.7%) were confirmed to have hearing loss, of whom 7 had mild hearing loss and 26 had moderate to profound hearing loss. "Absence of skilled attendant at birth and severe neonatal jaundice" were among the factors associated with the permanent hearing loss.

Genetic Hearing Loss

Epidemiologic studies in the United States have shown that approximately 1 in 1000 to 2000 children are born with or present in early childhood with severe or profound hearing impairment, of whom approximately half have a genetic cause (Parving, 1983; Newton, 1985). Marazita and colleagues (1993) reported that the incidence of profound early-onset deafness was present in 4 to 11 per 10,000 children. Of these, 37.2% of the cases were attributed to sporadic causes and 62.8% to genetic causes (47.1%, recessive; 15.7% dominant). Recent studies have suggested that approximately 50% of moderate to profound, congenital, or early-onset hearing loss is genetic in origin. A genetic hearing impairment may occur in isolation (nonsyndromal) or in association with other features (syndromal). Nonsyndromal hearing impairments (70%) occur as a single gene disorder due to an autosomal dominant gene, X-linked gene, or mitochondrial inheritance. For instance, adult-onset progressive hearing impairment can be caused by mutations in a single gene. Syndromal hearing impairments (30%) result from chromosomal or single gene causes. A syndrome is defined as multiple anomalies in a person, with all of the anomalies having a single cause, which may be a genetic mutation, chromosomal abnormality, teratogen, or some extrinsic factor. There are more than 400 known syndromes with hearing loss as one of the anomalies. In the case of a syndrome, hearing loss may be just one of several problems. A few of the syndromes associated with hearing loss are Usher syndrome, Pendred syndrome, and Turner syndrome.

Data from the Annual Survey of Deaf and Hard of Hearing Children and Youth for the years 2003 to 2007 conducted by the Gallaudet Research Institute consistently showed that genetic/hereditary/familial factors accounted for the largest percentage of hearing impairment/deafness than any other etiological factor. The incidence ranged from 21.8% in 2003-2004 to 23.6% in 2007-2008. During the years 2004-2005, 2005-2006, and 2006-2007 the incidence rates were 22.7%, 23%, and 23.3% respectively (Gallaudet Research Institute, January 2005; December 2005; December 2006; December 2007; November 2008).

Based on data from the 1989-1990 Annual Survey of Hearing Impaired Children and Youth (Nuru, 1993) reported that the incidence of genetic hearing loss varied across races and ethnic groups. Similarly, the 1991-1992 Annual Survey of Hearing Impaired Children and Youth (Schildroth, 1994) indicated that heredity as a causative factor was the highest among white (72%) children and youth when compared with peers from the Hispanic (14%), African American (10%), Asian and Pacific Islander (2%), and other (2%) communities.

Parving (1996) summarized the incidence of hearing impairment in children that was attributed to genetic causes based on 14 surveys conducted internationally. The incidence of genetic hearing impairment reported in these surveys varied from 9% to 54%, whereas 16% to 42% of the children had hearing impairment of unknown origin. Parving suggested that it was likely that the variation in the proportion of genetic hearing impairment reflected true differences in the genetic expression in the different populations. In the United States, autosomal recessive nonsyndromal hearing impairment is estimated to occur in 1 of 1000 children (Morton, 1991), whereas in England and Denmark, it is reported to occur in 0.7 of 1000 children (Davis & Parving, 1994). However, in Sichuan, China, it was estimated that the prevalence rate of genetic hearing loss was 0.28% (Liu et al, 2001).

Cultural practice in a community affects the incidence of genetic hearing impairment. In some cultures, consanguineous marriages are an accepted practice. Al-Shihabi (1994) reported that the incidence of hearing impairment was 12.9 per 1000 in offspring in consanguineous marriages but 3.1 per 1000 births in nonconsanguineous marriages in the same geographic area. This suggested that autosomal recessive hearing impairment was a monogenic disease. The Sultanate of Oman in the Arabian Peninsula is still predominantly tribal. Al Khabori and Patton (2008) reported on a retrospective analysis of 1400 questionnaires (which the ear-nose-throat [ENT] staff completed at the time of mandatory hearing screening administered when a child first started school) on the etiology of deafness in Omani children collected between 1986 and 2000. They observed that 70% of children with deafness were from parents of consanguineous marriages. Among consanguineous families, 70.16% were first-cousin marriages, 17.54% were second-cousin marriages, and 10.86% were from the same tribe. In addition, 45% of the total cohort had other family members with hearing loss. There was a greater chance of other relatives having a hearing loss in the consanguineous group (29.7%) than in the nonconsanguineous group (15.3%). In most cases, the affected relative was a sibling with deafness (67.8%) indicating a high frequency autosomal recessive transmission.

Mueller (2000) reported that investigations of the recurrence of hearing impairment in children born to hearing-impaired or deaf couples have indicated that there are approximately 100 genes that may be responsible for nonsyndromal sensorineural hearing impairment or deafness. During the past 8 years, 28 autosomal recessive, 30 autosomal dominant, and 5 X-linked genes for nonsyndromal sensorineural hearing impairment or deafness have been cloned. The gene known as *GJB2* (Gap Junction Beta 2), or *Connexin 26* or *CX26,* which is located on chromosome 13, accounts for approximately 50% of nonsyndromic sensorineural hearing loss. *GJB2* produces a protein called connexin 26, which creates channels between cells through which small molecules diffuse. It has been suggested that this protein may be involved in maintaining potassium levels in the cochlea. The hearing loss associated with mutations in *GJB2* varies in severity, generally ranging from moderate to profound, although most range from severe to profound hearing loss. *GJB2* mutations were identified first in 1997. Since then, more than 90 *GJB2* mutations have been reported. It is now known that three specific mutations (35delG, 167delT, 235delC) are responsible for the majority of *GJB2*-related hearing loss. 35delG is more prevalent in whites of Northern European descent as well as persons from the Mediterranean and Middle Eastern regions. 167delT is found in the Ashkenazi Jewish population, and 235delC is observed primarily in Asian populations (Palmer et al., 2003). By testing for this gene, it is possible to identify the cause of deafness in 20% to 40% of persons with hearing impairment or deafness of unknown etiology. For instance, Morell and colleagues (1998) reported that the 167delT mutation had only been identified in the Ashkenazi Jewish population. On the other hand, the 35delG mutation in *Connexin 26* has been shown to account for nonsyndromal sensorineural hearing impairment or deafness in Western Europe and North America (Estivill et al., 1999; Lench et al., 1998; Zelante et al., 1997). To examine the influence of 35delG on autosomal recessive nonsyndromic hearing loss, Mahdieh and Rabbani (2009) conducted a meta-analytical review. They reported mean carrier frequency for this gene to be 1.89 for Europeans, 1.52 for Americans, 0.64 for Asians, 1 for Oceania, and 0.64 for African populations. Further, they reported that the carrier frequency was highest in southern Europe and lowest in eastern Asia.

Researchers from around the globe have been investigating the role of *GJB2* in hearing loss in their countries and communities. Löppönen and associates (2003) examined *Connexin 26* mutations and nonsyndromic hearing impairments in northern Finland, and observed that 21.1% of the hearing impaired children they examined had *CX26* mutations. Mutation 35delG was the cause of hearing impairment in 86.7% of the children. The carrier frequency for the mutation 35delG was 1 of 78, whereas that for mutation M34T was 1 of 26. Batissoco and associates (2009) determined the frequencies of *GJB2* mutations and *GJB6* deletions in the Brazilian population. They screened 300 persons with hearing impairment, who did not have known deafness syndromes. The most frequently found mutation, 35delG, was seen in 23% of familial and 6.2% of sporadic cases. The second most frequently occurring mutation was a deletion in the *GJB6* gene (GJB6-D13S1830).

Propst and coworkers (2006) examined the relationship between ethnicity and mutations in the *GJB2* and *GJB6* genes in multicultural patients enrolled in a pediatric cochlear implant program in Canada. Nine different *GJB2* mutations were identified in persons from 14 different countries. About 78% of all identified pathogenic *GJB2* mutations were 35delG. The researchers observed that individuals of African, Caribbean, and East Indian descent had different *GJB2* mutations compared with other individuals who were tested. Gravina and associates (2010) examined the prevalence of *GJB2* mutations and *GJB6* deletions in Argentinean children with nonsyndromic deafness. They observed that the most frequently found *GJB2* mutation was 35delG, and the second most common mutation was deletion GJB6-D13S1830. The frequency of the deletion was as high as that "found in Spain from where Argentina has received one of its major immigration waves." Teek and colleagues (2010) studied the prevalence of 35delG and M34T mutations in the *GJB2* gene in children with early-onset hearing loss as well as within the general population of Estonia. Based on their data, they concluded that in Estonian children with early-onset hearing loss, the most common *GJB2* mutations were 35delG and M34T. In the general population, 1 of 22 persons carried the 35delG mutation, and 1 of 17 carried the M34T mutation. Siem and associates (2010) reported that *GJB2* mutations were a common cause of hearing impairment in Norwegian children with cochlear implants; 35delG mutation accounted for 85% of mutations. Similarly, Cama and colleagues (2009) found that 35delG was one of the most frequent (64%) mutations in their patients from the Veneto region in Italy.

Unlike the European researchers, investigators from China and Japan found the 235delC mutation to be the most prevalent. Chen and coworkers (2009) enrolled 115 cochlear implant patients for mutation screening to ascertain whether *GJB2* mutations were the major causes of deafness in Chinese cochlear implant recipients. They reported that 36.5% of their cochlear implant recipients and 41% of nonsyndromic deafness patients had *GJB2* mutations. They found 11 variations in the *GJB2* gene; the 235delC mutation was the most prevalent mutation. Similarly, Hayashi and associates (2011) conducted mutation screening and direct sequencing for *GJB2* in 126 Japanese children who had been implanted. They also observed 10 different mutations, but the one that was most prevalent (44.8%) was the 235delC mutation.

Although a lot more is known about genetic hearing loss today than ever before, there is a lot more that remains to be learned. For instance, although 400 different syndromes have been identified, the reasons for variations in the degree of penetrance, and differences in the age of onset in different persons, are unknown as yet. Some individuals with syndromes also carry the *GJB2* mutation. Whether or not and to what degree this mutation affects the degree of penetrance or the age of onset are unknown.

Congenital Cytomegalovirus

CMV is a member of the herpes virus family; it is a lifelong, latent infection that may become reactivated periodically. Recurrent infection may be due to reinfection with a new strain or to reactivation. According to the CDC (2010a), CMV is found in all geographic locations and socioeconomic groups and infects 50% to 85% of adults in the United States by 40 years of age. CMV infection is more widespread in developing countries and in areas of lower socioeconomic conditions.

Grosse and coworkers (2008) conducted a systematic review of studies of children with congenital CMV to ascertain the frequency of bilateral moderate to profound sensorineural hearing loss. They reported that about 14% of children with congenital CMV infection developed sensorineural hearing loss, and 3% to 5% developed bilateral moderate to profound sensorineural hearing loss. Further, they estimated that congenital CMV was probably the etiology in 15% to 20% of all children with bilateral moderate to profound sensorineural hearing loss. Fowler and Bopanna (2006) reported that 22% to 65% of symptomatic and 6% to 23% of asymptomatic children with congenital CMV have hearing loss, ranging from unilateral high-frequency to profound bilateral loss.

Colugnati and colleagues (2007) used seroprevalence data from the Third National Health and Nutrition Examination Survey to estimate the incidence of CMV among the general U.S. population and among pregnant women. They reported that their computations indicated that an infected person transmits CMV to nearly two susceptible people. What was most significant was the racial disparity; the force of infection (incidence in seronegative individuals) was significantly higher among non-Hispanic blacks (5.7) and Mexican Americans (5.1) than among non-Hispanic whites (1.4). The force of infection was significantly higher in the low household income group (3.5) than in the middle (2.1) and upper (1.5) household income groups. They estimated that approximately 27,000 new CMV infections occur annually among seronegative pregnant women in the United States. They advocated for accelerating research to develop vaccines to reduce CMV transmission.

Schildroth (1994) reported that the number of children with CMV as a cause of hearing impairment has increased every year since the question was first included in the Annual Survey of Hearing Impaired Children and Youth conducted by Gallaudet University during the 1985-1986 school year. Although the 1991-1992 survey data showed that CMV cases were reported in all four regions of the country, the South reported 45% of the cases. Schildroth (1994) specified that Texas, North Carolina, and California reported almost one fourth of the CMV cases, and the large number of cases in Texas accounted for much of the survey's CMV overrepresentation in the South. This large number reported by Texas was attributed to this state's emphasis on early identification of hearing impairment. Schildroth (1994) reported that 88% of the CMV group had severe to profound hearing impairment, and 98% of the CMV children had bilateral hearing impairment. The ethnic breakdown from the survey showed that 72% of the CMV children were white, 16% were African American, 8% were of Hispanic origin, 2% were from the Asian and Pacific Islander group, and 2% were identified in the "other" category. This was consistent with the U.S. Department of Education's (2000) observation that in California, Texas, and New York, minority children with hearing impairments made up a large percentage of children in special education classrooms. Furthermore, according to the U.S. Census Bureau (2001), African American, Hispanic, and American Indian children were more likely to live in poverty and have less access to health care. At the same time, the CDC (1999) reported that CMV is more widespread in areas of lower socioeconomic conditions. Disparities in risk for the infection, access to health care, and higher incidence of poverty place minority children at a greater risk for hearing impairment.

In Milan, Italy, Barbi and associates (2003) retrospectively examined CMV DNA in stored samples of neonatal dried blood of 130 children with hearing loss that was greater than 40 dB HL. Their data suggested that 20% to 30% of all deafness cases were caused by CMV and that 40% of deafness cases with an unknown cause were also due to congenital CMV.

DNA specimens from preserved umbilical cords are available to anyone born in Japan. After examining DNA specimens from dried umbilical cords, Ogawa and associates (2007) reported that congenital CMV infection was identified in 15% of children with severe sensorineural hearing loss, all of whom developed their hearing loss by 2 years of age. These children had no obvious clinical abnormality at birth, and their viral loads were lower than those of children who were symptomatic at birth. Similarly, Mizuno and colleagues (2009) also conducted a retrospective diagnostic study by examining DNA of 45 children with sensorineural hearing loss. They detected CMV DNA in the preserved umbilical cords of three patients, all of whom had bilateral late-onset sensorineural hearing loss. The researchers reported that CMV DNA was not found in any patients with sudden sensorineural hearing loss or in those with enlarged vestibular aqueduct-associated sensorineural hearing loss. Further, they observed that hearing loss due to CMV was more asymmetrical than hearing loss due to other etiology.

Ahlfors and associates (1999) reported on a long-term study of maternal and congenital CMV infection in Sweden. They found 0.5% congenitally infected infants, 29.0% with transient neonatal symptoms, and 18.0% with neurologic symptoms by the age of 7 years. They observed that central nervous system disturbances in infants occurred after primary and secondary maternal infections. On the other hand, Balasubramaniam and colleagues (1994) reported that CMV was highly endemic in Malaysia. Congenital CMV was detected in 11.4% of infants, in comparison with congenital syphilis in 4.0%, congenital rubella in 3.7%, and congenital toxoplasma in 1.0% of infants. Furthermore, 10.4% of the infected cases had central nervous system deficits. They concluded that CMV appeared to be the most important cause of congenital infection in Malaysia.

De Paschale and coworkers (2009) ascertained the incidence and risk for infection during pregnancy in 2817 women in an urban area of Northern Italy, who had anti-CMV immunoglobulin G (IgG) and IgM antibody screening between 2005 and 2007. The prevalence of anti-CMV IgG antibodies was 68.3%. The screening helped to identify 13 cases of primary infection in pregnant women, who were then referred for serological testing and intervention. The researchers indicated that such screening though controversial was very useful because once CMV is identified, intervention can be planned and implemented.

Kenneson and Cannon (2007) reviewed studies that reported results of systematic CMV screening in fetuses and live-born infants. The overall birth prevalence of congenital CMV infection was 0.64% but varied a lot between populations examined by the researchers. Both maternal seroprevalence and birth prevalence were higher in populations that were examined at birth than prenatally, suggesting that the time of examination should be considered when determining the prevalence of this disease. The rate of transmission to infants born to infected mothers was 32% for primary infections and 1.4% for recurrent infections.

A few studies have suggested that there may be a relationship between maternal seropositivity for CMV and the clinical features of CMV infection. The enzyme-linked immunosorbent assay is the most commonly available serologic test for measuring antibody to CMV. The result can be used to determine whether maternal antibody is present in an infant. Stagno and colleagues (1982) compared the prevalence of congenital CMV infection in a Chilean population with low-income, middle- and upper-class populations in Birmingham, Alabama. Although the incidence was higher in the highly seroimmune Chilean (1.7%) and low-income Birmingham (1.9%) groups than in the less immune middle- and upper-class group (0.6%), 407 autopsies did not attribute neonatal deaths to CMV in the Chilean group, whereas 1.0% of infant deaths in the Birmingham groups were attributed to CMV. The investigators concluded that despite an apparent lack of protection against intrauterine transmission, maternal immunity reduces the risk for severe fetal infection. Similarly, Morita and coworkers (1998) reported a low incidence (1.6 of 100,000 births) of symptomatic CMV disease in Japan. Major clinical manifestations were observed in 38% to 50% of the symptomatic neonates. Sequelae such as hearing impairment, mental retardation, and motor disability developed in 71% of survivors, whereas 35% of infected infants died or had severe disability. The investigators attributed the lower frequency of clinical findings at birth to the higher seroprevalence of pregnant women in Japan than in Europe and the United States.

Sickle Cell Disease

Sickle cell disease (SCD), also known as sickle cell anemia, is a group of inherited blood disorders. When sickle cell hemoglobin deoxygenates while passing through blood vessels, it polymerizes, becomes fibrous-like and causes the red blood cells (erythrocytes) to become rigid and change shape to look like sickles. These altered cells die early, which results in a constant shortage of erythrocytes. Further, sickled erythrocytes tend to form clumps, and as they travel through smaller blood vessels, they block the blood vessels, resulting in lack of oxygen to tissue and causing extreme pain or crises, stroke, permanent organ damage, anemia, and acute chest pain syndrome (CDC, 2009a).

The most common types of SCD include (1) HbSS, or sickle cell anemia, in which the person inherits two sickle cell genes, one from each parent, which is typically the most severe form of the disease; (2) HbSc, a milder form of the disease, in which the person inherits one sickle cell gene and one abnormal gene from an abnormal type of hemoglobin called "C"; (3) HbS β-thalassemia, in which the person inherits one sickle cell gene and one gene for β-thalassemia, another type of anemia. A few other rare types of sickle cell disease are HbSD, HbSE, and HbSO, in which the person inherits one sickle cell gene and one gene from an abnormal type of hemoglobin. The severity of these rare types varies, and the symptoms and complications are similar to those of HbSS. Finally, the sickle cell trait (HbAS) is acquired when one inherits one sickle cell gene and one normal gene. Persons who have the sickle cell trait do *not* have any symptoms of the disease and live a normal life. However, they can pass the disease on to their offspring (CDC, 2009a).

SCD affects people of many racial and ethnic groups. Although the severity of the disease varies from person to person, complications are often life-threatening. Unfortunately, this disease occurs more frequently among persons who have limited access to comprehensive health care because of social, economic, cultural, and geographic barriers. Besides the United States, SCD is particularly common among those whose ancestors come from sub-Saharan Africa, Saudi Arabia, India, and the Mediterranean countries, such as Greece, Turkey, and Italy.

The CDC (2010b, 2010c, 2010d) estimated that in the United States, approximately 70,000 to 100,000 persons are affected by SCD. It affects ethnic groups differently; SCD occurs in 1 out of every 500 African American births, and in 1 out of every 36,000 Hispanic American births. The sickle cell trait occurs in about 1 in 12 African Americans. The WHO (2008) estimated that about 7% of the world population carries an abnormal hemoglobin gene. Around the globe, about 300,000 to 500,000 children are born with clinically significant hemoglobin disorders each year, and about 80% of affected children are born in developing countries. Approximately 70% of these children are born with SCD, whereas the rest are born with thalassemia syndromes. In low- and middle-income countries, 50% to 80% of children with SCD and 50,000 to 100,000 children with thalassemia major die annually. According to the CDC (2010c), in Brazil and Columbia, South America, approximately 1500 to 3000 children born each year have SCD. In sub-Saharan Africa, the incidence is 1% to 3% of newborns, whereas in the United Kingdom, more than 200 babies are born annually with SCD. In the Middle East, approximately 6000 children are born with SCD, and at least 50% of these children are born in Saudi Arabia.

Balgir (2007) reported that the exact number of persons with SCD is unknown in India. He was of the opinion that previous estimates (24,34,170 carriers, 1,21,375 homozygotes) were very low, and he estimated that in the State of Orissa alone there were 3 to 4 million people suffering from hemoglobinopathy. The combined average allele frequency of the three most predominant abnormal hemoglobins (HbD0, HbE, HbS) is 5.35% in India.

Neurologic symptoms are frequently present in persons with SCD. The vaso-occlusive nature of the disease may cause damage to the auditory mechanism and hearing loss may be reported. Gentry and colleagues (1997) screened

100 young subjects with SCD for hearing loss. Twelve percent of the children failed the screening; although this failure rate is higher than reported prevalence rates, the researchers recommended routine screening of hearing as the first step in the audiological management of children with SCD.

Middle ear effusion in children with SCD has been reported by several researchers, who have also reported the presence of hearing loss that was sensorineural in origin (MacDonald et al., 1999; Alabi et al., 2008). Liu and colleagues (2009) reported on a child with SCD who had sensorineural hearing loss, resulting from labyrinthitis ossifications possibly due to an infection, inflammation, or "destructive insult to the membranous labyrinth." Reports of the existence of unilateral or bilateral, mild sensorineural hearing loss in children with SCD have been published around the world. Piltcher and colleagues (2000) in Southern Brazil, Al-Dabbous and associates (1996) in Saudi Arabia, Onakoya and coworkers (2002) in Nigeria, and Tsibulevskaya and colleagues (1996) in Kenya have all reported observing sensorineural hearing loss in some persons with SCD. The prevalence ranged from 19% to 66%. However, these data should be interpreted with caution because the subjects ranged in age from children to adults; some hearing loss could be attributed to presbycusis and/or noise exposure. Elola and associates (2009) also assessed the auditory function of 112 cases of sickle cell anemia in Côte d'Ivoire. They observed that 17% of the cases presented a hearing loss of 30-65 dB HL. Further, they reported the incidence of different types of the disease; the SCD form had an incidence of 47%, the HbSS form 37%, and the HbS β-thalassemia form 16%. Whereas 58% of cases demonstrated sensorineural hearing loss, 42% of the cases had mixed hearing loss.

Distortion product otoacoustic emissions (DPOAEs) have been used to study auditory function in persons with SCD. Downs and coworkers (2000) reported that the amplitudes of DPOAEs were significantly larger in children with SCD than children with normal hemoglobin. Stuart and colleagues (2006) compared DPOAEs in normal-hearing children with homozygous SCD, who were receiving hydroxyurea (HDU) treatment, a matched group of children with SCD, who were not on HDU, and children with normal hemoglobin. They observed increased DPOAE amplitudes in children with SCD, who were not taking HDU. Children who were taking HDU had DPOAE amplitudes that were similar to those of the normal children. These findings were interpreted to suggest that HDU not only reduces the symptoms of SCD but may also play a role in inhibiting or preventing cochlear pathology and hearing loss.

De Castro and coworkers (2010) used brainstem auditory evoked response (BSER) audiometry to check neural integrity, electrophysiologic thresholds, and P300 to analyze auditory selective attention in 40 patients with SCD and matched normal subjects. They observed hearing loss in 16 ears (20%) and there was a statistically significant reduction in the I-V interpeak latency in the SCD group, indicating the presence of cochlear abnormality. On the other hand, normal values were observed for P300 latency and amplitude suggesting that the central auditory system was normal. These researchers had excluded individuals with comorbidities from the study; their observations indicated the presence of cochlear pathology with normal neural function in the SCD group.

Jovanovic-Bateman and Hedreville (2006) studied 79 homozygote and heterozygote sickle cell anemia patients and a control group of 40 persons. They observed that both genders and haplotypes were affected equally. Nineteen (47.2%) HbSC patients, 17 (43.59%) HbSS patients, and 3 (7.5%) members of the control group had sensorineural hearing loss (>20 dB HL at two or more frequencies). Nineteen (52.78%) patients had bilateral hearing loss, 5 (13.89%) had unilateral hearing loss in the right ear, and 12 (33.33%) had unilateral hearing loss in the left ear. During BSER testing, 13 (25.35%) patients, 8 of whom had HbSS, demonstrated a prolonged I-V (III-V) interpeak latency. The researchers concluded that the hearing loss in the HbSS patients was neural in origin and had an earlier onset, whereas that in the HbSC patients was cochlear in origin and had a later onset. Most of their patients had the Benin haplotype. The researchers explained that the relatively high incidence of sensorineural hearing loss in their patients was possibly due to their "specific haematological profile and to the original geographical distribution of the disease in the tropics."

Although a gradual onset of sensorineural hearing loss is typical of SCD, there are several reports of sudden sensorineural hearing loss in children and adults with SCD (Whitehead et al., 1998; Garcia et al., 2002; Ondzotto et al., 2002; Mace et al., 2009). One of the causes of sudden hearing loss in persons with SCD is a labyrinthine hemorrhage. Whitehead and colleagues (1998) have suggested that a hemorrhagic sudden hearing loss in a patient with SCD indicates "a sickling crisis of the labyrinthine capillary bed either in the distribution of the anteroinferior cerebellar artery or a branch of the basilar artery, which should be considered equivalent to other intracranial sickling effects." Ondzotto and associates (2002) were of the opinion that the cause of sudden deafness in their 30-year-old patient with sickle cell anemia was obliteration of the terminal auditory artery resulting in anoxia of the cochlea. On the other hand, Mace and coworkers (2009) reported the case of a 7-year-old child with sickle cell anemia who developed profound bilateral sensorineural hearing loss over a period of 5 days. During the preceding weeks, the child had presented inflammatory markers and ophthalmologic disease. The diagnosis included "a vaso-occlusive or inflammatory aetiology such as Cogan's syndrome."

Diabetes

Diabetes is known to negatively affect hearing. There are significant racial and ethnic disparities in the prevalence of diabetes. According to data from the CDC (2011b), compared with non-Hispanic white adults, the risk for diagnosed diabetes was 18% higher among Asian Americans, 66% higher among Hispanics, and 77% higher among non-Hispanic blacks. Among Hispanics compared with non-Hispanic white adults, the risk for diagnosed diabetes was about the same for Cuban Americans and for Central and South Americans, 87% higher for Mexican Americans, and 94% higher for Puerto Ricans.

Cheng and colleagues (2009) examined change in the prevalence of hearing impairment over three decades in adults with and without diabetes using data from the National Health and Nutrition Examination Surveys (1971-1973, 1999-2004). They reported that among 25- to 69-year-old persons without diabetes, the prevalence changed from 24.4% to 22.3%; however, for adults with diabetes, the prevalence changed from 28.5% to 34.4%. The researchers concluded that persons with diabetes had a higher prevalence of hearing impairment, and they did not achieve the same reduction in hearing impairment over three decades, as persons without diabetes.

Bacterial Meningitis

Bacterial meningitis remains a serious threat to global health; it accounts for approximately 170,000 annual deaths worldwide. It is estimated that as many as 450 million people across Africa are at risk for contracting meningitis. During the 2009 epidemic season, 88,199 suspected cases and 5352 deaths were reported (WHO, 2010d, 2010e).

On December 6, 2010, the WHO (2010d, 2010e) started a nationwide campaign to introduce a new meningococcal A conjugate vaccine in Burkina Faso, Mali, and Niger. This vaccine induces a higher and more sustainable immune response against group A meningococcus. It is expected to provide long-term protection, to reduce infection and transmission, is available at a lower price, and is "particularly effective in protecting children under two years of age, who do not respond to conventional polysaccharide vaccines." This is the first vaccine designed specifically for Africa, and it is hoped that by targeting the 1- to 29-year-old group, it will help to eliminate meningococcal A in the meningitis belt.

Data from the Gallaudet Research Institute's Annual Survey of Deaf and Hard of Hearing Children and Youth for the years 2003 to 2006 indicated that meningitis was among the five most frequently reported etiological factors for hearing loss and deafness. However, it appeared that the incidence was showing a declining trend (1483 cases in 2003-2004; 1291 cases in 2004-2005; 1197 cases in 2005-2006). Additionally for each of these years, the number of cases of meningitis was highest in the southern region of the United States and the lowest in the northeast (Gallaudet Research Institute, January 2005, December 2005, December 2006). It was not possible to provide data for subsequent years because the Survey has been revised, and different types of data are being collected and reported.

The CDC (2009b, 2010a) reported that three common clinical forms in which meningococcal disease occurs in the United States are meningitis (50% of cases), blood infection (30% of cases), and pneumonia (10% of cases); other forms account for the remaining 10% of cases. The onset and course of the disease are rapid, with a fatality rate of 10% to 14%. Further, 11% to 19% of the survivors have serious sequelae, including deafness, neurologic deficits, or limb loss. Annually, 1000 to 2000 cases of invasive meningococcal disease occur in the United States; 20% of the affected persons are 14 to 24 years of age, and 16% are infants younger than 1 year. Currently, in the United States, there is no licensed vaccine that protects against serogroup B meningococcal disease.

MacNeil (2009) provided data from 1999 to 2008 on the incidence of meningococcal disease (types B, C, Y) in children younger than 5 years and projected these to the U.S. population. A comparison of sequelae in children at hospitalization showed that for children younger than 5 years, who had contracted serogroup B meningococcal disease, the incidence of hearing loss was 10.7%, whereas the incidence was 12% when data for serogroups C and Y were combined. For children older than 5 years, the incidence of hearing loss was 17.6% when serogroup B had been contracted, whereas the incidence was 9.7% when data for serogroups C and Y were combined. Further, regardless of the age group, more children had hearing loss than the other two sequelae (necrosis and hemiplegia).

Boswell (2003) reported on the increase in the incidence of meningitis among cochlear implant recipients in 2002. As of May 2003, 118 cochlear implant recipients, 63 cases abroad and 55 cases in the United States (including five deaths), had developed bacterial meningitis. Approximately 50% of the cases of meningitis were attributed to an electrode design that included a positioner that placed the electrode in close proximity to the auditory nerve. However, it was observed also that even without implants, children with hearing loss had a higher incidence of meningitis than children of the same age in the general population.

Hearing loss or deafness is often found as a sequela to meningitis. Tan and associates (2010) described a patient in Singapore with *Streptococcus suis* meningitis, who developed permanent deafness from hemorrhagic labyrinthitis as shown on magnetic resonance imaging. The patient had suffered a relapse despite a 7-week course of antibiotics. Worsøe and associates (2010) investigated the frequency and severity of hearing loss retrospectively in 343 Danish patients, who survived pneumococcal meningitis, and they also identified risk factors for developing hearing loss. Of

240 patients who were tested audiometrically, 129 (54%) had hearing loss, and 50 (39%) of these 129 patients had not been suspected of having a hearing loss at discharge. Of the 240, 16 (7%) had profound unilateral hearing loss, and another 16 (7%) had bilateral profound hearing loss. Risk factors that were found to be significant for hearing loss included advanced age, presence of comorbidity, severity of meningitis, low cerebrospinal fluid (CSF) glucose level, high CSF protein level, and a certain pneumococcal serotype. The researchers suggested that hearing loss is fairly common after pneumococcal meningitis and recommended that all survivors be tested audiologically before discharge.

Trotman and colleagues (2009) described the clinical features and outcomes of pneumococcal meningitis in 25 Jamaican children. Four of the children had SCD; 2 of these children were first diagnosed with SCD during hospitalization for meningitis, and 1 of these children died. Only eight of the 25 children survived, of whom 3 were found to have hearing loss. One of the recommendations made by the researchers was that as a policy, children who were high risk, such as those with SCD, should be administered conjugate pneumococcal vaccine.

Edmond and associates (2010a) reviewed papers published between 1980 and 2008 to (1) examine the risks for major and minor sequelae caused by bacterial meningitis, (2) estimate the distribution of the different types of sequelae, and (3) compare risk by region and income. After reviewing 132 selected papers, they concluded that regardless of the type of bacteria, the risk for a major sequela was twice as high in the African (25.1%) and Southeast Asia (21.6%) regions compared with the European region (9.4%). Low-income countries, where the burden of bacterial meningitis is the greatest, had the highest risk for long-term disabling sequelae. The researchers were of the opinion that most reported sequelae could have been prevented if the children had been vaccinated with Hib, pneumococcal, and meningococcal vaccines.

The CDC (2000, 2009c, 2010e) reported that there were 123,658 cases of meningococcal disease with 21,830 deaths in West African countries during 1996 and 1997. More typically, the incidence is 2% during epidemics and 0.5 to 5.0 per 100,000 cases worldwide for endemic disease. There is a mortality rate of 10% to 15%. Of patients who recover, 10% have permanent hearing impairment or other sequelae.

To examine disabling sequelae and quality of life in children with bacterial meningitis in urban Senegal, Edmond and associates (2010b) followed children from Dakar, Senegal, who were on the pediatric bacterial meningitis surveillance system. The researchers classified disabling sequelae and the quality of life of these children, and they compared the sequelae with an age- and community-matched group. They followed 66 cases and 66 controls and found that the odds of a major sequela were three times greater in cases with meningitis (65.1%) than in the control group (40.9%). Hearing loss was the most common sequela in the cases (51.8%); other sequelae were cognitive deficits (40%), seizures (21.2%), and motor deficits (21.2%). Of these, 34.9% of the cases had multiple impairments. In children who had previously had pneumococcal meningitis, the risk for a major sequela was 79.2%; in cases with *Haemophilus influenzae* type b, the risk was 59.1%; and in those who had meningococcal meningitis, the risk for a major sequela was 54.6%. The total quality-of-life scores were significantly lower in cases with meningitis than in controls. The researchers concluded that children with bacterial meningitis are at high risk for developing complex multiple impairments, many of which could be prevented with the use of new conjugate vaccines against *H. influenzae* type b, pneumococcus, and meningococcus.

Sensorineural hearing impairment is the most common complication of bacterial meningitis. Typically, the hearing impairment is mild to profound and bilateral. In a few cases, some recovery of hearing has been reported. For instance, Guiscafre and colleagues (1984) reported that 22 of 32 children with bacterial meningitis in Mexico recovered normal hearing. Vienny and associates (1984) examined 51 children with bacterial meningitis in Switzerland and reported that 35 children had normal hearing, 11 children showed transient abnormalities in the auditory brainstem response, and 5 children had permanent sensorineural hearing loss. The investigators observed occurrence of deafness during the early phase of the disease, with a crucial phase in the first 2 weeks during which hearing improved or worsened.

Human Immunodeficiency Virus

Human immunodeficiency virus (HIV) is a retrovirus that causes acquired immunodeficiency syndrome (AIDS). The incidence of HIV/AIDS shows geographic variation between regions in the world. According to UNAIDS (2010), of the 33.3 million persons living with HIV in 2009, 22.5 million persons lived in sub-Saharan Africa, 4.1 million lived in South and Southeast Asia, 1.5 million lived in North America, 1.4 million lived in Central and South America, 820,000 lived in Western and Central Europe, 770,000 resided in East Asia, 460,000 lived in the Middle East and North Africa, 240,000 lived in the Caribbean, and 57,000 lived in Oceania (UNAIDS, 2010).

Matkin and coworkers (1998) reported that pediatric AIDS patients are susceptible to infections and neurologic complications that can compromise auditory function. According to Bankaitis and Schountz (1998), ototoxicity and opportunistic infections associated with HIV/AIDS are potential causes of sensory hearing loss among HIV/AIDS cases. Ototoxicity has been associated with antiretroviral drugs, antifungal agents, antineoplastic drugs, immune modulators, and aminoglycoside antibiotics. The severity of the resulting hearing impairment varies from mild to profound depending on the patient's sensitivity, size of the dosage, and length of time the drug is taken. Besides ototoxicity, sudden-onset sensorineural hearing impairment associated with direct infection of the central nervous system, such as AIDS encephalopathy or subacute encephalitis, has also been reported. Opportunistic infections of the central nervous system, such as cryptococcal meningitis and tuberculous meningitis, also have been associated with deafness.

Palacios and colleagues (2008) assessed the auditory and vestibular systems in 23 children infected with HIV type 1 at a pediatric hospital in Mexico. Their mean age was 4.5 years. Twelve children older than 4 years, 5 months were assessed using pure tone audiometry; 4 children demonstrated hearing loss, of whom 2 had conductive hearing loss. ABR audiometry was administered to all 23 children; 6 children demonstrated conductive hearing loss, whereas 2 demonstrated sensorineural hearing loss. Most children with conductive hearing loss had a history of acute or chronic suppurative otitis media. Abnormally long interwave intervals were observed in 3 children (4 ears), abnormal morphologies were observed in 4 children (7 ears), and abnormal amplitudes were observed in 11 children (17 ears). Six children, who were administered vestibular tests, showed asymmetrical caloric and rotatory tests. Although the differences were not significant, the researchers reported a pattern of more frequent audiological abnormalities in "patients with more prolonged HIV-1 infections, higher viral loads, or lower absolute CD4+ cell counts."

To ascertain the degree and type of hearing loss in patients infected with HIV and to determine the type of relationship if any between the hearing loss and the severity of the disease itself, Wang and coworkers (2006) assessed the hearing of 350 HIV-infected patients at a university hospital in Zhengzhou, China. They reported that 159 cases (45.4%) in the HIV-infected group had hearing loss, compared with 69 cases (19.7%) in the control group. Of the 159 cases, 56 had sensorineural hearing loss, 34 had conductive hearing loss, and 69 had mixed hearing loss. The degree of hearing loss varied; 49 cases demonstrated mild hearing loss, 69 demonstrated moderate hearing loss, and 41 had severe hearing loss. Although the researchers found no relationship between the hearing loss and the severity of the disease, they did report that "the hearing loss was dominant at high frequencies in HIV infected patients." Similarly, Khoza and Ross (2002) examined the prevalence, as well as the type, degree, and configuration, of hearing loss, the type of onset of hearing loss, and the relationship if any between the hearing loss and the progressive stage of the disease. The prevalence rate was reported to be as high as 23%. Their subjects demonstrated conductive and sensorineural hearing loss, ranging from "slight" to profound. Although Khoza and Ross did not find a pattern of hearing loss at specific frequencies, and they did not observe a relationship between the degree of hearing loss and the progression of

the disease, they did observe an increase in the incidence of sensorineural hearing loss with deterioration of the patient's immunological status.

Chandrasekhar and coworkers (2000) also tried to quantify the incidence of ear disease in 50 patients infected with HIV who were outpatients at a university hospital in New Jersey. Their subjects were volunteers with a mean age of 40 years, who had had the disease for a mean duration of 3.5 years. Eighteen percent of the patients fell in category CDC-A, 38% in CDC-B, and 44% in CDC-C. Otologic complaints in these patients included aural fullness (34%), dizziness (32%), hearing loss (29%), tinnitus (26%), otalgia (23%), and otorrhea (5%). The researchers found abnormal tympanometric findings in 21% of the patients. Further, many patients demonstrated high frequency sensorineural hearing loss; patients in categories CDC-B and CDC-C demonstrated worse hearing than CDC-A patients at three frequencies. The researchers reported that patients who complained of hearing loss had significantly worse otoacoustic emission results and greater hearing loss at all frequencies except 1000 Hz. They reported that the incidence of ear disease in patients who were infected with HIV was about 33%; otitis media was the most frequent finding. Patients who had a more severe form of the disease had more severe sensorineural hearing loss, and otopathology was frequently found in patients with complaints of the ear.

One of the treatment options reported in the literature to improve the quality of life for persons with HIV, who develop profound sensorineural hearing loss bilaterally, is cochlear implantation. Roland and associates (2003) evaluated the efficacy of cochlear implantation in seven HIV-infected patients and correlated the results with a pathophysiological mechanism of HIV-associated hearing loss. Although there was variability in performance, the group performance was reported to be good. There were no surgical or postoperative complications. The researchers concluded that patients with HIV benefit from cochlear implantation without additional risks, and the good performance of their subjects supported the hypothesis that the mechanism of HIV-associated deafness involved "infiltration, malfunction, and premature degeneration of the hair cells and supportive cells of the cochlea." Vincenti and colleagues (2005) reported on a profoundly deafened person, who was HIV infected, who underwent cochlear implantation. Four years after the surgery, the patient had not experienced any complications and had regained open-set speech perception.

Persons who are deaf or hard of hearing make up approximately 10% of the U.S. population. Although exact figures are not available, estimates of the number of HIV/AIDS cases among the Deaf vary from 2640 to 7000 (Gaskins, 1999). It has been speculated that the higher figure is probably more realistic than the lower estimate. In fact, there has been great concern that this group is very vulnerable to this disease and is disproportionately affected. However, there is a paucity of research on the prevalence, incidence, mode of infection, and intervention in this group. Several researchers have commented on factors that contribute to risk behaviors among the Deaf and hard of hearing (Bat-Chava et al., 2005; Winningham et al., 2008; Hanass-Hancock & Satande, 2010). The most frequently cited factors include different communication strategies, such as ASL, that are not used by persons who hear normally, especially medical and health care workers; high incidence of alcohol and substance abuse in the Deaf and hard of hearing community; higher incidence of child abuse in this group compared with persons with normal hearing; limited knowledge of HIV/AIDS transmission and less access to information and services; and lack of intervention materials and approaches developed for this population that take into consideration the different modes of communication used by persons who are deaf or hard of hearing.

One factor that has been investigated by a few researchers is the extent of knowledge that persons who are deaf or hard of hearing have regarding HIV/AIDS. Heuttel and Rothstein (2001) administered a survey to undergraduate students who were deaf and those with normal hearing, to ascertain their knowledge and sources of information regarding HIV/AIDS. The deaf students earned significantly lower scores than their normal-hearing peers. Also, although students with normal hearing relied more on teachers, television, and reading materials to obtain information on HIV/AIDS, students who were deaf relied more on friends and family for the information, which may have been more prone to factual errors. Similarly, Groce and coworkers (2007) compared knowledge about HIV among a group of Nigerians who were deaf and those with normal hearing. They also attempted to determine how effectively HIV/AIDS information was reaching persons who were deaf. They found significant differences between the two groups in the level of understanding of how AIDS is spread and in the resources available. They recommended developing educational materials and including the Deaf community in HIV awareness programs.

Bat-Chava and colleagues (2005) used focus groups and individual interviews to investigate knowledge about HIV/AIDS and possible barriers to education and prevention of this disease in persons with hearing loss. They observed that persons who were oral deaf and those who were hard of hearing were more knowledgeable about HIV/AIDS than deaf sign language users, and that adolescents who were deaf were more knowledgeable than adults who were deaf. The differences between the groups were interpreted to indicate differences in the levels of education and proficiency in English. Additionally, the researchers reported that individuals living in urban areas and in larger deaf communities were more exposed to information on HIV/AIDS than those who did not. It should be noted that in this study all participants reported having difficulty in communicating with medical providers, which restricts the information they can

obtain from them. Bisol and colleagues (2008) examined knowledge of HIV/AIDS as well as health-related attitudes and behaviors in adolescents who were deaf and those who had normal hearing in southern Brazil using a computerized questionnaire. They provided "simultaneous video translation of questions" in Brazilian sign language. They observed that participants who were deaf scored lower on knowledge of HIV/AIDS, and that those who had normal hearing reported more sexual activity. Additionally, the responses of adolescents who were deaf were indicative of a high incidence of sexual abuse, and a large number of them reported having friends who had AIDS.

Persons who are deaf are more vulnerable to HIV infection for many reasons but especially because of the challenges they face in communication. Prevention intervention messages must be tailored to identify high-risk behaviors and promote perceived susceptibility. It is equally important to present the materials using diverse media and technology (e.g., visual presentations, Internet, social networks, discussion boards, listservs) to reach as many persons as possible. Use should be made of community-based organizations, the "Deaf Grapevine," and Deaf clubs to identify HIV-risk behaviors and to relay factual information toward reducing the incidence of such behaviors and the risk for HIV infection (Winningham et al., 2008).

Presbycusis

A gradual decline in hearing has been regarded as an inevitable consequence of the normal aging process. Life expectancy in the United States and around the globe has increased. According to the WHO (2011), by 2025 there will be approximately 2 billion persons in the world who will be older than 60 years, and the world's population will have a greater proportion of older rather than younger persons. As persons live longer, there is growing emphasis on extending not merely the years of life but also the quality of life. Unfortunately, presbycusis or age-related hearing loss leads to isolation, dependence, and frustration, and negatively affects communication, social interaction, and the quality of life; that is, it is a leading cause of years lived with a disability. It has been estimated that 25% of persons aged 65 to 75 years and 70% to 80% of persons older than 75 years have hearing impairment as a direct consequence of aging. De Sousa and associates (2009) examined the prevalence of presbycusis and associated high-risk factors. After reviewing charts of 625 patients in a Brazilian hospital, they reported a prevalence of 36.1% in their subjects who ranged in age from 40 to 86 years, of whom 85.5% were males and 14.5% were females. The risk factors identified in this group were age, gender, diabetes mellitus, and heredity.

Presbycusis is a hearing loss that is typically insidious, bilaterally symmetrical, and sensorineural; the hearing loss starts in the high frequencies, and may gradually involve all the frequencies. Hearing loss impairs the elderly person's ability to understand conversational speech in quiet because many consonants are high-pitched sounds. Temporal processing is affected also; therefore, the older person has difficulty understanding speech in a complex, noisy environment (Pichora-Fuller & Souza, 2003). A number of pathophysiological processes underlying age-related changes have been examined, including heredity, environmental factors, and medical conditions. Loss of or damage to hair cells from exposure to everyday noise over a period of time, loss of or reduced blood supply, and loss of nerve fibers and neural elements, all contribute to presbycusis. Gopinath and colleagues (2010) examined the dietary intake to identify modifiable risk factors that could slow or prevent presbycusis. They observed that subjects who had two or more servings of fish per week had a significantly reduced risk (42%) of developing presbycusis compared with those who had a lower intake. Further, persons who consumed one to two servings of fish per week had a reduced risk for a progression of hearing loss. They also observed that there was an inverse association between intake of long-chain n-3 polyunsaturated fatty acid (PUFA) and prevalent as well as incident hearing loss. They concluded that dietary intervention with n-3 PUFAs could prevent or delay the development of presbycusis.

Dillon and associates (2010) reported on hearing impairment in Americans who were 70 years and older; non-Hispanic whites and Mexican Americans had a higher prevalence of hearing problems than non-Hispanic blacks. Lee and colleagues (2005) analyzed pure tone thresholds at conventional and extended frequencies in 188 persons (91 females, 97 males), 60 to 81 years of age, to study longitudinal changes in thresholds and the effects of other factors on thresholds. They reported that hearing thresholds increased by approximately 1 dB HL per year in persons who were 60 years and over. Age, gender, and initial threshold levels apparently affected the rate of change.

Demeester and associates (2009) conducted a study aimed at describing the audiometric shape in persons between 55 and 65 years of age. They examined audiograms of 1147 subjects (549 males, 598 females) and reported that 37% of the subjects showed flat audiograms, 35% demonstrated high frequency gently sloping audiograms, and 27% showed high-frequency steeply sloping configurations. The flat configuration was more prevalent in females, whereas the high frequency steeply sloping configuration was more common in males. History of noise exposure did not influence the configuration. Further, females with a flat configuration had the greater hearing loss. Subsequently, Demeester and colleagues (2010) described the heritability of the audiometric shape and the familial aggregation of different types of presbycusis in healthy Flemish persons, who were 50 to 75 years old. A total of 342 siblings of 64 families participated in the study. Audiometric shape was mathematically quantified to measure, size, slope,

concavity, percentage of frequency-dependent and frequency-independent hearing loss and "bulge depth." They observed high heritability estimates and reported that risk ratios for total hearing loss (size), uniform hearing loss (percentage of frequency-dependent hearing loss), and bulge depth were suggestive of a higher heredity for severe types of presbycusis than for moderate or mild types. The researchers suggested that separating the parameter total hearing loss into two parameters, uniform hearing loss and nonuniform hearing loss, could lead to the discovery of different genetic subtypes of presbycusis. Further, they recommended the use of the parameter bulge depth instead of concavity to classify subjects into "susceptible" or "resistant" to noise exposure.

Treatment options for presbycusis, depending on the type and severity of hearing loss, include fitting amplifying and/or assistive devices, adaptation of the environment, training communication partners, middle ear implantation, electric acoustic stimulation (use of a hearing aid and cochlear implant together in the same ear), cochlear implantation, and aural (re)habilitation (Sprinzl & Riechelmann, 2010). Recently, Salami and associates (2010) evaluated the efficiency and applicability of water-soluble formulation of CoQ10 (Q-TER((R))) in persons with presbycusis. Their preliminary data on the use of this drug in Italy with persons who had presbycusis have been promising. They observed improvement in air and bone conduction thresholds at 1000, 2000, 4000, and 8000 Hz.

Auditory Neuropathy Spectrum Disorder

A discussion of the etiology would be incomplete without mentioning auditory neuropathy spectrum disorder (ANSD), or auditory neuropathy/auditory dyssynchrony as the disorder used to be called. Although its incidence is low, this disorder has received much attention during the past decade. In fact, the JCIH 2007 Committee expanded the definition of hearing loss to include neural hearing loss (auditory neuropathy/dyssynchrony). In 2008, a group of professionals, including audiologists, met in Como, Italy, for the Guidelines and Development Conference on the Identification and Management of Children with Auditory Neuropathy. One of the outcomes of this conference was a consensus to change the terminology that is used to refer to this type of hearing impairment to ANSD. It is characterized by absent or abnormal auditory brainstem response, intact or near-intact otoacoustic emissions and cochlear microphonics, and poor speech perception that is much worse than what one would expect on the basis of the pure tone audiogram. This suggests normal outer hair cell function with impaired or absent conduction of synchronous signals by the auditory nerve. The pathogenesis of ANSD is not definitely known. It appears that the underlying abnormality possibly may be in the inner hair cells, the nerves of the primary auditory pathway, the connecting synapses, or a combination of these

(Keats, 2007). Persons with ANSD may have normal hearing or hearing loss that may range from mild to severe. Absent middle ear muscle reflexes has been another characteristic mentioned often.

According to Keats (2007), this disorder has been observed in 10% to 15% of the Deaf population and in 40% of babies in NICUs. The 2007 JCIH recommended separate hearing screening protocols for infants admitted to the NICU and those in well-baby clinics because it has been reported that infants admitted to NICUs are at high risk for neural loss. Babies admitted to the NICU for more than 5 days are to have ABR included as part of their hearing screening to ensure that neural hearing loss is identified. Kirkim and colleagues (2008) attempted to determine the frequency of ANSD in the Western Anatolian region of Turkey. They reported that in their universal newborn hearing screening program, the incidence of the disorder was 0.44%. Similarly, Kumar and Jayaram (2006) examined the prevalence of this disorder in Mysore, India, and reported that 1 in 183 persons with sensorineural hearing loss had this disorder.

Although a clear cause-and-effect relationship has not been established, several factors have been linked to this disorder after children who were diagnosed with ANSD experienced health problems prenatally, paranatally, or postnatally, such as jaundice, premature birth, low birth weight, and hypoxia or anoxia. For instance, Saluja and associates (2010) reported that 6 of the 13 (46%) neonates with severe jaundice that they observed had audiological findings of acute ANSD. Typically, environmental factors such as hypoxia result in a mild form of ANSD, whereas genetic abnormalities result in a more severe form of the disorder (Keats, 2007). Since ANSD runs in some families, a genetic predisposition has not been ruled out. Additionally, some persons have ANSD as well as neurological disorders unrelated to the auditory system, as in Charcot-Marie-Tooth syndrome. Roche and coworkers (2010) reported on 118 children with ANSD who had computed tomographic and magnetic resonance imaging (MRI) studies available for a retrospective review. They reported that 28% of the children showed "cochlear nerve deficiency" and other positive central nervous system findings on the MRI. Huang and colleagues (2010) used MRIs to determine whether cochlear nerve deficiency was associated with brain or inner ear abnormalities in 103 children with ANSD. They found that cochlear and hindbrain abnormalities are significantly more common among persons with ANSD with bilateral cochlear nerve deficiency than those with at least one intact cochlear nerve.

Debate continues on the most effective treatment for infants, children, and adults with ANSD. Professionals differ in their opinions regarding the benefits of technology in persons with ANSD. Hearing aids, cochlear implants, and other technologies (e.g., FM systems) have been advocated, but their benefits for children with neural hearing loss are variable. Similarly, there are different philosophies about how best to communicate and educate children with ANSD; the use of sign language, speechreading, and listening skills have all been advocated. Rance and Barker (2009) compared speech and language abilities of 10 children with ANSD who received cochlear implants with those of 10 age-matched children with ANSD who used hearing aids and 10 age-matched cochlear implant users with sensorineural hearing loss. At the end of 17 months, assessments indicated that the performance of children in the three groups was similar. The researchers suggested that children should not automatically be considered to be candidates for cochlear implants. Rather, in making a recommendation the clinician should consider each child's auditory capacity, that is, the child's potential to use audition to support understanding of speech and production of speech. In summary, all options should be kept open for every child and the best option should be determined based on the needs of the individual child and family.

WORLDWIDE HEARING SERVICES

Rapid technological advances over the past couple of decades have brought about substantial changes in amplification instruments and assistive devices. As digital technology picked up momentum, it brought about new ways of processing acoustical signals and revolutionized acoustic amplification. Hearing aids today combine amplification with advanced signal processing to enhance the speech signal. Current signal processors have features that allow for noise reduction, feedback cancellation, speech enhancement, self-adapting directional inputs, acoustic scene analysis, and monitoring of data. The most exciting and promising development has been the introduction of Bluetooth technology. Numerous excellent textbooks, websites, and published articles are available that provide detailed information regarding amplification and assistive devices in developed countries. This section, therefore, focuses only on information regarding the status of hearing care in developing countries primarily in the Southeast Asia region.

According to the WHO (2007), about 50% of hearing impairment in the world population is preventable. Considering the impact hearing loss has on the development of communicative skills in children, the quality of life of the person with hearing impairment, the economic toll society pays for it, and the emotional burden born by the individual and the family, the WHO saw the need to assess the prevalence of deafness and hearing impairment, the nature of ear diseases in specific regions, the availability of facilities, activities and trained personnel in ear and hearing care, and prevention measures in use (national policy and legislation), if any, in developing countries. To formulate a regional strategy for prevention of ear disease and deafness and to measure its progress, it was necessary to assess the basic infrastructure in the region. Accordingly, a questionnaire was developed based on the WHO protocol used previously, it was field-tested, and then mailed to member countries. The data that were gathered were examined, and it was recommended that a national ear and hearing care policy be developed in all countries.

In 1998, the WHO collaborated with the Christian Blind Mission (CBM) to hold a Workshop on Needs and Technology Assessment for Hearing Aid Services in Developing Countries. CBM is an international Christian development organization committed to improving the quality of life of people with disabilities in low-income regions of the world. Data before the group at the workshop indicated that current production of hearing aids worldwide was one tenth of the global need, and 75% of the annual production was distributed to North America and Europe, with only 25% to the rest of the world. There was an urgent need to provide amplification devices and related services that were both affordable and appropriate to the developing countries despite limited resources in terms of skilled clinicians, trained staff, and finances. One of the outcomes of the WHO-CBM Workshop was a recommendation to assemble an expert working group to develop guidelines containing requirements and recommendations for hearing aids and associated services toward ensuring that what was provided to developing countries was appropriate and affordable. This group, Hearing Aids Working Group (HAWG), assembled in 1999 and set up guidelines that were minimum requirements and recommendations for hearing aids and associated services; the purpose of the guidelines was to provide guidance to manufacturers, distributors, policy makers, and service providers (WHO, 2004). The WHO recommended that developing countries use the guidelines to set up programs to provide hearing aid services in their individual countries, but before implementing such a program, each country was urged to conduct a pilot project to determine the costs of services, fine-tune the model of service delivery, and ascertain the impact as well as effectiveness of such services.

The HAWG took into consideration the extreme shortage of professionals trained to provide ear care and hearing aid services and included in the guidelines different levels of service delivery using trained nonprofessional staff to help build capacity. The guidelines provided specific responsibilities and specified the content of the training that staff members should receive for each level of service. For specific details regarding the content of the training at each level, the reader is referred to the original document, *Guidelines for Hearing Aids and Services for Developing Countries,* which is available online at www.who.int/pbd/deafness/activities/hearing_care/en/.

The *Guidelines* recognize various levels of providing services according to the resources of the country. Services at the *primary level* are to be provided by *primary health workers* who may be community volunteers, or nurse practitioners/clinical assistants, or primary health care workers with special

training and skills. Services at the *secondary level* are provided by *audiology/audiometric technicians*, who are required to have at least secondary school education and some previous experience in working with persons with hearing impairment. It is recommended that persons identified (to have a hearing loss) at the secondary level be tested at the tertiary level. *Audiologists* provide services at the *tertiary level*. Besides conducting assessments and fitting hearing aids for all ages, audiologists manage, monitor, and evaluate programs and train personnel at lower levels. *Physicians* and *specialists/otolaryngologists* in hospitals also serve at the tertiary level. Some specialists have training in audiology also. *Earmold technicians and hearing aid repair technicians* also work at the tertiary level.

The guidelines specify that a hearing test should precede fitting a hearing aid, and both should be done by a person with the appropriate training, who should maintain appropriate records of rendered services. Hearing aid users, family members (if appropriate), and teachers should be provided easily understood instructions regarding the hearing aid, its care and maintenance, its use, and troubleshooting in case of minor problems. All instructions must be given by a secondary level person in a format that is easily understood, using a combination of verbal instructions in the local language, brochures, information sheets, pictorial instructions, and demonstrations. Hearing aid users may require repeated instructions. Follow-up should be provided by primary or secondary level personnel, preferably in the person's own community. Replacement batteries and ear molds, as well as maintenance and repair of hearing aids, should be affordable and easily accessible (WHO, 2004).

Available services should include raising awareness, identification and assessment, hearing aid fitting, support for users of hearing aids, and training. To raise awareness of problems caused by hearing loss, information regarding its detection and prevention should be disseminated among specific groups in society, including persons with hearing loss, parents, teachers, community and national leaders, health care, educational, and other service providers, policy makers, and administrators. Programs designed to raise awareness should plan activities at three levels: national level, provincial or district level, and local community level (WHO, 2004).

In the Southeast Asia region, less than 10% of persons who need hearing aids actually receive them. There is a tremendous shortage of distributors and manufacturers in Nepal and Sri Lanka. The 2001 data on patients fitted with hearing aids in Bangladesh indicated that 223 hearing aids were fitted on children younger than 5 years, 1438 units were fitted on persons ranging from 5 to 60 years, and 48 units were fitted on persons older than 60 years. In fact, data from the region showed that, with the exception of India, where 50% of the hearing aids were fitted on children younger than 5 years, the majority of hearing aids were fitted on adults. This indicates that a large number of children who should be fitted with hearing aids are not provided amplification. Another concern is the price of hearing aids. Although the prices have gone down over the years (e.g., $25 to $85 for a body aid, $58 to $1300 for a behind-the-ear hearing aid in Sri Lanka), hearing aids are still far beyond the means of the needy population of this region. Additionally, significant costs are involved in the maintenance of hearing aids and replacement of batteries, and these are frequently not available (WHO, 2007).

Organizations such as Worldwide Hearing, Impact, and Godisa are looking at creative ways to make hearing aids and hearing care more affordable and available. For instance, batteries are very expensive in developing countries and are often not easily available. Godisa, a nonprofit enterprise in Botswana, facilitates affordable access of batteries to persons with hearing impairment by providing Solar Aid battery chargers. In some countries, the private health care sector has started to collaborate with the public sector and assumes a greater role. There is considerable overlap in the area of work of agencies, such as WHO, UNICEF, UNESCO, and UNESCAP, which could be coordinated to work toward a common cause. Capacity building at the level of human resources, infrastructure, and financial resources must occur. Enhancing the capacity of existing infrastructure, establishing new infrastructure, and ensuring optimal performance as well as good clinical practice and management will serve to build capacity. An important initiative, *Worldwide Hearing (WW Hearing),* is geared toward making hearing aids available to all those who need them. It is looking at the possibility of bulk purchase of hearing aids and other equipment for a Purchasing Consortium. Purchasing large quantities of basic hearing aids would help to substantially lower the cost of individual units. The drawback of bulk purchasing, although not insurmountable, is that the purchaser typically must ensure that each unit is working satisfactorily and return faulty units to the manufacturer within a specified number of days. Hearing aids can be purchased in bulk by countries, districts, or regions. Another initiative, a regional forum, provides a mechanism for cooperation among the countries of the Southeast Asia region toward preventing deafness and providing ear and hearing care. The regional forum, which includes representatives from selected governments, professional organizations, nongovernmental organizations, Hearing International, and WHO, is doing collaborative work in the region. Communication, cooperation, and collaboration among national governments, professionals, communities, bilateral and multilateral agencies, and the private sector are critical if ear and hearing care disparities are to be eliminated (WHO, 2007).

AUDITORY REHABILITATION

To be effective, auditory rehabilitation services must be responsive to the different needs of the individuals being served. Personal and family context should be a fundamental part of any evaluation or treatment. Besides assessments and fitting hearing aids, the clinician must consider the use of assistive listening devices, management of the acoustical environment, and provision of individual or group rehabilitation, including counseling (Gatehouse, 2003).

Laplante-Lévesque and colleagues (2010) used shared decision making in auditory rehabilitation. They discussed four options (hearing aids, group communication program, individual communication program, no intervention) with adults who had acquired hearing impairments and identified seven categories of factors that influenced their rehabilitation decisions: convenience, expected adherence and outcomes, financial costs, hearing disability, nature of intervention, other people's experiences, recommendations and support, and preventive and interim solution.

Although hearing aids are not the only intervention available, and it is known that auditory rehabilitation can reduce the deleterious consequences of hearing impairment, very few audiologists integrate auditory rehabilitation in their hearing aid fitting protocol. Gatehouse (2003) advocated for the use of a holistic approach that was responsive to individual needs. Structured enquiry is critical to ascertain the problems that are experienced, the environments in which they occur, and their effect on daily life. To be effective, intervention must be selected on the basis of the disability that is experienced, individual expectations, attitudes and motivation, family needs and expectations, comorbidity, and individual priorities. In addition to amplification and assistive devices, based upon individual needs, intervention should include counseling, and activities to enhance speech perception and communication. The ultimate goal of intervention should be improvement of individual quality of life.

Many developing countries have no aural habilitation or rehabilitation programs. At the most, they may have schools for children with hearing impairment in which sign language is the predominant mode of communication. Such schools are frequently overcrowded, poorly maintained, and dependent on charitable donations. The prevalent culture is one of noninclusion, which isolates the person from society, often rendering the person incapable of earning a decent means of livelihood (Olusanya, 2006).

Sign Language

ASL was derived from French Sign Language. It is used by the Deaf in the United States as well as by Deaf persons in English-speaking parts of Canada and some regions of Mexico. Also, ASL is used together with indigenous sign languages in countries such as the Philippines, Malaysia, and Singapore. Many countries have developed their own sign languages (e.g., United Kingdom, Israel, Australia, Russia), and many Spanish-speaking countries have their own version of Spanish Sign Language (e.g., Mexican Sign Language, Columbian Sign Language). To facilitate communication at international meetings, a committee of the World Federation of the Deaf selected signs that were most understandable in different sign languages and developed the International Sign Language (ISL), or Gestuno, which in Italian means "the unity of sign language." Fifteen hundred ISL signs were published in a book. ISL does not have a concrete grammar; persons communicating in it use features common to most sign languages in addition to ISL signs. For more information on ISL and sign languages used in other countries, the reader should visit www.library.gallaudet.edu/Library/Deaf_Research_Help/Research_Guides_ (Pathfinders).

Although the World Wide Web provides access to information to millions of people, it can be difficult for some sign language users because of the heavy use of text and static images. Fels and colleagues (2006) described a system that allows sign language–only Web pages to be created and linked through a video-based technique called *sign linking*. Use of this technique allows users to easily navigate sign language information.

Cochlear Implants

Cochlear implants are neural prostheses that have revolutionized the treatment of persons with deafness and severe hearing loss. Cochlear implants improve most recipients' ability to communicate and are considered safe and effective for appropriately selected adults and children with severe to profound sensorineural hearing loss. These biomedical electronic devices convert sound into electrical current that stimulates the auditory nerve, resulting in the sensation of sound. In 1985, the U.S. Food and Drug Administration (FDA) approved the first cochlear implant for use in postlinguistically deafened (hearing loss > 100 dB HL) adults aged 18 years and older, who did not benefit from the use of amplification. By 2000, the FDA approval had extended the implantable age to 12 months, and broadened the general hearing criteria. During the subsequent years, advances in technology allowed implants to stimulate different portions of the auditory nerve based on sound frequencies in the incoming signal. At this time in many developed countries, the issues are whether to implant the child or adult with unilateral or bilateral implants and whether to implant the two ears simultaneously or sequentially.

According to the FDA, as of April 2009, 188,000 people worldwide had cochlear implants, including persons in China, Malaysia, India, Egypt, Saudi Arabia, and South America. In the United States, approximately 41,500 adults and 25,500 children have been implanted. Gallaudet Research Institute's Annual Survey of Deaf and Hard of Hearing Children and Youth has several questions pertaining to cochlear implants. Data from 2003 through 2008 surveys are reported in Table 11-4. In the 2007-2008 survey, a new question was added to ascertain the number of children and youth with binaural implants; 15.4% of respondents indicated that they had bilateral implants. In 2003 to 2004 and 2004 to 2005, geographically, the largest numbers of students with unilateral or bilateral implants were located in the South; however from 2005 through 2008, the largest number of students with cochlear implants were in the northeast. The smallest number of students with

TABLE 11-4 Number and Percentage of Children and Youth with Unilateral or Bilateral Cochlear Implantation Who Use or Do Not Use Their Cochlear Implants

	2003-2004	2004-2005	2005-2006	2006-2007	2007-2008
Have not had a cochlear implant (CI)	33,578 (90.4%)	32,021 (88.8%)	33,698 (87.9%)	31,895 (87.1%)	31,239 (86.3%)
Have had a CI	3575 (9.6%)	4051 (11.2%)	4642 (12.1%)	4609 (12.6%)	4969 (13.7%)
Implant still used	3118 (91.3%)	3544 (91.8%)	4088 (92.1%)	4092 (92.5%)	4303 (92.4%)
Implant no longer used	297 (8.7%)	316 (8.2%)	352 (7.9%)	333 (7.5%)	355 (7.6%)
Implant used in classroom	2194 (89.7%)	3,001 (90.2%)	3834 (91.9%)	3971 (92.2%)	4260 (92.2%)
Implant not used in classroom	251 (10.3%)	325 (9.8%)	340 (8.1%)	334 (7.8%)	362 (7.8%)
Have had 2nd implant	No data	No data	No data	No data	406 (15.4%)
Have not had 2nd implant	No data	No data	No data	No data	2231 (84.6%)

From Gallaudet Research Institute (January 2005, December 2005, December 2006, December 2007, November 2008). Regional and National Summary Report of Data from the 2003-04, 2004-05, 2005-06, 2006-07, 2007-08 Annual Survey of Deaf and Hard of Hearing Children and Youth. Washington, DC: GRI, Gallaudet University.

cochlear implants for each year of the survey (2003 through 2008) were in the West.

Twenty-five years after the initial FDA approval, disparities continue to exist in the rate of implantation in multicultural groups. The Gallaudet Research Institute (1998) reported that less than 16% of all deaf minorities combined had implants. Among the minorities, the American Indians seemed to be the least likely to obtain cochlear implants. Stern and colleagues (2005) examined the epidemiology of 124 children who underwent cochlear implantation in 1997 and observed a disparity among children of different ethnic groups and socioeconomic status. White and Asian children were implanted at higher rates than Hispanic and black children. Further, they observed that implanted children came from homes with higher median incomes. Fortnum and associates (2002) reported epidemiologic data for 17,160 children in the United Kingdom with permanent bilateral hearing loss greater than 40 dB HL. They reported that more children who were profoundly impaired and who came from affluent families had implants than did children from less affluent families.

Insufficient funds may not be the only factor restricting patient access to cochlear implants. Weinick and coworkers (2000) analyzed data from the Household Component of the 1996 Medical Expenditure Panel Survey collected in the United States to ascertain the differences, if any, in access to and use of health care services. They observed that Hispanic children (17.2%) were 3 times as likely and African American children (12.5%) were twice as likely as white children (6%) to lack a usual source of health care. Adjusting for health insurance and other socioeconomic measures had no effect on these outcomes. However, when language of interview was added to the variables, they observed a difference; children whose interview was conducted in English were 2.6 times more likely to have a usual source of care than children whose interview was conducted in Spanish. After further analysis the data indicated that Hispanic children whose interview was conducted in Spanish were only 27% as likely as white children to have a usual source of care. The researchers interpreted the results to suggest that the marked Hispanic disadvantage in children's access to health care may be related to language ability (i.e., the family members' ability to communicate in English) and suggested that there was a need for interpreters and bilingual health care providers.

Developed countries vary in their policies regarding financial support for cochlear implants. In countries such as Norway, the process of implantation involves no cost to parents (Simonsen et al., 2009), whereas in other developed countries, expenses are paid by the family, private insurance, a governmental agency, or a nongovernmental organization. In developing countries, the issue is whether to use meager resources to fit more persons with hearing aids, thereby impacting more lives, or to spend funds on cochlear implantation and positively affect one person.

Teleaudiology

Teleaudiology is a term that was coined from the term *telemedicine*, which is " . . . the use of telecommunications technology for medical diagnostic, monitoring, and therapeutic purposes when distances separate the users." Telemedicine used to deal exclusively with medical applications by physicians using advanced technology; however, since the passage of the 1997 Comprehensive Telehealth Act, the term *telehealth* has been used to refer to services delivered by nonphysicians as well as physicians. *Telepractice* is the application of telecommunications technology to deliver professional services at a distance by linking clinician to client or vice versa for assessment, intervention, or consultation (ASHA, 2005a, 2005b). The impact of teleaudiology could be tremendous during the next decade; with the help of telecommunications technology, many underserved areas, both in the United States and around the globe, could receive quality hearing care promptly without traveling long distances or waiting for weeks, months, or longer. Besides the provision of clinical services (hearing screening, assessment, fitting hearing aids, mapping cochlear implants, treatment and management, counseling), teleaudiology has the potential for use in educating and training health care professionals, paraprofessionals, parents, and the community at large, especially in areas around the world where there is a paucity of trained service providers. Teleaudiology offers the potential to provide services to underserved populations as well as to culturally and linguistically diverse populations.

The Agency for Healthcare Research and Quality (2001) has described three basic models of telepractice:

1. Store-and-forward (asynchronous), in which clinical data collected at a remote site are electronically transmitted (e.g., via Internet) to a main location (e.g., transmission of audiologic data, ABRs, OAEs)

2. Clinician interactive (synchronous), which is conducted in real time for diagnosis or treatment through interactive audio or video. Remote control computing is another form of synchronous telepractice in which remote control software allows the audiologist to control computers and peripherals at a remote site.

3. Self-monitoring and testing, in which the patient provides data to the provider without an on-site facilitator. Data are collected in the patient's home, residential care facility, and so forth.

During the past couple of decades, applications of telehealth in the areas of communicative disorders have been sporadically described. Vaughn (1976) developed "tel-communicology"; a full range of services were provided using a telephone and previously mailed educational materials. Kully (2000) provided therapy to persons with fluency disorder. Ricker and colleagues (2002) surveyed patients with traumatic brain injury regarding their rehabilitation needs, and Krumm and associates (2002) used it for diagnostic audiology, hearing aid fitting, and counseling. The American Speech-Language-Hearing Association (ASHA, 2002) conducted a survey to ascertain the use of telepractice among its membership and found that 11% of its members were using it.

The Interdisciplinary Technical Assistance Center (n.d.) reported on several telepractice projects: (1) the Marion Downs Center has used telehealth/tele-education since 2007 and in 2009 initiated the Co-LEND project; (2) Children's Medical Services started a pilot teleaudiology project in Gallup, New Mexico, to reduce delays in the provision of evaluations to the pediatric population; (3) Wisconsin Sound Beginnings has partnered with the Marshfield Clinic to provide hearing-related care for home-birth populations and underserved remote areas; and, (4) North Carolina's Teleaudiology Project is directed toward making diagnostic services available within 2 hours of place of residence and increasing the percentage of babies completing diagnostic evaluations by 3 months of age. Some other projects that have been reported include one in North Dakota, to improve follow-up of infants identified through their EHDI program (Rural Assistance Center, 2010), and East Carolina University's telehealth program, which has developed a system to conduct real-time pure tone audiometry at a distant site using a palmtop or desktop computer, the Internet, and a commercially available audiometer (Givens & Elangovan, 2003).

Polovoy and Crowley (2009) reported on international collaboration and the use of telepractice to administer aural rehabilitation services to 10 children with hearing loss in La Paz, Bolivia. Polovoy (2008) reported on three teleservice programs:

1. The use of real-time telepractice in Ontario, Canada, to perform diagnostic ABRs in remote communities on infants who do not pass their hearing screening. The Infant Hearing Program does this through the Ontario Telemedicine Network that connects remote communities in Ontario with medical services.

2. Children's Hospital in St. Petersburg, Florida, maintains 12 outreach centers and offers remote cochlear implant mapping to children in Florida. Many of these children reportedly come from disadvantaged and nontraditional families; by bringing cochlear implant services closer to the family's home through telepractice, the probability of successful intervention is increased.

3. Secure store-and-forward telepractice in Alaska has greatly reduced the amount of time a patient must wait to see an otolaryngologist and has reduced patient travel costs significantly. In the telepractice model, the audiologists fly to the villages several times a year and use high-definition video otoscopes to take pertinent images of the auditory system. The images, OAE, tympanometry data, and patient's history are transmitted electronically to the ENT specialists in Anchorage so that treatments are prescribed promptly. Reportedly, telepractice

has been very effective "in facilitating medical clearance for hearing aids, assessing the need for surgery, surgical follow-up, and assessing the urgency of conditions." Further, it was reported that of the 2000 audiology patients seen annually, one third were being seen through telepractice.

Recently (April 4, 2010), TeleAudiology Network (www.teleaudiology.org), a nonprofit, nongovernmental organization, whose mission is to improve hearing health of persons throughout the globe with the help of telemedicine technology, successfully conducted its "first transatlantic real-time hearing test"; a patient in South Africa was administered an audiological test by an audiologist in Dallas, Texas, with the help of an "innovative audiometer, specially designed with telemedicine capabilities." The goal of the TeleAudiology Network is to link hearing professionals and villages in need of services. Thus, through the online platform, the network will link clinics in villages without hearing services to audiologists who are willing to volunteer their services. The Network also links villages to sponsors who want to donate funds to finance telemedicine audiometers. In developed countries where audiology is well established, teleaudiology may be used to reach isolated and remote communities, such as in Alaska, Appalachia, and Canada (Swanepoel et al., 2010.)

International Education in Audiology

Throughout the world, there has been a drop in mortality rates and an increase in life expectancy, which has resulted in increased attention on the impact of disabilities on the quality of life. With the increasing incidence of hearing loss and deafness, there has been a much greater demand for professionals educated to provide hearing health care. According to the WHO (2006), there was one audiologist per 0.5 to 6.25 million people in developing countries, whereas in developed countries, there was one audiologist per 20,000 persons. In developing countries, deafness and hearing impairment may not be viewed as a significant problem and preventive and rehabilitative options are not always given priority because of the paucity of financial and technical resources. Additionally, many audiologists educated in developing countries find better employment opportunities and immigrate to developed countries. Therefore, there is a tremendous need for hearing health care providers in developing countries, but in developed countries, there has also been a growing demand for more audiologists.

Goulios and Patuzzi (2008a, 2008b) conducted a survey to ascertain the state of audiology in the world. Of the 123 countries (representing 92% of the total world population) to whom their questionnaire was distributed, 62 countries (representing 78% of the total world population) responded. Of the respondents, 86% indicated that they had insufficient number of audiologists. Only Argentina, Belgium, Denmark,

Germany, Italy, The Netherlands, and Poland indicated that they had a sufficient number of audiologists. Sixty-eight percent of respondent countries reported having established audiology education programs; however, there was significant diversity in minimal entry-level requirements and preparation. Although countries like Denmark have a 2-year technical college diploma program, countries such as South Africa and the United Kingdom have 4-year baccalaureate programs. Other countries, such as Australia, Canada, and New Zealand, have 2-year postgraduate master's degree programs, whereas the United States has 4-year postgraduate doctoral degree programs. Furthermore, in many European and South American countries, a medical degree followed by postgraduate training in audiology is required. The number of supervised clinical practicum hours required in different countries varies from none to more than 1000 hours. Despite these differences in educational requirements, there are significant similarities in the scope of practice. Additionally, although audiologists are the primary professionals conducting basic audiological assessments in 62% of the respondent countries, there is considerable variability among countries for the provision of services for other disorders, such as auditory processing disorders, tinnitus, vestibular disorders, and so forth; audiologists, ENT specialists, neurologists, and other professionals are providing these services.

It is evident that there is a tremendous need for audiologists around the world. To contain this need, a multifaceted approach is indicated.

- There must be increased attention paid to the prevention of hearing loss by increasing public awareness of the impact of hearing loss and deafness on communication and the quality of life, and to making the public more aware of the profession of audiology.
- There must be increased use of technology, at least in developed countries, to provide distance education and clinical supervision, to provide clinical services to areas that are underserved at home and abroad, and to educate the public regarding prevention of hearing loss.
- Arrangements could be made between audiology programs in different countries to allow the exchange of students and faculty for mutually acceptable periods of time.
- Corporations, nongovernmental organizations, and civic groups must be encouraged to provide grants and seed funds for educational programs toward building capacity, and to clinical agencies for technology to expand services to unserved communities.
- To assist in the provision of education and services, national and international professional groups and governmental and nongovernmental organizations should facilitate the adoption of developing countries and underserved and unserved communities by educational programs in audiology and speech-language pathology as well as by service providers (hospitals, centers, individuals).

- Further, educational programs should facilitate and encourage graduating students to provide a few weeks or months of clinical service in unserved or underserved communities in their own or a developing country.

DISCUSSION QUESTIONS

1. You are responsible for developing an educational program on hearing loss for persons who live below the poverty line in your community or state. (a) What steps will you take to select communities that you intend to target, and to set up education sessions? (b) List materials that you will develop for your oral presentation to a group and materials that you will distribute to participants during your presentations. (c) Describe in detail the contents of the materials that you will develop for both the presentation and distribution. (d) What steps will you take to ensure that you meet the needs of persons from different cultures?

2. A 62-year-old African American woman has a severe to profound sensorineural hearing loss. She has been fitted with binaural behind-the-ear hearing aids. Her aided speech discrimination scores are 78% in the left ear and 68% in the right ear. Her own speech is well articulated, but she tends to talk rather loudly. She lives at home with her retired husband who is a couple of years older than her but reportedly "hears well." She has two married children and four grandchildren who live in the same city. She has a friendly disposition but has difficulty communicating at the community's general hospital where she provides volunteer service, where she must communicate for the major part of the day with patients, their families, and hospital personnel. List the elements of an appropriate aural rehab program for her and describe in detail the steps you plan to take to alleviate her activity limitations and participation restrictions.

3. Discuss the relationship between CMV and hearing impairment. (a) Why did the JCIH (2007) recommend frequent testing of children with congenital CMV? (b) How is CMV acquired in adults and in infants (i.e., what is the mode of transmission)? (c) What is the impact of reactivation compared with initial infection on mother and baby? (d) How can CMV be prevented? (e) What damage does CMV cause in the auditory system? (f) What is the rate of CMV infection nationally, in your state, and in your community? (g) Does CMV differentially affect persons of different ethnic groups? If yes, how and why?

4. Prepare a proposal to develop and implement a hearing care program in a developing country. Describe in detail the resources that you will use and the steps that you will take to establish relationships and to develop and implement the program.

REFERENCES

Abdel-Hamid, O., Khatib, O., Aly, A., et al. (2007). Prevalence and patterns of hearing impairment in Egypt: A national Household survey. *Health Journal, 13* (*5*). Available at: www.emro.who.int/Publications/ EMHJ/1305/article21.htm.

Agency for Healthcare Research and Quality. (2001). *Telemedicine for the Medicare population.* Rockville, MD: Author.

Agrawal, Y., Platz, E., & Niparko, J. (2008). Prevalence of hearing loss and differences by demographic characteristics among US adults: Data from the National Health and Nutrition Examination Survey, 1999-2004. *Arch Intern Med, 168* (*14*), 1522-1530.

Ahlfors, K., Ivarsson, S. A., & Harris, S. (1999). Report on a long-term study of material and congenital cytomegalovirus infection in Sweden. Review of prospective studies available in the literature. *Scandinavian Journal of Infectious Diseases,* 31 (*5*), 443-457.

Alabi, S., Ernest, K., Eletta, P., et al. (2008). Otological findings among Nigerian children with sickle cell anemia. *Int J Pediatr Otorhinolaryngol, 72* (*5*), 659-663.

Al-Dabbous, I., Al Jam'a, A., Obeja, S., et al. (1996). Sensorineural hearing loss in homozygous sickle cell disease in Qatif, Saudi Arabia [Abstract]. *Ann Saudi Med,* 16 (*6*), 641-644.

Al Khabori, M., & Khandekar, R. (2004). The prevalence and causes of hearing impairment in Oman: A community-based cross-sectional study. *International Journal of Audiology, 43,* 486-492.

Al Khabori, M., & Patton, M. (2008). Consanguinity and deafness in Omani children. *International Journal of Audiology, 47,* 30-33.

Al-Shihabi, B. A. (1994). Childhood sensorineural hearing loss in consanguineous marriages. *Journal of Audiological Medicine 3,* 151-159.

American Speech-Language-Hearing Association (2002). Survey report on telepractice use among audiologists and speech-language pathologists. Available at: www.asha.org.

American Speech-Language-Hearing Association (2005a). Audiologists providing clinical services via telepractice [Position Statement]. Available at: www.asha.org/policy.

American Speech-Language-Hearing Association (2005b). Audiologists providing clinical services via telepractice [Technical Report]. Available at: www.asha.org/policy.

Attias, J., Al-Masri, M., AbuKader, L, et al. (2006). The prevalence of congenital and early-onset hearing loss in Jordanian and Israeli infants. *International Journal of Audiology, 45,* 528-536.

Australian Hearing. (n.d.) Hearing loss in Australia. Retrieved from: www .hearing.com.au/upload/media-room/Hearing-loss-in-Australia.pdf.

Balasubramaniam, V., Sinniah, M., Tan, D. S., et al. (1994). The role of cytomegalovirus (CMV) infection in congenital disease in Malaysia. *Medical Journal of Malaysia, 49* (*2*), 113-116.

Balgir, R. (2007). Epidemiology of sickle cell disease. *Internet Journal of Biological Anthropology, 1*(*2*). Available at: www.ispub.com/ostia/ index.php?xmlFilePath=journals/ijba/vol1n2/sickle.xml.

Bankaitis, A., & Schountz, T. (1998). HIV-related ototoxicity. *Seminars in Hearing, 19,* 155-163.

Barbi, M., Binda, S., Caroppo, S., et al. (2003). A wider role for congenital cytomegalovirus infection in sensorineural hearing loss. *Pediatr Infect Dis J, 22*(*1*), 39-42.

Barfield, W., Manning, S., Kroelinger, C., Martin, J., & Barradas, D. (2010). Neonatal intensive-care unit admission of infants with very low birth weight–19 States, 2006. *MMWR Morbidity and Mortality Weekly Report, 59*(*44*), 1444-1447.

Barnes, P., Adams, P., & Powell-Griner, E. (2008, January 22). Health characteristics of the Asian adult population: United States, 2004-2006.

Advance Data for Vital and Health Statistics, No. 394. Hyattsville, MD: National Center for Health Statistics.

Bat-Chava, Y., Martin, D., & Kosciw, J. (2005). Barriers to HIV/AIDS knowledge and prevention among deaf and hard of hearing people. *AIDS Care, 17*(*5*), 623-634.

Batissoco, A., Abreu-Silva, R., Braga, M., et al. (2009). Prevalence of GJB2 (connexin-26) and GJB6 (connexin-30) mutations in a cohort of 300 Brazilian hearing-impaired individuals: Implications for diagnosis and genetic counseling. *Ear and Hearing, 30*(*1*), 1-7.

Bevilacqua, M., Alvarenga, K., Costa, O., & Moret, A. (2010). Universal newborn screening in Brazil. *International Journal of Pediatric Otorhinolaryngology, 74*(*5*), 510-515.

Bisol, C., Sperb, T., Brewer, T., et al. (2008). HIV/AIDS knowledge and health-related attitudes and behaviors among deaf and hearing adolescents in Southern Brazil. *American Annals of the Deaf, 153*(*4*), 349-356.

Boswell, S. (2003, September 23). Cochlear implant recipients have increased risk of meningitis. *ASHA Leader.*

Brennan, S., Gombac, I., & Sleightholm, M. (2006). *Participation and Activity Limitation Survey, 2006.* Available at: www.statcan.gc.ca/ pub/89-628-x/89-628-x2007002-eng.pdf.

Bubbico, L., Tognola, G., Greco, A., & Grandori, F. (2008). Universal newborn hearing screening programs in Italy: Survey of year 2006. *Acta Otolaryngol, 128*(*12*),1329-1336.

Cama, E., Melchionda, S., Palladino, T., et al. (2009). Hearing loss features in GJB2 biallelic mutations and GJB2/GJB6 digenic inheritance in a large Italian cohort. *International Journal of Audiology, 48,* 12-17.

Centers for Disease Control and Prevention (1999). *Cytomegalovirus (CMV) infection.* Atlanta: Author.

Centers for Disease Control and Prevention (2000). *Meningococcal disease.* Atlanta: Author.

Centers for Disease Control and Prevention (2004, January 30). Economic costs associated with mental retardation, cerebral palsy, hearing loss, and vision impairments, United States, 2003. *MMWR Morbidity and Mortality Weekly Report, 53*(*03*), 57-59.

Centers for Disease Control and Prevention (2009a). *Sickle cell disease: Facts.* Atlanta: Author.

Centers for Disease Controle and Prevention (2009b). *Factsheet: Meningococcal diseases and meningococcal vaccines.* Atlanta: Author.

Centers for Disease Control and Prevention (2009c). *Meningitis in other countries.* Atlanta: Author.

Centers for Disease Control and Prevention (2009d). *Factsheet: Meningococcal diseases and meningococcal vaccines.* Atlanta: Author.

Centers for Disease Control and Prevention (2009e). *Meningitis in other countries.* Atlanta: Author.

Centers for Disease Control and Prevention (2010a). *Congenital CMV trends and statistics.* Atlanta: Author. Available at: www.cdc.gov/cmv/ trends-stats.html.

Centers for Disease Control and Prevention (2010b). *Sickle cell disease–Data and statistics.* Atlanta: Author.

Centers for Disease Control and Prevention (2010c). *World sickle cell day: 100 Years of research.* Available at: www.cdc.gov/Features/ SickleCell/.

Centers for Disease Control and Prevention (2010d, March 5). Identifying infants with hearing loss – United States, 1999-2007. *MMWR Morb Mortal Weekly Reports, 59*(*8*), 220-223.

Centers for Disease Control and Prevention (2011a). *Hearing loss in children.* Available at: www.cdc.gov/ncbddd/hearingloss/data.html.

Centers for Disease control and Prevention (2011b). *National diabetic fact sheet.* Available at: www.cdc.gov/diabetes/pubs/estimates11.htm#4.

Chambers, J., Shkolnik, J., & Perez, M. (2003). Total expenditures for students with disabilities, 1999-2000: Spending variation by disability. Report. Special Education Project (SEEP). Available at: www.eric.ed.gov/ERICWebPortal/search/detailmini.jsp?_nfpb=true&_&ERICExtSearch_SearchV.

Chandrasehkar, S., Connelly, P., Brahmbhatt, S., et al. (2000). Otologic and audiologic evaluation of human immunodeficiency virus-infected patients. *American Journal of Otolaryngology, 21*(1), 1-9.

Chen, D., Chen, X., Cao, K., et al. (2009). High prevalence of the connexin 26 (GJB2) mutation in Chinese cochlear implant recipients. *Journal of Otorhinolaryngology, 71*(4), 212-215.

Cheng, Y., Gregg, E., Saaddine, J., et al. (2009). Three decade change in the prevalence of hearing impairment and its association with diabetes in the United States. *Preventive Medicine, 49*(5), 360-364.

Coenraad, S., Goedegebure, A., van Goudoever, J., & Hoeve, L. (2010). Risk factors for sensorineural hearing loss in NICU infants compared to normal hearing NICU controls. *International Journal of Pediatrics and Otorhinolaryngology, 74*(9), 999-1002.

Colugnati, F., Staras, S., Dollard, S., & Cannon, M. (2007). Incidence of cytomegalovirus infection among the general population and pregnant women in the United States. *BMC Infectious Diseases, 7*, 71. Doi: 10.1186/14712334771.

Dammeyer, J. (2010). Prevalence and aetiology of congenitally deafblind people in Denmark. *International Journal of Audiology, 49*, 76-82.

Davis, A., & Parving, A. (1994). Towards appropriate epidemiology data on childhood hearing disability: A comparative European study of birth-cohorts 1982-1988. *Journal of Audiological Medicine, 3*, 35-47.

De Castro, S., Magalhães, I., Toscano, R., Gandolfi, L., & Pratesi, R. (2010). Auditory-evoked response analysis in Brazilian patients with sickle cell disease. *International Journal of Audiology, 49*(4), 272-276.

Demeester, K., van Wieringen, A., Hendrickx, J., et al. (2009). Audiometric shape and presbycusis. *International Journal of Audiology, 48*, 222-232.

Demeester, K., van Wieringen, A., Hendrickx, J., et al. (2010). Heritability of audiometric shape parameters and familial aggregation of presbycusis in an elderly Flemish population. *Hearing Research, 265*(1-2), 1-10.

De Paschale, M., Agrappi, C., Manco, M., et al. (2009). Incidence and risk of cytomegalovirus infection during pregnancy in an urban area of northern Italy. *Infectious Diseases in Obstetrics and Gynecology,* Doi: 10.1155/2009/206505.

De Sousa, C., de Castro, Jr., N., Larsson, E., & Ching, T. (2009). Risk factors for presbycusis in a socio-economic middle-class sample. *Brazilian Journal of Otorhinolaryngology, 75*(4), 530-536.

Dillon, C., Gu, Q., Hoffman, H., & Ko, C. (2010). *Vision, hearing, balance, and sensory impairment in Americans aged 70 years and over: United States, 1999-2006* . NCHS data brief, no 31. Hyattsville, MD: National Center for Health Statistics.

Downs, C., Stuart, A., & Holbert, D. (2000). Distortion product otoacoustic emissions in normal-hearing children with homozygous sickle cell disease. *Journal of Communication Disorders, 33*(2) 111-127.

Durieux-Smith, A., Fitzpatrick, E., & Whittingham, J. (2008). Universal newborn hearing screening: A question of evidence. *International Journal of Audiology, 47*, 1-10.

Edmond, K., Clark, A., Korczak, V., et al. (2010a). Global and regional risk of disabling sequelae from bacterial meningitis: A systematic review and meta-analysis. *Lancet Infect Dis, 10*(5), 317-328.

Edmond, K., Dieye, Y., Griffiths, U., et al. (2010b). Prospective cohort study of disabling sequelae and quality of life in children with bacterial meningitis in urban Senegal. *Pediatric Infectious Disease Journal, 29*(11), 1023-1029.

Elola, A., Hien, F., Ouattara, M., et al. (2009). Major sickle cell anemia and hypoacusia: About 112 cases in Yopougon, Côte d'Ivoire [Abstract]. *Bulletin de la Societe de Pathologie Exototique, 102*(3), 173-174.

Engdahl, B., & Eskid, A. (2007). Birthweight and the risk of childhood sensorineural hearing loss. *Paediatric and Perinatal Epidemiology, 21*(6), 495-500.

Estivill, X., Fortina, P., & Surrey, S. (1999). Connexin-26 mutations in sporadic and inherited sensorineural hearing deafness. *Lancet, 387,* 394-398.

Fels, D., Richards, J., Hardman, J., & Lee, D. (2006). Sign language web pages. *American Annals of the Deaf, 151*(4), 423-433.

Fortnum, H., Marshall, D., & Summerfield, A. (2002). Epidemiology of the UK population of hearing–impaired children, including characteristics of those with and without cochlear implants – audiology, aetiology, comorbidity and affluence. *International Journal of Audiology, 41*(3), 170-179.

Fowler, K., & Boppana, S. (2006). Congenital cytomegalovirus (CMV) infection and hearing deficit. *J Clin Virol, 35*(2), 226-231.

Fu, C., Chen, G., Dong, J., & Zhang, L. (2010). Prevalence and etiology of hearing loss in primary and middle school students in the Hubai province of China. *Audiology & Neurotology, 15*(6), 394-398.

Gallaudet Research Institue (1998). Who and where are our children with cochlear implant? Available at: http://gri.gallaudet.edu/Cochlear/ASHA.1997/.

Gallaudet Research Institute (January 2005). *Regional and National Summary Report of Data from the 2003-2004 Annual Survey of Deaf and Hard of Hearing Children and Youth.* Washington, DC: GRI, Gallaudet University.

Gallaudet Research Institute (December 2005). *Regional and National Summary Report of Data from the 2004-2005 Annual Survey of Deaf and Hard of Hearing Children and Youth.* Washington, DC: GRI, Gallaudet University.

Gallaudet Research Institute (December 2006). *Regional and National Summary Report of Data from the 2005-2006 Annual Survey of Deaf and Hard of Hearing Children and Youth.* Washington, DC: GRI, Gallaudet University.

Gallaudet Research Institute (December 2007). *Regional and National Summary Report of Data from the 2006-2007 Annual Survey of Deaf and Hard of Hearing Children and Youth.* Washington, DC: GRI, Gallaudet University.

Gallaudet Research Institute (November 2008). *Regional and National Summary Report of Data from the 2007-2008 Annual Survey of Deaf and Hard of Hearing Children and Youth.* Washington, DC: GRI, Gallaudet University.

Garcia, C., Sebastián, G., Morant, V., & Marco, A. (2002). Presentation of 2 cases of sudden deafness in patients with sickle-cell anemia and trait. *Acta Otolaryngologica, 53*(5), 371-376.

Gaskins, S. (1999). Special population: HIV/AIDS among the Deaf and hard of hearing. *Journal of the Association of Nurses in AIDS Care, 10,* 75.

Gatehouse, S. (2003). Rehabilitation: Identification of needs, priorities and expectations, and the evaluation of benefit. *International Journal of Audiology, 42,* 2S77-2S83.

Gentry, B., Davis, P., & Dancer, J. (1997). Failure rates of young patients with sickle cell disease on a hearing screening test. *Perceptual and Motor Skills, 84*(2), 434.

Givens, G., & Elangovan, S. (2003). Internet application to tele-audiology: "Nothin' but Net." *American Journal of Audiology, 12,* 59-65.

Gopinath, B., Flood, V., Rochtchina, E., McMahon, C., & Mitchell, P. (2010). Consumption of omega-3 fatty acids and fish and risk of age-related hearing loss. *American Journal of Clinical Nutrition, 92*(2), 416-421.

Goulios, H., & Patuzzi, R. (2008a). Audiology education and practice from an international perspective. *International Journal of Audiology, 47,* 647-664.

Goulios, H., & Patuzzi, R. (2008b). Education and practice of audiology internationally: Affordable and sustainable education models for developing countries. In B. McPherson and R. Brouillette (Eds.), *Audiology in Developing Countries* (pp. 51-67). New York: Nova Science.

Gravina, L., Foncuberta, M., Prieto, M., et al. (2010). Prevalence of DFNB1 mutations in Argentinean children with non-syndromic deafness: Report of a novel mutation in GJB2. *International Journal of Pediatric Otorhinolaryngology, 74*(3), 250-254.

Groce, N. Yousafzai, A., & Van der Maas, F. (2007). HIV/AIDS and disability: Differences in HIV/AIDS knowledge between deaf and hearing people in Nigeria. *Disability and Rehabilitation, 29*(5), 367-377.

Grosse, S. (2007). Education cost savings from early detection of hearing loss: New findings. *Volta Voices, 14*(6), 38-40.

Grosse, S., Ross, D., & Dollard, S. (2008). Congenital cytomegalovirus (CMV) infection as a cause of permanent bilateral hearing loss: A quantitative assessment. *Journal of Clinical Virology, 41*(2), 57-62.

Guiscafre, H., Benitex-Diaz, L., Martinez, M., & Munoz, O. (1984). Reversible hearing loss after meningitis. *Annals of Otology, Rhinology and Laryngology, 93,* 229-232.

Hanass-Hancock, J., & Satande, L. (2010). Deafness and HIV/AIDS: A systematic review of the literature. *African Journal of AIDS Research, 9*(2), 187-192.

Harrison, M., & Rousch, J. (2002). Information for families with young deaf and hard of hearing children: Reports from parents and pediatric audiologists. In R. Seewald and J. Gravel (Eds.), *A Sound Foundation Through Early Amplification. 2001. Proceedings of the 2nd International Conference* (pp. 233-250). Great Britain: St. Edmundsbury Press.

Hayashi, C., Funayama, M., Li, Y., et al. (2011). Prevalence of GJB2 causing recessive profound non-syndromic deafness in Japanese children. *International Journal of Pediatric Otorhinolaryngology, 75*(2), 211-214.

Helzner, E., Cauley, J., Pratt, S., et al. (2005). Race and sex differences in age-related hearing loss: The health, aging and body composition study. *Journal of the American Geriatric Society, 53*(12), 2119-2127.

Heuttel, K., & Rothstein, W. (2001). HIV/AIDS knowledge and information sources among deaf and hearing college students. *American Annals of the Deaf, 146*(3), 280-286.

Huang, B., Roche, J., Buchman, C., & Castillo, M. (2010). Brain stem and inner ear abnormalities in children with auditory neuropathy spectrum disorder and cochlear nerve deficiency. *American Journal of Neuroaudiology, 31*(10), 1972-1979.

Interdisciplinary Technical Assistance Center. (n.d.). Telehealth and teleaudiology webinar. Speed Linkage Presenters. Available at: www .aucd.org/itac/template/page.cfm?id=709

Joint Committee on Infant Hearing (2000). Year 2000 position statement: Principles and guidelines for early hearing detection and intervention programs. *American Journal of Audiology, 9,* 9-29.

Joint Committee on Infant Hearing (2007). Year 2007 position statement: Principles and guidelines for early hearing detection and intervention programs. Retrieved from: www.asha.org/docs/html/PS2007-00281. html.

Jovanovic-Bateman, L., & Hedreville, R. (2006). Sensorineural hearing loss with brainstem auditory evoked responses changes in homozygote and heterozygote sickle cell patients in Guadeloupe (France). *Journal of Laryngology and Otology, 120*(8), 627-630.

Keats, B. (2007, February 13). Genetics and auditory neuropathy/dyssynchrony. *The ASHA Leader.*

Kenneson, A., & Cannon, M. (2007). Review and meta-analysis of the epidemiology of congenital cytomegalovirus (CMV) infection. *Reviews in Medical Virology, 17*(4), 253-276.

Khoza, K., & Ross, E. (2002). Auditory function in a group of adults infected with HIV/AIDS in Gauteng, South Africa [Abstract]. *South African Journal of Communication Disorders, 49,* 17-27.

Kirkim, G., Serbetcioglu, B., Erdag, T., & Ceryan, K. (2008). The frequency of auditory neuropathy detected by universal newborn hearing screening program. *International Journal of Pediatrics and Otorhinolaryngology, 72*(10), 1461-1469.

Korver, A., Konings, S., Dekker, F., et al. (2010). Newborn hearing screening vs later hearing screening and developmental outcomes in children with permanent childhood hearing impairment. *Journal of the American Medical Association, 304*(15), 1701-1708.

Krumm, M., Ribera, J., & Froelich, T. (2002). Bridging the service gap through audiology telepractice. *The ASHA Leader, 7,* 6-7.

Kully, D. (2000). Telehealth in speech pathology: Applications to the treatment of stuttering. *Journal of Telemedicine and Telecare, 6*(Suppl. 2), 39-41.

Kumar, U., & Jayaram, M. (2006). Prevalence and audiological characteristics in individuals with auditory neuropathy/auditory dys-synchrony. *International Journal of Audiology, 45,* 360-366.

Laplante-Lévesque, A., Hickson, L., & Worrall, L. (2010). Factors influencing rehabilitation decisions of adults with acquired hearing impairment. *International Journal of Audiology, 49,* 497-507.

Lee, F., Matthews, L., Dubno, J., & Mills, J. (2005). Longitudinal study of pure-tone thresholds in older persons. *Ear and Hearing, 26*(1), 1-11.

Lench, N., Houseman, M., & Newton, V., et al. (1998). Connexin-26 mutations in sporadic nonsyndromal sensorineural deafness. *Lancet, 351,* 415.

Lin, H., Shu, M., Chang, K., & Bruna, S. (2002). A universal newborn hearing screening program in Taiwan. *International Journal of Pediatrics and Otorhinolaryngology, 63*(3), 209-218.

Lin, C., Huang, C., Lin, Y., & Wu, J. (2004). Community-based newborn hearing screening program in Taiwan. *International Journal of Pediatrics and Otorhinolaryngology, 68*(2), 185-189.

Liu, B., Saito, N., Wang, J., et al. (2009). Labyrinthitis ossificans in a child with sickle cell disease: CT and MRI findings. *Pediatric Radiology, 39*(9), 999-1001.

Liu, X., Xu, L., Hu, Y., et al. (2001). Epidemiological studies on hearing impairment with reference to genetic factors in Sichuan, China. *Annals of Otology, Rhinology, and Laryngology, 110*(4), 356-363.

Löppönen, T., Väisänen, M., Luotonen, M., et al. (2003). Connexin 26 mutations and nonsyndromic hearing impairment in northern Finland. *Laryngoscope, 113*(10), 1758-1763.

MacDonald, C., Bauer, P, Cox, L., & McMahon, L. (1999). Otologic findings in a pediatric cohort with sickle cell disease. *International Journal of Pediatric Otorhinolaryngology, 47*(1), 23-28.

Mace, A., Ferguson, M., Offr, M., et al. (2009). Bilateral profound sudden sensorineural hearing loss presenting a diagnostic conundrum in a child with sickle cell anaemia. *Journal of Laryngology and Otology, 123*(7), 811-816.

MacNeil, J. (2009, October). *Epidemiology of meningococcal disease in infants and young children.* Paper presented at Meeting of the Advisory Committee on Immunization Practices (ACIP), CDC, Atlanta, GA.

Mahdieh, N., & Rabbani, B. (2009). Statistical study of 35delG mutation of GJB2 gene: A meta-analysis of carrier frequency. *International Journal of Audiology, 48,* 363-370.

Marazita, M., Ploughman, L., Rawlings, B., et al. (1993). Genetic epidemiological studies of early-onset deafness in the U.S. school-age population. *American Journal of Medical Genetics, 46,* 489-491.

Martinez-Cruz, C., Poblano, A., Fernández-Carrocera, L. (2008). Risk factors associated with sensorineural hearing loss in infants at the neonatal intensive care unit: 15-year experience at the National Institute of Perinatology (Mexico City). *Archives of Medical Research, 39(7),* 686-94.

Mathews, M., & MacDorman, M. (2010, April 30). Infant mortality statistics from the 2006 period linked birth/infant death data set. *National Vital Statistics Report, 58(17).* Hyattsville, MD: National Center for Health Statistics.

Matkin, N., Diefendorf, A., & Erenberg, A. (1998). Children: HIV/AIDS and hearing loss. *Seminars in Hearing, 19,* 143-153.

McPherson, B. (2008). Audiology: A developing country context. In B. McPherson & R. Brouillette (Eds.), *Audiology in Developing Countries* (pp. 6-20). New York: Nova Science.

Mehra, S., Eavey, R., & Keamy, D., Jr. (2009). The epidemiology of hearing impairment in the United States: Newborns, children, and adolescents. *Otolaryngology, Head and Neck Surgery, 140(4),* 461-472.

Mencher, G. (2000). Challenge of epidemiological research in the developing world: Overview. *Audiology, 39(4),* 178-183.

Mencher, G., & Madriz, A. (2000). Prevalence of sensorineural hearing loss in children in Costa Rica. *Audiology, 39(5),* 278-283.

Meuwese-Jongejeugd, A., Vink, M., van Zanten, B., et al. (2006). Prevalence of hearing loss in 1598 adults with an intellectual disability: Cross-sectional population based study. *International Journal of Audiology, 45(11),* 660-669.

Millar, W. (2005). Hearing problems among seniors. Statistics Canada. *Health Reports, 16(4).*

Mitchell, R. (2006). How many deaf people are there in the United States? Estimates from the Survey of Income and Program Participation. *Journal of Deaf Studies and Deaf Education, 11(1),* 112-119.

Mizuno, T., Sugiura, S., Kimura, H., et al. (2009). Detection of cytomegalovirus DNA in preserved umbilical cords from patients with sensorineural hearing loss [Abstract]. *Eur Arch Otorhinolaryngol, 266(3),* 351-355.

Mohr, P. E., Feldman, J., Dunbar, J., McConkey-Robbins, A., Niparko, J., Rittenhouse, R., & Skinner, M. (2000). The societal costs of severe to profound hearing loss in the United States. *International Journal of Technology Assessment in Health Care, 16(4),* 1120-1135.

Morell, R., Kuir, H., & Hood, L. (1998). Mutations in the connexin 26 (GJB2) among Ashkenazi Jews with nonsyndromic recessive deafness. *New England Journal of Medicine, 339,* 1500-1505.

Morita, M., Morishima, T., Yamazaki, T., et al. (1998). Clinical survey of congenital cytomegalovirus infection in Japan. *Acta Paediatrica Japan, 40(5),* 2-6.

Morton, N. E. (1991). Genetic epidemiology of hearing loss. *Annals of the New York Academy of Sciences, 630,* 16-31.

Morzaria, S., Westerberg, B., & Kozak, F. (2004). Systematic review of the etiology of bilateral sensorineural hearing loss in children. *International Journal of Pediatrics and Otorhinolaryngology, 68(9),* 1193-1198.

Mueller, R. (2000). Genetics of hearing loss. *Seminars in Hearing, 21(4),* 399-408.

National Institute on Deafness and Other Communication Disorders. (1993, March 1-3). *Early identification of hearing impairment in infants and young children.* NIH Consensus Statement. [Online]. 11(1), 1-24.

Neumann, K., Nawka, T., Hess, M., et al. (January 2009). Quality assurance of a universal newborn screening: Recommendations of the German Society of Phoniatrics and Pediatric Audiology. *PubMeds 57(1),* 17-20.

Newton, V. E. (1985). Aetiology of bilateral sensorineural hearing loss in young children. *Journal of Laryngology and Otology Supplement, 10,* 1-57.

Nuru, N. (1993). Multicultural aspects of deafness. In D. Battle (Ed.). *Communication disorders in multicultural populations* (pp. 291-292). Boston: Butterworth-Heinemann.

Ogawa, H., Suzutani, T., Baba, Y., et al. (2007). Etiology of severe sensorineural hearing loss in children: Independent impact of congenital cytomegalovirus infection and GJB2 mutations. *Journal of Infectious Disease, 195(6),* 782-788.

Okhakhu, A., Ibekwe, T., Sadoh, A., & Ogisi, F. (2010). Neonatal hearing screening in Benin City. *International Journal of Pediatric Otorhinolaryngology, 74(11),* 1323-1326.

Olusanya, B. (2006). Early hearing detection and intervention in developing countries: Current status and prospects. *Volta Review, 106(3),* 381-418.

Olusanya, B., Wirz, S., & Luxon, L. (2008). Community-based infant hearing screening for early detection of permanent hearing loss in Lagos, Nigeria: A cross-sectional study. *Bulletin of the World Health Organization, 86,* 956-963. Doi: 10.2471/BLT.07.050005.

Olusanya, B. (2011). Predictors of early-onset permanent hearing loss in malnourished infants in Sub-Saharan Africa. *Research in Developmental Disabilities, 32(1),* 124-32.

Onakoya, P., Nwaorgu, O., & Shokunbi, W. (2002). Sensorineural hearing loss in adults with sickle cell anemia [Abstract]. *African Journal of Medical Science, 31(1),* 21-24.

Ondzotto, G., Malanda, F., Galiba, J., et al. (2002). Sudden deafness in sickle cell anemia: A case report [Abstract]. *Bulletin de la Societe de Pathologie Exotique, 95(4),* 248-249.

Palacios, G., Montalvo, M., Fraire, M., et al. (2008). Audiologic and vestibular findings in a sample of human immunodeficiency virus type-1 infected Mexican children under highly active antiretroviral therapy. *International Journal of Pediatric Otorhinolaryngology, 72(11),* 1671-1681.

Palmer, C., Martinez, A., Fox, M., et al. (2003). Genetic testing and the early hearing detection and intervention process. *The Volta Review, 103(4),* 371-390.

Parving, A. (1983). Epidemiology of hearing loss and aetiological diagnosis of hearing impairment in childhood. *International Journal of Pediatric Otorhinolaryngology, 5,* 151-165.

Parving, A. (1996). Epidemiology of genetic hearing impairment. In A. Martini, A. Read, & D. Stephens (Eds.). *Genetics and hearing impairment* (pp. 73-81). San Diego: Singular Publishing Group.

Pastor, P., Reuben, C., & Loeb, M. (2009, November 4). Functional difficulties among school-aged children: United States, 2001-2007. *National Health Statistics Reports,* No. 19. Hyattsville, MD: National Center for Health Statistics.

Pichora-Fuller, M., & Souza, P. (2003). Effects of aging on auditory processing of speech. *International Journal of Audiology, 42,* 2S11-2S16.

Piltcher, O., Cigana, L., Friedriech, J., et al. (2000). Sensorineural hearing loss among sickle cell disease patients from southern Brazil. *American Journal of Otolaryngology, 21(2),* 75-79.

Polovoy, C. (2008, June 17). Audiology telepractice overcomes inaccessibility. *The ASHA Leader.*

Polovoy, C., & Crowley, C. (2009, June 16). Aural rehabilitation telepractice: International project links NY student clinicians, Bolivian children. *The ASHA Leader.*

Pratt, S., Kuller, L., Talbott, E., et al. (2009). Prevalence of hearing loss in Black and White elders: Results of the Cardiovascular Health Study. *Journal of Speech, Language and Hearing Research, 52(4),* 973-989.

Propst, E., Stockley, T., Gordon, K., et al. (2006). Ethnicity and mutations in GJB2 (connexin 26) and GJB6 (connexin 30) in a multi-cultural Canadian paediatric cochlear implant program. *International Journal of Pediatric Otorhinolaryngology, 70(3),* 435-444.

Quinn, S., & Rance, G. (2009). The extent of hearing impairment amongst Australian indigenous prisoners in Victoria, and implications for the correctional system. *International Journal of Audiology, 48,* 123-134.

Rance, G., & Baker, E. (2009). Speech and language outcomes in children with auditory neuropathy/dys-synchrony managed with either cochlear implants or hearing aids. *International Journal of Audiology, 48,* 313-320.

Ricker, J., Rosenthal, M., Garay, E., et al. (2002). Telerehabilitation needs: A survey of persons with acquired brain injury. *Journal of Head Trauma Rehabilitation, 17(3),* 242-250.

Robertson, C., Howarth, T., Bork, D., & Dinu, I. (2009). Permanent bilateral sensory and neural hearing loss of children after neonatal intensive care because of extreme prematurity: A thirty-year study. *Pediatrics, 123(5),* 797-807.

Roche, J., Huang, B., Castillo, M., Bassim, M., Adunka, O., & Buchman, C (2010). Imaging characteristics of children with auditory neuropathy. *Otology and Neurotology, 31(5),* 780-788.

Rohlfs, A., Wiesner, T., Drews, H., et al. (2010). Interdisciplinary approach to design, performance, and quality management in a multicenter newborn hearing screening project: Introduction, methods, and results of the newborn hearing screening in Hamburg (Part I). *European Journal of Pediatrics, 169(11),* 1353-1360.

Roland, J., Alexiades, G., Jackman, A., et al. (2003). Cochlear implantation in human immunodeficiency virus-infected patients. *Otology and Neurotology, 24(6),* 892-895.

Rural Assistance Center (2010). Teleaudiology: Taking diagnostics to the infant. Retrieved from: www.raconline.org/success/success_details .php?success_id=641.

Russ, S., Poulakis, Z., Barker, M., et al. (2003). Epidemiology of congenital hearing loss in Victoria, Australia. *International Journal of Audiology, 42,* 385-390.

Salami, A., Mora, R., Dellepiane, M., et al. (2010). Water-soluble coenzyme Q10 formulation (Q-TER((R))) in the treatment of presbycusis. *Acta Otolaryngologica, 130(10),* 1154-1162.

Saluja, S., Agarwal, A., Kler, N., & Amin, S. (2010). Auditory neuropathy spectrum disorder in late preterm and term infants with severe jaundice. *International Journal of Pediatric Otorhinolaryngology, 74(11),* 1292-1297.

Schildroth, A. N. (1994). Congenital cytomegalovirus and deafness. *American Journal of Audiology, 3,* 27-38.

Schildroth, A., & Hotto, S. (1995). Race and ethnic background in the Annual Survey of Deaf and Hard of Hearing Children and Youth. *American Annals of the Deaf, 140,* 96-99.

Schmitz, J., Pillon, J., Le Clerq, S., et al. (2010). Prevalence of hearing loss and ear morbidity among adolescents and young adults in rural southern Nepal. *International Journal of Audiology, 49,* 388-394.

Schoenborn, C., & Heyman, K. (2009). *National Health characteristics of adults aged 55 years and over: United States, 2004-2007.* Health statistics reports: No. 16. Hyattsville, MD: National Center for Health Statistics.

Shargorodsky, J., Curhan, S., Curhan, G., & Eavey, R. (2010). Change in prevalence of hearing loss in US adolescents. *Journal of American Medical Association, 304(7),* 772-778.

Siem, G., Fagerheim, T., Jonsrud, C., et al. (2010). Causes of hearing impairment in the Norwegian paediatric cochlear implant program. *International Journal of Audiology, 49,* 596-605.

Simonsen, E., Kristoffersen, A., Hyde, M., & Hjulstad, O. (2009). Great expectations: Perspectives on cochlear implantation of deaf children in Norway. *American Annals of the Deaf, 154(3),* 263-273.

Smith, A. (2008). Demographics of hearing loss in developing countries. In B. McPherson & R. Brouillette (Eds.), *Audiology in Developing Countries* (pp. 21-50). New York: Nova Science.

Sprinzl, G., & Riechelmann, H. (2010). Current trends in treating hearing loss in elderly people: A review of the technology and treatment options. A mini-review. *Gerontology, 56,* 351-358. doi:10.1159/000275062

Stagno, S., Dworsky, M., Torres, J., et al. (1982). Prevalence and importance of congenital cytomegalovirus infection in three different populations. *Journal of Pediatrics, 101(6),* 897-900.

Statistics Canada (2009). *Facts on hearing limitations.* Retrieved from: www.statcan.gc.ca/pub/89-628-x/2009012/fs-fi/fs-fi-eng.htm.

Stern, R., Yueh, B., Lewis, C., Norton, S., & Sie, K. (2005). Recent epidemiology of pediatric cochlear implantation in the United States: Disparity among children of different ethnicity and socioeconomic status. *Laryngoscope, 115(1),* 125-131.

Stuart, A., Jones, S., & Walker, L. (2006). Insights into elevated distortion product otoacoustic emissions in sickle cell disease: Comparison of hydroxyurea-treated and non-treated young children. *Hear Res, 212(1-2),* 83-89.

Sun, X., Wei, Z., Yu, L., et al. (2008). Prevalence and etiology of people with hearing impairment in China [Abstract]. *Zhonghua Liu Xing Bing Xue Za Zhi, 29(7),* 643-646.

Swanepoel, de W., Clark, J., Koekemoer, D., et al. (2010). Telehealth in audiology: The need and potential to reach underserved communities. *International Journal of Audiology, 49,* 195-202.

Swanepoel, De W., Louw, B., & Hugo, R. (2007). A novel service delivery model for infant hearing screening in developing countries. *International Journal of Audiology, 46,* 321-327.

Tan, J., Yeh, B., & Seet, C. (2010). Deafness due to haemorrhagic labyrinthitis and a review of relapses in streptococcus suis meningitis. *Singapore Med J, 51(2),* e30-e33.

Teek, R., Kruustük, K., Zordania, R., et al. (2010). Prevalence of c.35delG and p.M34T mutations in the GJB2 gene in Estonia. *International Journal of Pediatric Otorhinolaryngology, 74(9),* 1007-1012.

Tomasik, T. (2008). Risk factors of hearing impairment in premature infants [Abstract]. *Przegl Lek, 65(9),* 375-384.

Trotman, H., Olugbuyl, O., Barton, M., et al. (2009). Pneumococcal meningitis in Jamaican children. *West Indian Medical Journal, 58(6),* 585-588.

Tsibulevskaya, G., Oburra, H., & Aluoch, J. (1996). Sensorineural hearing loss in patients with sickle cell anemia in Kenya [Abstract]. *East African Medical Journal, 73(7),* 471-473.

Uilenburg, N., Kauffman-de Boer, M., van der Ploeg, K., et al. (2009). An implementation study of neonatal hearing screening in the Netherlands. *International Journal of Audiology, 48,* 108-116.

UNAIDS. (2010). *Report on the global AIDS epidemic* [On-line]. Available at: www.unaids.org/globalreport/default.htm.

U.S. Census Bureau (2001). *Current population survey, March 2000, Racial Statistics Population Division* [On-line]. Available at: www .census.gov.

U.S. Department of Education (2010). *Twenty-Ninth Annual Report to Congress on the Implementation of the Individuals with Disabilities Education Act, 2007.* Washington, DC: U.S. Government Printing Office.

U.S. Department of Health and Human Services (1990). *An assessment based on the health status indicators for the United States and each state.* Hyattsville, MD: Author.

U.S. Department of Health and Human Services (2001). *Healthy People 2010*. Hyattsville, MD: Author.

U.S. Department of Health and Human Services (2010). *Summary Health Statistics for U.S. Adults: National Health Interview Survey, 2009*. Hyattsville, MD. Author.

Vaughn, G. (1976). Tel-communicology: Health-care delivery system for persons with communicative disorders. *ASHA, 18*, 13-17.

Vienny, H., Despland, P., Lutschg, J., et al. (1984). Early diagnosis and evolution of deafness in childhood bacterial meningitis: A study using brain stem auditory evoked potentials. *Pediatrics, 73*, 579-586.

Vincenti, V., Pasanisi, E., Bacciu, A., et al. (2005). Cochlear implantation in a human immunodeficiency virus-infected patient. *Laryngoscope, 115(6)*, 1079-1081.

Wang, Y., Yang, H., & Dong, M. (2006). The hearing manifestations of 350 patients of AIDS. Published in Chinese [Abstract]. *Lin Chuang Er Bi Yan Hou Ke Za Zhi, 20(22)*, 1020-1021.

Weinick, R., Zurekas, S., & Cohen, J. (2000). Racial and ethnic differences in access to and use of health care services, 1977 to 1996. *Medical Care Research and Review, 57(Suppl. 1)*, 36-54.

Whitehead, R., MacDonald, B., Melhem, E., & McMahon, L. (1998). Spontaneous labyrinthine hemorrhage in sickle cell disease. *American Journal of Neuroaudiology, 19*, 1437-1440.

Williams, W. (2010). Australian Senate Community Affairs Reference Committee Inquiry into hearing health in Australia. Retrieved from: www.aph.gov.au/senate/committee/clac_ctte/hearing_health/report/c02.htm.

Winningham, A., Gore-Felton, C., Galletly, C., et al. (2008). Lessons learned from more than two decades of HIV/AIDS prevention efforts: Implications for people who are deaf or hard of hearing. *American Annals of the Deaf, 153(1)*, 48-54.

Wong, L., & McPherson, B. (2008, December 6). Universal hearing health care: China. *The ASHA Leader*.

World Health Organization (1998). *Report of a WHO/CBM Workshop, November 24-26. State of hearing & ear care in the south-east Asia region*. Available at: www.who.int.

World Health Organization (2001). *Prevention of deafness and hearing impairment* [On-line]. Available at: www.who.int.

World Health Organization (2004). *Guidelines for hearing aids and services for developing countries. Second edition, September 2004*. Available: www.who.int.

World Health Organization (2006). *Primary ear and hearing care training resource*. Available at: www.who.int.

World Health Organization (2007). *Situation review and update on deafness, hearing loss and intervention programmes. Proposed plans of action for prevention and alleviation of hearing impairment in countries of the south-east Asia Region*. Available at: www.who.int.

World Health Organization (2008). Report of a joint WHO-TIF meeting in Cyprus, 16-18, November, 2007. Available: www.who.int.

World Health Organization (2010a). *National programmes for prevention of deafness and hearing impairment*. Available at: www.who.int/pbd/deafness/activities/national_programmes/en/print.html.

World Health Organization (2010b). *Deafness and hearing impairment*. Available at: www.who.int/mediacentre/factsheets/fs300/en/.

World Health Organization (2010c). *Raising awareness–Community ear and hearing health*. Available at: www.who.int/pbd/deafness/activities/awareness/en/print.html.

World Health Organization (2010d). *Meningococcal meningitis*. Available at: www.who.int.

World Health Organization (2010e). *Revolutionary new meningitis vaccine set to wipe out deadly epidemics in Africa*. Available at: www.who.int.

World Health Organization (2010f). Global Epidemic. Available at: www.who.int/hiv/data/en/index.html.

World Health Organization (2011). *World health report. 2003*. Available at: www.who.int.

Wormald, R., Viani, L., Lynch, S., & Green, A. (2010). Sensorineural hearing loss in children [Abstract]. *Irish Medical Journal, 103(2)*, 51-54.

Worsøe, L., Cayé-Thomasen, P., Brandt, C., et al. (2010). Factors associated with the occurrence of hearing loss after pneumococcal meningitis. *Clin Infect Dis, 51(8)*, 917-924.

Xoinis, K., Weirather, Mavoori, H., et al. (2007). Extremely low birth weight infants are at high risk for auditory neuropathy. *Journal of Perinatology, 27(11)* 718-723.

Zelante, L., Gasparini, P., & Estivill, X. (1997). Connexin 26 mutations associated with the most common form of non-syndromic neurosensory and autosomal recessive deafness (DFNB1) in Mediterraneans. *Human Molecular Genetics, 6*, 1608-1609.

ADDITIONAL RESOURCES

McPherson, B., & Brouillette, R. (Eds.). (2008). *Audiology in developing countries*. New York: Nova Science.

Pascolini, D., & Smith, A. (2009). Hearing impairment in 2008: A compilation of available epidemiological studies. *International Journal of Audiology, 48*, 473-485.

Chapter 12

Assessment of Multicultural and International Clients with Communication Disorders

Toya Wyatt

THE CASE HISTORY INTERVIEW

The speech and language assessment process with clients from international culturally and linguistically diverse (CLD) backgrounds is the same as that for any client. According to Meitus and Weinberg's (1983) model of clinical service delivery, there are four functions associated with the diagnostic evaluation process: investigative, analytic, utilization, and accountability. Part of the *investigative function* involves the collection of historical information about a client and his or her communication status through case history interviews, referral reports, and testing.

In the case of CLD clients, the case history is crucial because it often serves as a primary source of data for clients who speak languages for which there are no existing assessment tools. The case history interview provides a rich source of data for determining how the family and client perceive their communicative ability compared with individuals from similar cultural-linguistic backgrounds using community standards.

A guiding principle in CLD assessments, as delineated in the American Speech-Language-Hearing Association (ASHA; 2004) knowledge and skills document for CLD populations, is the importance of determining "what is typical speech/language development in the client's/patient's speech community and communication environment" through interview with a parent or caregiver "on how the client's/patient's speech/language development compares to peers in his/her speech community." In addition, according to Battle (2000), culturally competent clinicians use "the case history for obtaining information about a client's culture, communication, speech history and life history" (p. 20).

The process of obtaining information through the case history interview, however, is a sensitive one. It is important to establish a positive information gathering and sharing climate by working to establish rapport and an atmosphere of mutual trust and respect (Haynes & Pindzola, 2008). This can be challenging when working with clients and families from differing cultural backgrounds because what is perceived as trust and respect in one group can differ from that in another group. The strategies and type of discourse interaction that are most useful for accomplishing this task can also vary.

One additional consideration when assessing bilingual and multilingual clients is the importance of using case history interview questions that provide a clear overview of (1) comprehensive language system and use patterns within and across all languages spoken, (2) relative communication strengths and weaknesses within each language spoken, and (3) the impact of any perceived communication difficulties on that client's ability to "communicate effectively in his/her speech community or family" (Battle, 2000, p. 21).

The purpose of this chapter is to provide an overview of key considerations that clinicians should take into account when obtaining the case history interview with CLD clients. It also provides examples of the types of questions that should be included when assessing the language skills of individuals who speak more than one language.

ESTABLISHING RAPPORT

One of the most important aspects of the case history interview process with any client or family member is how it begins, especially with clients from CLD and international backgrounds. During the opening phase of the assessment, it is important to establish a positive information gathering and sharing atmosphere by establishing rapport in an atmosphere of mutual trust and respect.

The communication strategies that are most useful for establishing rapport and trust can vary across different individuals and families. Individuals and families vary in preferred cultural communication style. Cultural beliefs regarding what is most appropriate to discuss or disclose can also vary. Finally, differences in family structure and roles can determine who is to be involved in the information sharing process, what roles different individuals play in the family, and who is given the primary responsibility for making decisions.

Culture and the Case History Interview

Personal, Social, and Cultural Identity

Personal, social, and cultural identity are factors that affect the overall communication process with clients and families. According to Ting-Toomey and Chung (2005), *personal identity* includes those unique attributes that are associated with one's "individuated self in comparison with those of others" (p. 87). *Social identity* includes various other forms of identity such as cultural or ethnic membership identity, gender identity, disability identity, or professional identity. *Cultural identity* is defined as the "emotional significance" that individuals attach to their "sense of belonging or affiliation with the larger culture" (Ting-Toomey & Chung, 2005, p. 93) and reflects the extent to which one identifies with a larger cultural group. All cultures and cultural groups have not only "shared rules for appropriate behavior" but also shared "values and beliefs" that help "to regulate interaction with other members of the community and with individuals form cultural backgrounds different from their own" (Saville-Troike, 1986, p. 48). This can include common beliefs about how, when, where, and with whom they should use certain types of language and communication styles.

Cultural Identity Continuum

Families and individuals differ in their cultural or group affiliation even when they come from the same racial or ethnic background. Individuals will also differ in their degree of cultural identity salience (Ting-Toomey & Chung, 2005), which includes the strength of one's cultural group affiliations, allegiance and loyalty to a given group, unique individual personal identities, and differences in the degree of acculturation. Individuals within the same cultural community "may differ in the extent to which they chose to adhere to a set of cultural patterns" (Hanson, 2004a, p. 4). Some people identify more strongly with a particular cultural group, some identify less strongly, and others identify with more than one group.

As a result, it is important not to make generalizations about a given individual or family as a result of their cultural background. Individuals and families from the same cultural and ethnic background will not always assume or display the cultural practices and beliefs generally associated with that group. For example, Gushue and colleagues (2010) caution that although the primacy of the family (a concept referred to as *familismo*) may be an important feature of Mexican culture in general, one has to consider the extent to which it is true for a particular family.

Acculturation

The level of acculturation plays a role in a person or family's social identity. Acculturation is the process by which individuals assume and adopt the values, beliefs, and norms of a more dominant, mainstream culture (Battle, 2002; Gushue et al., 2010). As individuals interact with and begin to spend more time with a new or different culture, they can move along a continuum as they adopt, adapt, and accept more mainstream cultural group norms and practices.

Multiple Cultural Identities

In today's global world culture, there are growing numbers of individuals who balance multiple cultural identities because of their multiracial heritage (Choi-Misailidis, 2010). These individuals may display a cultural affiliation that differs from that of individuals within each of their cultural affiliation groups. Their cultural affiliation may differ dependent on the extent to which there is congruence and disparity between their internal mixed race identity and their external multiracial heritage. For example, an individual who is both African American and Hispanic may affiliate with African American culture and cultural groups for some functions but with Hispanic culture for others. There may be some biracial African American and Hispanic individuals who identify almost completely with African American culture. Others may identify almost completely with Hispanic culture. Still others may identify with neither.

Another example of individuals who have to balance more than one cultural identity are those who self-identify as lesbian, gay, bisexual, or transgender (LGBT). They may identify not only with LGBT culture but also with the cultural identity linked to their ethnic-racial background. There is also the struggle for some LGBT individuals who are CLD to balance multiple or conflicting cultural norms, values, and beliefs—those of the LGBT community and those of the CLD community with which they affiliate (Wilton, 2010).

New Emerging Global Identities

One additional category that deserves some attention is that of today's young adult generation of "e.net'ers" (Ting-Toomey & Chung, 2005). According to Ting-Toomey and Chung (2005, p. 314), e.net'ers represent a new generation of individuals who are attempting to create a third identity. Their identity involves a fusion of individualism and collectivism and embraces both individual privacy and a longing for a sense of global belonging and connection that transcends traditional ethnic-cultural boundaries. They have a sense of communal belonging on a global level. A key contributing factor to this new emerging identity is the Internet, which allows users to develop relationships across the barriers of time, space, geography, and ethnic-cultural boundaries.

Although some e.net'ers retain some degree of loyalty to their traditional ethnic groups, they are more likely to have a more connections with their technoglobal social networks. Ting-Toomey and Chung (2005) explain that one of the outcomes is a generation that differs from that of their parents and grandparents with respect to traditional cultural values and norms. This can create culturally based communication tensions and challenges across the generations within families as well as in interactions between individuals who are more technology oriented and those who are not. Part of the tension can be attributed to differing perceptions between family members (e.g., teens and adults) of one's attentiveness and one's desire to interact socially with others when using technology (e.g., texting) in the presence of others (Jayson, 2010-2011).

Impact of Culture on the Communication Style and Interaction

Cultural identity carries with it certain beliefs, assumptions, and expectations about how individuals should communicate with others from the same as well as differing cultural backgrounds. Understanding some of the differences is crucial to the establishment of rapport and relationship with the individuals and families being assessed. The following are a few examples of the ways in which varying cultural values, beliefs, language use, and communication style issues affect the establishment of rapport and client-family-clinician interactions during the clinical process.

High-Context versus Low-Context Communication

Cultures differ in the amount of information that is transmitted through words vs. nonverbal contexts and communication (Lynch, 2004). These differences have often been described in terms of high-context and low-context communication. *High-context* communicators place more emphasis on the expression of meaning and intention through "explicit verbal messages" (Ting-Toomey & Chung, 2005, p. 169). They give less emphasis to the spoken word and pay more attention instead to nonverbal cues and messages as conveyed by facial expression, body movement, gestures, environmental clues, and other body language cues or subtle "vibes" (Hecht, 1989, cited in Lynch, 2004). Pause, silence, and tone of voice are other examples of nonverbal communication devices used to convey meaning and intent. There is also a greater expectation placed on the listener to "read between the lines" (Ting-Toomey & Chung, 2005). According to Crystal (1989, as cited in Chan & Lee, 2004), there are some communities where pride and value are placed on one's ability to "know" intuitively what others are thinking and feeling without the benefit of words. For example, in the Korean community, *nun-chi* (reading the eyes) is an affective sense by which one is able to use external cues to assess genuine attitudes and emotional reactions about a given topic, proposal or situation.

Low context communicators, on the other hand, focus more on the use of explicit verbal messages (Ting-Toomey & Chung, 2004) and precise, direct, verbal communication with less processing of nonverbal cues and movement and explicit verbal messages (Lynch, 2004).

Asian, American Indian, Arab, Latino, and African American communities are examples of cultures that have typically been characterized as using high context in communication style (Lynch, 2004). Persons from European countries such as Germany, Switzerland, Denmark, and Sweden tend to be at the more extreme ends of low-context communicators. Persons from countries such as the United States, Canada, Australia, and the United Kingdom, although less extreme, also tend to be on the low-context end on this continuum of communication, perhaps because of their European roots. In some cultures, such as American culture, males also tend to be low-context in communication style, whereas females tend to be high context (Ting-Toomey & Chung, 2004).

Greetings

One of the ways that clinicians attempt to establish rapport with clients and family members is through greetings. Greetings can vary cross-culturally with respect to how they are done, with whom they are done, and the order in which they are done.

Shaking hands is a common form of greeting and departure and is an important part of social etiquette in many places throughout the world (Kulwicki, 2003). Even though handshaking may be used as a typical form of introduction, it may not be as "hearty" in some places in the world as it is in the United States (p. 63). For example, among the Navajo, the handshake is lighter than one would expect elsewhere and is "more of a passing of hands" (Lynch, 2004; Still & Hodgins, 2003).

In contrast, shaking hands as a way of greeting may be uncomfortable to Southeast Asians. In India, for example, individuals are greeted with a handshake known as *wai*, in which one brings the palms of the hand together and raises them to the chest or tip of the nose while lowering the head (Lynch, 2004). In Japanese culture, the traditional greeting is a bow with the "depth of the bow, its duration, and the number of repetitions" reflecting "the relative status of the parties involved and the formality of the situation" (Sharts-Hopko, 2003, p. 220).

The order and manner in which greetings and introductions are made can also be important. According to Matsuda (1989), when greeting and making introductions in many Asian cultures, it is important to know the client's status and position. When meeting Asian parents for the first time, professionals should identify themselves and their title and position through formal introduction. Chan and Lee (2003) recommend greeting members of Asian families in order of age beginning with the oldest. It is also typical to greet male members first.

Terms of Address

When meeting a client and family members for the first time, terms of address can also be equally important to establish rapport. Although the use of first names is often used in contemporary American culture as a way of establishing rapport with clients, there are a number of cultural groups with whom the continued use of a person's last name or the use of a title (e.g., Mr., Mrs., or Dr.) with a first or last name would be the best social protocol. For example, it is best not to address African American family members by their first name "unless given permission" to do so (Glanvillle, 2003; Willis, 2004). A common practice for addressing persons within Appalachian communities is through the use of a title with the first name, such as "Miss Elizabeth" or "Mr. William." Zoucha and Zamarripa (2008) also emphasize the importance of formality when addressing elderly members of Mexican families and state that being overly familiar by "using first names may not be appreciated early on in the establishment of a professional relationship with the families."

One additional consideration related to the use of terms of address are the various ways throughout the world to refer to married women. In some French Canadian communities, such as Quebec, married women are required by law keep their maiden name throughout their lifetime. It is therefore not uncommon for children of French Canadian parents to have differing surnames. One child may carry the mother's surname, another may have the father's surname, and others may have hyphenated or nonhyphenated combinations of both names in any order (Couto-Wakulczyk et al., 2003). In some Chinese and Korean cultures (except in Hong Kong and Taiwan), women also do not take on their husband's name after they marry (Chan & Lee, 2003; Wong, 2003). In some Hispanic cultures, the naming practice for married women is complex. According to Purnell and Paulanka (2003), in Hispanic communities married women are likely not only to take on their husband's surname but also to retain both of her parent's surnames, resulting in an extended name such as La Senora Roberta Rodriguez (husband's surname) de Malena (mother's maiden name) y Perez (father's surname).

Changes in naming practices have also occurred in contemporary American culture over the last couple of decades. As a result, it is not uncommon for women in contemporary American culture to keep their maiden name or use a hyphenated version of both her maiden and married surnames. Given the range of different names and preferred titles, clinicians need to be careful about what form of address to use in the case history interview. One of the best solutions is to always check on how individuals wish to be addressed at the beginning of the interview or double-check the titles and names used by significant others completing the initial paperwork for an assessment.

Beginning the Interaction

Once initial greetings have been made, professionals need to consider how they will begin the interview. There are some cultures in which clients may be ready to begin fairly quickly after some brief preliminary introductions and greetings. For example, according to Jezewski and Sotnik (2005), in American culture after a brief greeting, conversations immediately move to the primary business at hand. In other cultures, there is a great value placed on establishing a personal relationship first. In Arab cultures, for example, greetings, inquiries about well-being, pleasantries, and a cup of tea or coffee precede business (Kulwicki, 2003). When interacting with individuals of Mexican origin or heritage, Zoucha and Zamarripa (2008) suggest engaging in social talk before proceeding with the usual business as a means of encouraging open communication and sharing and establishing trust Similarly, Joe and Malach (2004) suggest that when beginning a conversation with American Indians, it is important first to engage in social talk. Doing such helps families get to know you as a person and are important as a means of establishing rapport.

Conversational Directness

Cultures can vary in the amount of directness used and expected during conversations. In some cultures, there is emphasis placed on directness and honesty with opinions expressed in a very open and direct manner. In others, where there is an emphasis on preserving group harmony and preserving face, a more indirect communication style may be used and valued (Chan & Lee, 2004; Hanson, 2004).

This difference can have a very important impact on how topics are addressed and on the types of responses given to questions. Individuals who use a more indirect style of communicating may, for example, sometimes say "yes" and use a negative head nod indicating "no" (i.e., telling the speaker what he or she wants to hear rather than giving a truthful answer). They may also be noncommittal or hesitant to respond to a direct question if they are reluctant to do what is being asked or there is some form of disagreement with what is being expressed or asked. Such responses can be misinterpreted or evaluated as being evasive, devious, and dishonest by individuals who use a more direct conversational style (Chan & Lee, 2004).

Listener Acknowledgement, Agreement, and Disagreement

While nodding one's head up and down typically is a sign of understanding and agreement in mainstream American culture, the same gesture may mean that the listener understands the message (e.g., "I hear you speaking") but does not suggest agreement in some Asian, American Indian, Middle Eastern, and Pacific Island cultures There can also be differences in how individuals also signal what they have heard. For example, individuals from India signal that they have heard what is said by moving their head in a quick, horizontal, figure-eight pattern (Lynch, 2004).

Listener agreement or disagreement can also be signaled verbally through the use of words such as "yes" and "no," but there can be cross-cultural differences in how these two terms are used. According to Santos and Chan

(2004), even when Filipino Americans are privately opposed to an issue or question at hand, they may still say "yes" instead of "no" despite of their feelings, or use more ambiguous responses such as "maybe" or "I don't know," especially when conversing with someone they consider to be superior or when they feel that the truth may offend or embarrass.

In some Middle Eastern cultures, in which a direct "no" is viewed as being impolite, a weak "yes," "maybe," or "perhaps" may also replace a direct "no" (Sharifzadeh, 2003).

Eye Contact

The interpretation and use of eye contact is another communication behavior that can vary during conversation. In mainstream American, Irish and Cuban cultures, in which direct eye contact during conversation is valued, a person who does not maintain eye contact may be perceived as not listening, not being trustworthy, not caring, or being less than truthful (Purnell, 2003; Purnell & Paulanka, 2003). In Irish culture, not maintaining eye contact can be interpreted as a sign of disrespect, guilt, or evidence that one cannot be trusted (Wilson, 2003).

On the other hand, in some communities, the use of direct eye contact may be considered disrespectful. For example, in American Indian and Asian communities, respect for others, such as elders and individuals with knowledge, authority, or status, is shown by not making direct contact (Lynch, 2004).

There can also be situational variables that dictate whether or not direct eye contact is appropriate. Among the Amish (Wegner & Wegner, 2003), avoidance of eye contact and an overall demeanor of general reserve is most appropriate during interactions with non-Amish in public situations. In one-on-one contacts, however, Amish clients are more likely to display more openness and candor with unhesitating eye contact.

According to Purnell and Paulanka (2003), sustained eye contact in some communities (e.g., Mexican, Cuban, Puerto Rican, Iranian, Egyptian, Italian, and Greek) may bring on the "evil eye" or "bad eye," which is considered a contributing cause of disability.

Silence

The use of silence can vary across cultural communities (Jezewski & Sotnik, 2005; Ting-Toomey & Chung, 2005). In some mainstream American cultures, a little silence is tolerated during conversation, but prolonged silence is often viewed as "empty pauses" or "ignorant lapses." In Eastern Asian cultures, silence is viewed as "a sign of thoughtful respect, affirmation or cooperation." The Navajo stress the importance of providing sufficient time for elderly people to respond to questions through silence. Failure to provide sufficient time can lead to an inaccurate response or no response at all (Still & Hodgins, 2003).

Silence can also be used as a tool during conversation to establish formal distance as is done with the French and many Native American cultures with strangers. In contrast, talk is often used by mainstream Americans to "break the ice," with silence being reserved for use in intimate relationships (Ting-Toomey & Chung, 2005).

Facial Expression

Facial expressions can vary in use and interpretation. In traditional Chinese families, facial expressions, such smiling, are used extensively among family and friends but may be limited in formal situations (Wang & Purnell, 2008). Smiling can also be used by Asian communicators as an expression of apology for minor offenses, deference to authority figures, to mask difficult feelings and emotions (e.g., pain, distress, discomfort, anger, disapproval, disappointment), and to avoid conflict when insulted, threatened, or otherwise provoked (Chan & Lee, 2004). In the Vietnamese community, silence or the use of a "reluctant" smile can be used as an expression of negative emotion (Nowak, 2003, p. 329).

In German culture, smiling is reserved for friends and family and may not occur during introductions. In settings (e.g., work) and situations that are considered to be serious (e.g., dealing with illness), the most appropriate response is one that is reserved, with no smiling (Steckler, 2008).

Body Language

The use of body language (i.e., the extent to which it is publicly evident) can also vary across different cultural communities. Those from certain cultures can be very expressive in their use of body language during conversations, such as African Americans and Puerto Ricans (Juarbe, 2003; Willis, 2004). Others can be more reserved. For example, in Irish culture, a high degree of value is placed on humility and emotional reserve, which are considered virtues. Public displays of emotion and affection are also typically avoided (Wilson, 2003). In traditional Japanese culture, value is placed on control over body language, making it difficult for some service providers to detect and interpret emotions such as anger and dismay (Sharts-Hopko, 2003).

Tone of Voice

Tone of voice is another channel through which emotions can be expressed differently cross-culturally. In some cultures, such as those in the Middle East, the manner and tone in speaking are just as important as what is said (Kulwicki, 2003).

Self-Disclosure

Cultural socialization influences can also impact the extent to which an individual self-discloses personal information to others. According to Ting-Toomey & Chung (2005), verbal self-disclosure of personal information involves some degree of "trust-risk." For example, in some African American families and communities, individuals "openly" express feelings to trusted friends of family; however, in others, what happens within the family is viewed as private and is not appropriate for discussion with strangers (Glanville, 2003). African Americans may be suspicious and cautious with health care practitioners that they do not know As a result, clinicians may find that some African American clients and families may initially be a little less willing to share personal information openly with health care practitioners that they do not yet know.

It can also take nontribal health care providers a long time to get Navajos to self-disclose because they "generally do not share inner thoughts and feelings with anyone outside of their clan" (Still & Hodgins, 2003). According to Wegner and Wegner (2003), people of Appalachian culture and heritage and who reside in that region of the United States do not easily trust or share their thoughts or feelings with outsiders.

In Filipino culture, the group status membership of an individual plays a significant role in determining the amount and type of sharing done. The degree and the nature of the sharing are dependent on insider or outsider status (Pacquiao, 2003).

In some cases, the amount of sharing and disclosure may be tied to the topics being discussed. Mexican Americans generally express their inner beliefs, feelings, and emotions once they get to know and trust a person.

The establishment of a personal relationship with service providers is equally important in Middle Eastern communities where a high value is placed on privacy. There may be a resistance to disclosing personal information to strangers, especially when it relates to familiar disease and conditions. As a result, persons from the Middle East "need to develop personal relationships with a health care provider before sharing personal information" (Kulwicki, 2003).

The history of a community can also play a role in the extent to which individuals disclose personal information with others. In Haiti, institutions that provide services for children with disabilities are often viewed as places of refuge from the public scrutiny and societal abuse that can occur against children with disabilities. Nongovernmental, religious, or foreign organizations that provide services are institutions in which Haitians place their faith owing to an expectation that these institutions will provide "miracles" because of stories of miraculous recoveries passed on by friends (Jacobson, 2005).

As a result of the long history of foreign invasions in Iran, people from Iran may hold a general suspicion of foreigners. The disclosure of personal information to strangers is generally perceived to have detrimental consequences. Not verbalizing one's thoughts to strangers is customary (Hafizi & Lipson, 2008).

Personal life experiences can play a role in any community. There will always be some individuals within communities who have witnessed or experienced personal life events that affect their overall willingness to trust. According to Short and associates (2010), a number of immigrants and refugees throughout the world, including those seeking asylum in the United States, have either survived, witnessed, or experienced acts of torture and abuse in their home countries. For example, according to statistics stated by Short and associates (2010), approximately one third of the world's refuges are survivors of torture, and more than 80 percent have experienced torture. Such experiences will obviously affect a family or individual's willingness to disclose during the case history interview, especially when individuals are coming from countries where issues such as war, violence, torture, poverty, imprisonment, and poor living conditions have been an issue.

The current social climate of a country can also affect the general willingness of individuals from certain communities to disclose. Issues such as increased discrimination or acts of hatred or violence aimed toward a certain ethnic group, evolving immigration policies, and attitudes toward immigrant groups and communities cannot be underestimated in their potential impact on the disclosure process. One such group in the United States is Muslim Americans in the aftermath of the attacks in New York on 9/11 and the subsequent years of war in the Middle East.

Attitudes toward Disability and Disorder

The case history interview process often involves personal questions about the nature and perceived causes of an individual's communication and swallowing difficulties. Responses to these questions and the amount of disclosure that occurs can vary as a function of culturally influenced beliefs and attitudes toward health, illness, disability, and disorder. Culture can also affect how individuals and communities react to, as well as accept, disorder and disability. The following are examples of the various ways in which these beliefs can affect the case history interview and general assessment process.

Perceived Causes

A key issue that can affect disclosure of information is the cultural beliefs about disabilities that can exist across communities. In many places of the world, such as Italy, various beliefs about the role of the "evil eye" in causing disability continue to exist (Hillman, 2003). Some cultural communities believe that disabilities are the result of punishment for past sins (Miller, 2005). In Samoa, a child born with a disability may be attributed to a poor relationship with God within the family (Mokuau & Tauili'ili, 2004). A summary of possible beliefs about the causes of disorder, disability, and illness can be found in Table 12-1.

Reactions and Acceptance

Where there is the belief that a disability is the result of punishment for past wrongs or sins, families may conceal family members with a disability (Miller, 2005). In Samoa, for example, because of the possibility of public embarrassment

TABLE 12-1 Traditional Beliefs about Perceived Causes of Disorder, Disability, and Illness

Belief	Culture	References
Punishment for past sins, transgressions in a previous life, bad deeds or sins committed by ancestors	Arab	Kulwicki (2008)
	Guatemalan	Ellis & Purnell (2008)
	Thai	Ross & Ross (2008)
	Chinese	Liu (2005)
	Jamaican	Miller (2005)
	Mexican	Santana-Martin & Santana (2005)
	Vietnamese	Hunt (2005)
	African American	Willis (2004)
	Filipino	Santos & Chan (2004)
	Southeast Asian	Jacob (2004); Groce & Zola (1993)
Trial that builds strength or cleanses past sins or wrongs	Arab	Ebrahim, as cited in Kulwicki (2008)
God's will or fate	Mexican	Santana-Martin & Santana (2005)
	Filipino	Santos & Chan (2004)
	Appalachian	Huttlinger & Purnell (2008)
Blessing or gift from God	Israeli Arab	Kulwicki (2008)
	Filipino	Pacquiao (2008)
Doing something wrong or improper self-care during pregnancy	Korean	Kip-Ripnow (2005)
	Filipino	Santos & Chan (2004)

and guilt and possible public scrutiny and ridicule, some families hide their children with a disability from the public (Mokuau & Tauili'ili, 2004). In Korea, children with disabilities are often stigmatized and kept out of the public or abandoned because of the lack of support services and prohibitive cost of care (Purnell & Paulanka, 2003).

Cultural views of disability may have a negative effect on self-disclosure during the assessment. In places where there is less acceptance of disability or significant stigma or shame, it may be difficult to obtain detailed information about a client's history and ability to communicate. Families

may also be less than truthful about all of the conditions surrounding the child and family. They may also be reluctant to come forward to seek services and clinical support.

Attitudes about Language Use

Family and community beliefs about language use can also vary as a function of wider community and social attitudes in the mainstream as well as their own home community. In communities where the family's use of a native language or bilingualism is viewed negatively, they may be hesitant to respond to questions during the interview about the use of any language at home other than what they perceive to be the most socially acceptable or valued language. As a result, when probing about language use patterns, clinicians need to ensure that they convey a sense of sincere interest in understanding how all languages are used as well as an open supportive attitude toward multiple language use. If families and individuals feel that information about their language used will be accepted openly, they will be more willing to disclose.

Clinicians should also be sensitive to the fact that some parents believe or have been counseled that their use of more than one language or a language other than the majority language has contributed to a child's language delay. It is still the case that some professionals continue to counsel families against using more than one language even when research such as that cited in Kohnert (2008) clearly shows that learning more than one language does not confuse children and that children with language delays are just as capable as their monolingual peers of learning more than one language.

Family Structures and Networks

Types of Family Structures and Networks

In recent years, there have been changes in the types of family structures and networks around the world. The traditional family unit in the United States has typically been the nuclear family, consisting of a married man and woman with one or more unmarried children. This traditional family unit, however, is changing in the United States. (U.S. Census Bureau, 2009). Families are becoming more varied, including married and unmarried couples, both men and women living alone or living together with or without children; single parents with children; and blended families consisting of two parents who have remarried or who are not married to each other, with children from their previous marriages or relationships, and male and female same-sex parents. Along with these changes has been an increased acceptance of divorce, non-marital cohabitation, unmarried parenthood, permanent non-marriage and voluntary childlessness.

In many other parts of the world as well as with some cultural communities within the United States, the typical family unit has been the extended family unit, typically consisting of grandparents, aunts, uncles, cousins, nieces, and nephews (Ting-Toomey & Chung, 2005, p. 88). In extended family households, it is very common for family members across two or three generations to live within the same household or within close proximity of each other. According to the U.S. Census Bureau (2009), in the United States 3.6% of families are multigenerational. In some cultural communities, the extended family unit also included nonbiologic kin. For example in Hispanic communities, the extended family can include "biological relatives and non-biological members who may be considered brother, sister, aunt, or uncle" (Purnell & Paulanka, 2003, p. 20).

The inclusion of nonbiologic kin within the family unit is also common in same-sex partnerships. These families consist of *fictive* kin that provide family, cultural, and social support networks for gay, lesbian, bisexual, and transgender individuals.

Gender and Family Roles and Decision Making

During the past couple of decades, there has been a significant shift in perspectives on gender equity and equality in some countries such as the United States. As a result, males and females are more likely to have equal status in the child-rearing or elder care. Despite these changes, there are still many parts of the world where the male continues to serve as the primary family representative for any matters concerning the family. For example, in Iran, where the traditional culture is still patriarchal and hierarchical, the father has the greatest authority for all family decisions. In the absence of the father, the oldest son has the primary authority. Older male siblings also have the authority to make decisions for younger siblings even with the father present (Hafizi & Lipson, 2003, p. 181). In more acculturated families, the roles are more flexible (Hafizi, Sayyedi, & Lipson, 2008). In other cultures, it will be the female. In still others, the decision will be shared equally between the males and females. In some communities, it is the grandparents rather than the parents who have this primary responsibility. In Haitian communities, when an individual has a disability, decisions regarding the most appropriate type of intervention or rehabilitation plan are made by the entire family, with each member of the extended family being consulted before a final decision is reached (Jacobson, 2005).

The individual who represents the family publicly in certain settings may not be the one who is charged with the primary responsibility of decision making in private. For example, in Middle East cultures, the man's status as head of the family is evident in public even though in private the wife typically wields tremendous influence in matters pertaining to home and children (Kulwicki, 2003). Although decision making about health care–related matters is egalitarian among many Hispanics at home, the male in the family is usually the spokesperson for the family in public (Purnell & Paulanka, 2003).

BOX 12-1 Strategies for Communicating Effectively with Families from Diverse Backgrounds

- Use a communication style that is likely to be valued and/or used by the family (e.g., indirect vs. direct, with more silence and pause vs. talk).
- Be attentive to how one's own nonverbal and verbal communication style is likely to be perceived.
- Pay attention to others' nonverbal communication signals but be careful with interpretations of signals that can vary in meaning cross-culturally.
- Be sensitive to the ways in which questions are worded; review wording and topics with interpreters/translators or some other type of cultural broker in advance.
- Do advance readings on possible cultural communication style differences and health care beliefs, but keep the diversity that exists within communities in mind.

Because of their complexity and variety, the roles of each member of the family may be less clear to clinicians. Clinicians may need to determine the most appropriate decision maker by addressing questions to all involved and watching for the individual who appears to take the lead most often. Questions and concerns may be addressed primarily to the individual who holds the legal or guardianship responsibility while still considering the comments and concerns of other family member participants.

Clinical Implications

There are a number of clinical implications for clinicians conducting the assessment with clients from different cultural backgrounds given some of the issues addressed in this chapter. One of the best strategies for addressing some of these differences is being prepared for the case history interview by researching in advance some of the possible communication and other cultural issues that may potentially affect the process using some of the resources provided at the end of this chapter. Professionals can also work closely with interpreters, translators, and other professionals who can serve as cultural brokers that are familiar with the communication norms of the community of the families served. A summary of other suggestions for communicating effectively with families from diverse cultural backgrounds around the world are presented in Box 12-1.

CASE HISTORY INTERVIEW WITH BILINGUAL AND MULTILINGUAL CLIENTS

A key component of the case history interview with CLD clients involves the types of questions that are used and the ways questions are worded. The types of questions used with clients who speak more than one language are also key to determining important issues, such as the primary languages for assessment and intervention. Obtaining input from significant others also helps clinicians determine how well a client is able to communicate according to the standards of his or her community. The purpose of this section is to provide an overview of key considerations to be taken into account when interviewing bilingual clients.

Interviewing Primary Caregivers of Bilingual and Multilingual Children

There are a number of key topics and questions that should be addressed when interviewing caregivers of bilingual child clients. The following section contains a summary of key topic and question considerations for the case history interview with caregivers. A list of possible questions can also found in Appendix 12-1.

Languages Spoken at Home

The case history interview with parents or caregivers of bilingual children should include questions that help determine the child's primary, dominant, most proficient, and most frequently used language. Questions should also focus on the child's language use across different communication partners and contexts. This information is useful for determining the language for assessment and intervention. Assessment should be done in a child's most proficient language and the one used most. However, it is also useful to conduct at least some part of the assessment (e.g., informal language sampling) in any other languages used to obtain the most accurate description of relative language strengths and weaknesses within and across languages. As previously mentioned in the section on language attitudes, clinicians need to be mindful of the potential sensitivity of probing for information about language(s) used in the home, especially when the languages used differ from the majority language of a county or region.

Language Exposure

Even in those cases in which a child is primarily exposed to English, it is helpful to know something about other languages used in the home because they can still affect the vocabulary used by the child. It is common for bilingual and multilingual child speakers to have their early vocabulary and concepts coded in one language but not the other receptively, expressively, or both. It is also important to know something about the primary languages of instruction that have been used for educating the child as well as during any previous speech and language intervention services.

Ratings of Language Proficiency

Another topic that should be addressed during the interview is the perceived levels of relative language proficiency across and within all languages spoken and understood. In addition, when identifying the language the child speaks most often, clinicians should determine which language the child speaks best. However, given that levels of language proficiency can vary within the same language across different domains of language, it is important to ask for separate ratings of abilities in different communication modalities within all languages spoken (e.g., vocabulary, sentence production, storytelling, and conversation) and across different language modalities (e.g., speaking, listening, reading, and writing).

Course of Language Development in All Languages Spoken

The developmental progress of each language spoken should also be included. This can be obtained by identifying the age at which first words were spoken in each language, the age at which sentences were produced in each language, and the current average length of sentences in each language. Identifying the average number of words used by a child in sentences in each language can also help clinicians determine the strongest language.

Nature of Communication Difficulties Observed in All Languages Spoken

A key focus of any case history interview is the types of communication difficulties observed and experienced. The same information should be obtained for bilingual children. The difference from monolingual language speakers is that whatever is asked about one language should be asked about any others spoken. Identifying areas of difficulty in more than one language helps to support a diagnosis of true impairment. There is an interdependent relationship or common underlying proficiency between the L1 and L2 in bilingual speakers (Roseberry-McKibbin, 2008). As a result, difficulties in one language are likely show to be similar in the second. This suggests that true disorders are likely to be evident in all languages spoken. Although there can be differences in the way in which an underlying disorder is expressed owing to language-specific characteristics of each language, the underlying nature of the difficulties is likely to be the same. As a result, the bilingual Spanish-English speaking child who uses velar fronting in English (e.g., "tat" for "cat") is likely to display the same problem in Spanish (e.g., "tortuda" for "tortuga").

Perceptions of Family and Other Speech Community Members

Being familiar with community standards for identifying individuals at risk for articulation/phonology, resonance, voice, fluency, swallowing, and hearing/balance disorders is emphasized in ASHA's (2004) Knowledge and Skills Statement for Providing Culturally and Linguistically Appropriate Services.

Understanding the communication standards of the community are helpful for distinguishing true disorders from speech and language differences, particularly when there are no existing published norms or standards for that child's language. Obtaining information about the perceptions of others close to the child helps to provide information about the expectations and standards of the client's language community.

Interviews with Bilingual and Multilingual Adult Clients

The types of questions that should be asked of bilingual and multilingual adult clients with suspected communication disorders are similar to those that should be asked when evaluating child clients with a few exceptions and additions. (See Appendix 12-2 for sample bilingual adult topics and questions.) In addition to those questions recommended in Appendix 12-2, clinicians may also review questions that are included in the Language Experience and Proficiency Questionnaire (LEAP-Q) for assessing the language proficiency, profiles, and background of adult multilingual speakers (Marian et al., 2007).

Languages Used across Communication Environments and Partners

Similar to child clients, interviews with adult bilingual and multilingual speakers should include questions about the languages that they currently use in the home and other relevant communication environments. With adults, these environments include work, school, and social community. The types of communication partners should include the spouse, partners, children, grandchildren, family caregivers, extended family, caregivers, and others residing in the home.

With individuals using alternative augmentative communication (AAC) devices and other nonvocal forms of communication, gathering information during the case history interview on current language use will also help determine not only the decisions of what languages to include in the assessment but also decisions about possible languages to be used when selecting the type of vocabulary and symbols to be used on the AAC device. With AAC devices that have voice output, identifying languages that might be used over the phone when communicating with family and friends in a home country can be useful in determining the most appropriate languages for assessment and intervention.

History of Language Exposure and Use

In addition to determining current language use and exposure, it is useful to explore a client's language history (e.g., languages spoken from childhood to adulthood). Questions should focus not only on exposure languages but also on when, how, and where the exposure occurred. Understanding a client's language history helps clinicians understand the client's present level of language proficiency and can play a role determining the most appropriate language for assessment.

If clients feel comfortable enough to disclose, it is also useful to obtain information about the client's history of residence since birth. This provides information for understanding a client's history of language exposure. This type of information may be a sensitive issue dependent on the client's immigration or refugee status. However, asking the client to provide a narrative of their life journey with a question such as, "Can you give me a brief history of how you came to this country, starting with your country of birth?" can serve as a neutral means for eliciting this information. It may also provide an extended monologue that can serve as a rich source of data for assessing the client's grammatical, speech sound production, and voice and fluency skills.

It is important to determine family and community perceptions of past and current communication ability. Asking questions such as, "When you were growing up, did any of your family or friends ever make comments about your speaking or communication skills?" can be useful for evaluating a client's communication abilities with respect to an existing speech community standard. The same type of question can be asked about current skills. For example, "Does anyone in your family make comments about your communication skills?" When clients share comments, such as, "My mother told me I have to rest my voice," or "Yes, people say they have trouble understanding me," or "I used to be teased when I was younger," they help to identify communication concerns that are more likely disorders than differences.

Language Use across Communication Environments and Partners

In addition to determining which languages are used, it is also useful to obtain some information on the extent to which the different languages are spoken within each environment and the percentage of time each language is used in various environments. This helps to determine not only the most appropriate languages for testing but also the functional advantages and significance of providing intervention in more than one language. For adults who plan to return to employment after a stroke, it is important to identify the language that they will need to use in the workplace. Although clinicians may initially begin with intervention in the client's strongest language after the stroke, intervention should eventually transition to incorporate at least some of the language the client will need for job-related responsibilities.

Determining the extent to which languages are used for social activities is also relevant. If a key aspect of a client's social life is church, the clinician needs to identify the language that is most often used as a part of church activities. Practicing words, phrases, and functional sentences that are used within that context using the language used most in that setting is a good strategy for promoting functional and relevant communication skills.

Ratings of Language Proficiency

With adult clients, it is useful to obtain self-ratings of their perceived levels of language proficiency across all domains of communication (e.g., speaking, listening, reading, and writing). When assessing the language abilities of clients whose communication skills have changed over time as the result of some type of neurological injury (e.g., stroke, traumatic injury), it is useful to ask for self-ratings of perceived language ability in all languages spoken before the injury compared with abilities after the stroke.

Nature of Communication Difficulties in All Languages Spoken

With adult clients, it is important to obtain descriptions of communication difficulties in each of the key languages spoken, including related issues, such as when the problem was first noticed in each language. Descriptions of the types of difficulties experienced in both languages should also be provided.

Levels of Education and Languages of Instruction

As with all adult clients, it is important to determine a client's level of education to identify the most appropriate reading level for any reading assessment tasks. Adults who are literate in one language may not be so in another. Therefore, it may not always be possible to test written language abilities in all languages spoken. A client's bilingual literacy experiences are often shaped by the primary languages of instruction used in their formal education. It is useful to obtain information about the languages used in their education.

THE PROCESS

CURRENT ASSESSMENT MODELS AND FRAMEWORKS

A number of different factors have influenced current perspectives and clinical practice as they relate to assessment of CLD clients in the United States and worldwide. The following is a brief summary of the regulatory, professional association standards, and research-based influences that have the greatest impact on shaping best practice

perspectives and paradigms in populations primarily in the United States but increasingly for other parts of the world as well.

Assessment Models and Frameworks

Culturally and Linguistically Diverse Child Populations

A number of models, assessment frameworks, and principles have been proposed for assessing child CLD clients. A brief overview of some of the most recent can be found in Box 12-2.

Although each of the frameworks presented in Table 12-1 varies slightly in terms of specific recommended considerations, each framework emphasizes the importance of a comprehensive assessment that generates a variety data, uses a variety of procedures and measures, is conducted in each of the languages spoken or understood by the client, and includes the case history interview, review of written documentation, observation, and both formal and informal measures. They all emphasize a move away from sole reliance on standardized tools for determining the presence of disorder and a growing reliance on dynamic, process-based procedures. They also emphasize the importance of assessing all languages spoken and understood.

Culturally and Linguistically Diverse Adult Populations

To date, there have been relatively few proposed models and frameworks for assessing adult CLD clients. Those that have been proposed have focused primarily on adult populations with cognitive-communication impairments resulting from neurologically based conditions such as stroke, traumatic brain injury, and Alzheimer disease. They have also stressed the importance of using approaches that are similar in many ways to those used with children. For example, when working with clients with neurologically based cognitive-communication impairments, Langdon (2008) recommends a comprehensive case history interview that includes information about a client's language use, exposure, and preferences. According to Langdon, the interview also helps to provide a "sociocultural appraisal" (p. 221) of clients and family concerns, beliefs, attitudes, and desires as they relate to the clinical service delivery. This enables clinicians to identify some of the underlying cultural beliefs that may affect how clients and families respond to recommended treatment plans and approaches resulting from the assessment process.

Langdon (2008) also emphasizes the importance of conducting assessments in all languages spoken and understood by the client using culturally and linguistically appropriate assessment measures (e.g., those that are adapted

---

BOX 12-2 Culturally and Linguistically Diverse Assessment Models and Frameworks

"RIOT"*

- **Review** relevant documents (e.g., school and medical/health records), client background information (e.g., cultural, language, family, social), and previous therapy/testing results.
- **Interview** the client and/or significant others (e.g., family members, teachers, peers) about the client's communication skills and abilities.
- **Observe** the client in multiple contexts with multiple partners.
- **Test** the client using multiple forms of assessment (e.g., formal and informal, language sampling, classroom-based authentic assessments, dynamic assessment).

"GRASP IT!"†

- **Gather:** Gather the necessary information.
- **Review:** Examine what you find and determine what else is needed.
- **Ask:** Interview teachers, family members, and/or members of the community to provide you with information to help you determine the significance of the assessment results.
- **See:** Observe the student in multiple settings with different partners.
- **Proceed:** Determine the next step (e.g., information to help design effective instruction, need for additional English language development support).
- **Integrate:** Analyze the data and integrate all of the relevant data that has been reviewed.
- **Test:** Undertake formal and informal assessments to complete the picture.

"Ecologically Valid Assessment"‡

- Thorough case history interview
- Formal assessment in L1 and L2 using standardized tests as appropriate
- Informal assessments in L1 and L2 using checklists, criterion-referenced assessments, language sampling, authentic performance-based assessments
- Dynamic assessments
- Observation in naturalistic environments (e.g.,,, classroom, recess, lunch, library, home)
- Proficiency testing in L1 and L2 to determine level of language ability in both (e.g., BICs and CALP)

BICs, Basic interpersonal communication skills; CALP, cognitive academic language proficiency; L1, language 1; L2, language 2.
*Data from Cheng, L. L. (2012). Asian and Pacific American cultures. In D. E. Battle (Ed.), *Communication disorders in multicultural and international populations* (4th ed). Boston: Butterworth-Heinemann.
†Data from Lewis, N., Castilleja, N., Moore, B. J., & Rodriquez, B. (2010, July). Assessment 360°: A Panoramic framework for assessing English language learners. *Perspectives on Communication Disorders and Sciences in Culturally and Linguistically Diverse Populations, 17,* 37-56.
‡Data from Roseberry-McKibbin, E. (2008). *Multicultural students with special language needs: Practical strategies for assessment and intervention* (3rd ed). Oceanside, CA: Academic Communication Associates.

---

for or normed on the populations with which they are to be used). Medical data and records from relevant radiologic and technologic tests (e.g., computed tomography [CT] and magnetic resonance imaging [MRI]) are also recommended to help substantiate the presence of a disorder. Using medical information helps minimize the possibility of misdiagnosis owing to possible underlying cultural-linguistic differences.

According to Kohnert (2008), when assessing CLD adults, a holistic disability framework, such as the International Classification of Functioning, Disability, and Health (ICF) developed by the World Health Organization (2001) should be used. This framework is designed for use in classifying the functional impact of any type of disability on an individual's ability to participate in meaningful activities and daily interactions with others in their social and family networks. Family and social networks can include immediate family, friends, personal care providers, neighbors, community members, and health care providers.

Using the ICF model, clinicians can examine the follow-through case history interview and observation of interactions conducted in all languages spoken from a cross-cultural perspective:

1. The types of cultural communication patterns that exist among members of the client's social communication network, including the types of languages typically used during social interactions with the client
2. The specific attitudes and beliefs that are held by members of the support network on issues such as communication, language use, and disability
3. Social communication expectations that members have for that client and how well that individual is capable of performing in line with those expectations

The information generated from this type of assessment is particularly useful for identifying the components of disorder that go beyond culture and language to be targeted as part of an individual's intervention plan. It also helps to pinpoint possible cultural communication differences displayed by the individual and others in their social network that can affect successful communicative interactions and the intervention process in general.

Professional Association Knowledge, Skills Expectations

In 2004, ASHA published guidelines on the knowledge, skills, and competencies for providing culturally linguistically appropriate and responsive services. The document includes important culturally and linguistically appropriate considerations for assessing different disorder areas including language, articulation, resonance, voice, fluency, swallowing, and hearing and balance. They also provide guidelines for making distinction between a disorder and a difference. A summary of sample competencies related to the issue of CLD assessments can be found in Table 12-2.

Federal and State Special Education Mandates

Federal Mandates

The final regulations of the Individuals with Disabilities Education Improvement Act (IDEIA) (2006) commonly known as IDEA (Individuals with Disabilities Education Improvement Act PL 108-446) (2004) reinforce key principles associated with the assessment children with disabilities. The law has several provisions specifically tailored to

the assessment of CLD children (Sec. 300.304). Examples include the following:

1. Local educational agencies must not use any single measure or assessment as the sole criterion for determining whether the child has a disability and for determining the most appropriate educational setting or program [Sec. 300.304 (b) (2)].
2. When interpreting evaluation data to determine whether a child has a disability, public agencies are required to draw on information from a variety of sources, including aptitude and achievement tests, parent input, and teacher recommendations, as well as information about the child's . . . social or cultural background . . ." [Sec. 300.306 (c) (1) (i)].
3. Assessments must be administered in the child's native language or other mode of communication.
4. A child must not be determined to be a child with a disability if the determinant factor is limited English proficiency [Sec. 300.306 (a) (2) (iii)].
5. States can use other alternative research based procedures to identify children with specific learning disabilities (U.S. Department of Education, Office of Special Education Programs) (2006, October 4). This provides additional support for the use of assessments other than or in addition to standardized tests for making eligibility decisions.
6. Assessments under IDEIA are also to be conducted in the form most likely to yield accurate information on what the child knows and can do academically, developmentally,

TABLE 12-2 Knowledge and Skills Needed by Speech-Language Pathologists and Audiologists to Provide Culturally and Linguistically Appropriate Services

Area	Knowledge/Skill
Language	Recognizing "inherent cultural and linguistic biases" in test materials (5.2 A) Inherent problems using translated tests (5.2 C) Appropriate use of alternative assessments (5.2 D) Potential impact of cultural and linguistic bias on differential diagnosis (5.2 E)
Articulation and phonology	Current research and best practices in identification/assessment of articulation/phonological disorders in the client's language(s)/dialect(s) (7.0 A) Phonemic and allophonic variations of language(s)/dialect(s) spoken by the client (7.0 B) Differentiating between disorder, accent, dialect, transfer patterns, and typical development (7.0 C) Standards of the client's speech community Determining what is typical in the client's speech community (7.0 D)
Resonance, voice, fluency	Community standards of typical resonance, voice, and/or fluency patterns (9.0)
Swallowing	Community standards of typical swallowing/feeding patterns and preferences (10.0)
Hearing, balance	Culturally and linguistically appropriate assessment materials, tools, and methods (11.0 C) Inherent problems in using speech testing materials (e.g., word lists, speech discrimination lists) that have been translated (11.0 D) Influences of language and speech differences including issues related to bilingualism and dialectal differences on hearing evaluation decisions such as in speech recognition tests (11.0 E)

Adapted from American Speech-Language-Hearing Association. (2004). Knowledge and skills needed by speech-language pathologists and audiologists to provide culturally and linguistically appropriate services. Retrieved from www.asha.org/docs/html/KS2004-00215.html.

and functionally. For CLD child populations, this emphasizes the importance of considering what a child knows and needs not only for school but also for the home language environment.

Collectively, these mandates emphasize the importance of a comprehensive culturally appropriate assessment using various and alternative forms of assessment conducted in the native language of the child and taking into account possible other cultural-linguistic differences when making final eligibility decisions. The Act also requires states to track, monitor, and review on an ongoing basis ethnicity and race data for evidence of any disproportionality. This highlights the need for assessments not to overrefer and to be accurate in making final special education eligibility and placement decisions.

IDEIA also contains revised eligibility guidelines for identifying whether or not a child has a specific learning disability. According to IDEIA regulations 34 CFR 300.8 (c) (10), when attempting to determine whether a child has a specific learning disability, a state must permit the use of a process based on the child's response to scientific, research-based intervention. The regulations ushered in a new model of educational assessment, instruction, and intervention known as Response to Intervention (RTI). RTI is a multi-tiered approach that involves ongoing assessment, individualized instruction, and intervention tailored to meet specific student needs using research-validated methods of instruction that incorporate compensatory learning strategies and classroom environment accommodations as needed. It is now being used in many public school settings as a primary strategy for determining eligibility for special education services. (See Chapter 14 for a further discussion of RTI.)

Part of the impetus for this proposed model of intervention was the growing concern about the number of students being inappropriately identified as having a disability. This includes concerns about the overrepresentation of minority students in special education (Rudebusch, 2007). Ongoing and multitiered assessment, progress monitoring, and the use of individualized, curriculum-based and intensive research-based interventions are one way for achieving this goal.

State Mandates

Federal special education law has an impact on state educational regulations. As an example, the State of California has no reference to the use of standardized tests for determining a child's eligibility for services due to a language or speech disorder. Eligibility is instead defined fairly broadly as "difficulty understanding or using spoken language to such an extent that it adversely affects his or her educational performance" (California Education Code, Section 56333-56338, § 1). It establishes criteria, such as "inappropriate or inadequate acquisition, comprehension, or expression of spoken language such that the pupil's language performance level is found to be significantly below the language performance level of his or her peers" (California Education Code, Section 56333-56338, § 5). This enables assessors to use their own professional judgment in the assessment measures and procedures used.

The California and other state guidelines for selecting assessment materials and procedures mirror federal regulations. For example, under the state's educational code, tests are to be "selected and administered so as not to be racially, culturally, or sexually discriminatory" and "provided in the pupil's native language . . . unless it is clearly not feasible to do so" (California Education Code, Section 56320-56331, § 2).

Changing Assessment Perspectives and Paradigms

Since the early 1990s, there has been a paradigm shift in views about assessment in a number of different professional fields that have affect not only speech and language assessment but also educational and psychological assessment. Part of the driving force behind paradigm shift has been the need for more culturally sensitive procedures that can be used with an increasingly diverse client population.

Process-Dependent Measures

A major paradigm shift has been toward the use of process-dependent assessments. Processing tasks and assessments are always part of the recommended assessment battery with adult as well as child clients with cognitive-linguistic impairments, including those with suspected learning disability and language disorder.

Process-dependent assessments bypass some of the problems inherent in the assessment of CLD populations. Campbell and coworkers (1997) suggest that process-dependent measures can minimize the inherent bias of language assessment by minimizing the potential impact of prior experience and world knowledge on performance. They state that whenever "test-takers differ in their exposure to concepts, words, or activities" as a function of various ethnic, cultural or socioeconomic factors, any assessment tool that taps into their "existing store of knowledge runs the risk of confusing 'difference' with 'disorder.'" (Campbell et al., p. 520). In contrast to "knowledge-based" measures that rely more heavily on prior language knowledge and experience, process-dependent measures rely more heavily on psycholinguistic processing, which is less dependent on prior language knowledge and exposure. Campbell and coworkers (1997) compared the test performances of minority and nonminority subjects on one traditional knowledge-dependent and three processing-dependent language measures. Their results revealed significantly lower scores by minority participants than majority subjects on the knowledge-dependent measure but no differences between the two subject populations on the three processing-dependent measures.

Engle and associates (2008) had similar outcomes when comparing the performances of 20 Brazilian children from low-income families and children from families of higher socioeconomic status on measures of vocabulary and working memory. No significant group differences were found on the working memory measure. However, children from the lower socioeconomic group obtained significantly lower scores on measures of expressive and receptive vocabulary.

Fast-mapping or quick incidental learning tasks are examples of process-dependent measures that have been recommended for use with CLD populations. These tasks, which Hwa-Froelich and colleagues (2000) refer to as "language learnability tasks" focus more on language potential than static language knowledge.

Incidental word learning tasks have often been used to examine how quickly, easily, and well children are able to figure out the meaning of novel, nonsense, or unfamiliar words simply through exposure without any formal teaching. According to Brackenbury and Pye (2005), the use of incidental word learning tasks can be beneficial for assessing children from diverse backgrounds because, like other processing-dependent measures, they minimize the potential influence of factors such as sociocultural history, language differences, and socioeconomic status. Such tasks discriminate between children from diverse linguistic backgrounds with and without specific language impairment (Hwa-Froelich et al., 2000). Fast-mapping novel verb, real verb, and morpheme learning tasks have been proposed as a viable alternative method for assessing word knowledge in CLD children with possible semantic-based deficits (Hwa-Froelich & Matsuo, 2005; Johnson, 2010).

The *Diagnostic Evaluation of Language Variation (DELV) Norm Referenced* (Seymour et al., 2005), which is designed for differentiating difference from disorder in mainstream American English (MAE) and non-MAE speakers, contains subtests based on this fast-mapping procedure.

Dynamic Assessment

Dynamic assessment measures examine performance over time using a test-teach-retest paradigm to evaluate learning potential. Several researchers have proposed dynamic assessment as an alternative to traditional static language assessments for CLD clients (Peña et al., 1992; 2001). For example, Peña and colleagues (1992) compared the performance of African American and Puerto Rican Head Start preschool children on the *Expressive One Word Picture Vocabulary Test* (Gardner, 1979) following a brief 20-minute mediated learning/intervention session. They found significant improvement in test performance by typically developing children following a 20-minute intervention session. However, the children who were

predetermined to have possible underlying language learning difficulties based on classroom observations, parent and teacher feedback, and clinical judgment showed little improvement following the mediated intervention session, suggesting that their difficulties could not be attributed solely to differences in exposure, experience, or environment.

Similar research conducted by Roseberry and Connell (1991) and Hwa-Froelich and colleagues (2000) also found this method to accurately discriminate between children from differing cultural-linguistic backgrounds with and without language impairment. According to Rosa-Lugo and associates (2010), dynamic assessment can play a crucial role in identifying school-aged English language learners with possible language learning difficulties within the context of RTI methods of identification described in the next section.

General Best Practice Assessment Considerations for Culturally and Linguistically Diverse Clients

Each of the previously described assessment considerations is essential for best practice assessment procedures with CLD populations. They have implications for how to select, administer, score, and interpret formal as well as informal language assessment measures. The following is a summary of key considerations for bilingual, nonstandard, or mainstream dialect speakers as well as monolingual speakers of other languages both within the United States and in other parts of the world.

Reviewing and Selecting Appropriate Standardized Assessment Tests

Test Standardization Sample

For all clients, regardless of their cultural or linguistic background, clinicians need to carefully review the appropriateness of tests in light of their normative sample. Most speech and language tests published in the United States, for example, are normed on populations that mirror the demographic makeup of the United States, with the majority of individuals being from white, middle-class, MAE-speaking backgrounds. This means that individuals from other backgrounds are often in the minority or are not represented in the standardization sample. As a result, normative standards and acceptable test item responses are likely to be based primarily on the performance of majority group members. The performance of members in underrepresented groups is likely to be masked by that of the larger group. Therefore, simply including a small number of individuals from CLD backgrounds within the standardization sample is insufficient for making a test culturally and linguistically appropriate. In addition, most tests make no mention of the language-dialect status of participating subjects, making it difficult to determine a test's appropriateness for use with other populations.

A common problem that occurs when using standardized tests is test bias. Test bias can occur when using tests that contain items or theoretical frameworks based on research from other cultural-linguistic groups and can occur in a variety of forms. Research on the potential test bias of using certain vocabulary tests with African American children has been published (Champion et al., 2003; McCabe & Champion, 2010; Qi et al.; Restrepo et al., 2006; Stockman, 2000). Examples of possible test bias influences can be found in Table 12-3.

Because of test bias, clinicians should select tests that are specifically designed for and normed on the specific language population for which they are to be used. It is not enough to select a test that simply includes individuals from the cultural-linguistic community with whom it is to be used. For example, a test that includes a standardization sample comprised of only 5% American Indian does not make it appropriate for use with American Indians because the norms for test performance will continue to be based primarily on the performance of the largest majority group in the sample. This majority is usually white Americans.

Using a test that includes individuals who self-identify as a certain ethnic group (e.g., Hispanic/Latino) during the standardization process also does not make the test appropriate for use with all members of that population. Hispanic/Latino includes several subgroups such as Puerto Rican, Mexican American, Cuban American, and Salvadorian unless it is specifically normed with sufficient members of each sub group. The normative sample may not also differentiate between individuals from different socioeconomic backgrounds and geographic regions. Hispanics in the United States, like any other group, also differ in their language use and exposure patterns. Some are monolingual or predominantly Spanish speaking. Others are monolingual or predominantly English speaking. Others are more balanced in terms of their language use. In addition, there is diversity in the Spanish dialects spoken as well as regional differences in the sound and grammatical rules of each dialect. The Spanish used by Mexican Spanish speakers from Texas differs from that spoken by individuals in New Mexico, Florida, California, and New York. As a result, even tests that are designed for use with Spanish-speaking populations have to accommodate the different patterns of responses that might be produced by Spanish-speaking test takers from differing regional and dialect backgrounds. If a test is primarily normed on Hispanic groups in the United States, it may also not be appropriate for use with individuals who live in Hispanic/Latino communities outside of the United States.

As a result, of these differences, to the extent possible, clinicians should attempt to search for tests that are primarily normed on the specific cultural-language group with which they are to be used, while also accommodating possible dialect differences.

The administration manual should also provide detailed information on the demographic characteristics of the standardization sample (e.g., the cultural-racial-ethnic makeup, the language exposure and dominance of participating subjects, and dialects spoken). In cases in which the demographic makeup differs from that of the test taker, clinicians need to be cautious in making final clinical decisions based on test scores and consider including caution statements in their written reports about the accuracy of those scores. An example of a cautionary statement is as follows:

These results should be interpreted with caution given that the test was standardized on individuals from a different language background from X. As a result, test scores may not provide the most accurate assessment of his/her language ability.

TABLE 12-3 Common Forms of Test Bias

Type of Bias	Description
Linguistic bias	Can occur when using test items that assess speech sounds and grammatical rules/forms/structures that do not exist in the client's native language/dialect and/or that exist but operate differently within that language/dialect from the one in which a test is given
Format bias	Can occur when using testing procedures, formats, items, and vocabulary that are not familiar to the client due to differing cultural-linguistic experiences, exposure, and/or socialization influences
Value bias	Can occur when the scoring for test items give more credit, value, or weight/worth to responses that are acceptable/correct in some cultural-linguistic populations but not others
Situational bias	Can occur when the social/situational dynamics of the testing situation affect the responsiveness of clients (e.g., topic initiation or verbal elaboration) from certain cultural backgrounds due to differing sociocultural norms (rules for adult-child conversation)

Data from Taylor, O. L., & Payne, K. (1983). Culturally valid testing: A proactive approach. *Topics in Language Disorders, 3,* 8-20; Vaughn-Cooke, F. (1986). The challenge of assessing the language of non-mainstream speakers. In O. L. Taylor (Ed.), *Treatment of communicative disorders in culturally and linguistically diverse populations* (pp. 23-48). San Diego: College-Hill Press.

Alternatively, clinicians can provide a descriptive summary of test performance without reporting scores. This summary can include a brief overview of language strengths and weaknesses using an item analysis framework. An example of a report without scores is as follows:

Test scores are not reported because this test was primarily normed on individuals from a different language background and may therefore not provide the most accurate assessment of his/her ability. A descriptive analysis of test performance, however, revealed the following patterns of strength and weakness. X performed best on one-step (60% accuracy) compared with two- (40%) and three-step (20%) commands. . . .

Translated or Adapted Tests

When assessing bilingual and monolingual speakers, clinicians should use assessments that are specifically developed for use with the language and culture of the client. They should also select tests that include guidelines for scoring responses in languages other than English, code-mixed responses, and possible dialect-influenced variations. Information about the language exposure, use, and proficiency levels of individuals in the standardization sample should also be included.

In cases in which there is no existing test for a given language group, clinicians may consider developing or using a translated or adapted version of that test. Clinicians need to be careful, however, when selecting or using tests that are translations of existing tests for a number of different reasons, including those outlined in Box 12-3.

Published translated and adapted tests should meet accepted guidelines, such as those developed by the International Test Commission (ITC) originally developed in 1992 and revised in 2010 (ITC, 2010). The guidelines were intended for test developers and publishers; however, they apply to clinicians who may attempt to adapt or translate a published test for use with a particular population. Among the ITC Guidelines are the following:

C1: The effects of cultural difference that are relevant or important to the main purpose of the test or instrument should be minimized to the extent possible.

D1: Test developers and publishers should ensure that the adaptation process takes full account of the linguistic and cultural differences among populations for whom the adapted versions of the test or instrument are intended.

D2: Test developers or publishers should provide evidence that the language used in directions, rubrics, and items, as well as in the handbook, is appropriate for all cultural and linguistic populations for whom the test or instrument is intended.

D65: Test developers and publishers should ensure that data collected permit the use of appropriate statistical techniques to establish item equivalence between different language versions of the test of instrument.

E1: When the test of instrument is adapted for use with other populations, test developers and publishers should document changes to ensure the test and instrument are equivalent.

According to Kwan and coworkers (2010) and Hambleton and de Jong, (2003), there are a number of test equivalence issues that need to be taken into consideration, including *linguistic equivalence* (e.g., accurately worded using translation and back-translation procedures), *conceptual equivalence* (e.g., making sure that a certain concept or construct exists across different groups), *functional equivalence* (controlling for behaviors that may differ in interpretation across cultures), and *metric equivalence* (e.g., making sure that scores yield similar distributions across groups).

One way for establishing *conceptual or cultural equivalence* is to use a simultaneous process of translation whereby a tool is developed for use with more than one language in its first stage of development. Kim and colleagues (2005) used this method for establishing conceptual or cultural equivalence of American English and Spanish versions of the Pediatric GERD Caregiver Impact Questionnaire (PGCIQ). They used this method of translation with focus group input from both populations to create a tool that was less susceptible to cultural differences than one developed in one language and followed by translation into other languages. Their goal of using this approach was to reduce possible item and construct bias. Their strategy also addresses the ITC recommendation that test developers and publishers provide evidence that item content and stimulus materials are familiar to all intended populations.

The ITC recommendations also state that appropriate statistical techniques be applied to establish equivalence for different test versions and identify problematic components of a test that may be inadequate to one or more of the intended populations. A good example of how statistical

---

BOX 12-3 Common Problems Associated with Translated Tests

- Some translated tests are simple translations that do not modify test items, content, or format to adjust for possible cultural test bias influences.
- Some translated tests continue to use norms from the group on which the test was originally standardized.
- It is not always possible to translate certain grammatical structures or linguistic concepts into other languages.
- Translations can change the age or difficulty level of test items.
- Test items that are clinically significant in one language (e.g., that assess language structures and behaviors that serve as a sign of disorder in one language or dialect) may not be clinically significant for differentiating difference from disorder in another.

modeling can be used to assess and improve the validity of a translated measure can be found in the report by Mokkink and colleagues (2010), who used a graded response model to develop a valid and translation of the six scales from the Communication Profile for the Hearing Impaired into Dutch.

Another key recommendation is that the test adaptations take full account of linguistic and cultural differences among the populations for whom the adapted version is intended. There are a number of different ways that tests can be adapted. Items can be deleted, modified, or added. Adaptations in some cases can also include the use of different picture stimuli, making them more culturally relevant. For example, when developing an assessment measure to collect normative data on the narrative productions of Cantonese speakers, Pak-Hin and Law (2004) adapted pictures from two commonly used aphasia tests to reflect Chinese scenes. Adaptations like these ensure that test performance is not hindered by possible differences in cultural knowledge, exposure, or familiarity.

In other cases, adaptations can involve the more linguistic elements of an item such as the sound-syllable word structure. Ebert and associates (2008) discuss the importance of this when developing nonword repetition tasks in different languages. Even though the stimuli used for such tasks are nonmeaningful words, they still need to correspond to the language-specific phonotactic patterns of the target language. For example, when developing stimuli for a Spanish nonword repetition task, Ebert and associates (2008) noted the importance of using stimuli that used the most frequent syllable structure in Spanish (CV), contained sounds based on their overall frequency or occurrence in Spanish, and used patterns in which the penultimate syllable received primary stress. Because the average length of Spanish words is longer than that of English words, they stressed the importance of including stimuli up to five syllables long, in contrast to the maximum four-syllable length used in English nonword repetition tasks.

In some cases, clinicians may have to use tests or instruments normed for speakers of a majority language or dialect different from that of the client. In this case, clinicians may consider using test administration and scoring modifications such as those listed in Box 12-4. Testing modifications such as using alternative scoring of productions take normal dialect and language differences into account and may provide more accurate assessment of speech-language abilities. It can also decrease the likelihood that speakers are penalized for normal dialect differences, as was found by Laing (2003) in her study of African American English (AAE) child speakers' test performance on two standard articulation tests using two different modes of scoring (standard response vs. alternate response modes).

Caution should be used, however, when considering any of the modifications listed in the table because they can affect test item difficulty, validity, and reliability. Although modified testing procedures can be still be useful

---

BOX 12-4 Possible Test Administration and Scoring Modifications

- Increase the number of practice items to ensure that a client understands what they are being asked to do.
- Reword instructions/test item prompts (e.g., "point to" vs. "show") in a way that does not cue or change the type of knowledge that is being assessed if the client appears to be having difficulty understanding what you want him or her to do.
- Change the format of the item prompt (e.g., from a sentence completion format to a question format) in a way that does not cue or change the type of knowledge that is being assessed if the client appears to be having difficulty understanding what you want him or her to do. Example: "A ___ and ___ are alike because. . . ." → "How are a ____ and ____ alike?"
- Allow additional response time.
- Accept and score as correct any responses to items produced in a second less proficient language or dialect taking normal other language or dialect differences into account.
- Accept and score as correct any culturally appropriate responses.
- Translate any missed items presented in one language into the other language and then using a dual language or conceptual scoring approach with responses produced correctly in at least one language scored as correct.
- Allow the client to name items missed on a receptive vocabulary test to determine whether they would have known the item under a different label.
- Allow the client to explain why an "incorrect" answer was selected.
- Record all responses, including extra comments, revised responses, and explanations for later review by someone who is familiar with the cultural-linguistic norms of the client's community.
- Develop and use local norms for the cultural-linguistic community of the client.
- Continue testing above the ceiling to rule out item familiarity and other possible forms of test bias as a possible factor in the client's performance.

Data from Goldstein, B. (2000). *Resource guide on cultural and linguistic diversity.* San Diego: Delmar Learning; Kayser, H. (1998). *Assessment and intervention resource for Hispanic children.* San Diego: Singular; Peña, E. D., & Kester, E. S. (2004). Semantic development in Spanish-English bilinguals: Theory, assessment and intervention. In B. A. Goldstein (Ed.), *Bilingual language development and disorders in Spanish-English speakers* (pp. 105-130). Baltimore: Paul H. Brookes; Wyatt, T. A. (2002). Assessing the communicative abilities of clients from diverse cultural and language backgrounds. In D. E. Battle (Ed.), *Communication disorders in multicultural populations* (3rd ed) (pp. 415-450). Boston: Butterworth-Heinemann.

in providing information on what a client knows and is capable of producing, such modifications (except when specified as appropriate in the test manual) violate established testing procedures. It is not appropriate to report test scores but is instead more appropriate to either provide a criterion-referenced descriptive analysis of test performance or to include a caution statement regarding interpretation, reliability, and validity of testing outcomes. Before implementing, clinicians should therefore carefully review the test manual for instructions on whether modifications can be made and, if so, which and how. Any modifications used that differ from those recommended should be reported in the evaluation report with a descriptive, criterion-referenced description of test performance compared with scores and a careful description of the modifications or adaptations that were made.

Assessing Non–Mainstream Dialect Speakers

Test review and selection considerations for non–mainstream dialect speakers are similar to those used for bilingual and monolingual speakers of other languages when choosing an assessment measure for individuals who speak a dialect that differs from the mainstream or standard dialect. Key considerations include attempting to use tests that are specifically designed for use or appropriately normed on the dialect group with which it is to be used. Alternatively, clinicians can use tests that accommodate or provide information on possible dialect differences by providing separate scoring guidelines or criteria for differing dialect variations or by providing reference tables of possible dialect differences to be considered when scoring test items, as in the *Clinical Evaluation of Language Fundamentals,* 4th edition (Semel et al., 2003) Preschool Language Scale, 5th edition, by Semel and associates [2011] and the *Structured Photographic Expressive Language Test, 3rd Edition* (Dawson et al., 2003). Additional examples include the following:

- A special version of the CELF-4 for Australia and New Zealand that accommodates cultural and dialect differences between the English spoken in the United States and these two other countries.
- The *Diagnostic Evaluation of Language Variation (DELV) Screening Test* (Seymour et al., 2003b) and the *DELV—Norm Referenced* (Seymour et al., 2005) are measures for use with speakers from differing dialect backgrounds. The same is true of the *DELV-Criterion Referenced* which was published as an earlier version of the *DELV-Norm Referenced*. The *DELV Screening Test* and *DELV Criterion Referenced Test* were predominantly normed on African American child speakers who use AAE. African American and non-African American MAE speakers were also included in the standardization sample. The normative sample for the *DELV-Norm Reference* in contrast was based on the 2000 U.S. Census population in terms of gender, race/ethnicity, region, and

parental education. As a result, African American children only make up 16% of its sample. AAE child speakers make up 8%. The potential for cultural-linguistic test bias influences, however, is still minimal because this test has the same format and all but a few of the same items as the DELV Criterion-Reference. In addition, the test scoring performance of AAE and MAE speakers was found to be equivalent for both dialect groups across all age ranges on non-contrastive tasks during initial tryout research development. Sampling of 80 typically developing children from four different American English dialect backgrounds (Appalachian English, Cajun English, Southern English, and Spanish-Influenced English) revealed patterns of responses similar (all except the Spanish-Influenced English group) to those produced by MAE and AAE speakers on both the screening and norm-referenced tests (Seymour et. al., 2003, 2005). Collectively, these findings support the appropriateness of this test for use with speakers from a variety of different American English speaking backgrounds.

The following are additional ways that the DELV accommodates dialect differences. *DELV* test items control for possible dialect-based grammatical and speech sound differences by focusing on either non-dialect-specific or noncontrastive aspects of language use (aspects of grammar and phonology that operate similarly in MAE and AAE (Roeper, 2004; Seymour, 2004; Seymour et. al., 2003a, 2005). Test prompts, testing format, and picture stimuli were also designed to minimize potential cultural bias by ensuring that children in the standardization sample from both dialect groups responded to the prompts as desired. The test provides very specific cueing and prompting modifications for children who do not understand the task after basic instructions are given. In addition, as previously indicated, process-dependent fast-mapping novel and fast mapping real verb tasks were incorporated to control for possible differences in word exposure and familiarity (J. deVilliers, 2004; Seymour et al., 2005). There is also a subtest to assess narrative coherence and cohesion, which show a common developmental pattern across languages and dialects (P. deVilliers, 2004). The *DELV—Norm Reference* also provides scoring that can be adjusted for differences in parent education level.

One additional unique characteristic of the *DELV Screening Test* is that it not only provides information about a child's language disorder risk status (e.g., "lowest risk," "low to medium risk," "medium to high risk," or "highest risk"). It takes into consideration the range of linguistic variation that exists within dialect communities by generating a score that assesses degree of language variation (Seymour et al., 2003a). This score allows clinicians to identify whether a child displays strong variation or some variation from MAE or uses MAE.

Similar adjustments for possible dialect differences are also important for language tests that assess languages other than English. Examples of Spanish tests that make accommodations for possible dialect differences include the following:

- Wiig Assessment of Basic Concepts (WABC)—Spanish [Prueba de Conceptos Básicos Wiig] (Wiig & Langdon, 2006);
- The Expressive One-Word Picture Vocabulary Test, Spanish-Bilingual edition (Brownell, 2001);
- The Preschool Language Scale, Fourth Edition, Spanish (Zimmerman et al., 2002).

Assessing Culturally and Linguistically Diverse Infants and Toddlers

When assessing infants and toddlers who are in the earliest stages of language development (e.g., 0 to 3 years), the issue of test bias may be slightly less problematic because of the universal nature of many early speech and language developmental milestones (e.g., babbling, cooing, first communicative gestures, first words, and two word utterances). As a result, it is perhaps less of a problem to use a developmental assessment that focuses on such behaviors with a variety of different child language populations.

There are some communication behaviors, however, that can vary cross-culturally in use, frequency, age level, or nature. It is therefore important for a test that has equivalent language versions in two or more languages to make sure that items included on each version are appropriate for use with the specific language populations. One reason for this is that even when differing versions of a test include the same items, the tested behaviors may have occur at differing age ranges for different groups. For example, on the English version of the *Preschool Language Scale-Fourth Edition* (*PLS-4*) by Zimmerman and associates (2002), the ability to identify body parts is found in the 18- to 23-month age range. The same item, however, is found in the 24- to 29-month age range on the PLS-4 Spanish version (Zimmerman et al., 2002) of this test. Similar age level differences can be found with other later developing items such as identifying colors. There are also some test items and sounds that are assessed on the English version of the *PLS-4, English* but not the *PLS-4, Spanish,* and vice versa owing to normal language differences.

In some cases, it may be appropriate to give an assessment in more than one language to capture the full range of language ability. For example, Kohnert (2008) notes that although there are more than 50 different language versions of the *McArthur-Bates Communicative Development Inventories* (Finsen et al., 1993), it is may be best to use more than one language version with children who are bilingual and to combine the results from the different inventories to "capture the full extent of a child's language abilities" (p. 131).

Alternative Sources of Data

In those cases in which tests are not appropriate, clinicians may need to rely more heavily on other sources of assessment data beyond standardized tests. Other sources of data may include observations of communicative effectiveness during naturalistic interactions with speakers in all languages spoken, medical and educational record reviews, process-dependent and dynamic assessments, and speech-language sampling completed in all languages spoken by the client with or without the assistance of a trained interpreter and translator. For adult clients, the case history interview can be used as source of data by generating speech and language samples that can be analyzed for patterns of disorder and difference.

Another key source of data for clients with disorders resulting from underlying physical pathology or etiology is the use of instrumental, neurological, and other medical procedures that help diagnose the physical causes of the disorder. These procedures will be equally useful regardless of a client's cultural or language background. Examples include MRI, CT, modified barium swallow assessment, and videoendoscopy. Although instrumental procedures can be invaluable in helping clinicians to identify the source of a client's communication or swallowing difficulties and help to determine the presence of a true disorder or deficit, clinicians may find the use of and access to these technologies limited dependent on their geographic location. Clinicians may need to rely on more informal assessments, clinical observations, and family reports of prestatus and post-status abilities.

Additional Disorder-Specific Testing Considerations for Culturally and Linguistically Diverse Clients

The following are additional disorder-specific assessment considerations that should be taken into account when assessing individuals from CLD backgrounds.

Neurologically Based Cognitive-Communication Disorders

For CLD clients with neurologically based cognitive-communication disorders, Langdon (2008) recommends that clinicians look for culturally and linguistically appropriate assessment tools that can be used with diverse as well as mainstream clients. Cited examples include the *Reliable Assessment Inventory of Neuro-Behavioral Organization* (RAINBO) (Wallace, 1997), a comprehensive, culturally inclusive assessment system that includes 10 tests that examine a range of different cognitive, linguistic, pragmatic, oral-motor, and swallowing skills and includes adaptations for speakers of non-MAE dialects, including AAE, Hawaiian pidgin dialect, and Appalachian English as well as language influences from 28 other languages. The *Functional Assessment of Communication Skills* (FACS) (Frattali et al., 1995), also cited by Langdon (2008), is a functional outcomes measure designed to evaluate communication and swallowing skills and impairments in adults and adolescents who have incurred stroke and brain injury due to other causes. The FACS can be used to assess functional communication skills using items that are appropriate regardless of a client's age, gender, socioeconomic status, education, and vocational or cultural background.

Kohnert (2008), Langdon (2008), and Lorenzen and Murray (2008) all also suggest the use of aphasia and other cognitive-linguistic assessments that have been developed for or translated into languages other than English. Examples include the *Boston Aphasia Test* (Goodglass & Kaplan, 1983), which has been translated into 60 different languages and can be used with a computer program that can evaluate responses in more than 100 different languages and can facilitate comparisons across languages (Langdon, 2008; Lorenzen & Murray, 2008). Other examples include the *Alzheimer's Quick Test* (AQT) (Brown et al., 2009); *Assessment of Temporal-Parietal Function* (Wiig et al., 2002), *Cognitive-Linguistic Quick Test* (Helm-Estabrooks, 2001), and NEUROPSI—Attention and Memory (Ostroksy-Solis et al., 2005).

Fluency

When assessing individuals with suspected fluency disorders, the procedures are the same as with any client, with the exception that samples may need to be obtained in more than one language for comparison purposes. Individuals who are bilingual and multilingual can display similar as well as differing patterns of fluency and disfluency across languages spoken. The information that can be obtained from comparing performance across languages can be very helpful in distinguishing normal second-language disfluencies from true underlying disorder. Normal second-language disfluencies, such as interjection, revision, rephrasing, pause, and hesitation, are more likely to occur in the less proficient languages of the client, whereas true disorder-based disfluencies (e.g., prolongation, block, sound repetition) are more likely to be evident in a client's first or strongest language. To ensure that clients are identified as having a true stuttering disorder, clinicians need to obtain fluency samples in the client's strongest language. (See Chapter 9 for more information on assessment of fluency disorders.)

Voice and Resonance

A normal part of the voice assessment process is the evaluation of voice use (e.g., pitch, loudness, quality) across a variety of different speaking tasks (e.g., conversation, paragraph reading, verbal recitation and counting tasks, picture description). When assessing clients who speak more than one language, it is equally useful to evaluate voice and resonance patterns in all languages spoken by a client during conversational interactions with other speakers of those languages, keeping in mind the fact that voice use patterns can vary as a function of normal cross-cultural community influences. Observations across differing language situations should focus on those aspects of voice identified by the client as being of greatest concern to them as well as others in their family and community during the case history interview.

A common procedure that is often used to assess voice is having the client sing a familiar tune sometimes at very low intensity (e.g., softly) and in a falsetto register. Singing using a soft falsetto voice can often be diagnostic of swelling because it is difficult for a client who has edema of the vocal folds to sing. When working with any client, including those from diverse cultural and linguistic backgrounds, it is best to have the client select the song rather than having the clinician select it. This allows clinicians to use a task for which familiarity is eliminated as a possible mitigating factor in performance.

If singing is a regular part of a client's life (e.g., a frequent hobby, avocation, vocation, or cultural ritual), it is useful to obtain samples sung in the genre or style that the client typically sings (e.g., rock, opera, jazz, gospel, country, blues). It is important to remember that the type of singing done across world communities varies in nature and type, with each involving differing voice use patterns. A key focus of assessment should be on how a client's perceived or true voice difficulties affect the ability to use the voice within those contexts and traditions most relevant to the client's social and professional life. To accomplish this task, clients can be encouraged to bring in musical recordings that they can sing along with during the assessment.

Swallowing

When conducting swallowing assessments with individuals from diverse cultural and religious backgrounds, clinicians need to be sensitive to possible differences and restrictions in meal practices, feeding schedules, and food types owing to religious restrictions and cultural patterns that affect days and times concerning meals and feeding (Purnell, 2008; Tonkovich, 2002). There can also be differing cultural beliefs about the medicinal or spiritual qualities of certain foods that can affect a client's willingness to eat certain foods of combinations of foods during the assessment (Davis-McFarland, 2008). Dietary restrictions regarding permissible foods, such as pork and beef products, and religions practices regarding kosher foods for some Jewish persons are important considerations. In addition, religious holiday periods, such as Ramadan for persons who practice Islam, may restrict the time that person may eat. (See Chapter 14 for a discussion of religious beliefs that affect service delivery.)

Each of these possibilities should be taken into consideration when planning a dysphagia assessment by consulting family, cultural informants, and relevant literature of cultural food practices. The types of foods to be used during the assessment may then be adjusted to accommodate possible food restrictions.

Hearing

There are certain speech audiometry measures that can be affected by language differences. Factors such as degree of familiarity with words and sounds presented in a language other than the client's primary language can potentially affect an individual's ability to hear discriminating differences. Normal first language and dialect differences can also potentially affect an individual's ability to repeat certain words heard.

For example, if clients are asked to say a word that contains a sound not found in their native language, they may have difficulty hearing certain sound contrasts accurately and may also produce the word in a way that may signal a word different from the intended word. Sentence repetition tasks may also be difficult for clinicians to score if certain words are produced differently. Same-different word-pair contrasts may also be difficult for clients to accurately discern and produce in a less familiar language. Minimal English word-pair contrasts such as "back-bag" are likely to be particularly difficult to pronounce or discern by speakers of languages in which the /k/ and /g/ are allophonic versions of each other, one of the two sounds does not exist in that language, or final voiced sounds are frequently devoiced. In cases in which clients are asked to mark the word that they hear, language familiarity and differences can still affect client choices, especially when they are not fully familiar with the orthographic or symbolic written representation of sounds in that language. Some of the words typically used in English speech threshold testing may also be culturally less familiar to individuals who non-American English speakers (Ramkissoon, Proctor, Lansing, & Bilger, 2002). Using English spondee word lists with non-English speakers may be inappropriate because of the ways in which typical word-stress patterns vary across languages.

In light of these possible cultural-linguistic differences, audiologists conducting speech discrimination testing with clients who speak a language or dialect different from that on which certain assessment procedures are based should consider alternative testing measures such as using words that contain sound and syllable word stress patterns commonly found in the native language of the client being assessed. For example, according to Mattes and Omark (1991), trochaic stress patterns (words with stressed first syllables and unstressed second syllables) may be more appropriate to use with native Spanish speakers than spondee words, because trochaic word stress patterns occur more frequently in Spanish. Other possible modifications include using word lists translated into the language of the client and digit pair sequences (Ramkissoon et al., 2002). See Chapter 11 for more information on assessment of hearing disorders.

Augmentative Alternative Communication Assessments

When completing an assessment of symbol recognition and ability to access symbols with augmentative alternative communication clients, clinicians need to be familiar with possible differences in how certain concepts are represented in different world communities. According to Soto and colleagues (1997), it is also important to understand the nonverbal forms of communication that have meaning to a cultural group. They state, "not being aware of culturally meaningful forms of nonverbal communication would lead to misinformation about an individual's current communication skills" (Soto et al., 1997, p. 410).

When assessing the language comprehension and verbal expression skills of the bilingual AAC client, language exposure, proficiency, and use issues should be taken into account. This should be the case even when a client is considered to be "nonspeaking." Even when individuals are nonspeaking, they can display differing levels of receptive language exposure and proficiency between their first language (L1) and second language (L2). Knowing their strongest language of comprehension is essential when assessing conceptual knowledge or their ability to identify or select appropriate symbols. The possibility that concepts can be represented in L1 but not in L2, or that they can be represented one way in L1 and another way in L2, also means that clinicians need to be prepared to use all of the testing strategies recommended for other bilingual clients such as assessing items missed in one language in another language, using an interpreter or translator or bilingual administration and scoring of client responses.

Using Interpreters and Translators

According to ASHA's *Knowledge and Skills Needed by Speech-Language Pathologists and Audiologists to Provide Culturally and Linguistically Appropriate Services* (2004), clinicians need to possess "native or near-native proficiency in the language(s) spoken or signed by the client/patient." In those cases in which clinicians do not possess native or near-native proficiency in the languages spoken or signed by a client, they should use a trained interpreter or translator (ASHA, 2004). According to Langdon and Cheng (2002), the terms *interpretation* and *translation* are complementary terms that can differ in use dependent on the context. They are complex processes requiring in-depth knowledge of two languages and two cultures, familiarity with specific vocabulary, and understanding of procedures used in a given profession (ASHA, 2002). Interpretation is used to reference the oral transmission of information from one language to another, whereas translation is used to reference the written transmission. The two terms can also be used interchangeably; however, although they are related, they require different skills.

For the purposes of this chapter, the two terms will be used together to reference an individual who assists with the conveying of meaning across languages in one or both forms of communication.

Interpreter and Translator Skills, Abilities, and Competencies

Clinicians are responsible for ensuring that any assisting professionals or interpreters are adequately trained for the tasks to which they are assigned. In those cases in which there is no formal training program, interpreters and translators can be used but only if they receive some form of training and briefing on the client case before testing begins According to ASHA's *Tips for Working with Interpreters* (2010), there are four key stages involved with the using interpreters and translators during assessment: selection, briefing before the session, interaction during the session, and debriefing after the session. The interpreter or translator to be used should be proficient in both the language of the assessment and that of the client and understand the need for honesty, neutrality, and accuracy. Before the session, the clinician should ensure that the interpreter understands the goals and procedures of the assessment. During the session, the clinician should observe the interaction among the interpreter, the client, and the clinician to ensure that there is time to organize information and effectively translate both verbal and nonverbal responses. Finally, after the session, the clinician and the interpreter should discuss the client responses to clarify any remaining issues and any difficulties that were experienced during the session.

Sources for Interpreters and Translators

According to ASHA (1985) and Langdon and Cheng (2002), interpreters and translators used to assist with the assessment process can be recruited from a variety of different places and sources, including but not limited to schools, service agencies, community and health centers, churches, universities, community colleges, embassies, or international associations. In cases in which there are no other professional options, clinicians can also consider the use of age- or grade-level peers or other clients to assist with assessment. The least preferred option, but still a viable one when no other resources exist, is the use of family members, who should be trained to remain neutral during the session.

Differential Diagnosis The final step of the assessment process for CLD clients is the challenging task of distinguishing differences and variations that are the result of normal culturally or linguistically based influences from those associated with true disorder in clients who are either monolingual or bilingual speakers of other languages. The same applies to individuals who speak dialects of languages

different from those spoken by mainstream speakers and that of the clinician. When making the differential diagnosis, it is important to base decisions on multiple sources of assessment data using methods such as those discussed earlier in this chapter.

Analyzing Assessment Data

Focus on Language Universals

When analyzing assessment data from very young clients (ages 0 to 3 years), a key focus should be on universally shared aspects of speech, language, hearing, and swallowing ability that occur in typically developing individuals. This is an approach that can be used regardless of a child's cultural-linguistic background or community.

Focus on Productions in the Client's Strongest Language

Whenever possible, clinicians should focus on productions in the client's strongest, most proficient language. Using this approach provides a focus on what is most likely a true disorder as opposed to a language difference.

Take Cultural-Linguistic Influences into Account

In older speakers, clinicians need to rule out any productions in a client's second or other least proficient languages (L2) that may be due to normal first language influences (L1). Specifically, clinicians should avoid attributing the omission of certain sounds or grammatical forms in L2 that do not exist or that can be optionally absent in the client's L1.

Similar caution should be used when evaluating conversational discourse and narrative production skills. Cross-cultural narrative style differences can definitely affect how individuals engage in conversation and retell narratives. The differences may be in overall organization, structure, strategies for beginning and ending, and imbedding evaluative feedback (Champion, 1998; Champion, 2003; Gutierrez-Clellen, 2004; Gutierrez-Clellen & Quinn, 1993; Hyter & Westby, 1996; McCabe & Bliss, 2003; Taylor & Matsuda, 1988; Westby, 1994). Possible cross-cultural discourse style differences should also be taken into account when making decisions concerning normal versus unusual discourse and narrative style patterns. As reported by Terrell and associates (1992), clinicians can feel more confident identifying certain patterns of conversational and narrative discourse as a potential disorder when clients or caregivers have expressed concerns about an individual's ability to hold a conversation or tell a story to others in the same cultural community.

In addition to seeing normal L1 influences on productions in L2, clinicians may see productions in a client's L1 that are the result of reverse L2 influences. According to research by Goldstein and Iglesias as cited in Goldstein (2004), it was common to see this type of cross-linguistic effect in 4- to 6-year-old bilingual Spanish- and English-speaking children who substituted the English postvocalic, unstressed /r/ for the flap /r/ in Spanish words such as "flower" /flor/. Such differences are more likely to occur on sounds that are not mastered or acquired in L1 before the second is introduced or acquired in L2.

Some of these differences may also be related more to the issue of first language loss, attrition, and regress. Anderson (2004) provides examples of how patterns of language loss in Spanish-speaking children learning English as L2 can affect productions of lexical, morphological, mood, and syntax productions in Spanish. Common effects include lexical innovations whereby children create words based on English, such as *emtiar* (using a derivation of the English word "empty" instead of the Spanish word *vaciar*). Other examples include transferring English word order to Spanish language productions (e.g., *el grande vaso* vs. *el vaso grande*).

When analyzing productions in a client's second or least proficient language or dialect, clinicians need to rule out normal second language learning and potentially dialect- or language-influenced productions as a possible indicator of disorder. This means that in addition to knowing how the phonetic and grammatical inventories of the client's languages and dialects differ from each other, clinicians must be familiar with how possible patterns of normal L1 or first dialect influence might be displayed in the less proficient dialect or language (e.g., typical speech sound and grammar differences that one might expect to find).

Consider Language-Specific Developmental Norms

When assessing bilingual children, clinicians need to be familiar with the language-specific developmental expectations and norms for speakers from the same language. This is important because sounds and grammatical forms can differ across languages. For example, the trilled /r/ in Spanish, and the back fricative /χ/ in Arabic do not exist in English. Although languages such as Spanish requires mastery of both the masculine ("el") and feminine ("la") forms of articles, English has only one article form. Turkish uses the word *bir* ("one") as the indefinite article but has no definite article. In English and Afrikaans, adjectives come before nouns in sentences. In some languages, such as Spanish, adjectives follow the nouns they modify. In other languages, such as Romanian, the word order is more flexible (adjectives may follow the noun but often proceed it). In languages such as Navajo, the information conveyed by adjectives is included as part of the verb form or noun suffixes.

There are differing developmental orders of sound acquisition and mastery even on sounds shared with other languages. For example, Amayreh and Dyson (1998) found that that standard productions of /j/ were acquired with 75% accuracy in all tested word positions by Arabic-speaking children between the ages of 6 years and 6 years, 4 months living in or around Amman, Jordan. This compares to English, in which /j/ is acquired between the ages of 2 years, 4 months and 3 years, 6 months by English speakers according to previously published norms. The same can be true for grammatical forms. For example, the age at which Spanish-speaking children acquire copula verb forms *ser* and *estar* has been reported to be between 2 and 3 years (Anderson, 1995; Goldstein, 2000). This is earlier than the reported age of 4 years for English-speaking children (Owens, 2005).

Clinicians need to be mindful that the age of acquisition for different sounds can also vary as a function of dialect. Even within the same dialect, age differences can be found between speakers in different geographic regions. For example, according to Spanish normative data presented by Bedore (1999), using a criteria of 90%, /g/ was found to be acquired by Spanish-speaking children in California at 3 years, 3 months; between the ages of 4 and 4 years, 6 months in Mexico City; and by age 5 years, 11 months or later in Texas. Additional examples of dialect-based speech acquisition differences are documented by McLeod (2007) who has produced a comprehensive guide to speech acquisition in 12 English dialects and 20 other languages around the world.

Use Parent-Child Comparative Analyses

In cases in which there is little information available on a reference language, one could potentially use a parent-child comparative analysis of data similar to that proposed by Terrell and colleagues (1992). In a single-subject study of a young child with suspected language delays who spoke Ibo, they compared the English speech sound productions of the child to that of her father on a standardized test of articulation and in a conversational speech sample. A systematic process was then used to identify Ibo-influenced English speech production patterns produced by the father that were unmatched by his daughter, with possible developmental influences taken into account. A conversational language sample was also analyzed for differences in sentence word order, word choices, and overall logical structure. Results from this analysis helped to identify possible areas of difference due to a possible underlying disorder and to establish appropriate intervention goals.

Identifying Disorder

Using Language-Specific Criteria

Clinicians also need to be aware that the criteria for identifying language impairment may vary as a function of the language used. For example, in recent years, there has been attention to the various ways in which specific language impairment is revealed through the use of certain inflectional markers and forms in different languages such as Afrikaans (Southwood & van Hout, 2010), French (Thordardottir, 2008), Icelandic (Thordardottir & Namazi, 2007), and Cantonese (Wong et al., 2010). Findings from these studies suggest that certain morphosyntactic forms associated with speech-language impairment in English cannot always be used to identify impairment in other languages or that the types of forms to be used vary as a function of the language. Similar research has been conducted in French-speaking children with reading impairment (St-Pierre & Béland, 2010).

The appropriateness of using certain measures such as MLU has also been examined and found to not always be equally distinguishing between different language groups (Wong et al., 2010). In some languages, evidence of speech-language impairment can be identified through elements of grammar and language production and comprehension not typically studied or present in other language populations. Examples include lexical tone contrasts (Wong et al., 2009) and language-specific aspectual markers (Fletcher et al., 2005).

Using Dialect-Specific Criteria

When working with individuals who speak a dialect of language that is different from the community standard, clinicians should be guided by ASHA's position paper on social dialects (ASHA, 1983) and its technical report on American English dialects (ASHA, 2003). Specifically, according to the position statement, clinicians should only treat those features of characteristics of dialect that are true errors and not attributable to dialect. The focus of diagnosis should therefore be focused on the identification of speech sound and grammatical productions that cannot be attributed to normal dialect differences as well as aspects of communication that are universal across differing speakers.

One way to accomplish this is to use adapted scoring that gives credit for allowable dialect variations. Examples of how adapted scoring for AAE speaker responses can be used with standardized tests can be found in Terry, Jackson, Evangelou, and Smith (2010). Another method involves focusing on the non-dialect-specific and noncontrastive features that are shared with other dialects. Clinicians should focus on those speech sounds that make up the minimal core of sounds shared between dialects (Stockman, 1996; 2008). Seymour and associates (1998) and Oetting and Newkirk (2008) identified differences in non-dialect-specific sounds and grammatical forms that are clinically significant in distinguishing between typically developing and nontypically developing AAE and MAE speakers. A number of researchers such as Craig and Washington (1998), Horton-Ikard and coworkers (2005), Oetting and Newkirk (2008) and Oetting and colleagues (2010), identified commonly used language sample analysis measures that can be reliably used with speakers of different dialects, such as mean length of utterance

(MLU), mean syntactic length (MSL), c-unit analyses of complex sentence constructions and scores from the Index of Productive Syntax (IPSYN) (Scarborough, 1990).

Clinicians can also consider dialect-specific aspects of language if they have some understanding of the sound and grammar rule system for the client's dialect, including possible speech sound (e.g., allophonic) variations and dialect-specific variable rules and obligatory contexts. For example, according to Wyatt (1991, 1995), the copula (main) verb forms of be (is and are) can be variably absent in the sentences of young AAE child speakers (e.g., *He a cry baby*), as can be the case for older speakers owing to linguistic contextual factors, such as whether this verb is followed by a noun, verb, or adjective. The first-person singular form of this verb (e.g., *I am* five), as well as the past tense forms of this verb (e.g., *was* and *were*) copula, are also typically present (obligated) according to the research of Labov (1969) and Wolfram (1969). These same researchers note that this verb is obligated or required, similar to MAE, in the final position of clauses and sentences.

These findings suggest that when assessing the copula verb productions of AAE speakers, clinicians need to recognize that the absence of the copula in certain sentence contexts (e.g., nonfinal clause position) is acceptable if the intended form is *is* or *are,* but not if it is *am*, *was*, or *were*. This requires some knowledge of the dialect-specific constraints on certain grammatical form use that goes beyond understanding that certain grammatical forms can be variably absent. Similar considerations need to be taken into account when assessing phonological productions in any dialect. For example, Stockman (2006) found that some final voiceless stops (e.g., /t/) are variably absent more often than others, such as /p/ and /k/. As a result, she concludes that it is important not to consider all final consonant deletions as typical.

Additional Disorder-Specific Considerations

When attempting to make clinical decisions about testing outcomes in aspects of communication beyond phonology and language, clinicians should reference some of the disorder-specific recommendations made in other chapters in this text. Examples of some of the disorder-specific issues that clinicians may want to consider include the following.

Voice and Resonance

When analyzing results from voice testing, focus on aspects of voice that are less likely to vary as a function of cultural-linguistic community differences and are most likely to be the result of true underlying vocal pathology, such as excessive breathiness and hoarseness, keeping in mind that the term *excessive* is a subjective descriptor that can vary from person to person and across cultural communities. The perception of a voice difference, therefore, should be verified from the perspective of not only the clinician but also the client and significant others from their community through the case history interview.

When analyzing voice data according to established, norms clinicians need to also be cautious. Holland and DeJarnette (2002) reported evidence of ethnic-racial group differences in the use of certain voice parameters such as fundamental frequency. Although these differences have often been found not to be statistically significant, they do still suggest caution in making final clinical decisions about voice normalcy based on existing norms derived from research on other ethnic groups.

Similar caution should be used when interpreting results from instrumental assessments of nasal resonance because nasality can vary as a function of language-specific differences. Nasalance norms, based on measures of oral and nasal resonance initially conducted in English have been established for other languages as well, such as Spanish, Finnish, Flemish, German, and Thai (Hirschberg et al., 2006).

Fluency

When analyzing fluency in bilingual and CLD clients, there are a number of important factors to take into consideration in making a differential diagnosis of stuttering.

1. There can be cross-cultural variations in how hesitation, pause, and repetition are used as part of normal discourse across different cultural communities. The types of fillers and pauses that are used in differing languages can also differ (Montes, 1999; Muños-Duston, 1992).

2. Speakers may produce typical disfluencies, such as hesitation, pause, revision, and interjection, in L2 as the result of normal second language learning. Other nontypical disfluencies, such as sound and syllable repetitions, prolongations, and blocks, are more likely to be associated with true stuttering, especially when also evident in L1 (Ratner, 2004).

3. Caution should also be used when interpreting nonverbal communication, such as diverted eye gaze during sustained listening, as a sign of avoidance or secondary mannerisms in disfluency. Such nonverbal behavior could be associated with normal cross-cultural variations unless it is clearly associated with disfluency. Other behaviors, such as foot tapping, lip quivering, looking away, or turning one's body away during a moment of disfluency are more likely to be associated with true stuttering or avoidance behavior.

4. It is important to consider language-specific influences when analyzing patterns of disfluency in bilingual speakers. Cross-linguistic differences in language structure (e.g., syntactic structure) can play a role in how and where stuttering occurs as well as the frequency of stuttering on certain grammatical elements (Bernstein-Ratner

& Benitez, 1985). The elements that are stuttered can be similar as well as different across languages spoken by a client (Bernstein-Ratner & Benitez, 1985; Jayram, 1983). This latter factor suggests that analyses of disfluency patterns across languages can be of great value in making a differential diagnosis and also for identifying primary targets for intervention by looking for shared patterns of difficulty.

5. Clinicians need to be aware that code switching can be used as form of avoidance for some bilingual speakers (e.g., switching to the other language when difficulties are being experienced). As a result, it is important to pay close attention to patterns of code switching in bilingual clients.

Oral-Motor and Craniofacial Speech Disorders

Although there are certain aspects of speech production that are universally associated with oral motor and other physically or neurologically based speech disorders (e.g., apraxia, dysarthria, or craniofacial disorders), some types of difficulties associated with these problems in English speakers may not be so for speakers of other languages. For example, "weakened" productions of stops and fricatives (e.g., substituting a bilabial fricative for a labiodental fricative) that could serve as a sign of disorder in English would not be considered a problem in a Spanish. In Spanish, bilabial fricatives can serve as an acceptable speech sound variant for bilabial stops. Fricatives /f/ can be produced as the bilabial fricative /ɸ/ in a word such as *emfermo,* and /b/ can be produced as the bilabial fricative /β/ in the word *llave.* There are also some dialects of Spanish, such as Puerto Rican and Dominican Spanish, in which the /f/ is often produced as /Φ/ in word such as *café* (Goldstein, 2000).

Glottal stop and pharyngeal fricative sounds are common in the speech of individuals with unrepaired as well as repaired clefts (Shipley & McAfee, 2009). However, there are a number of languages in the world, such as Arabic, that contain these same types of sounds as part of their normal phonemic inventory (Amaryreh & Dyson, 1998). As such, these types of speech sound productions may not be as clinically distinctive in identifying disorder-based productions when used in speech samples conducted in that language or any other languages spoken by the individual.

CLOSING COMMENTS

In summary, there are a number of different cultural and linguistic considerations that clinicians need to keep in mind when conducting a speech and language assessment of any client. They are particularly important when doing an assessment with a client and family who speak a language other than that of the clinician or who have a cultural and linguistic background and experience the embodies one or more languages and cultures. These considerations apply not only to the overall frameworks for assessments used but also the specific types of formal as well as informal measures used. Cultural-linguistic considerations are equally important when analyzing data from the case history, observations, formal and informal testing, and making a final differential diagnosis. Above all, it is important to clearly distinguish between typical development and dialectal or language differences in the language and culture of the client from those factors that would indicate a true diagnosed disorder so that appropriate intervention strategies can be developed if necessary.

DISCUSSION QUESTIONS

1. How do you define yourself in terms of your own cultural identity? How does your cultural identification or affiliation differ from that of others in your family?

2. Have you ever personally experienced or witnessed some of the cross-cultural differences described in this chapter during interactions between yourself or another professional and clients? How did the differences affect the interaction process and how were they handled?

3. How might some of the cross-cultural communication style differences discussed in this chapter potentially affect the postassessment counseling process?

4. What type of impact, if any, might the emerging new e.net'er identity have on case history interview and counseling interactions between clinicians who ascribe to that identity and on clients and family holding more traditional views of cultural identity and technology?

5. According to ASHA's (2004) knowledge and skills document, one strategy or resource that clinicians can use for obtaining information about "what is typical in a client's speech community" is to use a cultural informant or broker. Think of a possible scenario in which it might be appropriate to use a cultural informant or broker or an actual past situation in which one could have used a cultural informant to prepare for the case history interview interaction. Who would that person be, and what kinds of questions would you ask to obtain the information needed to understand what is typical in a client's speech community?

6. Think of some recent challenges you have had or have witnessed other professionals having in assessing clients from other dialect and language backgrounds. What information or suggestions presented in this chapter would have been most useful in addressing those challenges?

7. What new steps do you feel you need to take most after reading this chapter in preparing for future assessments with CLD clients?

8. Examine the state education code, standards, and regulations for assessing CLD students in your state. Look for instances in which some of key guidelines for assessing CLD children under IDEIA are included in that code or regulation.

9. Assume that you have been asked to be part of a speech and language assessment team being sent to another country (pick a specific country). What types of knowledge and skills do you feel you would need to have before traveling to that country, and how would you go about acquiring them?

10. Review one child and one adult standardized test commonly used in the field and try to identify some of the items, pictures, and concepts on the test that might present some source of cultural or linguistic bias for a specific cultural or linguistic population either recently immigrated to the United States or living in some other part of the world.

REFERENCES

Ahluwalia, M. K., & Zaman, N. K. (2010). Counseling Muslims and Sikhs in a post-9/11 world. In J. G. Ponterotto, J. M. Casas, L. A. Suzuki, & C. M. Alexander (Eds.), *Handbook of multicultural counseling* (3rd ed.) (pp. 467-478). Thousand Oaks, CA: Sage.

Amayreh, M. M., & Dyson, A. T. (1998). The acquisition of Arabic consonants. *Journal of Speech-Language and Hearing Research, 41,* 642-653.

American Speech-Language-Hearing Association (1983, September). Social dialects (Position statement). *ASHA, 25,* 23-27. Available at: www.asha.org/docs/html/PS1983-00115.html.

American Speech-Language-Hearing Association (1989). Bilingual speech-language pathologists and audiologist: Definition [Relevant paper]. Available at: www.asha.org/docs/html/RP1989-00205.html.

American Speech-Language-Hearing Association (1985). Clinical management of communicatively handicapped minority language populations [Position statement]. Available at: www.asha.org/policy.

American Speech-Language-Hearing Association (2002).

American Speech-Language-Hearing Association (2003). American English dialects [Technical report]. Available at: www.asha.org/docs/html/TR2003-00044.html

American Speech-Language-Hearing Association (2004). Knowledge and skills needed by speech-language pathologist and audiologists to provide culturally and linguistically appropriate services. Available at: www.asha.org/docs/html/KS2004-00215.html.

American Speech-Language-Hearing Association (2010). Tips for working with interpreters. Retrieved February 1, 2011, from www.asha.org/practice/multicultural/issues/interpret.htm.

Anderson, R. T. (2004). First language loss in Spanish-speaking children: Patterns of loss and implications for clinical practice. In B. A. Goldstein (Ed.), *Bilingual language development and disorders in Spanish-English speakers* (pp. 187-211). Baltimore: Paul H. Brookes.

Anderson, R. T. (1995). Spanish morphological and syntactic development. In H. Kayser (Ed.), *Bilingual speech-language pathology: An Hispanic Focus* (pp. 41-73) San Diego: Singular.

Battle, D. E. (2000). Becoming a culturally competent clinician. *Perspectives: Special Interest Division 14: Communication Disorders and Sciences in Culturally and Linguistically Diverse Populations, 6,* 20-25.

Battle, D. E. (2002). Communication disorders in a multicultural society. In D. E. Battle (Ed.), *Communication disorders in multicultural populations* (3rd ed.) (pp. 3-31). Boston: Butterworth-Heinemann.

Bedore, L. M. (1999). The acquisition of Spanish. In O. L. Taylor, & L. B. Leonard (Eds.), *Language acquisition across North America: Cross-cultural and cross-linguistic perspectives* (pp. 157-207). San Diego: Singular.

Bernstein-Ratner, N., & Benitez, H. (1985). Linguistic analysis of a bilingual stutterer. *Journal of Fluency Disorders, 10,* 211-219.

Brackenbury, T., & Pye, C. (2005). Semantic deficits in children with language impairments: Issues for clinical assessment. *Language, Speech, and Hearing Services in Schools, 36,* 5-16.

Brown, J., Pengas, G., Dawson, K., et al. (2009). Self administered cognitive screening test (TYM) for detection of Alzheimer's disease: Cross-sectional study. *British Journal of Medicine, 338,* b2030.

Brownell, R. (2001). *Expressive one-word picture vocabulary test: Spanish-bilingual edition.* Novato, CA: Academic Therapy Publications. California Law: California Education Code (n.d.). Retrieved from www.leginfo.ca.gov/cgi-bin/calawquery?codesection=edc&codebody+&hits=20.

Campbell, T., Dollaghan, C., Needleman, H., & Janosky, J. (1997). Reducing bias in language assessment: Processing-dependent measures. *Journal of Speech, Language, and Hearing Research, 40,* 519-525.

Champion, T. B. (1998). "Tell me somethin' good": A description of narrative structures among African American children. *Linguistics and Education, 9,* 251-286.

Champion, T. B. (2003). *Understanding storytelling among African American children: A journey from Africa to America.* Mahwah, NJ: Lawrence Erlbaum Associates.

Champion, T. B., Hyter, Y. D., McCabe, A., & Bland-Stewart, L. M. (2003). A matter of vocabulary: Performances of low-income African American Head Start children on the Peabody Picture Vocabulary Test-III. *Communication Disorders Quarterly, 24,* 121-127.

Chan, S., & Lee, E. (2004). Families with Asian roots. In E. W. Lynch & M. J. Hanson (Eds.), *Developing cross-cultural competence: A guide for working with children and families* (3rd ed.) (pp. 219-298). Baltimore: Paul H. Brookes.

Choi-Misailidis, S. (2010). Multiracial-heritage awareness and personal affiliation (MHAPA): Understanding identity in people of mixed-race descent. In J. G. Ponterotto, J. M. Casas, L. A. Suzuki, & C. M. Alexander (Eds.), *Handbook of multicultural counseling* (3rd ed.) (pp. 301-311). Thousand Oaks, CA: Sage.

Couto-Wakulczyk, G., Moreau, D. , & Beckingham, A. C. (2003). People of French Canadian heritage. In L. D. Purnell, & B. J. Paulanka (Eds.), *Transcultural health care: A culturally competent approach* (2nd ed.) (pp. 160-175). Philadelphia: F. A. Davis.

Craig, H. K., Washington, J. A., & Thompson-Porter, C. (1998). Average c-unit lengths in the discourse of African American children from low-income, urban homes. *Journal of Speech, Language, and Hearing Research, 41,* 433-444.

Dawson, J. I., Stout, C. E., & Eyer, J.A. (2003). *Structured photographic expressive language test* (3rd ed.). Dekalb, IL: Janelle.

Davis-McFarland, E. (2008). Family and cultural issues in a school swallowing and feeding program. *Language, Speech, and Hearing Services in Schools, 39,* 199-213.

deVilliers, J. (2004a). Cultural and linguistic fairness in the assessment of semantics. *Seminars in Speech and Language, 25,* 73-90.

deVilliers, P. (2004b). Assessing pragmatic skills in elicited production. *Seminars in Speech and Language, 25,* 57-71.

Ebert, K. D., Kalanek, J., Cordero, K. N., & Kohnert, K. (2008). Spanish nonword repetition: Stimuli development and preliminary results. *Communication Disorders Quarterly, 29,* 67-74.

Ellis, T. A. , & Purnell, L. D. (2008). People of Guatemalan heritage. In L. D. Purnell & B. J. Paulanka (Eds.), *Transcultural health care: A culturally competent approach* (3rd ed.) (pp. 145-156). Philadelphia: F. A. Davis.

Engel, P. M. J., Santos, F. H., & Gathercole, S. E. (2008). Are working memory measures free of socioeconomic influence? *Journal of Speech, Language, and Hearing Research, 51,* 1580-1587.

Fenson, L., Dale, P. S., Reznick, J. S., et al. (1993). *The MacArthur Communicative Development Inventories: User's guide and technical manual.* San Diego: Singular.

Fletcher, P., Leonard, L. B., Stokes, S. F., & Wong, A. M. Y. (2005). The expression of aspect in Cantonese-speaking children with specific language impairment. *Journal of Speech, Language, and Hearing Research, 48,* 621-634.

Frattali, C., Thompson, C., Holland, A., Wohl, C., & Ferketic, M. (1995). *Functional Assessment of Communication Skills in Adults [FACS].* Rockville, MD: ASHA.

Gardner, M. F. (1979). *Expressive one word picture vocabulary test.* Novato, CA: Academic Therapy.

Glanville, C. L. (2003). People of African American heritage. In L. D. Purnell, B. J. Paulanka (Eds.), *Transcultural health care: A culturally competent approach* (3rd ed.) (pp. 40-53). Philadelphia: F. A. Davis.

Goldstein, B. (2000). *Resource guide on cultural and linguistic diversity.* San Diego: Delmar Learning.

Goldstein, B. (2004). Phonologicalal development and disorders. In B. A. Goldstein (Ed.), *Bilingual language development and disorders in Spanish-English speakers* (pp. 259-285). Baltimore: Paul H. Brookes.

Goodglass, H. & Kaplan, E. (1983). *Boston diagnostic aphasia test.* Philadelphia, PA: Lean & Ferbiger.

Granville, C. L. (2003). People of African-American heritage. In L. D. Purnell, B. J. Paulanka (Eds.), *Transcultural health care: A culturally competent approach* (2nd ed.) (pp. 40-53). Philadelphia, PA: F. A. Davis.

Groce, N. E., & Zola, I. K. (1993). Multiculturalism, chronic illness and disability. *Pediatrics, 91,* 1048-1055.

Gushue, G. V., Sciarra, D. T., & Mejía, B. X. (2010). Family counseling: Systems, postmodern, and multicultural perspectives. In J. G. Ponterotto, J. M. Casas, L. A. Suzuki, & C. M. Alexander (Eds.), *Handbook of multicultural counseling* (3rd ed.) (pp. 677-688). Thousand Oaks, CA: Sage.

Gutierrez-Clellen, V. (2004). Narrative development and disorders in bilingual children. In B. A. Goldstein (Ed.), *Bilingual language development and disorders in Spanish-English speakers* (pp. 235-256). Baltimore: Paul H. Brookes.

Gutierrez-Clellen, V., & Quinn, R. (1993). Assessing narratives of children from diverse cultural/linguistic groups. *Language, Speech, and Hearing Services in Schools, 24,* 2-9.

Hambleton, R. K., & de Jong, J. H.A.L. (2003). Advances in translating and adapting educational and psychological tests. *Language Testing, 20,* 127-134.

Hanson, M. J. (2004a). Ethnic, cultural and language diversity in service settings. In E. W. Lynch & M. J. Hanson (Eds.), *Developing cross-cultural competence: A guide for working with children and families* (3rd ed.) (pp. 3-18). Baltimore: Paul H. Brookes.

Hanson, M. J. (2004b). Families with Anglo-European roots. In E. W. Lynch & M. J. Hanson (2004). *Developing cross-cultural competence: A guide for working with children and families* (3rd ed.) (pp. 81-108). Baltimore: Paul H. Brookes.

Hafizi H., & Lipson, J. G. (2003). People of Iranian heritage. In L. D. Purnell, B. J. Paulanka (Eds.), *Transcultural health care: A culturally competent approach* (2nd ed.) (pp. 177-193), Philadelphia: F. A. Davis.

Hafizi, H., Sayyedi, M., & Lipson, J. G. (2008). People of Iranian heritage. In L. D. Purnell, & B. J. Paulanka (Eds.), *Transcultural health care: A culturally competent approach* (3rd ed.) (pp. 248-59). Philadelphia: F. A. Davis.

Haynes, W. O., & Pindzola, R. B. (2008). *Diagnosis and evaluation in speech pathology* (7th ed). Boston: Pearson Education, Inc.

Helm-Estabrooks, N. (2001). *Cognitive Linguistic Quick Test*. San Antonio, TX: The Psychological Corporation.

Hillman, S.M. (2003). People of Italian heritage. In L. D. Purnell, B. J. Paulanka (Eds.), *Transcultural health care: A culturally competent approach* (2nd ed.) (pp. 205-217). Philadelphia, PA: F. A. Davis.

Hirschberg, J., Bók, S., Juhász, M., et al. (2006). Adaptation of nasometry to Hungarian language and experiences with its clinical application. *International Journal of Pediatric Otorhinolaryngology, 70,* 785-798.

Holland, R. W., & DeJarnette, G. (2002). Voice and voice disorders. In D. E. Battle (Ed.), *Communication disorders in multicultural populations* (3rd ed.) (pp. 299-333). Boston: Butterworth-Heinemann.

Horton-Ikard, R., Weismer, S. E., & Edwards, C. (2005). Examining the use of standard English production measures in the language samples of African American toddlers. *Journal of Multilingual Communication Disorders, 3,* 169-182.

Hunt, P. C. (2005). An introduction to Vietnamese culture for rehabilitation service providers in the United States. In J. H. Stone (Ed.), *Culture and disability: Providing culturally competent services* (pp. 203-223). Thousand Oaks, CA: Sage.

Huttlinger, K. W., & Purnell, L. D. (2008). People of Appalachian heritage. In L. D. Purnell, & B. J. Paulanka (Eds.), *Transcultural health care: A culturally competent approach* (3rd ed.) (pp. 95-112). Philadelphia: F. A. Davis.

Hwa-Froelich, D. A., & Matsuo, H. (2005). Vietnamese children and language-based processing tasks. *Language, Speech, and Hearing Services in Schools, 36,* 230-243.

Hwa-Froelich, D. A., Westby, C. E., & Schommer-Aikins, M. (2000). Assessing language learnability. *Special Interest Division 14: Communication Disorders and Sciences in Culturally and Linguistically Diverse Populations Newsletter, 6,* 1-6.

Hyter, Y. D., & Westby, C. E. (1996). Using oral narratives to assess communicative competence. In A. G. Kamhi, K. E. Pollock, & J. L. Harris (Eds.), *Communication development and disorders in African American children: Research, assessment and intervention* (pp. 247-275). Baltimore: Paul H. Brookes.

Individuals with Disabilities Education Improvement Act PL 108-446 (2004). Washington, DC: U.S. Department of Education.

International Test Commission (2010). International Guidelines for Translating and Adapting Tests. Accesssed June 18, 2011, from www.intestcom.org.

Jacob, N. (2004). Families with South Asian roots. In E. W. Lynch & M. J. Hanson (Eds.), *Developing cross-cultural competence: A guide for working with children and families* (3rd ed.) (pp. 415-439). Baltimore: Paul H. Brookes.

Jacobson, E. (2005). An introduction to Haitian culture for rehabilitation service providers. In J. H. Stone (Ed.), *Culture and disability: Providing culturally competent services* (pp. 139-160). Thousand Oaks: Sage.

Jayram, M. (1983). *Journal of Communication Disorders, 16,* 287-297.

Jayson, S. (2010-2011, Dec. 30-Jan. 2). The year we stopped talking. *USA Today,* 1A-2A.

Jezewski, M. A., & Sotnik, P. (2005). Disability service providers as culture brokers. In J. H. Stone (Ed.), *Culture and disability: Providing culturally competent services* (pp. 37-64). Thousand Oaks: Sage.

Joe, J. R., & Malach, R. S. (2004). Families with American Indian roots. In E. W. Lynch & M. J. Hanson (Eds.), *Developing cross-cultural competence: A guide for working with children and families* (3rd ed.) (pp. 109-139). Baltimore: Paul H. Brookes.

Johnson, V. E. (2010). Fast mapping verb meaning from argument structure. *Topics in Language Disorders, 30,* 103-118.

Juarbe, T. C. (2003). People of Puerto Rican heritage. In L. D. Purnell, B. J. Paulanka (Eds.), *Transcultural health care: A culturally competent approach* (2nd ed.) (pp. 307-326). Philadelphia, PA: F. A. Davis.

Kayser, H. (1998). *Assessment and intervention resource for Hispanic children.* San Diego: Singular.

Kim, J., Keininger, D. L., Becker, S., & Crawley, J. A. (2005). Simultaneous development of the Pediatric GERD Caregiver Impact Questionnaire (PGCIQ) in American English and American Spanish. *Health and Quality of Life Outcomes, 3,* 5-12.

Kip-Ripnow, W. S. (2005). Disability and Korean culture. In J. H. Stone (Ed.), *Culture and disability: Providing culturally competent services* (pp. 115-138). Thousand Oaks: Sage Publications, Inc.

Kohnert, K. (2008). *Language disorders in bilingual children and adults.* San Diego: Plural.

Kulwicki, A. D. (2003). People of Arab heritage. In L. D. Purnell, B. J. Paulanka (Eds.), *Transcultural health care: A culturally competent approach* (2nd ed.) (pp. 90-105), Philadelphia: F. A. Davis.

Kulwicki. A. D. (2008). People of Arab heritage. In L. D. Purnell, & B. J. Paulanka (Eds.), *Transcultural health care: A culturally competent approach* (3rd ed.) (pp. 113-128). Philadelphia: F. A. Davis.

Kwan, K. K., Gong, Y., & Maestas, M. (2010). Language, translation, and validity in the adaptation of psychological tests for multicultural counseling. In J. G. Ponterotto, J. M. Casas, L. A. Suzuki, and C. M. Alexander (Eds.), *Handbook of multicultural counseling* (3rd ed.) (pp. 397-412). Thousand Oaks, CA: Sage.

Labov, W. (1969). Contraction, deletion, and inherent variability of the English copula. *Language, 45,* 715-762.

Laing, S. P. (2003). Assessment of phonology in preschool African American vernacular English speakers using an alternate response mode. *American Journal of Speech-Language Pathology, 12,* 273-281.

Langdon, H., W. (2002). *Interpreters and translators in communication disorders.* Eau Claire, WI: Thinking Publications.

Langdon, H. W. (2008). *Assessment and intervention for communication disorders in culturally and linguistically diverse populations.* Clifton, NY: Thomson Delmar Learning.

Langdon, H. W., & Cheng, L. L. (2002). *Collaborating with interpreters and translators.* Eau Claire, WI: Thinking Publications.

Lewis, N., Castilleja, N., Moore, B. J., & Rodriquez, B. (2010). Assessment 360. *Perspectives on Communication Disorders and Sciences in Culturally and Linguistically Diverse Populations, 17,* 37-56.

Lorenzen, B., & Murray, L. L. (2008). Bilingual aphasia: A theoretical and clinical review. *American Journal of Speech-Language Pathology, 17,* 299-317.

Liu, G. Z. (2005). Best practices: Developing cross-cultural competence from a Chinese perspective. In J. H. Stone (Ed.), *Culture and disability: Providing culturally competent services* (pp. 65-85). Thousand Oaks, CA: Sage.

Lynch, H. (2004). Developing cross-cultural competence. In E. W. Lynch & M. J. Hanson (Eds.), *Developing cross-cultural competence: A guide for working with children and families* (3rd ed.) (pp. 41-77). Baltimore: Paul H. Brookes.

Marian, V., Blumenfeld, H. K., & Kaushanskaya (2007). The Language Experience and Proficiency Questionnaire (LEAP-Q): Assessing language profiles in bilinguals and multilingual. *Journal of Speech, Language, and Hearing Research, 50,* 940-967.

Matsuda, M. (1989). Working with Asian parents: Some communication strategies. *Topics in Language Disorders, 9,* 45-53.

Mattes, L., & Omark, D. (1991). *Speech and language assessment for the bilingual handicapped* (2nd ed.). Oceanside, CA: Academic Communication Associates.

McCabe, A., & Bliss, L. S. (2003). *Patterns of narrative discourse: A multicultural, life span approach.* Boston: Pearson Education.

McCabe, A., & Champion, T. B. (2010). A matter of vocabulary II: Low-income African American children's performance on the Expressive Vocabulary Test. *Communication Disorders Quarterly, 31,* 162-169.

McLeod, S. (2007). *The international guide to speech acquisition.* Clifton Park, NY: Thompson Delmar Learning.

Meitus, I. J., & Weinberg, B. (1983). *Diagnosis in speech-language pathology.* Baltimore: University Park Press.

Miller, D. (2005). An introduction to Jamaican culture for rehabilitation service providers. In J. H. Stone (Ed.), *Culture and disability: Providing culturally competent services* (pp. 87-113). Thousand Oaks: Sage.

Mokkink, L. B., Knol, D. L., van Nispen, R. M. A., & Kramer, S. E. (2010). Improving the quality and applicability of the Dutch scales of the Communication Profile for the Hearing Impaired using item response theory. *Journal of Speech, Language, and Hearing Research, 53,* 556-571.

Mokuau, N., & Tauili'ili, P. (2004). Families with native Hawaiian and Samoan roots. In E. W. Lynch, & M. J. Hanson (Eds.), *Developing cross-cultural competence: A guide for working with children and their families* (3rd ed.) (pp. 345-371). Baltimore: Paul H. Brookes.

Montes, R. (1999). The development of discourse markers in Spanish interjections. *Journal of Pragmatics, 3,* 1289-1319.

Muñoz-Duston, E. (1992). Self-repetitions: Analyzing the Speech of Spanish and English bilingual children. Unpublished doctoral dissertation: Georgetown University.

Nowak, T. T. (2003). People of Vietnamese heritage. In L. D. Purnell, B. J. Paulanka (Eds.), *Transcultural health care: A culturally competent approach* (2nd ed.) (pp. 327-343). Philadelphia, PA: F. A. Davis.

Oetting, J. B., & Newkirk, B. L. (2008). Subject relatives by children with and without SLI across different dialects of English. *Clinical Linguistics and Phonetics, 22,* 111-125.

Oetting, J. B., Newkirk, B. L., Hartfield, L. R., et al. (2010). Index of productive syntax for children who speak African American English. *Language, Speech, Language, and Hearing Services in Schools, 41,* 328-339.

Ostrosky-Solis, F., Gómez Pérez, E., Matute, E., Rosseli, M., Ardila, A., & Pineda, D. (2005). *NEUROPSI-Attention and Memory.* San Antonio, TX: The Psychological Corporation.

Owens, R. E. (2005). *Language development: An introduction* (6th ed.). Boston: Pearson Education, Inc.

Pacquiao, D. F. (2003). People of Filipino heritage. In L. D. Purnell, & B. J. Paulanka (Eds.), *Transcultural health care: A culturally competent approach* (2nd ed.) (pp. 138-159). Philadelphia: F. A. Davis.

Pacquiao, D. F. (2008). People of Filipino heritage. In L. D. Purnell, & B. J. Paulanka (Eds.), *Transcultural health care: A culturally competent approach* (3rd ed.) (pp. 175-195). Philadelphia: F. A. Davis.

Pak-Hin, A. K., & Law, S. P. (2004). A Cantonese linguistic communication measure for evaluating aphasic narrative production: normative and preliminary aphasic data. *Journal of Multilingual Communication Disorders, 2,* 124-146.

Pearson, B. Z. (2004). Theoretical and empirical bases for dialect-neutral language assessment: Contributions from theoretical and applied linguistics to communication disorders. *Seminars in Speech and Language, 25,* 13-25.

Peña, E. D., & Kestrel, E. S. (2004). Semantic development in Spanish-English bilinguals: Theory, assessment and intervention. In B. A. Goldstein (Ed.), *Bilingual language development and disorders in Spanish-English speakers* (pp. 105-130). Baltimore: Paul H. Brookes.

Peña, E., Quinn, R., Iglesias, A. (1992). The application of dynamic methods to language assessment: A nonbiased procedure. *Journal of Special Education, 26,* 269-280.

Peña, E., Iglesias, A., & Lidz, C. S. (2001). Reducing test bias through dynamic assessment of children's word learning ability. *American Journal of Speech-Language Pathology, 10,* 138-154.

Purnell, L. D. (2003). People of Appalachian heritage. In L. D. Purnell, & B. J. Paulanka (Eds.), *Transcultural health care: A culturally competent approach* (2nd ed.) (pp. 73-89). Philadelphia: F. A. Davis.

Purnell, L. D. (2008). The Purnell model for cultural competence. In L. D. Purnell & B. J. Paulina (Eds.), *Transcultural health care: A culturally competent approach* (3rd ed.) (pp. 19-55). Philadelphia: F. A. Davis.

Purnell, L. D., & Paulanka, B. J. (2003). Transcultural diversity and healthcare. In L. D. Purnell, & B. J. Paulanka (Eds.), *Transcultural health care: A culturally competent approach* (2nd ed.) (pp. 8-39). Philadelphia: F. A. Davis.

Qi, C. H., Kaiser, A. P., Milan, S., & Hancock, T. (2006). Language performance of low-income African American and European American preschool children on the PPVT-III. *Language, Speech, and Hearing Services in Schools, 37,* 5-16.

Ramkissoon, I., Proctor, A., Lansing, C. R., & Bilger, R. C. (2002). Digit speech reception thresholds (SRT) for non-native speakers of English. *American Journal of Audiology, 11,* 23-28.

Ratner, N. B. (2004). Fluency and stuttering in bilingual children. In B. A. Goldstein (Ed.), *Bilingual language development and disorders in Spanish-English speakers* (pp. 287-308). Baltimore: Paul H. Brookes.

Restrepo, M. A., Schwanenflugel, P. J., Blake, J., et al. (2006). Performance on the PPVT-III and the EVT: Applicability of the measures with African American and European American preschool children. *Language, Speech, and Hearing Services in Schools, 37,* 17-27.

Roeper, T. (2004). Diagnosing language variations: Underlying principles for syntactic assessment. *Seminars in Speech and Language, 25,* 41-55.

Rosa-Lugo, L. I., Rivera, E., & Rierson, T. K. (2010). The role of dynamic assessment within the Response to Intervention model in school-age English language learners. *Perspectives on school-based issues, 11,* 99-106.

Roseberry, C. A., & Connell, P. J. (1991). The use of an inverted language rule in the differentiation of normal and language-impaired Spanish-speaking children. *Journal of Speech and Hearing Research, 34,* 596-603.

Roseberry-McKibbin, C. (2008). *Multicultural students with special language needs: Practical strategies for assessment and intervention* (3rd ed.). Oceanside, CA: Academic Communication Associates.

Ross, R., & Ross, J. (2008). People of Thai heritage. In L. D. Purnell, & B. J. Paulanka (Eds.), *Transcultural health care: A culturally competent approach* (3rd ed.) (pp. 355-371). Philadelphia: F. A. Davis.

Rudebusch, J. (2007). *LinquiSystems Guide to RTI (Response to Intervention).* East Moline, IL: LinguiSystems, Inc.

Santana-Martin, S., & Santana, F. O. (2005). An introduction to Mexican culture for service providers. In J. H. Stone (Ed.), *Culture and disability: providing culturally competent services* (pp. 161-186). Thousand Oaks: Sage.

Santos, R. M., & Chan, S. (2004). Families with Pilipino roots. In E. W. Lynch, & M. J. Hanson (Ed.) *Developing cross-cultural competence: A guide for working with children and families* (3rd ed.) (pp. 299-344). Baltimore: Paul H. Brookes.

Saville-Troike, M. (1986). Anthropological considerations in the study of communication. In O. L. Taylor (Ed.), *Nature of communication disorders in culturally and linguistically diverse populations* (pp. 47-72). San Diego, CA: College Hill Press, Inc.

Scarborough, H. S. (1990). Index of productive syntax. *Applies Psycholinguistics, 11*, 1-22.

Semel, E., Wiig, E. H., & Secord, W. A. (2003). *Clinical evaluation of language fundamentals* (4th ed.), San Antonio, TX: Psychological Corporation.

Seymour, H. N. (2004). A noncontrastive model for assessment of phonology. *Seminars in Speech and Language, 25*, 91-99.

Seymour, H. N., Bland-Stewart, L., & Green, L. J. (1998). Difference versus deficit in child African American English. *Language, Speech, and Hearing Services in Schools, 29*, 96-108.

Seymour, H. N., Roeper, T. W., & deVilliers, J. (2003a). *Diagnostic evaluation of Language Variation Criterion Referenced.* San Antonio, TX: Psychological Corporation.

Seymour, H. N., Roeper, T. W., & deVilliers, J. (2003b). *Diagnostic evaluation of Language Variation Screening Test.* San Antonio, TX: Psychological Corporation.

Seymour, H. N., Roeper, T. W., & deVilliers, J. (2005). *Diagnostic evaluation of Language Variation Norm-Referenced.* San Antonio, TX: Psychological Corporation.

Sharifzadeh, V. (2004). Families with Middle Eastern roots. In E. W. Lynch, & M. J. Hanson (Eds.), *Developing cross-cultural competence: A guide for working with children and families* (3rd ed.) (pp. 373-414). Baltimore: Paul H. Brookes.

Sharts-Hopko, N. C. (2003). People of Japanese heritage. In L. D. Purnell, & B. J. Paulanka (Eds.), *Transcultural health care: A culturally competent approach* (2nd ed.) (pp. 218-233). Philadelphia: F. A. Davis.

Shipley, K. G., & McAfee, J. G. (2009). *Assessment in speech-language pathology: A resource manual* (4th ed.). Clifton Park, NY: Delmar Cengage Learning.

Short, E. L., Suzuki, L., Prendes-Lintel, M., et al. (2010). Counseling immigrants and refugees. In J. G. Ponterotto, J. M. Casas, L. A. Suzuki, and C. M. Alexander (Eds.), *Handbook of multicultural counseling* (3rd ed.) (pp. 201-212). Thousand Oaks, CA: Sage.

Soto, G., Huer, M. B., & Taylor, O. (1997). Multicultural issues. In L. L. Lloyd, D. R. Fuller, & H. H. Arvidson (Eds.), *Augmentative and alternative communication: A handbook of principles and practices* (pp. 406-413). Boston: Allyn & Bacon.

Southwood, F., & van Hout, R. (2010). Production of tense morphology by Afrikaans speaking children with and without specific language impairment. *Journal of Speech, Language, and Hearing Research, 53*, 394-413.

St-Pierre, M. & Béland, R. (2010). Reproduction of inflectional markers in French-speaking children with reading impairment. *Journal of Speech, Language, and Hearing Research, 53*, 469-489.

Steckler, J. A. (2008). People of German heritage. In L. D. Purnell, & B. J. Paulanka (Eds.). *Transcultural health care: A culturally competent approach* (3rd ed.) (pp. 213-230). Philadelphia, PA: F. A. Davis.

Still, O., & Hodgins, D. (2003). Navajo Indians. In L. D. Purnell, & B. J. Paulanka (Eds.), *Transcultural health care: A culturally competent approach* (2nd ed.) (pp. 279-283). Philadelphia: F. A. Davis.

Stockman, I. J. (1996). The promises and pitfalls of language sample analysis as an assessment tool for linguistic minority children. *Language, Speech, and Hearing Services in Schools, 27*, 355-366.

Stockman, I. J. (2000). The new Peabody Picture Vocabulary Test-III: An illusion of unbiased assessment. *Language, Speech, and Hearing Services in Schools, 31*, 340-353.

Stockman, I. J. (2006). Alveolar bias in the final consonant deletion patterns of African American children. *Language, Speech, and Hearing Services in Schools, 37*, 85-95.

Stockman, I. J. (2008). Toward validation of a minimal competence phonetic core for African American children. *Journal of Speech, Language, and Hearing Research, 51*, 1244-1262.

Taylor, O. L., & Matsuda, M. M. (1988). Storytelling and classroom discrimination. In G. S. Donaldson, & van Dijk, T. A. (Eds.), *Discourse and discrimination* (pp. 206-220). Detroit: Wayne State University Press.

Taylor, O. L., & Payne, K. (1983). Culturally valid testing: A proactive approach. *Topics in Language Disorders, 3*, 8-20.

Terrell, S. L., Arensberg, K., & Rosa, M. (1992). Parent-child comparative analysis: A criterion-referenced method for the nondiscriminatory assessment of a child who spoke a relatively uncommon dialect of English. *Language, Speech, and Hearing Services in Schools, 23*, 34-42.

Terry, J. M., Jackson, S. C., Evangelou, E., & Smith, R. L. (2010). Expressive and receptive language effects of African American English on a sentence imitation task. *Topics in Language Disorders, 30*, 119-134.

Thordardottir, E. (2008). Language-specific effects of task demands on the manifestation of Specific Language Impairment: A comparison of English and Icelandic. *Journal of Speech Language Hearing Research, 51*, 922-937.

Thordardottir, E. T., & Namazi, M. (2007). Specific language impairment in French-speaking children: Beyond grammatical morphology. *Journal of Speech, Language, and Hearing Research, 50*, 698-715.

Ting-Toomey, S., & Chung, L. C. (2005). *Understanding intercultural communication.* New York: Oxford University Press.

Tonkovich, J. D. (2002). Multicultural issues in the management of neurogenic communication and swallowing disorders. In D. E. Battle (Ed.), *Communication disorders in multicultural populations* (3rd ed.) (pp. 233-265). Boston: Butterworth-Heinemann.

U.S. Census Bureau (2009). *American community survey, Puerto Rico community survey.* Washington, DC: U.S. Government Printing Office.

U.S. Department of Education, Office of Special Education Programs (2006, October 4). *Building the legacy: IDEA 2004. Topic: Identification of Specific Learning Disabilities.* Retrieved from http://idea.ed.gov/explore/view/p/%2Croot%2Cdynamic%2CTopicalBrief%2C23%2C.

U.S. Department of Education, Office of Special Education Programs (2007, February 2). *Building the legacy: IDEA 2004. Topic: Disproportionality.* Retrieved from http://idea.ed.gov/explore/view/p/%2Croot%2Cdynamic%2CTopicalBrief%2C7%2C.

Vaughn-Cooke, F. (1986). The challenge of assessing the language of nonmainstream speakers. In O. L. Taylor (Ed.), *Treatment of communicative disorders in culturally and linguistically diverse populations* (pp. 23-48). San Diego, CA: College-Hill Press.

Wallace, G. L. (1997). RANBO. The reliable assessment of neurobehavioral organization. Cincinnati, OH: University of Cincinnati Department of Communicative Disorders and Sciences.

Wang, Y. (2003). People of Chinese heritage. In L. D. Purnell, & B. J. Paulanka (Eds.), *Transcultural health care: A culturally competent approach* (2nd ed.) (pp. 106-121). Philadelphia: F. A. Davis.

Wang, Y., & Purnell, L. D. (2008). People of Chinese heritage. In L. D. Purnell, & B. J. Paulanka (Eds.), *Transcultural health care: A culturally competent approach* (3rd ed.) (pp. 129-144). Philadelphia, PA: F. A. Davis.

Wegner, A. F., & Wegner, M. R. (2003). The Amish. In L. D. Purnell, & B. J. Paulanka (Eds.), *Transcultural health care: A culturally competent approach* (2nd ed.) (pp. 54-72). Philadelphia: F. A. Davis.

Wiig, E. H., & Langdon, H. W. (2006). *Wiig Assessment of Basic Concepts-Spanish*. Greenville, SC: Super Duper Publications.

Wiig, E. H., Nielsen, N. P., Minthon, L., & Warkentin, S. (2002). Alzheimer's Quick Test. San Antonio, TX: The Psychological Corporation.

Willis, W. O. (2004). Families of African American roots. In E. W. Lynch, & M. J. Hanson (Eds.), *Developing cross-cultural competence: A guide for working with children and families* (3rd ed.) (pp. 141-177). Baltimore: Paul H. Brookes.

Wilson, S. A. (2003). People of Irish heritage. In L. D. Purnell, B. J. Paulanka (Eds.), *Transcultural health care: A culturally competent approach* (2nd ed.) (pp. 194-204). Philadelphia, PA: F. A. Davis.

Wilton, L. (2010). Where do we go from here? Raising the bar of what constitutes multicultural competence in working with lesbian, gay, bisexual, and transgender communities. In J. G. Ponterotto, J. M. Casas, L. A. Suzuki, & C. M. Alexander (Eds.), *Handbook of multicultural counseling* (3rd ed.) (pp. 313-323). Thousand Oaks, CA: Sage.

Wolfram, W. (1969). *A sociolinguistic description of Detroit Negro speech*. Washington, DC: Center for Applied Linguistics.

Wong, A. M., Ciocca, V., & Yung, S. (2009). The perception of lexical tone contrasts in Cantonese children with and without specific language impairment (SLI). *Journal of Speech, Language, and Hearing Research, 52*, 1493-1509.

Wong, A. M., Klee, T., Stokes, S. F., et al. (2010). Differentiating Cantonese-speaking preschool children with and without SLI using MLU and lexical diversity, *Journal of Speech, Language, and Hearing Research, 53*, 794-799.

Westby, C. E. (1994). The effects of culture on genre, structure, and style of oral and written texts. In G. Wallach, & K. Butler (Eds.), *Language learning disabilities in school-age children and adolescents* (pp. 180-218). New York: Macmillan College.

World Health Organization (2001). *International classification of functioning, disability and health: ICF*. Geneva: World Health Organization.

Wyatt, T. A. (1991). Linguistic constraints on copula production in Black English child speech. *Dissertation Abstracts International, 52*, 02B, 0781.

Wyatt, T. A. (1995). Language development in African American child speech. *Linguistics and Education, 7*, 7-22.

Wyatt, T. A. (2002). Assessing the communicative abilities of clients from diverse cultural and language backgrounds. In D. E. Battle (Ed.), *Communication disorders in multicultural populations* (3rd ed.) (pp. 415-459). Boston: Butterworth-Heinemann.

Zimmerman, I. L., Steiner, V. G., & Pond, R. E. (2002). *Preschool language scale: Spanish* (4th ed.) San Antonio, TX: Psychological Corporation.

Zimmerman, I. L., Steiner, V. G., & Pond, R. E. (2011). Preschool language scale (5th ed.). San Antonio, TX: Psychological Corporation.

Zoucha, R., & Zamarripa, C. A. (2008). People of Mexican heritage. In L. D. Purnell, & B. J. Paulanka (Eds.), *Transcultural health care: A culturally competent approach* (3rd ed.) (pp. 309-324). Philadelphia: F. A. Davis.

ADDITIONAL RESOURCES

The following resources provide excellent information on cross-cultural communication differences and beliefs that could potentially impact on the case history interview.

Culturegrams Online Database. Available at: www.culturegrams.com/products/onlineedition.htm.

Lynch, E. W., & Hanson, M. J. (2004). *Developing cross-cultural competence: A guide for working with children and their families* (3rd ed.). Baltimore: Paul H. Brookes.

Purnell, L. D., & Paulanka, B. J. (2008). *Transcultural health care: A culturally competent approach* (3rd ed.). Philadelphia: F. A. Davis.

Roseberry-McKibbin, C. (2008). *Multicultural students with special language needs: Practical strategies for assessment and intervention* (3rd ed.). Oceanside, CA: Academic Communication Associates.

Stone, J. H. (2005). *Culture and disability: Providing culturally competent services*. Thousand Oaks: Sage.

The following are recommended resources for investigating structure and rules of different languages:

Campbell, G. L. (1995). *Concise compendium of the world's languages*. London and New York: Routledge.

McLeod, S. (2007). *The international guide to speech acquisition*. Clifton Park, NJ: Delmar Thompson Learning.

UCLA Language Materials Project. Retrieved from www.lmp.ucla.edu.

Wikipedia's language website. Available at http://en.wikipedia.org/wiki/Wikipedia.

The following are recommended for information on working with interpreters and translators:

Langdon, H. W. (2002). *Interpreters and translators in communication disorders: A practitioner's handbook*. Eau Claire, WI: Thinking Publications.

Langdon, H. W., & Cheng, L. L. (2002). *Collaborating with interpreters and translators in communication disorders: A guide for communication disorders professionals*. Eau Claire, WI: Thinking Publications.

Bilingual Child Case History Interview

LANGUAGES USED IN THE HOME

1. Who lives at home with you and your child?
2. What language does your child use most?
   a. At home
   b. At school
3. What languages are used in your home or any other place when speaking with your child?

Name of Individual	Language 1	Language 2	Mixture of Both
Parent 1			
Parent 2			
Siblings			
Other family members at home			
Other relatives outside of home			
Peers			

4. What language does your child typically use when speaking to others?

Name of Individual	Language 1	Language 2	Mixture of Both
Parent 1			
Parent 2			
Siblings			
Other family members at home			
Other relatives outside of home			
Peers			

5. Which language do you feel your child uses best?

RATINGS OF PERCEIVED LANGUAGE PROFICIENCY

6. How would you rate your child's ability to speak?

Lang. 1:	Very good	Good	Fair	Poor
Lang. 2:	Very good	Good	Fair	Poor

7. How would you rate your child's ability to understand?

Lang. 1:	Very good	Good	Fair	Poor
Lang. 2:	Very good	Good	Fair	Poor

8. How would you rate your child's ability read (if relevant)?

Lang. 1:	Very good	Good	Fair	Poor
Lang. 2:	Very good	Good	Fair	Poor

9. How would you rate your child's ability write (if relevant):

Lang. 1:	Very good	Good	Fair	Poor
Lang. 2:	Very good	Good	Fair	Poor

RATINGS OF LANGUAGE ABILITY IN EACH LANGUAGE SPOKEN

10. How would you describe the child's vocabulary skills?

Lang. 1:	Very good	Good	Fair	Poor
Lang. 2:	Very good	Good	Fair	Poor

11. How would you describe the child's sentence production skills?

Lang. 1:	Very good	Good	Fair	Poor
Lang. 2:	Very good	Good	Fair	Poor

12. How would you describe your child's ability to hold a conversation?

Lang. 1:	Very good	Good	Fair	Poor
Lang. 2:	Very good	Good	Fair	Poor

13. How would you describe your child's ability to tell or retell stories (if age appropriate)?

Lang. 1:	Very good	Good	Fair	Poor
Lang. 2:	Very good	Good	Fair	Poor

14. How would you describe your child's ability to follow simple commands/instructions, such as "Brush your teeth"?

Lang. 1:	Very good	Good	Fair	Poor
Lang. 2:	Very good	Good	Fair	Poor

15. How would you describe your child's ability to follow complex commands/instructions, such as "Go to your room and get your green jacket out of the closet"?

Lang. 1:	Very good	Good	Fair	Poor
Lang. 2:	Very good	Good	Fair	Poor

16. How would you describe your child's pronunciation skills?

Lang. 1:	Very good	Good	Fair	Poor
Lang. 2:	Very good	Good	Fair	Poor

17. How well are you able to understand your child when he/she is talking?

Lang. 1:	Very well	Somewhat well	Not well
Lang. 2:	Very well	Somewhat well	Not well

18. How about other persons in the home?

Lang. 1:	Very well	Somewhat well	Not well
Lang. 2:	Very well	Somewhat well	Not well

19. How about other people outside of the home?

Lang. 1:	Very well	Somewhat well	Not well
Lang. 2:	Very well	Somewhat well	Not well

20. How about your child's friends?

Lang. 1:	Very well	Somewhat well	Not well
Lang. 2:	Very well	Somewhat well	Not well

21. How about your child's teachers at school?

Lang. 1:	Very well	Somewhat well	Not well
Lang. 2:	Very well	Somewhat well	Not well

CHILD'S LANGUAGE DEVELOPMENT

22. Did your child babble (e.g., make baby sounds like "baba" and "dada")?

23. At what age did your child say his/her first words?

24. What were his/her first words?
  a. Language 1 (ask for an example)
  b. Language 2 (ask for an example)

25. When did your child begin putting two words together?
  a. Language 1 (ask for an example)
  b. Language 2 (ask for an example)

26. When did your child start using sentences?
  a. Language 1 (ask for an example)
  b. Language 2 (ask for an example)

27. How long (e.g., number of words) are your child's sentences?
  a. Language 1 (ask for an example)
  b. Language 2 (ask for an example)

28. Does your child ever leave words out of sentences?
  a. Language 1 (ask for an example)
  b. Language 2 (ask for an example)

29. Does your child ever make any other types of mistakes in his/her sentences?
  a. Language 1 (ask for an example)
  b. Language 2 (ask for an example)

30. How does your child's language development compare with that of siblings and other children?
  a. His/her siblings when they were developing language
  b. His/her siblings when they were the same age that your child is now
  c. Other child family members or peers of the same age

Bilingual Adult Case History Interview

LANGUAGES USED WITHIN AND ACROSS DIFFERENT COMMUNICATION ENVIRONMENTS AND PARTNERS*

1. I'd like to start out by asking you a few questions about the languages you use in your home. First, who lives at home with you?
2. What percentage of the time would you say that you use each language with these individuals?

Name of Individual	Language 1	Language 2
Spouse		
Children		
Other relatives (e.g., parents, grandchildren)		
Other (specify)		

3. Are there any individuals who you talk with on a regular basis outside of the home?
   a. If yes, who?
4. What percentage of the time would you say that you use each of these languages with these individuals?

Name of Individual	Language 1	Language 2
Individual 1		
Individual 2		

5. What percentage of the time would you say that you use each of these languages within each of these environments?

Environment/ Activity	Language 1	Language 2	Both Used Equally
Home			
Work			
In the community while doing errands (e.g., shopping)			
School (if relevant)			

Environment/ Activity	Language 1	Language 2	Both Used Equally
On the phone with friends			
On the phone with relatives			
When socializing with others			

*Another alternative to the questions and charts used for questions #2 through #5 is to ask a question like, "on the average, how often do you use . . . " or "on a daily basis, how often do you use . . . " with a rating scale like "all the time," "sometimes," "rarely" vs. percentages for each listed individual and environment.

6. Overall, what language do you feel you use most?

RATINGS OF PERCEIVED LANGUAGE PROFICIENCY*

7. How well would you say that you speak?

Lang. 1:	Very good	Good	Fair	Poor
Lang. 2:	Very good	Good	Fair	Poor

8. How well would you say that you understand?

Lang. 1:	Very good	Good	Fair	Poor
Lang. 2:	Very good	Good	Fair	Poor

9. How well would you say that you read?

Lang. 1:	Very good	Good	Fair	Poor
Lang. 2:	Very good	Good	Fair	Poor

10. How well would you say that you write?

Lang. 1:	Very good	Good	Fair	Poor
Lang. 2:	Very good	Good	Fair	Poor

*Another way to rate responses to questions 7 to 10 is to provide the client with a rating scale like "on a scale of 1 to 5 with 1 being poor and 5 being very good, how would you rate your ability to (speak, understand, read, write) _____ language?"

11. Overall, what language do you feel you speak best?

DISORDER-SPECIFIC QUESTIONS

In addition to the above, clinicians should determine patterns of language difficulty across languages spoken, such as when the problem (e.g., stuttering) was first noticed in each language and whether the client experiences the same types of difficulties (e.g., difficulty coming up with words, difficulty getting the words out) in all languages spoken.

For clients with aphasia, traumatic brain injury, and other neurologic conditions, it is also useful to determine language use patterns and difficulties observed across different language modalities preonset (e.g., before a stroke) compared with postonset (immediately after the stroke and/or currently).

HISTORY OF LANGUAGE EXPOSURE AND RESIDENCE

I'd like to ask you a few questions about the languages that you used when you were growing up.

12. First, can you tell me where you were born?
13. How long have you lived in the United States?
14. What other places have you lived besides where you were born and the United States?
15. About how long did you live in each of these places?

Place of Residence	Length of Time	Approximate Dates
Place of birth		
United States		
Other location 1		
Other location 2		
Other location 3		

16. When you were growing up, what language(s) did you speak most:
    a. In your home?
    b. At school?
    c. With your friends outside of home and school?
    d. With anyone else outside of home and school?
17. When and how were you first exposed to:
    a. Language 1?
    b. Language 2?

18. Now I'd like to ask you a few questions about your education and schooling. Where did you attend:
    a. Elementary/primary school?
    b. Junior high school/middle school? (if relevant)
    c. High school/secondary school?
19. Have you had any schooling beyond high school? If yes, what type of schooling have you had (e.g., college, vocational training, adult education, adult language schooling)?
20. What was the primary language of instruction in:

Place of Schooling	Language 1	Language 2	Other
Elementary/primary school			
Junior high school/middle school			
High school/secondary school			
College 1			
College 2			
Other postsecondary school			

OTHER'S PERCEPTIONS OF COMMUNICATIVE DIFFICULTIES

21. When you were growing up, did anyone ever make any comments about your communication skills in:
    a. Language 1
    b. Language 2? (probe for types of comments made each language).
22. As an adult, does anyone in your family make any comments about your communication skills in:
    a. Language 1?
    b. Language 2?
23. How about others outside of your family, such as coworkers, colleagues, peers, in:
    a. Language 1?
    b. Language 2? (probe for types of comments made in each language)

Intervention for Multicultural and International Clients with Communication Disorders

Priscilla Nellum Davis and Tachelle Banks

With the increasing diversity of the U.S. population, speech-language pathologists (SLPs) have skills in cultural competence to ensure that they are able to meet the needs of children and adults with communication and swallowing disorders from diverse cultural and linguistic backgrounds. Professionals providing services need to be prepared to work with people from a variety of ethnic, racial, and cultural groups (American Speech-Language-Hearing Association [ASHA], 2008; 1985). The intervention chapter in previous editions of this book focused on cultural and linguistic diversity in the United States and included considerations for clinical practice, information for avoiding cultural conflicts in the clinic, the use of ethnographic interviews to learn about cultures, and guidelines for culturally relevant intervention procedures. Because of the increase in diversity in the United States and the need for information about clinical practice for communication disorders around the world, a more global perspective is addressed in this edition. Laws affecting persons with disabilities, best practices for intervention, and information about various cultures and religions are provided.

The increase in diversity resulting from immigration to industrialized countries all over the world has resulted in the need for changes in assessment and intervention for communication disorders. Many countries that did not provide clinical services for communication disorders as recently as 30 years ago are now seeking information, services, and training. Persons who immigrated to the United States and to other parts of the world are now seeking services for disorders. Issues for clinical intervention must recognize the increase in consumers who speak languages other than English and those who are learning English as a second language. The SLPs and audiologists must find ways to deliver services to persons from various cultures and those who speak various languages in order for assessment and intervention to be culturally and linguistically appropriate and for information to be disseminated around the world to people who need these services.

LEGAL ASPECTS OF INTERVENTION IN THE UNITED STATES

The No Child Left Behind (NCLB) Act (2002) seeks to correct achievement gaps that are most prevalent among students in specific subgroups, including those with disabilities, those with linguistic and cultural diversity, and those with economic disadvantage. The reauthorization of federal special education legislation through the Individuals with Disabilities Education Improvement Act (IDEIA, 2004) moved to align the accountability for learners with disabilities with the guiding principles of NCLB, which was signed into law in January 2002. This federal mandate was a major revision to the Elementary and Secondary Education Act (ESEA) of 1965. The law significantly challenged the status quo of public schools and established the U.S. Department of Education as a responsible party for increasing student achievement in public schools. Turnbull (2005) identified six primary principles of NCLB: accountability, highly qualified teachers, scientifically based instruction, local flexibility, safe schools, and parent participation and choice. IDEIA was reauthorized in 2004 with the intent of improving the existing legislation with a primary purpose of aligning the provisions of IDEIA with NCLB. Although the individual provisions of IDEIA are different from NCLB, the overall goals of the two are similar. The partnership of NCLB and IDEIA provides the opportunity for successful academic achievement for students with disabilities by implementing the systemic changes mandated by NCLB through the Individual Education Plans (IEPs) as regulated by IDEIA. In addition, IDEIA mandated the use of evidenced-based strategies to address concerns associated with the overidentification of culturally and linguistically diverse students, students from low-income families, and students in certain disability categories.

Overidentification and disproportionality of culturally and linguistically diverse children occur in special education, especially those identified with learning disability, mild mental retardation, and emotional behavior disorders. The disproportionality involves African American, Latino, and American Indian/Native American children, those from low-income families, and those learning English as a second language. Their identification as children in need of special education is often unrelated to a disability and is often related to poor instructional programs, language difficulty, and stress related to situations at school, in the family, or in the community. A new provision under IDEIA 2004 requires states to develop policies and procedures to decrease inappropriate identification of students with disabilities and to avoid and examine disproportionate representation by race and ethnicity. Schools are required to collect data to show the number of students in special education programs by race and ethnicity for each of the disability categories. Furthermore, if states identify a disproportionate number of students of color receiving special education services, they must follow through with procedures for analyzing and reporting the findings. This provision is linked to the 2004 IDEA Special Rule for eligibility determination: that a disability cannot be identified if the determining factor is a lack of instruction in reading or math or limited English proficiency (Wright & Wright, 2006). While ensuring access to high-quality instruction, the provision also ensures that students with limited English proficiency have sufficient time and instruction to acquire adequate English language skills. By providing both high-quality instruction and time to learn English, it will decrease incidents of misdiagnosis and overrepresentation of minority students, particularly students with limited English proficiency, in special education (Bowen, 2006).

Family-Centered and Culturally Responsive Services

An aim of all early intervention services and supports is responsivity to family concerns for each child's strengths, needs, and learning styles (Paul, 2007; Roth & Worthington, 2005). An important component of individualizing services includes the ability to align services with each family's culture and unique situation, preferences, resources, and priorities. The term *family centered* refers to a set of beliefs, values, principles, and practices that support and strengthen the family's capacity to enhance the child's development and learning (Boone & Crais, 2001; Dunst, 2001, 2004; IDEIA, 2004; Polmanteer & Turbiville, 2000). These practices are predicated on the belief that families provide a lifelong context for a child's development and growth (Beatson, 2006; Bronfenbrenner, 1992). The family, rather than the individual child, is the primary recipient of service delivery to the extent desired by the family. Some families may choose for services to be focused on the family, whereas others may prefer a more child-centered approach. Family-centered services support the family's right to choose who the recipient of the services is. Early identification and intervention efforts are designed and carried out in collaboration with the family, fostering their independence and competence and acknowledging their right and responsibility to decide what is in the best interest of their child (Dunst et al., 1993). Family-centered services emphasize shared decision making about referral, need for assessment and intervention, types of assessment and intervention approaches, methods for monitoring and sharing information with others important to the child and family, development of functional outcomes, and implementation of intervention. There is no single set of practices that is appropriate to meet the needs of all families. Family-centered early intervention practices respect family choices and decisions (Summers et al., 2005). Components of family-centered practices include offering more active roles for families in the planning, implementing, interpreting, and decision making in service delivery. Family-centered practices can maximize time and other resources, create closer alignment between family and professional decisions and plans, and increase decision making by families (Dunst, 2002; Summers et al., 2005).

All early intervention services and supports are directly influenced by the cultural and linguistic backgrounds of the family, child, and professionals. Every clinician has a culture, just as every child and family has a culture (ASHA, 2004). SLPs need to recognize their own as well as the family's cultural beliefs, values, behaviors, and influences, and how these factors might affect their perceptions of and interactions with others. Like all clinical activities, early intervention services are inherently culture bound because they reflect the beliefs, values, and interaction styles of a social group (Battle, 2002; Johnston & Rogers, 2001). Factors such as beliefs about child rearing, discipline, authority roles, and styles of communication, as well as views on disability and past experiences with health care or other professionals, can influence the family's interactions and decision-making process. In some cultures, for example, emphasis is placed on what a child can learn independently, whereas other cultures focus on what a learner can accomplish in collaboration with others. Therefore, different learning styles and values regarding means of teaching and learning necessitate different assessment and instructional approaches and strategies (Terrell & Hale, 1992; van Kleeck, 1994).

With the changing demographics in the United States and the differences that may occur between service providers and families in sociocultural characteristics (e.g., age, language, culture, race, gender, ethnicity, background, lifestyle, geography), it is important to gather information from families about the ways in which these factors may influence family-provider relationships and communication. For these reasons, some programs use cultural guides or cultural-linguistic mediators to facilitate communication and understanding between professionals and families (Barrera, 2000; Lynch & Hanson, 2004; Moore & Mendez,

2006). Moreover, from the perspective of "recommended practices" as well as policy (ASHA, 2004; IDEIA, 2004), all materials and procedures used in the provision of early identification and intervention services and supports should be culturally and linguistically appropriate for the individual child and family (ASHA, 2008a; National Association for the Education of Young Children [NAEYC], 2009).

Parental Involvement in Intervention

IDEIA (2004) (P.L. 108-446) ensures educational services for eligible infants, toddlers, children, and youth with disabilities. Under IDEIA, children with certain disabilities qualify for special education and related services designed to meet their unique needs and prepare them for further education, employment, and independent living. The law has specific provisions for ensuring that assessment and intervention are provided in a culturally and linguistically appropriate manner. Part B provides for children aged preschool through 21 years, including preparations for transition from school to community after age 21 years. Part C provides for infants and toddlers from birth through age 3 years. The law includes provisions to ensure parental participation in the decisions that are made regarding their child if they choose. If the native language of the parent is not English, the parents have the right to an interpreter for any and all sessions during which decisions are made regarding their child's educational program. They have the right to participate in meetings related to the provision of clinical special education and related services for their child; to be members of any group that decides whether their child is a "child with a disability" and meets eligibility criteria for special education and related services; to be members of the team that develops, reviews, and revises the IEP for their child; and to be members of any group that makes placement decisions for their child. As reauthorized in 2004, IDEIA gives parents the right to refuse special education and related services or simply to not respond to a request by the school district to develop an IEP for the child.

The culture and beliefs of the parents can play a part in the willingness of the parent to participate in intervention decision regarding their child. They may have come from a culture where special educational service for children with disabilities does not exist or is delivered in ways quite different from in the United States. Cultural differences in attitudes toward disabilities may lead to parental decision to refuse special education and related services as allowed for under the law (Middleton, 2009). Given that the status of having a disability gives rise to a child's right to special education and related services, a nexus is created between the connotations of "disability" and "special education." Caruso (2005) argues that newcomers and persons from certain racial and ethnic groups "are likely to be hostile to the idea of special education, which they often deem

stigmatizing." Cultural beliefs can reduce the use of disability services by some families. Some families prefer family care to care involving strangers. Some mistrust Western systems because of an inability to relate to or understand the system. Others hold perceptions that disabilities are ascribed and therefore cannot be treated with intervention (Dunnett & Schlossar, 2004). In addition, some families attach social stigmas to disabilities—this is a fourth factor that has been identified as having a possible effect on whether culturally and linguistically diverse families use disability services (Caruso, 2005).

Response to Intervention

The alignment of NCLB and IDEIA puts strong emphasis on achievement for all students. Specifically, NCLB and IDEIA focus on the improved achievement for students from low-income families, those from culturally diverse backgrounds, and English language learners (ELLs). Included in IDEIA is the suggested use of Response to Intervention (RTI) to increase the likelihood that all students will receive high-quality instruction and consequent progress monitoring before being referred for special education services. RTI is a comprehensive, multitiered strategy to enable early identification and intervention for students at academic or behavioral risk. It is an alternative to the discrepancy model for the identification of students with learning disabilities. It is an approach to providing services, interventions, and supports to struggling learners at increasing levels of intensity rather than waiting for a child to fail before offering help. It involves universal screening, high-quality instruction, and interventions matched to student need, frequent progress monitoring, and the use of child response data to make educational decisions. The approach uses early supports in three tiers before determining the need for special education and clinical intervention. The usual tiers are as follows: tier 1 includes intervention in the regular education classroom; tier 2 includes direct noncategorical, non–special education interventions such as after-school math and reading programs; and tier 3 includes special education with IEP. The RTI model presumes that if a child does not make adequate progress with intensive research-based instruction delivered in tiers 1 and 2, the child may require more individualized educational support and therefore will require special education or related services. It also presumes that if the child is able to make adequate progress with tier 1 or tier 2 supports, the child may not require special education or related services.

RTI has the potential to affect clinical intervention for culturally and linguistically diverse (CLD) children and ELLs by requiring the use of research-based practices based on individual children's specific needs. Instruction and interventions must consider a student's cultural background and experiences as well as linguistic proficiency (in both English and the native language) in order for instruction to be appropriate before determining that the child requires special education and related services as a child with a disability. RTI requires that clinicians consider students' life experiences, including their language proficiencies in their first and second languages, as well as the contexts in which they are taught in developing early intervention programs.

CULTURALLY AND LINGUISTICALLY DIFFERENT STUDENTS AND RESPONSE TO INTERVENTION

When deciding whether a practice is appropriate for implementation as part of an RTI model, the practice must have been validated with students with whom the interventions will be used. The RTI model is a promising practice when used with CLD students because of the implementation of universally appropriate strategies for all students, and it must include evidenced-based strategies and pedagogy. Before determining whether a strategy is evidence based for students identified as CLD, the research must clearly disaggregate CLD variables as well as additional contextual variables (Klinger & Bianco, 2006). However, children identified as ELLs are often not included in research samples because of their limited English proficiency, and this results in limited external validity. Therefore, a prescribed strategy may not be appropriate for CLD students (Klinger & Edwards, 2006).

To promote cultural sensitivity in the implementation of RTI, Klinger and Edwards (2006) discussed the importance of the role of the teacher and *teacher assistance teams* in providing early intervention for CLD children. The researchers offered several concerns regarding culturally responsive environments in the classroom, including (1) the knowledge of the teacher about second language acquisition; (2) the knowledge of the teacher about bilingual education and English as second language teaching methods; (3) the teacher's skill in effective intervention and assessment procedures for culturally and linguistically diverse students; and (4) the teacher's culturally responsive attributes.

Under the traditional model of RTI, teacher assistance teams are put in place to facilitate the referral process when students are unresponsive to evidence-based instruction. Klinger and Edwards (2006) stated that the makeup of the team should be diverse and include members with expertise in culturally responsive instruction and, if appropriate, expertise in English language acquisition and bilingual education. There should be a team member who can offer guidance with culturally sensitive ongoing assessment. Teams should have a wide range of meaningful intervention strategies available to them. Using a problem-solving approach, they should determine how to alter the support a student has been receiving and develop specific instructional objectives based on student performance data. An SLP should be a member of the team because of the SLP's expertise in language development and cultural and linguistic diversity.

INTERVENTION WITH ENGLISH LANGUAGE LEARNERS

Research has shown that instruction should be in the language used in the home in order to develop a firm foundation in the first language before the introduction of a second language. (See Chapter 7 for a further explanation of bilingual development and intervention for ELL children). Two approaches are recommended for intervention with ELLs: (1) provide intervention in the language of the child, and (2) provide intervention using the child's home language and the language of the school if the clinician knows both languages. For example, when introducing concepts such as colors, shapes, and body parts to preschool children, the clinician should use both the child's first language and English as a second language. Familiar preschool interactive activities can be used to increase receptive and expressive language skills, such as planting a seed. For example, goals should target words such as dirt, seed, water, cup, pour, window, and sun. The clinician can explain the activity in the child's language and then provide the English word. The child will be instructed to point to the item in the first language and then to another item in English. The child should be required to explain the concept in both languages. If the child is hesitant to speak, the clinician can allow more response time. The child may be going through the silent period, which may last from a month to a year. During this time, the child may be increasing receptive language skills.

Values of the child's culture should be taken into consideration. Information obtained in the ethnographic interview should help professionals provide services that will not cause cultural conflicts. Some cultures do not value competition, individualism, or self-fulfillment. Games that are competitive or require a winner may not be received well. Traditional reinforcers such as collecting tokens may not be effective for therapy. Parents should be consulted before selecting treatment plans and reinforcers, especially if food will be used as a reinforcer.

LANGUAGE SURVIVAL SKILLS FOR OLDER ENGLISH LANGUAGE LEARNERS

Language survival skills should be an immediate intervention goal for new older ELLs and CLD students. Survival skills should be taught immediately at the preschool, grade school, and high school ages. Suggestions for topics at each age level are provided.

Prevocational skills or survival skills for young children are similar to prerequisites often required for (1) kindergarten entry, such as being able to provide personal information (full name, address, phone, and names of parents); (2) grade school, such as time concepts, money, and survival safety; (3) middle and high school (grades 7 to 12), such as vocational skills and goals. Professionals should incorporate into therapy goals information about job advertisements, applications, interviews, and expected performance. Lessons targeting pragmatic skills are a necessity for classroom and vocational success. Children from diverse cultures often have language and nonverbal styles that are different from those of mainstream cultural groups. Topics that should be covered are eye contact, gestures and facial expressions, polite terms, and conversational discourse rules. Because idioms and slang are culture bound, special therapy sessions and classroom activities should be provided to teach idioms and slang common to the culture or geographical area. Examples of idiomatic expressions common to people in the United States and some Western cultures are "catch a plane," "hop a train," "butterflies in your stomach," "raining cats and dogs," "piece of cake," "costs an arm and a leg," "break a leg," "bite your tongue," "cry wolf," "dry run," "funny farm," "ride the short bus," "not playing with full deck," "high five," "kicking it," "bounce back," and "kick the bucket." These idioms may not be common to people outside the culture. Each geographic region may have different idiomatic expressions. Other suggestions about slang and business jargon may be sought from the students and members of the community (Roseberry-McKibbin, 2008a).

The following suggestions can be used by SLPs, classroom teachers, special education teachers, English as a second language teachers, and other professionals when providing intervention services to CLD children:

1. Do not emphasize language production immediately. Students may be encouraged to speak but should not be forced because they may be going through the silent period.
2. Speak slowly, allowing time for students to understand and process information.
3. Use frequent pauses between words, phrases, and sentences.
4. Use short, simple sentences.
5. Give examples. Use gestures, pictures, and visual aids to facilitate comprehension.
6. Allow extra time.
7. Avoid slang and idioms. Explain them when their use is unavoidable.
8. Give preferable seating for vision and hearing by placing students nearby.
9. Use the buddy system or assign a peer mentor for assistance in the classroom (adapted from Multicultural Speech Therapy, Wordpress.org, 2010a).
10. Use frequent checks for understanding instructions and content.

CULTURALLY DIVERSE FAMILIES IN EARLY INTERVENTION

Part C of the IDEIA provides for early intervention (EI) for children from birth to the age of 3 years who are diagnosed as having a physical or mental condition (with a high probability of resulting in a developmental delay), have an existing delay, are at risk for developing a delay, or have a special need that may affect their development or impede their education. The purpose of early intervention is to lessen the effects of the disability or delay. Services are designed to identify and meet a child's needs in five developmental areas: physical development, cognitive development, communication, social or emotional development, and adaptive development. A major goal of EI is to ensure that families who have children ages birth to 3 years with a diagnosed disability, developmental delay, or substantial risk for significant delay receive resources and supports that assist them in maximizing their child's development while respecting the diversity of families and communities.

The past two decades have seen a shift from direct services to the child toward services involving the families and caregivers as collaborators (Madding, 2000). This shift brings the primary focus of intervention to the level of the family system (Hanson & Lynch, 1995; Mahoney et al., 1999). The family system model relies on the education and empowerment of parents and caregivers to use strategies to improve their children's communication. The model is potentially culturally problematic if parents and EI providers do not share the same assumptions and understandings about their roles in the collaboration (Lowenthal, 1996; Lynch & Hanson, 2004; Madding 1996; Rivers, 2000; van Kleek, 1994). Differences in such assumptions can be influenced further by socioeconomic status of the families served by EI providers in early intervention settings. Specifically, issues such as parent education and literacy, availability of materials such as books and toys, and context such as the physical space accessible for child-focused activities also influence the focus of such services.

According to Peña and Fiestas (2009), families from diverse cultural backgrounds and lower socioeconomic levels are less pleased with early intervention services than their white families and families of higher socioeconomic levels. They cited the problem areas as differences in (1) parent education and training, (2) expectations or outcomes of intervention, (3) parent literacy, and (4) availability of space and material. Many of the Latina mothers in their study appeared uncomfortable using the techniques suggested in training. According to Madding (1999), Hispanic mothers in a center-based intervention program appeared uncomfortable playing on the floor with their children or using reciprocal interactions to improve their children's communication. The mothers appeared unconvinced of the value of using reciprocal interactions, a common strategy taught to parents to improve their children's communication. Likely, they did not see their role as that of an equal conversational partner with their children (Zayas & Solari, 1994). The parents reported they did not perceive their role to be playmate and teacher for their children, but rather they saw themselves as caretaker. The studies show that the use of common elicitation techniques suggested by SLPs for children with language delay may be contrary to child-rearing practices and communication styles in various cultures. Conflict may occur when practices for early intervention, such as teaching parents strategies for modeling communication development, are not congruent with those of the parents. The clinician should explain the purpose of the activity and its expected outcome.

Parents from some cultures view parental involvement in intervention differently from what some professionals expect. They may not feel comfortable participating in planning IEPs or in engaging in practice at home. Expecting parents to view themselves as service providers and parent-teachers may present a problem for those who do not see themselves in this role because of their cultural values. Some cultures do not feel that parents should "play" with children.

Parents from some groups, such as Asian and Pacific Islanders and Hispanics/Latinos, see the clinician as the utmost authority over the child's education or intervention program. They believe that parents are not supposed to interfere with this process and may regard clinicians who seek parental involvement as incompetent (Peña & Fiestas, 2009). It is important to explain that parental involvement is part of the intervention program. However, because the level of parental involvement varies with cultures, parents and caretakers should be involved in the clinical process according to their cultural values.

Developmental milestones, such as walking, drinking from a cup, eating solid foods, toilet training, and sleeping alone, are influenced by culture. Some cultures do not expect children to engage in equal conversational turn-taking with adults. Other cultures expect young children to have proto-conversations and real conversational dyads very early (Peña & Fiestas, 2009).

Access to materials and space may be challenging for low-income or culturally and linguistically diverse families. Toys, books, computers, electronic toys, and play materials are often used to stimulate development. If the parents cannot read aloud to their children because of their literacy level or because suitable books are not readily available in their home language, they may not be able to use the home language stimulation techniques suggested by the clinician. Using books without words or picture books may also not be appropriate if the story or events in the books are culturally unfamiliar or inappropriate to the family (Evans, 2004).

Successful evidence-based practices should be consistent with the family's culture, values, socioeconomic status, language, religion, and educational level. Cultural sensitivity and acceptance are also important. The professional should use direct and indirect intervention techniques. When visiting the homes, indirect approaches are recommended and should be based on routines. Routine-based approaches can highlight aspects of communication development that are important to the family. Use of the routine-based approach gives the family the opportunity to determine the appropriate outcome for the child. Examples of a routine-based approach include naming colors of clothing when getting dressed, naming the types of clothing, and addressing body parts by discussing where each article of clothing will be placed.

When visiting the home, the clinician should find out the rules of the household. Many cultures expect a visitor to remove shoes before entering the home. For persons from some cultures, it is unacceptable to consider providing intervention in the home.

The NAEYC (2009) has developed quality benchmarks for cultural competence for working with the families of young children. The initial concepts that define cultural competence for working with young children are especially important when providing intervention in the home of the family and include the following (pp. 3-4):

1. Acknowledge that children are nested in families and communities with unique strengths.
2. Identify and build on the strengths and shared goals between the professional and families.
3. Understand and authentically incorporate the traditions and history of the families and their impact on child-rearing practices.
4. Understand and support each child's development within the family as complex and culturally driven experiences.
5. Ensure that decisions and policies regarding all aspects of the intervention program embrace and respect the language, values, attitudes, beliefs, and approaches to learning of the family.
6. Ensure that the policies and practices in the intervention program build on and preserve the home language and dialects of the children and family.
7. Recognize that the family is expert in the home. Ensure that the boundaries of the family structure, roles for communication, and authority for decisions are adhered to.

LITERACY

Alphabet knowledge and phonologic awareness are strong predictors of successful literacy development in children. It is particularly important to recognize the role that phonologic awareness plays in ELLs who must learn to read both in their native language (L1) and in their second language

(L2). Recent research reported by Ford (2009) has shown that, for ELLs, phonologic awareness in the L1 predicts successful literacy acquisition in both L1 and L2. In other words, phonologic awareness skills developed in L1 transfer to L2 and facilitate L2 literacy development. Phonologic awareness skills developed in one language can transfer to another language, even while those skills are still in the process of being developed (Cisero & Royer, 1995). Although this is often an advantage, ELLs may inappropriately generalize their first language's rules of syntax, spelling, phonology, or pragmatics to their second language, resulting in an adverse effect on L2 literacy acquisition (Bialystok, 2002; Brice & Roseberry-McKibbin, 2001). Based on a study of the connection between L1 language phonologic skills and L2 reading with 92 Spanish-speaking first-graders, Gottardo (2002) found that the strongest predictors of English word reading ability were L1 and L2 phonologic processing, L1 reading, and L2 vocabulary.

The closer the phonologies of L1 and L2 are to each other the greater the likelihood that transfer of skills will be positive rather than negative because children are more adept at manipulating the sounds and patterns that exist in their native language (Bialystok, 2002). For example, if both L1 and L2 are alphabetic languages, transfer will be facilitated, although positive transfer has also been documented between languages with very different orthographies, such as Cantonese and English (Gottardo et al., 2001). An important factor here may be the type of phonologic skill in question. As Durgunoglu (2002) notes, "there are certain literacy concepts and strategies that can be universal and operate across languages. These insights and skills need to be acquired only once and apply in all languages of LLs. However, there are also language-specific concepts and knowledge; for example, orthographic patterns that are specific to a language" (p. 192).

The goal of literacy training is to increase phonologic awareness, reading, writing, and spelling abilities. Phonologic awareness is a necessary foundation for a variety of skills including reading, writing, and spelling. The best strategies for improving phonologic awareness incorporate direct phonologic instruction. Direct phonologic instruction has been proved effective with monolingual and bilingual children. Roseberry-McKibbin (2008b) concluded that junior high school and high school students, regardless of their first language, who received specific phonologic awareness intervention showed improvement in their reading ability. Roseberry-McKibbin (2007) reported that ELL students of all ages who were poor readers and spoke English as their second language and who received direct, specific phonologic awareness intervention showed improvement in their ability to analyze the phonologic construct of words. Phonologic awareness strategies have also been effective in accent reduction.

Children who are CLD and ELLs have several major challenges to succeeding in school. They are often learning a second or third language while they are attempting to master academic skills appropriate for their grade level. An additional challenge will be placed on the child who has a language or learning disability. Children who are CLD and ELLs and are learning another language need extra support in preliteracy skills such as phonologic awareness. Measurable gains were achieved in one semester by children receiving this support.

Professionals are also encouraged to help CLD and ELL students focus on reading comprehension, create a culturally diverse environment, and develop reading strategies. These students may benefit from interactive book reading with discussions about what was been read, small group tutoring, and participation in reading groups. Younger children may enjoy read-aloud programs at the library and interactive computer programs. Numerous free read-along and read-aloud programs are available online. One program has famous people reading aloud with captions below (www.storylineonline.net/).

LITERACY INTERVENTION

Cummins (1984; Cummins et al., 2007) has looked at the development of literacy in second language learners for many years. He made a distinction between conversational language (formerly referred to as *basic interpersonal communicative skills,* or BICS), discrete language skills, and academic language (formerly known as *cognitive academic language proficiency,* or CALP). Conversational language, the language used by all native speakers of the language, is cognitively undemanding and contextual and is the language used in informal settings, such as on a playground or café. Academic language is more complex, abstract, and decontextualized, requiring a higher level of cognition necessary for academic instruction and textbooks. Cummins suggests that language learners need 1 to 3 years to develop conversational language in L2 if they have sufficient exposure to the second language. He further suggests that ELL students need at least 5 to 7 years to acquire academic language in L2. If they do not have a strong language base in discrete language skills in L1, they may require as many as 7 to 10 years to acquire academic language in L2 to support literacy. Instruction and intervention in L1 need to be direct and effective, and the child needs adequate exposure to L2 to develop academic language proficiency and literacy.

A strong base in discrete language skills is necessary for the student to progress in literacy and the academic arena. These skills involve knowing the specific rule-governed aspect of L2, which can be developed through direct instruction or intervention and by immersion in a literacy-rich home and school environment. The discrete language skill intervention focuses on phonologic awareness, letter recognition, letter-sound relationships, and, most important, vocabulary development. A typically developing child should be able to make the transition to L2 with the direct instruction and immersion in 5 to 7 years. However, if the child has a disorder, the transition may take longer and will require more direct intervention.

Roseberry-McKibbin (2008b) provided several suggestions for encouraging literacy skills in CLD students: (1) have students listen to books on tape, which may be available from the local library; (2) encourage students to share their language, cultural heritage, and songs in their primary language; (3) show interest in the students' primary language and culture; (4) use maps of the world to locate countries of origin; (5) help students find culturally appropriate reading material for use at home; and (6) when possible, employ tutors or teaching assistants who speak and understand the students' primary language and culture to help with comprehension. The SLP should collaborate with classroom teachers to promote the success of students with learning disabilities within the classroom setting.

A strategy presented by Roseberry-McKibbin (2008b) is the *preview-view-review technique* for working with ELL students, which may be used to increase comprehension, fluency, and vocabulary. Strategies are provided to teach students to preview reading material by reading the title, examining the table of contents, and looking through graphic information for determining the main idea and gathering clues about the book contents. In the view phase, the professional reads the book aloud, and the student follows along. Strategies and techniques used allow opportunities for the professional to stop and explain material, define difficult words, allow students to ask questions, help students visualize what is being read, and predict what happens next. In the review phase, the student reads the title and headings, asks questions, and summarizes information previously read. This technique and similar ones are used with students who are monolingual or bilingual and with those who have various dialects of English but are in need of specific literacy intervention.

Components of a balanced literacy program include the following: teacher read-alouds, shared reading, guided reading, language activities, independent reading, shared writing, interactive writing, guided writing, and independent writing. An example of a preschool activity that helps children develop phonologic awareness and literacy incorporating all these components is having the clinician read aloud a book about popcorn and targeting the /p/ sound. The book is read first in the child's L1 and then in English (L2). Children may be given bubble wrap to pop and produce the /p/ sound. Popcorn popped in a popcorn popper can also be used. When children hear the popcorn pop, they are encouraged to make the /p/ sound. The clinician asks, "What sounds do you hear? Can you make those sounds?" The children may be asked to draw pictures of the popcorn, and the popcorn can be used in an art activity. Using a digital or video camera, the clinician may take pictures of the activity so that students can make sentences describing the activity. The clinician writes the sentences or stories

that the students make up about the activity, creating a storybook. The children and clinician can read the story or sentences from the storybook about popcorn together, emphasizing the target sound /p/. The children can write a sentence about the activity. Each student's story or sentence can be written next to the student's photograph. Students can listen for the /p/ sound in different positions of the word.

In summary, intervention strategies should provide direct instruction in phonemic awareness early in kindergarten through third grade to reduce the likelihood of continued reading problems through high school for ELL and CLD students. Professionals should modify or customize reading programs to fit the needs of a child who has deficits in early reading skills. These programs may be adapted for children from diverse cultures in order to design effective reading programs for those students who have difficulties in their early years. It has been determined that effective results can be achieved from programs of 12 weeks' duration with an intensity of twice a week for 20 minutes (Schuele & Boundreau, 2008).

SELECTING CULTURALLY APPROPRIATE LITERATURE

When developing literacy with CLD clients, the clinician should use culturally appropriate literature that is relevant and meaningful to the client. Multicultural literature represents a cultural group through accurate portrayal and rich detail of the culture (Yokota, 1993, p. 157). Such literature appears in different genres, which together present a multitude of perspectives about the lives, culture, and contributions of each group to American society. Many criteria can be used to evaluate multicultural literature. The same criteria can be used to evaluate the appropriateness of multicultural toys. Some of the more important criteria include whether the culture is portrayed correctly; whether the setting is accurately portrayed, especially in historical texts; whether proper language is used; and whether the author is using offensive language or prejudiced tones. According to Agosto (1997), multicultural literature should be of high quality and carefully selected according to the following principles, which were condensed and combined with the guidelines presented by Shioshita (1997):

1. *Accuracy.* Details presented in the story, such as language, dress, foods, customs, values, and holidays, should be accurate. Thoughts and emotions should be portrayed authentically and should be historically correct for the time period portrayed.

2. *Respect.* The characters in the literature should be treated with respect in language, appearance, and absence of stereotypes based on race, ethnicity, and gender. Illustrations should be positive and worthwhile and should not demean or ridicule, oversimplify, or generalize characters. The illustrations should be appropriate to

the culture or race being depicted. The leaders or persons in power should be fairly represented in terms of race, ethnicity, and gender.

3. *Purpose.* The author should present an important message in addition to providing interesting positive information or a story about a culture or value.

4. *Quality.* The book should be well written and presented with a high-quality style. Has the book or author won any literacy awards?

5. *Language.* The language, dialect, and terminology used should be current and appropriate to the time period and should be free from pejorative terms unless germane to the story.

6. *Settings and illustrations.* Books should include accurate settings free from stereotype. For example, the settings should accurately describe the housing germane to the story and should not depict that all Native American people lived in a teepee or all Africans live in grass huts in the jungle. Illustrations should show differences among members of an ethnic group. All members should not look alike.

7. *Author.* Authors should have extensive authentic knowledge about the culture that they depict in the text. Some people believe that writers should belong to the culture that they write about.

8. *Sensitivity.* Did the text handle controversial and difficult issues with sensitivity, such as real-life issues that clients are facing (for example, characters who are biracial or who are being reared in a single-parent or same-sex family–single-sex family)?

CREATING CULTURALLY APPROPRIATE PHYSICAL ENVIRONMENTS

Creating environments that are inviting and welcoming for all clients is key to providing culturally appropriate clinical services. The following is a list of suggested strategies that clinicians may use to create culturally responsive environments that are inviting and positive for all.

1. Use materials and content that reflect central aspects of the cultures of the clients served.

- Current and relevant bulletin boards that display positive and purposeful activities and events involving culturally diverse people. Include, for example, newspaper articles reporting newsworthy events or accomplishments that involve people of color, photographs of community leaders from culturally diverse backgrounds, historical events with culturally diverse themes. Posters and other visual displays should reflect an appreciation for diversity.

- Printed materials such as in-house publications, newsletters, brochures, and websites should reflect the population served. Materials about families in information libraries such as videos and handouts should be both adult and child focused. Traditional and nontraditional families should be included.

- Images of people with a range of abilities and body types engaged in a variety of activities.

2. Use welcome signage in different languages, including the languages of the clients served.

- For example, if the signs explaining that all visitors need to first sign in at the office are only in English, Spanish-speaking clients may be unable to follow the appropriate process.

3. Present clinical instructions in the language of the clients.

- Kohnert and associates (2005) recommend that SLPs provide services to CLD children with language impairment in a manner that effectively supports the development of the home language even when it is not the language used in the school or the community.

- For young children, services should be provided in the language spoken in the home. This technique incorporates the use of the family in the language learning process and shows respect for and value of the native language (Texas Speech and Hearing Association, 2010).

- The clinician should learn some key words or phrases, such as greetings or simple instructions, in the client's first language.

- If sign language is going to be taught, the clinician must be aware that some hand shapes are offensive gestures in some cultures.

- Some English sounds may have articulation placements that are offensive gestures. An effort was made to teach a Portuguese speaker the correct placement of the voiceless /th/ sound. The speaker said placing your tongue between your teeth in that manner was a lewd gesture in the part of Brazil where she lived.

4. Use language appropriate for the clinical setting.

- Use person-first language, such as the "child with a learning disability" rather than the "learning-disabled child."

- Use language that avoids perpetuating stereotypes, for example, avoiding phrases such as "sitting Indian style."

- Use gender-neutral language and terms that include nontraditional families such as "parent," "caregiver," "guardian," and "partner" rather than "mother" and "father."

5. Provide clinic materials and objects that represent various cultures.

- Toys, dolls, magazines, and books that represent the cultures of the clients should be available in the clinic area as well as the waiting area.

- Dolls' clothing should reflect accurately people's current daily lives. They may also focus on national dress of other countries. Both male and female dolls should be provided.

- Artwork and cultural displays, including the children's own work, should be drawn from a range of cultural traditions.

- Objects used for holiday celebrations should be secular, rather than religious, in order to respect the various religions of clients. For example, Christmas and Hanukkah decorations can focus on snowmen; Halloween can focus on fall and harvest; and Easter can focus on spring, rather than symbols of Christian religions.
- A variety of cooking and eating utensils from various cultures may be used in the preschool language room for play, such as chopsticks, forks, spoons, spatulas, rice bowls, wooden bowls, plates, woks, tortilla presses.
- Clothing for dress up should include play and work clothes, such as uniforms, pants, dresses, batik, saris, kimonos, serapes, kente cloth, ponchos, tunics, scarves, moccasins, and sandals. Consider that because of religious and cultural beliefs, some parents may not want their girls to wear pants and their boys to wear any clothing considered feminine.
- Musical instruments from around the world should be available, such as cymbals, guitars, harmonicas, xylophones, keyboards, triangles, bagpipes, accordions, castanets, conch shells, brass bells, rattles, wooden flutes, maracas, gourds, and bongo drums.
6. Display calendars that show special holidays and events from different cultures.
- For example, each month on the calendar recognizes different cultures, such as Spanish Culture Month, Native American Culture Month, Black History Month, and Womens' History Month.
- Objects or materials recognizing these themes may be displayed.
7. Music used in the waiting area and in the therapy session should be culture neutral or reflect the cultures of clients served.
- Music is integral to all groups and can be incorporated into therapy activities.
8. Music should reflect the culture and can be used for teaching different language concepts.
9. Physical space should be appropriate.
- Space should be large enough for the intervention session and to accommodate persons who may accompany the client. In some cultures, several members of the family may accompany the client and will expect to be present during the session.
- Physical space should be provided for family privacy as appropriate.

PLAY

Concepts and rules of play differ among cultures. Play allows children to practice skills needed as adults, such as following directions and working with others. How one plays and the value of play vary with cultures. Parmar and colleagues (2004) conducted a comprehensive study of the ethnotheories of play and learning with Asian and Euro-American parents. The Euro-American parents believed in the value of play for the cognitive and educational benefit of their children and thus engaged in and facilitated play with their children and provided them with numerous toys. The Asian mothers, on the other hand, believed more strongly in the early academic development of their children and were less likely to engage in or facilitate play with their children. They provided them with significantly fewer toys and were more likely to engage the children in preliteracy activities such as alphabet, numbers, and computer and reading activities. In New Guinea, games are not played competitively, as they are in the United States; rather, they are played until both sides reach equality. In Japan, caregivers do not stress independence; rather, they stress the importance of a group. In the Navajo culture, cheating in play is not viewed as bad (Rettig, 1995).

Ethnicity, gender, and poverty differences are critical variables that affect how and when children play together. Understanding how children discover cultural differences will assist with engineering environments and creating opportunities for play between children who are culturally different. Young children recognize differences based on ethnicity and gender, although gender is usually the first difference that children notice. For instance, between the ages of 3 and 4 years, children notice color and racial differences and are likely to start believing stereotypes (Rettig, 1995). Considering the impact of social and educational variables, professionals need help in structuring how they create and teach in a culturally diverse setting.

PLANNING AND ASSESSING CULTURAL DIVERSITY AND PLAY

Play could improve student empowerment as well as encourage students to engage more in therapy (Juelis, 2009). The relationship between play and culture in the therapy setting is noteworthy because of the number of culturally diverse clients receiving therapy.

Play is a way children learn about new cultures. Educational programs must include a positive awareness of cultural diversity (Rettig, 1995). It is important that students learn about cultural differences and that professionals build learning opportunities that center around cultural diversity. Table 13-1 provides guidelines for informal assessment of play environments for all children.

DIVERSE RELIGIONS AND CULTURE AND INTERVENTION

Religion has an influence on all aspects of culture. Where a particular religion is dominant, the culture will reflect the values of that religion. The following factors are important in the delivery of clinical services to those who hold certain religious beliefs. The information presented is not meant to be all inclusive or to apply to all persons who observe the religion and culture. In all religions, there is a continuum of

TABLE 13-1 Informal Assessment for Evaluating Play Environments for All Children

Creating Culturally Diverse Play Environments for All Children	Yes	No
Are diverse perspectives and cultures integrated into toys, textbooks, and other therapy materials?		
Are diverse perspectives portrayed without bias or stereotypes?		
Is the classroom religion neutral? Do therapy materials include appropriate information about religion only when religion is integral to the context of the subject? Is there consideration for those who do not follow a particular religion or religious holiday?		
Do therapy materials include various cultures represented by families in the school and community?		
Are therapy materials selected that allow all students to participate and feel challenged and successful?		
Does the professional model incorporate respect for, and inclusion of, people who are different (e.g., religion, race, language, abilities, disabilities, income level)?		

those who practice the religion according to strict beliefs and those who only loosely practice the religion. It is important to determine where clients are on that continuum before making generalizations about their observance or practice. The practices are intended as a guide to assist the clinician in determining the most culturally appropriate mode of service delivery.

Hindu and Buddhist Religion and Culture

1. Hindus believe that all life is sacred; therefore, they do not eat fish, chicken, shellfish, or any animal that is killed and eaten. Most Buddhists and Hindus are vegetarians and eat diets of vegetables and grains. Meats are not included in the diet. Meat should be avoided in activities, especially beef, because cows are thought to be sacred. Stories that depict killing animals should be avoided. References to fast-food restaurants where hamburgers are primarily served and the use of toys and items made and named for these restaurants should be avoided. Expressions such as "holy cow" may be inappropriate.

   Intervention and assessment materials should be reviewed to ensure that they do not contain items that may be offensive. Because monkeys and snakes are thought to be sacred, stories in children's books with monkeys and snakes with human characteristics should be avoided (Trofimov, 2007). The /s/ is often referred to as the "snake" sound. When children are misbehaving or acting silly, these behaviors may be referred to as "monkey shines."

2. No photographs or audio- or video tapes should be taken of female Hindu clients without their permission. Photographs of women are to be looked at only by male family members or other women.

3. Strict rules govern the relationship between the sexes for Buddhists and Hindus. In some countries, men and women are not permitted to work together, and unmarried male and females may not touch each other. Opposite-sex clinicians would not be permitted to work with some Hindus. Handshaking is not a common gesture between men and women. Clinicians should not extend their hand unless the client extends his or her hand first. Women often put their palms together at the waist and present a slight bow of the head for a greeting.

4. The head is the purest body part because it contains the human spirit. Patting a child's or adult's head is a great offense in some countries (Kok et al., 1997). Explanations should be given when touching the head is required in intervention. Permission should be granted before engaging in any activity that involves touching the head, including placing earphones or headsets for intervention activities.

5. Buddhists celebrate a special 3-day holiday in August. New Year's Day, the first day of the first month of the lunar calendar, is a holiday on which devout worshipers go to the shrine to pray. The third, fifth, and seventh birthdays of children are important celebrations for Buddhists. Some families may travel to shrines on these birthdays to pray for the development of the young child.

Islam

Islam was founded in the seventh century in the Empire of the Caliphs, which stretched from Spain and Morocco across the Middle East to central Asia. People who practice the religion of Islam are called Muslims or Moslems. There are nearly 1.57 billion Muslims in the world today and 2 to 10 million in the United States (Sacirbey, 2010). They form the majority, but not all, of the population in the Middle East. Countries such as North Africa, India, and Saudi Arabia and Southeast Asian nations such as Pakistan, Malaysia, and Indonesia practice Islam. Islam is the fastest-growing religion in the United States, largely because of the increased immigration of people from the Middle East and the conversion of many African Americans to Islam (Nasir, 2010).

Followers of Islam believe that God gave his final revelation to the prophet Mohammed, who they believe to be the last in a succession of prophets, including Moses and Jesus. The *Koran,* the holy book containing Mohammed's revelations, is believed to be the full expression of the divine will for human life. Followers of Islam believe in the strength of the family and children and that wealth and children are the ornaments of this life (University of Virginia, 2000).

Muslims follow the lunar calendar, which is based on the phases of the moon. Each New Year begins on the second new moon after the winter solstice or any time between January and March.

Ramadan is a month-long observance of dedication and self-control. Because the time of Ramadan is determined by the lunar calendar, it begins on a different date each year on a solar or a Christian calendar. During Ramadan, no food or drink is consumed from sunrise to sunset. Children are not required to participate until they are 8 or 9 years of age, although some may participate for certain portions of the day. Children from the age of 8 or 9 years through adolescence are expected to participate from sunrise to sunset. Those who are ill or who have medical concerns are permitted to not observe Ramadan at all or to participate on a limited basis. A large feast is held on Eid al-Feter to mark the end of the month of Ramadan. Schools and businesses may be closed during this time.

The following practices have been suggested for consideration by SLPs by Muslims from India, Kuwait, Saudi Arabia, Pakistan, and Africa currently living in the United States. Islam has laws for almost every aspect of life. Many rules of Islam are confused with Shariah law. Shariah is the code of law derived from the *Koran* and from the teachings and example of Mohammed and is only applicable to Muslims; "under Islamic law there is no separation of church and state" (Princeton University, 2010). Rules of Shariah law may affect verbal and nonverbal communication in the intervention setting. Because many Muslims are from different cultural and geographic regions, some of the following information may be based on culture, Shariah law, and religion (Nasir, 2010):

1. No pork or food products containing pork should be used in clinical activities. Items such as bacon and sausage should not be included when discussing breakfast foods. Consideration should be given to this belief by avoiding stories in therapy such as *The Three Little Pigs* and *Charlotte's Web.*

2. Adult clients may observe Ramadan and will not consume food or water during the day of the month-long observance. Although those with health problems are excused from the practice, many may wish to observe the fast on a limited basis. Children and adults who are ill are not required to participate in the observance, but some alteration in family patterns during the holiday period may still exist. It is considered rude for non-Muslims to eat in the presence of Muslims who are fasting. Therefore, clinical activities in adult groups during Ramadan should not involve food and drink unless permission is given by those practicing Islam.

3. Activities using violence or advocating hunting for sport should be avoided. Animals are killed only for food, and religious teachings dictate how animals should be killed. Giving animals humanlike characteristics and other forms of anthropomorphism is discouraged by some Muslims. For example, stories that use animals as characters, such as a talking cat, may be taboo.

4. Activities about dressing and clothing should be used carefully. Some devout Muslim women cover their arms, do not wear revealing clothes, and often cover their faces. This is not the practice in all Muslim countries. Activities involving dressing or bathing dolls without clothing should be avoided, unless previously discussed with parents and clients. Teaching body parts using anatomically correct dolls should be avoided. The use of cosmetics is discouraged (i.e., lessons teaching face parts by using lipstick and eye shadow with female clients should be avoided). If clothing naming is an objective, ask parents for proper names and types of clothing.

5. Friday is the Muslim Sabbath; it is called Jum'a. Some Muslims have restricted Jum'a celebrations to begin at 1:00 PM on Friday afternoons. Others may celebrate Jum'a at a different time, depending on the time zone. Some Muslims agree to diagnostic and intervention sessions on Friday, and others do not. Devout Muslims pray five times daily, with special prayers at sunrise, noon, and sunset.

6. Islamic religions and laws allow no physical contact between men and women in public. Women, traditionally, do not give orders or instructions to men. However, in medical and therapy settings, this may not be the case if the professional is a female. If services for a female client by a male clinician are accepted, strict rules may require that a parent or a male family member be present at all times.

7. Home visits are not encouraged. Because some Muslims view the home as private, business activities are not to be conducted in the home by outsiders. Some parents prefer to come to the clinic rather than have the clinician visit them at home. Friends, usually people of the same religion, may make unannounced visits. Outsiders, people who are not Muslims, are expected to wait for an invitation or to make an appointment.

8. Use of the left hand to pass items is considered rude. When passing out therapy materials during intervention, the right hand should be used only. Avoid giving or receiving with the left (Columbus Travel Media Ltd., 2010). When using heavy items, the left hand may be used under the elbow to support the right hand. When handing items to someone, place the item in the

person's hand, not on the table or counter. To place therapy materials, papers, and instrumentation on the counter is considered rude and offensive. When sitting during therapy session, the soles of the feet should not point toward your companion.

9. Same-sex relationships and adultery are illegal and carry the death penalty. They do not recognize rights for gay or lesbian persons. Discussion of nontraditional single-sex couples or families should be avoided.

There are several nonverbal behaviors that also should be avoided:

1. It is considered impolite to point to a person with the index finger or to beckon someone with the fingers.
2. The right fist should never be smacked into the left palm.
3. Do not pass an item with your foot or show the bottom of the foot when sitting. The foot is considered unclean (Columbus Travel Media Ltd., 2010).

Judaism

Judaism is the religion of approximately 15 to 17 million people worldwide. There are more than 5.7 million people who practice Judaism in the United States. Judaism is the oldest religion of the Western world and the first to teach monotheism. It was founded on the laws and teachings of the Hebrew Bible, or Old Testament, and of the Talmud. Christianity and Islam are both derived from Judaism, even though they both differ in many basic beliefs and practices. Because Jewish people do not recognize one single authority, they have found it possible to differ about their religion practices and still remain Jewish. Today these differences are expressed through four major religious groups: Hasidic, Orthodox, Conservative, and Reformed.

Hasidic Judaism and Orthodox Judaism are two distinct branches of Judaism. Persons who practice Orthodox Judaism strictly adhere to the teachings of the Written Law (the Torah) and Oral Law (the Talmud). Those who practice Orthodox Judaism represent a branch of Judaism that resists most change and are the most devout. They believe that they are observing the law as handed down to Moses on Mount Sinai. They observe all laws of the faith, including kosher dietary restrictions such as not eating pork or shellfish. They do not allow meat and dairy products to be served on the same dishes or to be served in the same meal. Many who practice Orthodox Judaism maintain two separate sets of dishes: one for meat meals and one for dairy meals. Serving foods such as pizza and other cheese and meat dishes would not be acceptable.

People who practice Judaism observe the Sabbath starting at sundown on Friday. Persons who practice Orthodox Judaism observe many restrictions on the Sabbath, including all forms of work, riding in automobiles, and pushing elevator buttons. They also observe holy days, including Rosh Hashanah, Yom Kippur, Succoth, Shemini Atzeret,

Simchat Torah, Hanukkah, Passover, and Shavuoth. Each holiday begins at sunset of the day before the holiday.

Persons who practice Conservative Judaism accept Jewish law as the primary Jewish expression of all time. They observe many, but not all, Jewish holy days and may observe the dietary restrictions only during the major holy days (e.g., Passover, Yom Kippur, Rosh Hashanah, and Hanukkah).

Those who practice Reformed Judaism are the largest and fastest-growing Jewish movement (Rich, 2010). They may not follow all kosher dietary restrictions or strictly observe the rules of the Sabbath. They observe only the major holy days, such as Yom Kippur, Rosh Hashanah, Passover, and Hanukkah.

As with any religion, the actual practice is on a continuum from those who adhere strictly to the major tenets of the religion to those who follow the practices at their own discretion.

The information may not apply to all groups but should serve as a guide during clinical services to those who practice any form of Judaism.

USING CULTURAL PARAMETERS AS GUIDELINES IN INTERVENTION

A question commonly used by health care professionals is, "Is there something that we should know about your culture and religion that would affect your treatment?" This question can be used in the clinic, classroom, and work place. Tomoeda and Bayles (2002) described nine basic cultural parameters that can have profound effects on the practice of speech-language pathology and audiology. They are the value placed on the individual versus the group, views of time and space, roles of men and women, concepts of class and status, values, language, rituals, the significance of work, and beliefs about health. These parameters apply to adults as well as children. The following topic discussions are adapted from Tomoeda and Bayles (2002):

1. *Individual versus the group.* Do the decisions made support the group or the individual? In classroom and work settings, some people work better in groups, whereas other would prefer to work alone. Decisions regarding intervention may be made by a single family member or the group.
2. *Views on time and space.* Intervention scheduling may be affected by the client's concept of time. In the clinic where planning and adhering to strict schedules are important, some cultures, such as Native American/Indigenous Americans, Hispanic/Latino, and African American, are more event oriented and view time as more "elastic." Space in the clinic is important. People from Hispanic cultures touch more and stand in closer proximity, whereas people from some European cultures require more space during interactions.
3. *Gender issues.* Many cultures and religious groups, such as Muslims, Hindu, and others, have specific rules

for male and female interaction, touching, giving orders, receiving therapy, dressing, speaking, and education. Intervention sessions with adults, such as swallowing and adult language therapy sessions, may require the presence of a male.

4. *Concepts of class and status.* In America, social class typically is defined by income, job prestige, and level of education; status refers to one's place of respect within a society. Countries such as India have social classes or "caste" systems; Asian cultures value education, respect, and titles; and some Native American cultures are not impressed with degrees and titles but value their relationship to their clan or tribe.

5. *Values.* Relationships, respect, and courtesy are important to most cultures. Family values should be respected and validated for effective service delivery to be provided.

6. *Rituals.* Rituals or ceremonies are accepted ways of commemorating meaningful historical events, life changes, and renewing commitment to shared values. Many rituals are rooted in religion. The impact of these rituals regarding scheduling, attendance, and compliance to therapy are discussed in the topic clinical services, religion, and culture.

7. *Language.* Communication is the essential parameter for SLPs and audiologists. Knowledge of both verbal and nonverbal language is important. The language of instruction is important for effective service delivery.

8. *Significance of work.* Americans are defined by their work. A common question to ask a person who has just been introduced to you in an informal setting is, "What do you do?" People in many other cultures are defined by the groups to which they belong and their role in the community. Sensitivity should be exercised when asking this question to a person who may be jobless or unable to perform a previous job. Sensitivity should also be given to women who may not work outside of the home or whose primary work is to care for the children and the home.

9. *Beliefs about health.* Cultural differences exist for causes of disabilities, intervention, and choice of service provider and delivery. Some cultures may not seek intervention for problems that you cannot see such as learning disabilities. Health care providers such as spiritualists, folk healers, herbalists, or witch doctors may be chosen over Western medical professionals. The clinician should ask the clients specific questions regarding their views about their problem, its cause, its appropriate treatment, and their expectations from the treatment process. By becoming aware of differences in cultural attitudes toward health, disability, and illness the professional will discover how these differences affect attitudes toward augmentative and alternative communication devices, surgery, aggressive medication, feeding, tracheotomy tube placement, and so forth (Moxley et al., 2004).

GUIDELINES FOR CULTURALLY RELEVANT INTERVENTION

Bull and colleagues (2000) identified teaching guidelines for working with culturally diverse populations. These guidelines can be adapted for the multicultural clinical setting. For successful intervention, the following guidelines should be observed:

1. *Present clear explanations of objectives.* The clinician should make sure that the client understands the objective of the assessment and treatment program. Asians prefer that the professional assume authority and provide clear and full information, such as what will be provided by and what is expected from each person attending the meeting, therapy session, or conference.

2. *Use methods and procedures that do not violate the beliefs of the client.* A cultural informant could be used to assist the clinician in selecting culturally appropriate methods and materials. Clinicians should respect a client's religious and spiritual beliefs and values, including taboos.

3. *Be flexible in selecting materials and activities.* Asian parents may prefer a direct, structured session rather than indirect therapy where games and play are used. Clinicians should be willing to vary the therapy content and teaching style as needed. The learning environment should allow the client to be creative and motivated to take communication risks in the setting. Although an organized training program is desired, clinicians should be willing to change the content and activities as the situation dictates. Clinicians should adapt materials to the needs of the particular client. Chinese parents expect children to be disciplined and courteous while learning. Play therapy may not be valued.

4. *Be flexible in scheduling.* Be flexible in scheduling therapy because of religious holidays or practices. American Indians/Native Americans, African Americans, and some Hispanic groups have an elastic concept of time (e.g., they believe they have kept the appointment if they arrive 5 to 15 minutes after the scheduled appointment time or any time within a flexible time period; they may consider it permissible to arrive between 2:00 and 3:00 PM for a 2:00 PM appointment). Therefore, they may arrive late for an appointment without apologizing. Flexibility can also be exercised in the therapy session. Be flexible in allowing family members to participate in sessions. Broaden your concept of family to include extended family (cousins, uncles, aunts) and nontraditional families such as nonmarried heterosexual or gay or lesbian couples (Riquelme, 2004).

5. *Interact with clients according to their perception or expectation.* In some cultures, the clinician's showing enthusiasm, vigor, or confidence is a sign of competence. In

other cultures, touching, showing enthusiasm, using elevated pitch, and "gushing" over babies may be offensive. Some Native Americans/Indigenous Americans do not permit hugging, kissing, and excessive handling of their babies by strangers. Hugging and patting children on the head are forbidden in some Asian cultures and some religions. Parents from India place a mark on their infant's forehead to remind you not to compliment the baby.

6. *Be businesslike and task oriented.* Clients need to feel that the clinician has a purpose for activities and lessons. Use examples from real-life situations to show the importance of the lesson and how to use the new information appropriately.

7. *Understand the dimensions of the cultural identity of the client.* Understand the centrality of ethnicity, culture, and race to the client. To some clients, their home culture is very important to them and their lives. They may travel frequently to the home country and continue many of the cultural practices of the home country. Others may be more interested in assimilating to the culture of the mainstream, adopting many of the customs and practices of the mainstream. Some clients are "flattered" when asked to share information about their culture and may become "empowered" and feel welcomed when asked about their home country. Others are less willing to discuss their past or their home country because of the situations in their home country. Because this dimension of centrality of culture varies with each individual, it is important to assess this dimension with every client (Santiago-Rivera et al., 2002).

8. *Be sensitive to seating and placement in the treatment session.* Some clients feel that the clinician is positive when they are permitted to stand or sit close to the clinician. Others may find close proximity to be intimidating.

9. *Preview and review lessons.* Repetition and variety have been suggested as key factors to aid learning. Explain the goal and purpose of the intervention session. Review concepts discussed. The review may help clarify any concepts that are not clear. Clients from some cultures are taught to review by repeating material themselves. Including the client as a participant in the review process can reinforce main points and give an opportunity for feedback when clarification is needed.

10. *Use multiple levels of questions or cognitive discourse.* Knowledge and use of different styles is important to increase the client's repertoire of useful language. Simplification of adult speech, repetition of phrases, expansions, and filling in omissions are ways that adults interact with young children. Knowledge of cultural activities and various speaking needs should be used to demonstrate different pragmatic aspects of language. Specific to dysphagia, the individual's

learning style and daily routine mu[...]
Treatment recommendations are som[...]
rectly to the patient; at other times, i[...]
include extended family. Consider m[...]
mendations in addition to supplying [...] ...priately
translated materials.

CONCLUSION

The inclusion of cultural diversity into intervention is a concept that has gained widespread support. According to the Individuals with Disabilities Education Act (2004), knowledge of various cultures is necessary to provide more effective service delivery. Cultural competence is a goal for all individuals providing intervention. Intervention strategies used, as well as the clinical environment, should create a feeling of inclusion that reflects the recognition and appreciation of cultural and linguistic diversity. By using a culturally competent approach to service provision, intervention becomes more relevant and interesting to clients (Lynch & Hanson, 2004). Additionally, this approach promotes understanding of other groups and reduces potential cultural conflicts. Because each client presents a unique set of cultural variables, addressing every possible source of cultural conflict that could occur in the therapy process is beyond the scope of this chapter. However, the culturally competent clinician should make every attempt to know each client as an individual and to avoid forming stereotypes or using formulaic approaches to the intervention strategies for clients.

REFERENCES

Agosto, D. (1997). Criteria for evaluating multicultural literature. In A. F. Ada & S. Silva (Eds.), *Gathering the sun: An alphabet in Spanish and English.* New York: Lothrop, Lee & Sheppard.

American Speech-Language-Hearing Association (2008a). Communication facts: Focus on culturally and linguistically diverse populations—2008 edition. Available at: www.asha.org/research/reports/multicultural.htm.

American Speech-Language-Hearing Association (2008b). Roles and responsibilities of speech language pathologists in early intervention: Guidelines [Guidelines]. Available at: www.asha.org/policy.

Barrera, I. (2000). Honoring differences: Essential features of appropriate ECSE services for young children from diverse sociocultural environments. *Young Exceptional Children, 3,* 17-24.

Battle, D. E. (2002). *Communication disorders in multicultural populations.* Boston: Butterworth-Heinemann.

Beatson, J. E. (2006). Preparing speech-language pathologists as family-centered practitioners in assessment and program planning for children with autism spectrum disorders. *Seminars in Speech and Language, 27,* 1-9.

Bialystok, E. (2002). Acquisition of literacy in bilingual children: A framework for research. *Language Learning, 52,* 159-199.

Boone, H., & Crais, E. (2001). Strategies for achieving family-driven assessment and intervention planning. In *Young exceptional children monograph series, No. 3.* Missoula, MT: Division for Early Childhood of the Council for Exceptional Children.

Bowen, S. K. (2006). Assessment and students with disabilities: Issues and challenges with educational reform, Rural Special Education Quarterly. Retrieved December 29, 2010, from http://findarticles.com/p/articles/mi_qa4052/is_200607/ai_n17182649/.

Brice, A., & Roseberry-McKibbin, C. (2001). Choice of languages in instruction. Teaching Exceptional Children, 33, 10-16.

Bronfenbrenner, U. (1992). Ecological systems theory. In R. Vast (Ed.), Six theories in early child development (pp. 187-249). Philadelphia: Jessica Kingsley.

Bull, K. S., Montgomery, D., & Kimball, S. L (2000). Working with culturally diverse students. In Oklahoma State University (Ed.), Quality University instruction: A teaching effectiveness training program. Stillwater, OK: Oklahoma State University.

Caruso, D. (2005). Bargaining and distribution in special education. Cornell Journal of Law and Public Policy, 14, 171-195.

Cisero, C. A., & Royer, J. M. (1995). The development and cross-language transfer of phonological awareness. Contemporary Educational Psychology, 20, 275-303.

Columbus Travel Media Ltd. (2010). Brunei History and Culture. Retrieved October 24, 2010, from www.worldtravelguide.net/brunei/history-and-culture#ixzz13KPDbCzI.

Cummins, J. (1984). Bilingual education and special education: Issues in assessment and pedagogy. San Diego: College Hill.

Cummins, J., Brown, K., & Sayer, D. (2007). Literacy, technology, diversity: Teaching for success in changing times. Boston: Allyn & Bacon.

Durgunoglu, A. Y. (2002). Cross-linguistic transfer in literacy development and implications for language learners. Annals of Dyslexia, 52, 189-204.

Dunnett, M., & Schlosser, S. (2004) Opening doors: Disability experiences in Bosnia and Australia. Harris Park, NSW, Australia: Multicultural Disability Advocacy NSW.

Dunst, C. J. (2001). Participation of young children with disabilities in community learning activities. In M. J. Guralnick (Ed.), Early childhood inclusion: Focus on change (pp. 307-336). Baltimore: Brookes.

Dunst, C. J. (2002). Family-centered practices: Birth through high school. Journal of Special Education, 36, 139-147.

Dunst, C. J. (2004). Revisiting "rethinking early intervention." In M. A. Feldman (Ed.), Early intervention: The essential readings (pp. 262-283). Oxford, UK: Blackwell.

Dunst, C. J., Trivette, C. M., Starnes, L., et al. (1993). Building and evaluating family support initiatives: A national study of programs for persons with developmental disabilities. Baltimore: Brookes.

Elementary and Secondary Education Act (ESEA) of 2002, P.L. 107-110.

Evans, G.W. (2004). The environment of childhood poverty. American Psychologist, 59, 792.

Ford, K. (2005). Fostering literacy development in English Language Learners. Retrieved January 15, 2011, from www.colorincolorado.org/article/12924.

Gottardo, A. (2002). The relationship between language and reading skills in bilingual Spanish-English speakers. Topics in Language Disorders, 22, 46-70.

Gottardo, A., Yan, B., Siegel, L. S., & Wade-Woolley, L. (2001). Factors related to English reading performance in children with Chinese as a first language: More evidence of cross-language transfer of phonological processing. Journal of Educational Psychology, 93, 530-542.

Hanson, M. J., & Lynch, E. W. (1995). Early intervention: Implementing child and family services for infants and toddlers who are at risk and disabled (2nd ed.). Austin, TX: PRO-ED.

Individuals with Disabilities Education Act (IDEA; 2004), Federal Register, Volume 71, No. 156 Part V, Department of Education, 34 CFR part 300.

Individuals with Disabilities Education Improvement Act of 2004, 20 U.S.C. §1400 et seq.

Johnston, P. H., & Rogers, R. (2001). Early literacy development: The case for "informed assessment." In S. B. Neuman & D. K. Dickinson (Eds.), Handbook of early literacy research (pp. 377-389). New York: Guilford.

Juelis, J. (2009). Parallels between cooperative play and multicultural education. Dissertation, University of Washington, 2009. Ann Arbor: UMI, 2009.AAT 3370503. Print.

Klinger, J. K., & Bianco, M. (2006). What is special about special education for English language learners? In B. G. Cook & B. R. Schirmer (Eds.), What is special about special education? (pp. 37-53). Austin, TX: PRO-ED.

Klinger, J. K., & Edwards, P. (2006). Cultural consideration with response-to-intervention model. Readings Research Quarterly, 41, 108-117.

Kohnert, K., Yim, D., Nett, K., et al. (2005). Intervention with linguistically diverse preschool children: A focus on developing home language(s). Language, Speech, and Hearing Services in Schools, 36, 251-263.

Kok, T., Peng, T. K., Charles, L., et al. (1997). Multicultural Singapore. Retrieved November 2010, www.thinkquest.org/pls/html/think.site?p_site_id=11518.

Lowenthal, B. (1996). Training early interventionists to work with culturally diverse families. Infant-Toddler Intervention, 6, 145-152.

Lynch, E. W., & Hanson, M. J. (2004). Developing cross-cultural competence: A guide for working with young children and their families (3rd ed.). Baltimore: Brookes.

Madding, C. C. (1999). Mamá y hijo: The Latino mother-infant dyad. Retrieved from Multicultural Electronic Journal of Communication Disorders, 1, at: www.asha.ucf.edu/madding3.html.

Madding, C. C. (2000). Maintaining focus on cultural competence in early intervention services to linguistically and culturally diverse families. Infant-Toddler Intervention, 10, 9-18.

Mahoney, G., Kaiser, A., Girolametto, L., et al. (1999). Parent education in early intervention: A call for a renewed focus. Topics in Early Childhood Special Education, 19, 131-140.

Middleton, R. T. (2009). Interaction of immigrant culture and the law: Focus on parental discretion under IDEIA of 2004. Journal of Immigrant and Refugee Studies, 7, 370-392.

Moore, S., & Mendez, C. (2006). Working with linguistically diverse families in early intervention: Misconceptions and missed opportunities. Seminars in Speech and Language, 27, 187-198.

Moxley, A., Mahendra, N., & Vega-Barachowitz, C. (2004, April 13). Cultural Competence in Health Care. The ASHA Leader.

Nasir, I. S. (2010). An Imam explains Islam. Retrieved October 31, 2010, from www.cyborlink.com/besite/indonesia.htm.

National Association for the Education of Young Children (NAEYC) (2009). Quality benchmarks for cultural competence project. Washington, DC: Author.

No Child Left Behind (2002). P. L. 107-110: An Act to Close the Achievement Gap with Accountability, Flexibility, and Choice So That No Child Is Left Behind. Retrieved January 17, 2011, from www2.ed.gov/policy/elsec/guid/states/index.html#nclb.

Parmar, P., Harkness, S., & Super, C. (2004). Asian and Euro-American parents ethnotheories of play and learning: Effects on pre-school children's home routines and school behaviors. International Journal of Behavioral Development, 28, 97-104.

Paul, R. (2007). Language disorders from infancy through adolescence (3rd ed.). St. Louis: Mosby.

Peña, E., & Fiestas, C. (2009, October, 10). Talking across cultures in early intervention: Finding common ground to meet children's communication needs. *Perspectives on Communication Disorders and Sciences in Culturally and Linguistically Diverse Populations, 16,* 79-85.

Polmanteer, K., & Turbiville, V. (2000). Family-responsive individualized family service plans for speech-language pathologists. *Language, Speech, and Hearing Services in Schools, 31,* 4-14.

Princeton University (2010). WordNet: A lexical database of English. Retrieved September 15, 2010, from http://wordnet.princeton.edu/.

Rettig, M. (1995). Play and cultural diversity. *Journal of Educational Issues of Language Minority Students, 15,* 1-9.

Rich, T. (2010). JewFAQ: Answering Jewish frequently asked questions for more than a decade. Retrieved August 5, 2010, from www.jewfaq.org/index.htm.

Riquelme, L. F. (2004, April 13). Cultural competence in dysphagia. ASHA Leader.

Rivers, K. O. (2000). Working with caregivers of infants and toddlers with special needs from culturally and linguistically diverse backgrounds. *Infant-Toddler Intervention, 10,* 61-72.

Roseberry-McKibbin, C. (2007). *Language disorders in children: A multicultural and case perspective.* Boston: Allyn & Bacon.

Roseberry-McKibbin, C. (2008a). *Increasing language skills of students from low income backgrounds.* San Diego: Plural.

Roseberry-McKibbin, C. (2008b). *Multicultural students with special language needs.* Oceanside, CA: Academic Communication Associates.

Roth, F., & Worthington, C. K. (2005). *Therapy resource manual for speech-language pathology.* Boston: Delmar-Thompson.

Sacirbey, O. (2010). Muslims launch survey of American mosques. The Pew Forum on Religion and Public Life. Retrieved October 24, 2010, from http://pewforum.org/Topics/Religious-Affiliation/Muslim/.

Santiago-Rivera, A. L., Arredondo, P., & Gallardo-Cooper, M. (2002). *Counseling Latinos and la familia: A practical guide.* Thousand Oaks, CA: Sage Publications.

Schuele, C. M., & Boundreau, D. (2008, January). Phonological awareness intervention: Beyond the basics. *Language Speech and Hearing Services in Schools, 39,* 3-20.

Shioshita, J. (1997, September-October). Beyond good intentions: Selecting multicultural literature. *Children's Advocate Newsmagazine, Action Alliance for Children.*

Summers, J. A., Hoffman, L., Marquis, J., et al. (2005). Relationship between parent satisfaction regarding partnerships with professionals and age of the child. *Topics in Early Childhood Special Education, 25,* 48-58.

Terrell, B. Y., & Hale, J. E. (1992). Serving a multicultural population: Different learning styles. *American Journal of Speech-Language Pathology, 1,* 5-8.

Texas Speech and Hearing Association (2010). Taskforce on cultural and linguistic diversity. Retrieved October 25, 2010, from www.txsha.org/_pdf/CLD_Corner/Linguistically%20Diverse%20Populations.pdf.

Tomoeda, C. K., & Bayles, K. A. (2002, April 2). Cultivating cultural competence in the workplace, classroom, and clinic. *ASHA Leader.*

Trofimov, Y. (2007). Snakes have divine power in Hinduism. Retrieved October 24, 2010, from http://superhindus.wordpress.com/?s=snakes.

Turnbull, A. P., Summers, J. A., Turnbull, R., et al. (2005). Family and supports and services in early intervention: A bold vision. *Journal of Early Intervention, 29,* 187-206.

University of Virginia (2000). The Koran at the Electronic Text Center, University of Virginia. Available at: http://etext.lib.virginia.edu/koran.html.

van Kleeck, A. (1994). Potential cultural bias in training parents as conversational partners with their children who have delays in language development. *American Journal of Speech Language Pathology, 3(1),* 67-78.

Wordpress.org. (2010a). Best practices for ELL students with speech-language disorders. Retrieved September 21, 2010, from http://multiculturalspeechtherapy.com.

Wordpress.org. (2010b). Supporting an ELL/special education student. Retrieved September 21, 2010, from http://multiculturalspeech-therapy.com/?p=97.

Wright, W. D., & Wright, P. D. (2006). *Special education law* (2nd ed.). Hartfield, VA: Harbor House Law Press.

Yokota, J. (1993). Issues in selecting multicultural children's literature. *Language Arts, 70,* 156-167.

Zayas, L. H., & Solari, F. (1994). Early childhood socialization in Hispanic families: Context, culture, and practice implications. *Professional Psychology: Research and Practice, 25,* 200-206.

ADDITIONAL RESOURCES

American Speech-Language-Hearing Association: Cultural competence checklist: Policies and procedures. Available at: www.asha.org/uploadedFiles/Cultural-Competence-Checklist-Policies-Procedures.pdf#search=%22multicultural%22.

American Speech-Language-Hearing Association: Cultural competence checklist: Service delivery. Available at: www.asha.org/uploadedFiles/Cultural-Competence-Checklist-Service-Delivery.pdf#search=%22multicultural%22.

Brown, J. E., & Doolittle, J. (2008). Framework for response to intervention with English language learners. National Center for Culturally Responsive Educational Systems: A practitioner brief. Available at: www.nccrest.org/professional/culturally_responsive_response_to_intervention.html.

E. H. Butler Library: For a listing of more than 3000 appropriate literature by cultural groups, including African, African American, Asian, Latino, Gay and Lesbian, Multiethnic, Irish, Jewish, Middle Eastern, Native American, Religions, Russian, and Women, see http://library.buffalostate.edu/collections/bard.php.

Chapter 14

Multicultural and International Research on Communication Disorders: Past, Present, and Future

Constance Dean Qualls

Research is a systematic way of knowing and thinking, has its own vocabulary, and can be learned and used by anyone (DePoy & Gitlin, 2011). The prevailing definition for scientific research is the ". . . systematic, empirical, amoral, public and critical investigation of natural phenomena. It is guided by theory and hypotheses about the presumed relations among phenomena" (Kerlinger & Lee, 2000). The purposes of research are to gain scientific knowledge by developing, testing, and generating theories. In communication sciences and disorders (CSD), goals of research are to (1) understand the processes (structural and functional) and products (i.e., speech, language, voice, fluency) of normal and disordered human communication and swallowing; (2) reveal how these processes and products vary as a result of development, difference, disorder, or decline; and (3) determine the best approaches, strategies, techniques, and tools for preventing, assessing, and treating communication, swallowing, and hearing disorders. Research must *inform clinical practice* so that clinicians working with individuals with speech, language, hearing, and swallowing disorders will have what they need (i.e., research data or other types of evidence, resources) to make the best clinical decisions for their clients. To accomplish these goals, it is imperative that researchers and clinical practitioners (audiologists and speech-language pathologists [SLPs]) work together. There is mounting interest and motivation in bridging the pervasive gap between the two groups in communication sciences and disorders. However, much more work needs to be done.

In 2009, the Science Advisory Board of the American Speech-Language-Hearing Association (ASHA, 2010) defined *clinical practice research* for communication sciences and disorders as research ". . . designed to produce knowledge that will help prevent, identify, assess, and treat communication and related (e.g., swallowing and balance) disorders." The concept of clinical practice research is key, precisely because of the growing movement toward

demonstrating clinical and health outcomes for improving the communication and swallowing status of U.S. citizens and those around the globe. There is also increasing pressure to provide evidence for the effectiveness of speech-language pathology services to third-party payers. Federal funding agencies, such as the National Institutes of Health (NIH), have increased their focus on this type of research, otherwise termed *translational, bench-to-bed,* and so forth. Further, given the seemingly persistent health disparities and academic achievement differences that exist among and between the growing racial-ethnic populations in the United States that can lead to communication and swallowing disorders, it will be important for CSD researchers to focus efforts on increasing the knowledge base in these populations. Clinical practice research is just one method by which this can be done.

MULTICULTURAL/MULTILINGUAL RESEARCH: WHAT IS IT AND WHY DO IT?

Multicultural research investigates the interaction and impact of cultural variables (age, race-ethnicity, gender, religion, socioeconomic status) on behavioral phenomena, such as literacy development, augmentative-alternative device use, and post-stroke aphasia and swallowing. In CSD, race-ethnicity is the defining cultural variable that distinguishes multicultural from nonmulticultural research. So, why is there a need for multicultural research in CSD? There are seven core reasons for increasing research in multicultural populations: (1) population shifts; (2) lack of information; (3) misinformation; (4) misrepresentation of information; (5) understanding local and cultural myths; (6) evidence-based practice; and (7) third-party payers.

First, in the United States, the growing numbers of individuals from culturally and linguistically diverse populations dictate the need for research to inform clinical services for these individuals. Individuals who identify with the Hispanic/Latino community speak a variety of Spanish "in-languages," depending on their country of origin. These in-languages are Cuban, Puerto Rican, Central/South American, Mexican, Dominican, Salvadorian, and Caribbean. The 2010 Census reported the development of messages for several new language audiences, including Asian (Bangladeshi: Bengali; Hmong: Hmong; Laotian: Lao; Thai: Thai; and Pakistani: Urdu), Armenian (Armenian), Iranian (Farsi), Greek (Greek), Portuguese-speaking Africans (Continental Portuguese), and Brazilians (Brazilian Portuguese) (Table 14-1). The number of other nonnative English language communities in the United States continues to grow; at some point, some of these individuals will require audiology or speech-language services. Multicultural research is needed to help clinicians understand the best ways to assess and treat disordered communication, swallowing, and hearing in these individuals.

Second is the general lack of information that accurately represents communication and swallowing behaviors not only across race-ethnicity, age, and gender but also across skill, education, acculturation, and socioeconomic levels and within and across cultural groups. Third, there is misinformation in some of the published research that needs to be debunked or corrected, or in which another perspective would provide valuable insight on the topic. Additional research will provide the necessary illumination to allow consumers to see the broader picture, gain more complete knowledge, and, thus, make better decisions about communication and swallowing disorders in individuals from a range of cultural and linguistic backgrounds. Fourth, researchers interpret the results of their studies from their own view of the world. If their world view reflects only limited life experiences with nonmainstream individuals such as through television and print media and movies, it is possible that they may show bias when interpreting behaviors or misrepresent behaviors based on such limited exposure. Fifth, multicultural research can confirm or disconfirm local and cultural myths about communication and swallowing disorders, family and community involvement in matters of education and health care, and so forth, and provide a platform for developing the relationship between the clinician and the client and family.

Sixth, cumulative multicultural research findings can significantly inform evidence-based practice, not only about client preferences but also about the differences between typical and disordered speech production, for example, and "best practices" for assessment and treatment. Finally, third-party payers increasingly are requiring information about treatment efficacy, effectiveness, and outcomes (e.g., Is this an effective treatment? Will this treatment be effective for most patients? Did the consumers feel they benefited from therapy?) to determine whether they will continue to pay for services or whether they will pay for others to get similar services. Because of known disparities in health care, multicultural research is needed to ensure that high-risk populations such as African Americans and Hispanics/Latinos show reasonable progress in therapy for communication and swallowing disorders. Knowing the importance of conducting multicultural research is one thing; however, a number barriers or challenges must be overcome to effectively engage in this type of research.

A major challenge is recruiting persons from culturally and linguistically diverse backgrounds to participate in research. The NIH charges researchers to ethically and responsibly include women and minorities in research samples unless there is a compelling reason not to, for example, when investigating heart disease in white men. In CSD, researchers largely depend on convenience samples (i.e., individuals who volunteer) to investigate phenomena. However, because of a number of factors such as historical (e.g., unethical practices, as seen in the Tuskegee Syphilis Study), educational (e.g., potential participants are wary because of the to lack of understanding of the process), sociocultural (e.g., low levels of acculturation, lack of trust, beliefs about the value of participation or how this information might be used against the client or family), economic (e.g., lack of transportation, time constraints), and so forth, many individuals from culturally and linguistically diverse populations do not readily volunteer to participate in research studies. Hence, there is a substantial body of literature examining approaches to encourage participation of these individuals.

In 2006, Yancey and colleagues reviewed 95 studies published over a 6-year period that described methods for increasing minority (African American, Hispanic/Latino, and Native American) enrollment and retention in research.

TABLE 14-1 New Languages for Which Messages Were Prepared for the 2010 Census

Audience	Language
Asians	
Bangladeshi	Bangla/Bengali
Hmong	Hmong
Laotian	Lao
Thai	Thai
Pakistani	Urdu
Armenian	Armenian
Iranian	Farsi
Greek	Greek
Portuguese-speaking Africans	Continental Portuguese
Brazilians	Brazilian Portuguese

Data from the U.S. Census Bureau. (2010). Available at: http://2010.census.gov/2010census/index.php.

These 95 studies represented more than three times the average annual output of scholarly work in this area during the prior 15-year period. Twenty of the 95 studies analyzed the efficacy or effectiveness of recruitment and retention strategies. The review revealed that four primary factors warrant serious consideration when recruiting and retaining research participants from culturally and linguistically diverse populations, including the following: (1) sampling approach and identification of targeted participants, (2) community involvement and nature and timing of contact with prospective participants, (3) incentives and logistics, and (4) cultural adaptations. Recruitment research suggests that the use of a multiple-strategies approach is best when recruiting individuals from culturally and linguistically diverse backgrounds to participate in research. Qualls (2002) used and reported on a multiple-strategies approach for her language and aging study. She effectively recruited and retained 80 African American participants for her study using the strategies outlined in Box 14-1. Qualls noted that these same strategies will likely be effective across multicultural populations.

A second major challenge has to do with the researcher's minimal exposure to diversity during professional preparation. In the United States, CSD academic programs inconsistently include multicultural issues and populations in the curriculum (Stockman et al., 2008); further, when this information *is* included, it may be insufficient to ensure that potential and future researchers feel comfortable asking questions and interpreting results to make good decisions about multicultural populations. Stockman and coworkers (2008) conducted a survey of 731 CSD university program administrators and faculty using a 49-item questionnaire to determine instructional strategies reported for multicultural/multilingual issues. The respondents were generally committed to multicultural instruction; however, the reported strategies (e.g., infusion vs. dedicated course) varied, with infusion without a dedicated course as the dominant model

in most programs. The authors acknowledged the inherent bias in these self-reported results; that is, the findings may be skewed to reflect ". . . what participants desire to believe or do as opposed to what they actually believe and do" (Stockman et al., p. 254). Further, faculty members commented on the small numbers of racially and ethnically diverse students in their CSD programs. The implications of this research for the current discussion suggest that CSD students graduating from many master's level programs, and, likely, many CSD faculty members, are not adequately trained to evaluate and conduct research in multicultural or international populations. On the other hand, it appears that, when multiculturalism is of interest, more focused and complete inclusion of multicultural issues may take place in doctoral training programs. Still, the numbers of doctoral-level personnel and doctoral students conducting research in this area continue to be small, although this is becoming a growing area of interest for CSD researchers.

This chapter speaks to the status of multicultural, multilingual, and international research in the context of the past, present, and future. The historical perspective considers how far research in multicultural populations has come, but only in specific content areas such as the impact of African American English (AAE) dialect on children's language for academic success. Methodological and ethical issues will be discussed as well. Next is a summary of the current literature in multicultural, multilingual, and international populations, revealing the dearth of research in this area. The last part of the chapter focuses on the future of multicultural, multilingual, and international research in communication sciences and disorders.

THE PAST: A HISTORICAL PERSPECTIVE OF RESEARCH IN MULTICULTURAL POPULATIONS IN THE UNITED STATES

The historical origins of multicultural research in CSD date back to the 1980s when there was significant public interest in and controversy about the dialect of English spoken by school-aged African American children. Wolfram captured the essence of the debate about AAE in the following statement:

No variety of English has been more closely scrutinized over the past half-century than African American English. We have learned much about its historical development and structural description, and its status as a legitimate variety of English is unquestioned. At the same time, it remains embedded in enduring controversy, due no doubt to the sensitivity of race and ethnicity in American society.

—Dr. Walt Wolfram (Sociolinguist), July 2007
(see Center for Applied Linguistics Homepage)

Early CSD research on AAE espoused the deficit hypothesis; that is, researchers compared the language of African American children relative to white middle-class

---

BOX 14-1 Strategies for Recruiting African Americans to Research

- Invite the individual to be a participant.
- Let the individual know that her/his input is important and necessary for the research.
- Speak to groups of individuals/family members.
- Be willing to contact individuals more than once.
- Provide a variety of information-yielding sources.
- Be flexible and go to the participant, if necessary.
- Ensure the participant is comfortable.
- Share information throughout the process.
- Encourage the participant to ask questions.

From Qualls, CD. (2002). Recruitment of African American adults as research participants to a language in aging study: Example of a principled, creative, and culture-based approach. *Journal of Allied Health, 31,* 241-246.

children, the prototypical normative group in language research (Stockman, 2010). Study designs compared the groups on tests that were standardized on the white middle class, with no consideration or accommodation for the cultural and linguistic experiences of the African American children. The results, not surprisingly, showed performance differences (using test scores) between the groups, with the African American children scoring lower than the whites. The results were then interpreted to mean that the African American children were deficient and that they had speech or language problems that need to be corrected. Stockman pointed out, however, the stark difference in the type of language research conducted with white children during the same time period. The research designs involved observing very young children who were followed over time using longitudinal methods that were ecologically valid (i.e., "home-elicited samples of natural verbal interactions with familiar adults" [Stockman, 2010, p. 25]) to determine normal developmental milestones. Unlike the studies with the African American children, these studies were reasoned and theoretically motivated (e.g., development stage theory [Piaget]; Chomsky's biologic, cognitive, and social experiences). The different approaches to investigating language development and use in African American and white middle-class children yielded different information about the groups and set the stage for significant and enduring debate about African American children's use of AAE. Stockman proposed that research employing the deficit view distracted researchers from answering questions about language development and use in African American children.

At some point, researchers began to understand the futility of the deficit hypothesis and shifted to a difference view for understanding African American children's language. Stockman (2010) discusses the impetus for this shift, stating that the convergence of the following four factors led researchers to adopt the difference approach:

1. *Expanding frameworks for investigating language.* Researchers included cultural and linguistic aspects of language that legitimized AAE (i.e., phonological, grammatical, syntactic, and pragmatic rules govern the dialect). Researchers began to develop theories to explain African American children's language, including the universal generative view of language and the theory of universal grammar.

2. *Litigation of minority language use in schools.* As a result of the Ann Arbor Black English Case, teachers were to identify children who used black English and to use that information to teach them how to read.

3. *Professional recognition of cultural and linguistic diversity.* There was a growing acceptance for and an increased focus on diversity within communication sciences and disorders at all levels, including research, clinical practice, education and training, and advocacy. Continuing challenges for researchers were to ask the right questions, employ appropriate research designs, recruit and treat

participants responsibly, and judiciously interpret the findings.

4. *Increased diversity of U.S. populations.* Demographic population shifts increased the range of culturally and linguistically different persons served by the professions, including individuals from around the world and individuals who speak more than one language.

THE PRESENT: STATE OF RESEARCH IN MULTICULTURAL/MULTILINGUAL AND INTERNATIONAL POPULATIONS

African Americans

Child Language Research

The current state of knowledge about the speech, language, and swallowing disorders in African Americans is extremely limited, with the exception of child language. According to Stockman (2010), researchers have spent the past 25 years investigating AAE and assessment and intervention issues in African American children. Research designs and sample sizes have varied, as have the type of language sampled and whether or not the focus was developmental. Descriptive and comparative studies have largely been employed, and the results have yielded information about *all* language domains. Specifically, researchers have examined syntactic, morphologic, phonological, semantic, and pragmatic and discourse (narratives) development in African American children. Also, the developmental patterns have differentiated typical populations from atypical ones. Intracultural, intercultural, and cross-cultural studies have matched study participants and groups on critical variables; any differences observed were interpreted from a difference perspective (Stockman, 2010).

Assessment research in African American children has dealt with identifying major sources of cultural variation (Stockman, 2010), identifying atypical AAE speakers, understanding the impact of standardization on performance, identifying within-group differences (e.g., gender, socioeconomic status) in performance, and determining the utility of standardized tests for distinguishing difference from disorder. Other research has investigated whether test scores are differentially affected by eliminating failed responses that may be due to a dialect. To negate the impact of bias on standardized tests, some researchers have established their own local or adult norms for assessing African American children's language, others have modified the phonetic context of the sound on standardized articulation tests, and others have used different formats (e.g., embedded in an activity) or contexts (e.g., thematic context) in which to present test items (Stockman, 2010). The Diagnostic Evaluation of Language Variation (DELV; Seymour et al., 2003) is the only valid test in CSD designed to diagnose spoken language impairments in children regardless of the dialect of English they speak.

Researchers have also used a variety of nonstandardized language assessment procedures to investigate African American children's language (see Stockman, 2010). These include analyzing spontaneous speech samples in various contexts (e.g., at home or at school; with sibling or with parent) or a combination of spontaneous speech samples and elicited speech samples, dynamic assessment (mediated test-teach-retest strategy), and fast-mapping (incidental learning) assessment.

Compared with assessment research, the research on interventions to modify the African American child's language-disordered behaviors is noticeably missing (Stockman, 2010). Rather, the emphasis is largely on helping African American children achieve literacy for academic parity (Champion & Rosa-Luga, 2010; Terry et al., 2010). For example, Terry and colleagues (2010) examined associations among dialect variation, literacy skills (phonological awareness, vocabulary, and word recognition), and school context in first graders who were racially, linguistically, and socioeconomically diverse. Their results showed that, overall, African American AAE and white standard American English (SAE) speakers were equivalent on the literacy tasks, although the groups showed differences in particular aspects of reading literacy. This study used comparative and descriptive methods, collected and analyzed data using inferential statistics, offered theoretical explanations for their findings, and demonstrated the complexity of research investigating multiple variables.

Speech Disorders Research

Augmentative and Alternative Communication Use

Augmentative and alternative communication (AAC) has gained a lot of attention in research during the past 15 years; yet, very little attention has been given to the influence of cultural variables. Goode (2006) compiled a bibliography of the research on diversity issues in the use of assistive technology. The review of the literature showed that African Americans wanted their children to fit in to their communities and not to appear different by using an AAC device. In addition, low-socioeconomic status individuals, regardless of race-ethnicity, felt that attending to basic needs (e.g., health care, getting food for their family, work, and transportation) was more important than the communication goals professionals were working on with their child. The research strategy commonly used to understand cultural influences in AAC use is descriptive. Parette (1998; see Parette et al., 2006) proposed an AAC decision-making model that included six issue areas within the context of the child's family: acculturation, culture, service system concerns, technology features, child characteristics, and ethnicity. Some of the existing research paradigms are now being tested with different racial-ethnic groups, for example, the effects of parent instruction on the symbolic communication of children using AAC during storybook reading (Binger et al., 2008; Kent-Walsh et al., 2010).

Stuttering and Fluency Disorders

Proctor and colleagues (2008) investigated the prevalence of stuttering in African American preschoolers using a three-pronged research strategy: (1) face-to-face interaction with each child, (2) teacher reports on each child, and (3) parent reports on each child. The researchers noted the extant literature in this area, citing conflicting and confusing findings and no prior research on preschoolers in this population. The two primary research strategies used were (1) questionnaire completed by principal and teachers or the school SLP and (2) investigator interview and observation. Three of the nine studies reported data samples between 49,263 and 199,839; the others reported between 400 and 6000 students. Seven different U.S. states were represented across the nine studies. Data analysis employed nonparametric statistics. The results showed that African American preschoolers are not overrepresented in the stuttering population for their age group.

Blood and associates (2009) examined the influence of race-ethnicity in children who stutter with coexisting disorders using a questionnaire that was sent to SLPs. In this type and prevalence comparative study, measures of risk, relative risks, and odds ratios for racial-ethnic differences among groups were calculated. The results showed that African American children who stutter showed a higher risk for comorbidities than non-Hispanic white, Hispanic/Latino, and Asian children who stutter.

Voice and Its Disorders

Using the identical research protocol used in their stuttering prevalence study (see earlier), Duff and colleagues (2004) investigated the prevalence of voice disorders in African American and white preschoolers and found no difference in prevalence as function of age, gender, or race-ethnicity. Mayo and associates (2006) investigated different aspects of voice in African Americans as well as other culturally and linguistically diverse groups' knowledge of voice disorders, race-based nasalance, and velopharyngeal closure timing characteristics. Mayo and coworkers (2007) and Xue and colleagues (2006) investigated race-based morphologic differences in vocal tract dimensions that influence formant frequency differences in vowel sounds void of specific language or dialect. This line of research aimed to prove that race plays a significant role in voice and speech production.

Acquired Neurogenic Disorders

The research on acquired neurogenic communication and swallowing disorders has largely not included African Americans and, therefore, the information on this population for this area of practice is limited (see Chapter 8).

A notable exception is the research done by Ulatowska and her colleagues. In their studies, African Americans were most often equally represented along with whites in a series of studies investigating narratives in aphasia (Olness et al., 2002, 2010; Streit Olness et al., 2005; Ulatowska & Olness, 2001; Ulatowska et al., 2000, 2011). Other studies by these researchers investigated language impairment, functional communication, and discourse measures in African American aphasic and normal adults (Ulatowska et al., 2001), interpretation of fables and proverbs by African Americans with and without aphasia (Ulatowska et al., 2001), and the relationship between discourse and Western Aphasia Battery performance in African Americans with aphasia (Ulatowska et al., 2003). Notably, Ulatowska and colleagues used both cross-cultural and intracultural group designs to examine phenomena.

Other research has examined the performance of African Americans and whites on tests of aphasia. For example, Molrine and Pierce (2002) compared the language performance of neurologically intact African Americans and whites on three tests of aphasia, including the Boston Diagnostic Test of Aphasia (BDAE), Minnesota Test for Differential Diagnosis of Aphasia (MTDDA), and Western Aphasia Battery. Ulatowska and associates (2003) examined the relationship between discourse measures and performance on the Western Aphasia Battery in African Americans with aphasia. The Molrine and Pierce (2002) normative study reported equivalent results between the groups on the test batteries. The Ulatowska and associates (2003) study found no significant, meaningful relationships between the discourse measures under study and the standardized test, with the caveat that the discourse measures provided a more naturalistic assessment of language in this population. Similar to the first study, in the third study, race-ethnicity did not significantly influence the outcome. In each of the studies, the sample size was small, although this is not atypical for research in individuals with speech and language impairments. However, no additional research to date has been published to answer these same or similar questions (see issues of replication under Future of Research in Communication Sciences and Disorders).

Wertz, Auther, and Ross (1997) investigated severity, improvement, and rate of improvement in aphasia between African Americans and whites. They found no differences on the variables between the groups in the first year post-onset. It is possible that these initial findings explain why subsequent studies on severity, rate of improvement, and aphasia treatment outcomes conducted or reviewed by Wertz and his colleagues make no distinction between racial-ethnic groups on these variables, although the Veterans Administration serves many African American war veterans (e.g., de Riesthal & Wertz, 2004; Ross & Wertz, 2003; Wertz et al., 2009).

Hispanics/Latinos

Child Language Research

Decoupling research on Hispanics/Latinos and research on bilingualism is difficult at best. The concept of bilingualism, however, is not restricted to Spanish and English speakers. In CSD, most of the research on individuals who speak more than one language has been limited to the language of Hispanics/Latinos who speak a variety of Spanish dialects, depending on the region of the world in which they have roots. Hispanics/Latinos make up the fastest growing and largest minority population in the United States, with the majority of individuals who are natives of Mexico. As a result, researchers are vigorously seeking ways to ensure that young, developing speakers of Mexican Spanish who are simultaneously learning English will have the necessary skills to be academically successful. For example, researchers in CSD are testing culture-free or culture-neutral tasks such as nonword repetition to differentiate language impairment and typical language development (e.g., Gutiérrez-Clellen & Simon-Cereijido, 2010; Summers et al., 2010); they are determining predictors of young children's language ability on the Bilingual English Spanish Assessment (BESA), a forthcoming standardized measure of language ability (Bedore et al., 2010), and identifying culturally appropriate methods for working with children with language-learning disabilities and their families within the framework of evidence-based practice (Kummerer, 2010). Research findings by both Gutiérrez-Clellen and Simon-Cereijido (2010) and Summers and colleagues (2010) show that the clinical accuracy of the nonword repetition task will vary depending on the language used; namely, the Spanish- and English-speaking bilingual children repeated the nonwords with greater accuracy when presented in Spanish (L1) than when presented in English (L2).

Kohnert and Medina (2009) examined the peer-reviewed literature that reported on investigations of performance in bilingual learners and children with communication disorders over a 30-year period. The purpose of the review was to identify trends, clinical implications for evidence-based practice, and gaps in the evidence. The researchers described the databases searched, operationalized *key terms* (e.g., bilingualism, second language, multilingualism, language impairment), described in detail *inclusion* and *exclusion criteria* (e.g., they included only investigations reported on original data from human subjects with a focus on spoken languages; they excluded studies that did not include both bilingual children and children with communication disorders, and eliminated adult survey data), and identified the peer-reviewed journals where the studies were published. Their final database was 64 articles from 34 different journals; however, most of the articles were published in two journals, the *Journal of Speech, Language, and Hearing Research* and *Applied Linguistics*. The focus of the studies reviewed included grammar (topic of the majority of the studies), phonology/phonological awareness, pragmatics, nonlinguistic processing, language learning, language processing, narrative features, information processing measures (speed and accuracy), and performance on a standardized assessment. The bilinguals were mostly Spanish and English speakers, although other bilingual combinations were studied (e.g., Arabic-Swedish, Urdu-Norwegian, Turkish-Dutch). The methods used varied and included single case studies, single-subject designs, and large group designs that were correlational, descriptive, comparative, or experimental. Approximately 72% of the studies investigated children with language impairment, whereas 19% of the studies investigated speech sound disorders, including articulation and phonological impairments. No studies included in the sample directly investigated bilingualism and stuttering.

Next, the researchers combined the evidence on second language learners (L2) and language impairment (a substantial proportion of the database) to answer empirical questions in this area. This was done to answer basic clinical questions. See Table 14-2 for the clinical questions and tentative responses gleaned from the article. Following a discussion of differential diagnosis using 32 (or half) of the studies, the authors provided conclusions, limitations, and future research needs. They pointed out that this review of studies was not a critical review of the literature in this area; rather, the purpose was to provide a global view

to illuminate trends. The authors suggested that SLPs can use the information provided to make clinical decisions for evidence-based practice.

Assessment

The research on assessment of bilingual speakers converges to suggest that three major factors must be taken into account, including (1) differential proficiency in the different languages spoken, (2) the association between languages, and (3) individual differences. These factors reveal the inadequacy of existing standardized tests of language for understanding and differentiating normal and disordered language in bilingual children. Kohnert (2010) described three standards of comparison as well as experimental tasks used to investigate whether or not the bilingual language learner presents with a difference versus a disorder. The standards of comparison were monolingual comparisons, bilingual comparisons, and within-in child comparisons. Studies that compared developing L2 learners with monolingual children with language impairments showed similarities between the groups because of the vulnerability of the grammatical aspects of language, with little or no consideration for language experience, distributed lexical-semantic knowledge, and other factors. Generally, these types of comparisons are not clinically useful because of the high incidence of false-positive results for L2 learners, for example, on a single vocabulary test or a nonword repetition task. On the

---

TABLE 14-2 Clinical Questions Answered by the Research

Question	What the Research Says
Can children with communication disorders learn two languages? Are they disadvantaged relative to monolingual speakers with similar impairments? Will changing the environment so that only one language is used improve short- or long-term outcomes for affected children?	Children with communication disorders can be bilingual. Developing bilingual children may present with a range of communication disorders; the relative level of skill in each language may vary. A bilingual environment does not, in and of itself, put children with a communication disorder at a disadvantage. When bilingualism is inherent in a child's life circumstances, clinical recommendations and actions that plan for long-term gain are considered best practices.
Do gains made in a treated language transfer to an untreated language?	For the most part, yes in speech sound disorders research; however, cross-language generalizations include the nature and severity of the disorder, the type of therapy used, the particular aspect of language considered (e.g., phonology or grammar), the modality (e.g., expressive or receptive), the typologic similarities between the languages, the child's developmental stage, and the child's level of skill in each language.
Will treatment in the home language (L1) for sequential bilingual children help or hinder progress in L2? Does treatment in a single language produce superior outcomes in bilingual treatment?	Bilingual treatment (e.g., treating and reaching criterion in L1 followed by treating L2) is superior to single language treatment; bilingual treatment results in faster gains on targeted tasks and may show better generalization to other tasks than treatment in a single language.
How can we separate bilingual children with speech or language impairments from their typically developing peers?	More research is needed to disentangle the areas of overlap and divergence between typical L2 learners and monolingual or bilingual children with language impairments.

From Kohnert, K., & Medina, A. (2009). Bilingual children and communication disorders: A 30-year research retrospective. *Seminars in Speech and Language, 30,* 219-233.

other hand, bilingual-to-bilingual (i.e., bilingual learners with and without language impairments) comparisons across a range of tasks (i.e., measures of grammar, nonword repetition, morphological tasks) effectively differentiate children with language disorders and their typically developing peers (Gutierrez-Clellen & Simon-Cereijido, 2010). Kohnert suggested that the diagnostic value of bilingual comparisons should be underscored as the standard of performance. The data on within-group comparisons account for individual variability and have been investigated using limited training tasks such as fast mapping (the child is taught new information and tested on the task or item at a later time; see Hwa-Froelich & Matsuo, 2005) and dynamic assessment (involves guided support for learning; see Pena, 2000). Researchers have found that both of these tasks provide a better indication of the child's potential for change in both languages and the level of support needed for change to occur. The research in this area, although not definitive at this time, provides guidance for differential diagnosis. To fully understand the utility of the existing assessment models and tasks for capturing the language behaviors of bilingual children, much more research is needed.

Intervention

Compared with assessment, intervention research has received much less attention in CSD. A major paradigm shift in the past decade is that the focus of what needs to done to help bilingual children with language impairments has moved from *which language to support* to *how best to support both languages* (Kohnert, 2010). The difficulty is that there exists little empirical evidence on the effectiveness of treatment for supporting the development of more than one language. Few studies have investigated generalization as a means of attempting to understand cross-linguistic associations. Most of the studies have been single-subject designs with small numbers of study participants. Nevertheless, there is some preliminary evidence for transfer of language skills across languages and language contexts (Kohnert, 2010; Kohnert & Medina, 2009). Kohnert and Derr (2004) presented two models of intervention for bilingual children with language impairments: the Bilingual Approach and the Cross-Linguistic Approach. The Bilingual Approach capitalizes on the dual languages by directing attention to improving the child's communicative competence in both languages. The Cross-Linguistic Approach targets training in each language at separate times and focusing on the unique features of each language. Aspects of each intervention have been studied in only a limited number of studies.

Speech Disorders Research

Augmentative and Alternative Communication Use

AAC researchers often employ single-subject experimental designs to determine the efficacy of interventions for children and their caregivers. Single-subject designs,

sometimes referred to as time series research, are experimental and typically include small numbers (<10) of participants. In these designs, the participant (e.g., child who uses AAC) serves as his or her own control, treatments (independent variable) can consist of one or more variables, multiple treatments (or probes within a treatment) can be administered simultaneously, and treatments can be introduced or faded at different times in the study. McReynolds and Kearns (1983) noted that "[s]ingle-subject designs are particularly well suited for AAC intervention as these designs allow for the establishment of experimental control with participants who are from heterogeneous populations" (as cited in Binger et al., 2008, p. 327). To date, much of the focus of AAC research has been (1) on the AAC speaker and (2) on the AAC speaker's conversational partners. Very little research has focused on understanding AAC use by children (and their caregivers) from culturally and linguistically diverse backgrounds. Binger and colleagues (2008) investigated the efficacy of teaching Latino parents to support the multisymbol message productions of their children who require AAC. Using a single-subject, multiple-probe research design, the Latino parents were trained on a particular cognitive strategy instructional approach (*Read, Ask, Answer* [RAA]; see Kent-Walsh et al., 2004) to engage their children who were AAC users during reading activities. Importantly, the researchers conducted a focus group before the experimental portion of the study. This allowed them to understand the diversity across Latinos, how levels of acculturation varied in the group, and the cultural considerations that needed to be factored into the experiment. Because of the high levels of acculturation of their participants ($N = 3$), minimal adjustments were required. The parents successfully learned the strategy, and the children increased their use of the multisymbol messages during reading activities.

Stuttering and Fluency Disorders

Van Borsel and coworkers (2001) reviewed the literature on stuttering and bilingualism, citing that clinicians who serve these individuals will likely encounter some unique challenges. Similar to other areas within CSD, the literature based on this topic is sparse and highly diverse relative to the methods and the findings. Although not a critical review of the literature, this review yielded some useful information to guide SLPs in their clinical practice and stimulates thinking about research questions that, hopefully, will be investigated and answered by future researchers. They found the following evidence in their review:

1. Consistent with the same hypothesis, bilinguals who stutter do so in both languages.
2. Consistent with the difference hypothesis, bilinguals who stutter show differential stuttering behaviors in each language.
3. Particular to bilingual learners, stuttering behaviors may be uneven between the languages; for example,

there may be differing degrees of severity between the languages.

4. Balanced bilinguals (equal proficiency in both languages) may show differences in the nature and severity of stuttering between languages.

Lim and associates (2008) provided additional evidence for the findings in the Van Borsel and colleagues (2001) review. They examined these questions in 30 English and Mandarin speakers to determine the influence of language dominance. The Lim study found equivocal frequency and severity of stuttering across the languages in adults and determined that stuttering severity was influenced by language dominance. In the English-dominant and Mandarin-dominant speakers, L2 (Mandarin and English, respectively) was more severe.

A key diagnostic issue for clinicians is distinguishing disfluencies related to stuttering from those related to learning a second language; hence, the child should be assessed in both languages (Mattes & Omark, 1991, cited in Van Borsel et al., 2001). In their research investigating coexisting speech and language disorders in children who stutter, Blood and colleagues (2009) found that males are especially susceptible to comorbidities and that this might also be affected by racial or ethnic background. This is yet another consideration for assessment, although caution against stereotyping is warranted.

Acquired Neurogenic Disorders

The scant research on individuals who are bilingual and who have neurogenic communication disorders is concentrated almost exclusively in the area of aphasia with Spanish-English or English-Spanish bilinguals. Research designs vary from case studies to single-subject designs to within- and between-group comparisons, depending on the focus of the research, much of which has been on recovery patterns (Lorenzen & Murray, 2008; see also Chapter 8) and assessment with much less attention to treatment.

Bilingualism

Muñoz and Marquardt (2008) examined performance on the Bilingual Aphasia Test (BAT; Paradis, 1987) in neurologically intact adult bilingual speakers of English. The BAT is the most widely used test for assessing aphasia in bilingual adults; however, the results must be interpreted relative to the influences of language proficiency, educational attainment, and structural differences between languages (i.e., dialect) (Muñoz & Marquardt, 2008). The participants were 22 Mexican American bilingual Spanish and English speakers with a mean grade level of 12 years. The researchers determined each individual's bilingualism status using measures of language history (questions on the BAT), language use (a questionnaire; see Muñoz et al., 1999), and language proficiency (self-ratings and a test of verbal fluency).

Centeno and Cairns (2010) found that daily use frequency of Spanish verbs strongly affects verb repetition in bilingual persons with agrammatic aphasia. This study used precision matching that included six Venezuelan individuals with agrammatic aphasia matched with six neurologically intact Venezuelan Spanish speakers on age, education level, and Spanish dialect. The researchers interpreted their findings to mean that, in aphasia, representational knowledge of word structure is not entirely lost; rather, limited processing resources may limit productive expression.

A different question was answered in a prior study (Centeno, 2007) using the same research protocol. In that study, Spanish speakers with agrammatic aphasia performed better when repeating structurally simple verb endings, analogous to verb forms that are acquired early in life and employed frequently in the oral discourse of Spanish-speaking individuals.

Using a single-subject, experimental, multiple baseline design, Edmonds and Kiran (2006) investigated generalization of semantically related items within and across dual languages in three persons with bilingual aphasia. The multiple baseline design uses repeated-measures design within the same individual and allows for replication (not comparisons) within and across individuals. Kiran and Roberts (2010) used the same research design to extend Edmonds and Kiran's findings. Four patients (two Spanish-English speakers and two French-English speakers) with post-stroke anomia were treated using the semantic feature analysis approach. Whereas individual results varied, overall, the patients showed gains in their naming abilities and those gains were attributable to the treatment (Kiran & Roberts). The investigators point out that researchers continue to be challenged in using existing theoretical models to explain the language behaviors of persons with aphasia who are also bilingual.

Asians and Pacific Islanders and Native Americans

Noticeably missing in the neurogenic disorders literature is research-based information on Asians and Pacific Islanders and Native Americans. Despite the fact that Asians and Pacific Islanders are one of the fastest growing populations in the United States, virtually no attention has been afforded this population by researchers in communication sciences and swallowing disorders. The majority of the existing research investigates incidence and prevalence in the context of racial-ethnic disparities (Braun & Browne, 1998; Chow et al., 2000; Gonzalez-Fernandez et al., 2008). Whereas this information is useful as a first step, empirical questions and the answers about prevention, identification, assessment, and treatment of communication, swallowing, and hearing disorders need to be addressed in these populations.

Chow and coworkers (2000) investigated utilization of Alzheimer's disease community resources among Asians and whites in California. They found that Asian, Filipino, and Pacific Islander elders subscribe to dementia evaluation services at much lower rates than their white counterparts and cited language barriers as a major source of differences for this underuse. Another factor suspected to affect underuse by Asians is the possible low or late reporting of dementia symptoms by their caregivers. This may occur because, from a cultural standpoint, Asians see the aging process as prestigious, in contrast to the American view of aging. For swallowing, Gonzalez-Fernandez and associates (2008) found that among African Americans, Asians, and whites, Asians were more likely to have dysphagia following stroke. The researchers used a case-control, comparative design that tapped into two large statewide databases.

One article described the cultural implications of posttraumatic aphasia treatment of a Native American male in Northern Arizona (Huttlinger & Tanner, 1994). After being seen by an SLP for mainstream therapy with minimal success, the patient and his family decided that incorporating their cultural practices in the rehabilitation process would be more effective, but mostly more satisfying for the patient. They discuss the tenets of culture care theory and implications for its use for aphasia rehabilitation. To date, no research exists on this approach to aphasia treatment in CSD.

International Research

Child Language Research

Globally, researchers are investigating various aspects of children's speech and language development and disorders. Of particular interest is the nexus between bilingualism and specific language impairment (Gutierrez-Clellen et al., 2008; Tsai & Chang, 2008) and serving bilingual children with speech and language impairments (Jordaan, 2008). Using a narrative task, Gutierrez-Clellen and colleagues (2008) investigated the production of English verb morphology in Spanish- and English-speaking bilingual children with and without specific language impairment (SLI) and in English-speaking monolingual children with and without SLI. The bilingual and monolingual children with SLI showed equivocal accuracy that distinguished them from their bilingual and monolingual typically developing peers. Tsi and Chang (2008) investigated the personal narratives of 12 Taiwanese boys: 6 with SLI and 6 deemed to be typically developing. It has been suggested that narrative production serves as an index of linguistic and cognitive abilities. The children with language impairments scored within normal limits on intelligence tests before the experimental task. All children produced three personal narratives elicited by the researchers using the Conversational Map Elicitation procedure (for a full

description of this procedure, see Peterson & McCabe, 1983). The narratives were transcribed using CHILDES (MacWhinney, 2000). The Mandarin-speaking children with SLI had greater difficulty producing clear, coherent narratives than their typically developing peers. These results were consistent with research findings in the United States. From a research perspective, Paradis (2010) stated that "[p]arallels between typically developing L2 children and monolingual children with SLI raise issues for maturational models of SLI, and at the same time, parallels between monolinguals and bilinguals with SLI raise issues for limited processing capacities theories" (p. 248).

Jordaan (2008) administered a survey to SLPs around the world to establish (1) biographic data on bilingual children on caseloads, (2) language profiles and proficiency of the SLPs serving bilingual children with speech and language impairments, (3) the SLPs' justification of services to the children, and (4) SLPs' assessment of parental attitudes toward maintaining the home language. The researcher used a quantitative, descriptive survey method that was administered by e-mail. Ninety-nine SLPs provided data from 13 countries, including Israel, Malta, Belgium, India, Canada, the United States, England, Sweden, Malaysia, Bulgaria, Denmark, Iceland, and South Africa. The returned surveys provided data on 158 bilingual children who had a variety of communication disorders; the majority, 150 (95.5%), exhibited developmental language delay. The overarching results of this study showed that clinical practice with bilingual children is not necessarily based on the evidence from the literature and that there is a general lack of bilingual intervention as well as lack of support for the development of L1.

Speech Disorders Research

Stuttering and Fluency Disorders

Investigations of stuttering have been reported by researchers in Sweden (Johannisson et al., 2009), the United Kingdom (Ayre & Wright, 2009), South Africa (Klompas & Ross, 2004), and Brazil (Juste & Andrade, 2011). Johannisson and coworkers (2009) obtained normative data on the Communication Attitude Test (CAT-S) from 220 typically developing Swedish children. The purposes of this study were to establish norms for age, sex, and size of community, to investigate aspects of test reliability (e.g., internal consistency, item analysis), and to perform a qualitative analysis of the responses. The Swedish children scored slightly higher on the CAT-S than their counterparts in other countries; the researchers determined that the test is reliable and valid and can be used for comparison with children with speech disorders. The Wright and Ayre Stuttering Self-Rating Profile (WASSP) is a clinical assessment tool used to illuminate change in adult clients, to plan therapy, and as a research tool to evaluate and compare therapy approaches (Ayre & Wright, 2009). The authors reported the findings from an international survey that was administered to the UK Special

Interest Group in Disorders of Fluency 6 years after publication of the WASSP using postal mailings and e-mail. Respondents were largely from the United Kingdom (80%), and all respondents reported that the WASSP was brief, easy to administer, and useful as an assessment and outcome measure. The authors stated that the forthcoming revised WASSP will incorporate the World Health Organization International Classification of Functioning, Disability and Health (ICF; 2010) framework; an adolescent version is also being developed. Klompas and Ross (2004) investigated the life experiences of South African adults who stutter using interview methods. Most of their participants felt that their stuttering negatively affected their academic performance, chances for promotion, and self-esteem, but not their social and family life. Most viewed speech therapy positively, although they expressed that stuttering evoked feelings of frustration and anger. Relative to research and theory for greater illumination of these issues for persons who stutter, Klompas and Ross suggested replicating this study with larger numbers of participants, testing a more ethnically representative sample, and situating cultural differences within the South African context. To determine age effects, Juste and de Andrade (2011) investigated the types of disfluencies observed in stuttering in fluent Brazilian Portuguese–speaking individuals across the life span. The number of stuttering-like disfluencies (much greater frequency in persons who stutter) and the nature of those disfluencies differentiated the stutterers from the nonstutterers.

Voice and Its Disorders

A group of researchers from New York, Brazil, England, and Canada conducted a systematic review of the content development in quality of life measures ($N = 9$) for patients with voice disorders (Branski et al., 2008). The authors acknowledged the importance of these tools for tracking disease progression, determining treatment effectiveness, informing intervention, and shaping patient expectations. Nevertheless, none of the quality-of-life instruments reviewed and currently being used (e.g., Voice Handicap Index) meet the current standards for instrument development. The bottom line is that these widely used instruments demonstrate deficient psychometric properties and, therefore, that clinicians and researchers must question their clinical utility. Australian researchers Oates and Winkworth (2008) attempted to find common ground in the research literature for hyperfunctional voice disorder, also known as *muscle tension dysphonia*. Two areas of agreement emerged: (1) hyperfunctional voice disorder is associated with increased perilaryngeal musculoskeletal activity, and (2) hyperfunctional voice disorder must be viewed relative to the multifactorial nature of the disorder (e.g., psychosocial, sensory factors). In another study, Vieira and coworkers (2009) reviewed the research questions and methods used in clinical studies of voice and the larynx published in Brazilian and international journals of speech-language

pathology and otorhinolaryngology. They found that the studies largely used weak methods and designs (i.e., case series, cross-sectional study, case study) that fail to meet the needs of the projected outcomes (i.e., diagnostic evaluation, treatment).

Acquired Neurogenic Disorders

SLPs around the world have the common goal of adopting evidence-based practice that focuses on treatment efficacy and effectiveness and clinical outcomes. The ICF (World Health Organization, 2001) model provides a framework within which they can accomplish these goals. Australian researchers Brunner and associates (2008), for example, investigated speech-language pathology outcomes for their stroke patients across two settings: inpatient rehabilitation and rehabilitation in home programs. The method involved ratings of patient outcomes from 10 SLPs; analyses included parametric and nonparametric methods. Results showed that rehabilitation outcomes for aphasia and swallowing therapy were equivalent between the settings, regardless of whether the patient received treatment in more than one modality (e.g., aphasia and dysphagia versus aphasia alone). However, greater gains were seen in individuals who were less than 75 years of age and in those who showed fewer restrictions on participation and increased distress levels. Additionally, greater gains were shown in swallowing compared with aphasia.

Another aspect of clinical outcomes deals with patient satisfaction. Fourie (2009) explored the therapeutic relationship between SLPs and their patients with acquired neurogenic communication and swallowing disorders in Ireland. This was a qualitative study that used grounded theory to analyze interviews from 11 adult females and males who presented with a variety of disorders, including glossectomy and articulation difficulties, laryngectomy and voice difficulties, dysphonia, dysarthria, and dysphagia. Action coding (any label containing a verb; e.g., the therapist made me feel comfortable) was used to label the line-by-line responses of the participants, and a computer software program identified and grouped "code families," which the researcher used to describe trends in the data. The substantive theory of *Restorative Poise* was used to explain the participants' responses, which included discussion of the interplay between therapeutic quality (understanding, gracious, erudite, and inspiring) and therapeutic actions (confident, soothing, practical, and empowering). Fourie's participants demonstrated understanding of and valued the therapeutic relationship as essential to positive clinical outcomes. This type of research is important because it contributes to the literature on patient outcomes, in particular, patient satisfaction and quality of life following stroke and cancer. Regarding assessment, researchers are testing the psychometric properties of existing tests of language and cognition in a range of populations. For example,

Kong (2011) found that main concept analysis is a valid measure for assessing discourse production in Cantonese speakers with aphasia, whereas Mupawose and Broom (2010) found that the Cognitive-Linguistic Quick Test is an appropriate assessment tool for diagnosing cognitive-linguistic deficits in South African adults with HIV.

FUTURE OF RESEARCH IN COMMUNICATION SCIENCES AND DISORDERS: WHERE DO WE GO FROM HERE?

Generally, the existing body of literature on multicultural/multilingual and international populations appears to provide an impressive collection of information for assessing and treating individuals with communication and swallowing disorders. In reality, there is much more work to do. Although the presentation of literature in this chapter is not in the least exhaustive, it does offer clear guidance for future studies dealing with multicultural/multilingual and international issues in communication sciences and disorders.

1. Incidence and prevalence data on communication and swallowing disorders are severely limited, particularly for individuals who are from culturally and linguistically diverse backgrounds. To date, virtually no research exists on language development and disorders in the Native American population as well as other populations (e.g., Aboriginals in Australia). Epidemiologic data will, importantly, aid CSD researchers as these data provide evidence for the need to conduct research with these populations, and also support the data on health disparities in underserved populations in the United States.

2. There is a need for additional research establishing typical and atypical speech and language development across the life span and across *all* language communities. This information can help to establish normative behaviors that can be used for comparisons when disorder is present. Further, these data will offer the flexibility of making within-group comparisons that will highlight the insidious heterogeneity in multicultural/multilingual and international populations.

3. There is a critical need for more research on the influence of racial-ethnic and linguistic diversity on the different aspects of speech and language and on those characteristics of language and communication that distinguish different racial-ethnic groups, particularly with regard to communication disorders.

4. There is a need to construct new and to refine existing theories, research designs (e.g., qualitative designs), methods, and tools (e.g., genetic tests) that can appropriately and accurately identify and explain communication and swallowing behaviors in multicultural/multilingual and international populations.

5. There is a need for *all* CSD researchers to understand, value, and employ both qualitative and quantitative research designs and methods for gaining knowledge about communication and swallowing and their related disorders in multicultural/multilingual and international populations.

6. Research on assessment and treatment approaches, techniques, and tools should take into account culture-dependent and culture-independent variables. Additional research is warranted to increase significantly the number of assessment tools that are appropriate for use with multicultural/multilingual and international populations.

7. Treatment research in these populations is noticeably missing. Researchers should test specific treatment techniques and approaches within and across multicultural/multilingual and international populations and use adequate numbers of participants when doing so. For example, with few exceptions, much of the research literature in CSD includes small numbers (e.g., proportional to the population) of multicultural/multilingual individuals. Further, when individuals from culturally and linguistically diverse backgrounds do participate, the researcher may not report this demographic because of oversight, perceived lack of importance to the goals of the study, or publication page limits. With many peer-reviewed journals available online, page limits may no longer be a factor.

8. Doctoral programs in CSD need to increase their focus on training student researchers about the relevance of including individuals from culturally and linguistically diverse backgrounds in their research, engaging in ethical and social responsibility when conducting research in multicultural/multilingual populations, posing culturally appropriate research questions, and judiciously interpreting their findings.

9. Significantly greater numbers of studies are needed to determine the influence of race-ethnicity on swallowing disorders and acquired neurogenic disorders of speech and language and cognition.

10. Bilingual research in CSD requires much more focused attention, for example, on the terminology, the variables, and interpretation of the findings.

SUMMARY AND IMPLICATIONS

This chapter discussed multicultural/multilingual research in CSD. Considering the increasing emphases on evidence-based practice and cultural competence, it is imperative that researchers in the field move quickly to investigate the identified gaps in knowledge. This chapter provides a framework for determining what research is needed and why, as well as the multicultural and multilingual issues that must be considered in the research paradigm. Generally, much more research is needed that includes adequate numbers of individuals from multicultural and multilingual populations around the world. Comparative designs should oversample or recruit equal numbers of individuals within and across groups and equate the groups on extraneous variables that could possibly skew the results if not well controlled. Researchers must create or adopt new ways of collecting data using current and future technologies. As population shifts occur, societal norms will dictate the use of different technologies in CSD research. Research paradigms should be equivalent across multicultural/multilingual groups: this speaks to replication, not typically done in CSD (Muma, 1992). Muma (1992) randomly selected published studies in the *Journal of Speech and Hearing Disorders* and the *Journal for Speech and Hearing Research* over a 10-year period and found that direct replications constituted 4% of a sample of 271 studies; derived studies constituted 6% of the sample. He urged researchers to consider the implications, suggesting that there were possibly 50 to 250 false findings in his sample and that these unknown false findings could be misdirecting the field. Replication studies are vital to all fields because they confirm or disconfirm the existence or persistence of phenomena. Efficacy and outcomes research must increasingly include individuals who are multicultural and multilingual, particularly because patient populations are composed of these individuals.

DISCUSSION QUESTIONS

1. Design a research study examining the influences of race-ethnicity and culture on narrative production in Native Americans with aphasia.
2. Discuss the significance of single-subject designs for understanding individual differences when conducting efficacy research with multicultural populations.
3. Explain the factors that need to be considered when conducting speech and language research in a global context.
4. Discuss the implications of *not* involving multicultural/multilingual and international individuals in research in CSD.

REFERENCES

Ayre, A., & Wright, L. (2009). WASSP: An international review of clinical application. *International Journal of Speech-Language Pathology, 11,* 83-90.

Bedore, L. M., Peña, E. D., Gillam, R. B., & Ho, T. (2010). Language sample measure and language ability in Spanish-English bilingual kindergarteners. *Journal of Communication Disorders, 43,* 498-510.

Blood, G. W., Blood, I. M., Kreiger, J., O'Connor, S., & Qualls, C. D. (2009). Double jeopardy for children who stutter: Race and coexisting disorders. *Communication Disorders Quarterly, 30,* 131-141.

Binger, C., Kent-Walsh, J., Berens, J., et al. (2008). Teaching Latino parents to support the multi-symbol message productions of their children who require AAC. *Augmentative and Alternative Communication, 24,* 323-338.

Branski, R. C., Cukier-Blaj, S., Pusic, A., et al. (2008). Measuring quality of life in dysphonic patients: A systematic review of content development in patient-reported outcomes measures. *Journal of Voice, 24,* 193-198.

Braun, K. L., & Browne, C. V. (1998). Perceptions of dementia, caregiving, and help seeking among Asian and Pacific Islander Americans. *Health & Social Work, 23,* 262-274.

Brunner, M., Skeat, J., & Morris, M. E. (2008). Outcomes of speech-language pathology following stroke: Investigation of inpatient rehabilitation and rehabilitation in the home programs. *International Journal of Speech-Language Pathology, 10,* 305-313.

Centeno, J. G. (2007). Canonical features in the inflectional morphology of Spanish speaking individuals with agrammatic speech. *Advances in Speech Language Pathology, 9,* 162-172.

Centeno, J. G., & Cairns, H. S. (2010). Assessing frequency effects on verb inflection use by Spanish-speaking individuals with agrammatism: Theoretical and clinical implications. *International Journal of Speech-Language Pathology, 12,* 35-46.

Champion, T. B., Rosa-Lugo, L. I. (2010). A preliminary investigation of second- and fourth grade African American students' performance on the Gray Oral Reading Test. *Topics in Language Disorders, 30,* 145-153.

Chow, T. W., Ross, L., Fox, P., et al. (2000). Utilization of Alzheimer's disease community resources by Asian-Americans in California. *International Journal of Geriatric Psychiatry, 15,* 838-847.

DePoy, E., & Gitlin, L. N. (2011). Introduction to research: Understanding and applying multiple strategies (4th ed.). St. Louis: Elsevier.

de Riesthal, M., & Wertz, R. T. (2004). Prognosis for aphasia: relationship between selected biographical and behavioural variables and outcome. *Aphasiology, 8 (10):* 899-915.

Duff, M. C., Proctor, A., & Yairi, E. (2004). Prevalence of voice disorders in African American and European American preschoolers. *Journal of Voice, 18,* 348-353.

Edmonds, L., & Kiran, S. (2006). Effect of semantic naming treatment on crosslinguistic generalization in bilingual aphasia. *Journal of Speech, Language, and Hearing Research, 49,* 729-748.

Fourie, R. J. (2009). Qualitative study of the therapeutic relationship in speech and language therapy: Perspectives of adults with acquired communication and swallowing disorders. *International Journal of Language & Communication Disorders, 44,* 979-999.

Gonzalez-Fernandez, M., Kuhlemeier, K. V., & Palmer, J. B. (2008). Racial disparities in the development of dysphagia after stroke: Analysis of the California (MIRCal) and New York (SPARCS) inpatient databases. *Archives of Physical Medicine and Rehabilitation, 89,* 1358-1365.

Gutierrez-Clellen, V., & Simon-Cereijido, G. (2010). Using nonword repetition tasks for the identification of language impairment in Spanish-English children: Does the language of assessment matter? *Learning Disabilities Research & Practice, 25,* 48-58.

Gutierrez-Clellen, V., Simon-Cereijido, G., & Wagner, C. (2008). Bilingual children with language impairment: a comparison with monolinguals and second language learners. *Applied Psycholinguistics, 29,* 3-19.

Head, K., Weeks, R., Stroud, A., & Coll, A. M. (2007). A survey of dysphagia screening practices across England and Wales. *International Journal of Therapy and Rehabilitation, 14,* 409-417.

Huttlinger, K. W., & Tanner, D. (1994). The peyote way: Implications for culture care theory. *Journal of Transcultural Nursing, 5,* 5-11.

Hwa-Froelich, D., & Matsuo, H. (2005). Vietnamese children and language-based processing tasks. *Language Speech and Hearing Services in Schools, 36,* 230-243.

International Classification of Functioning, Disability and Health (ICF). Retrieved December 19, 2010, from www.who.int/classifications/icf/en/.

Johannisson, T. B, Wennerfeldt, S., Havstam, C., et al. (2009). The Communication Attitude Test (CAT-S): Normative values for 220 Swedish children. *International Journal of Language and Communication Disorders, 44,* 813-825.

Jordaan, H. (2008). Clinical intervention for bilingual children: an international survey. *Folia Phoniatrica and Logopedics, 60,* 90-105.

Juste, F. S., & de Andrade, C. R. F. (2011). Speech dysfluency types of fluent and stuttering individuals: Age effects. *Folio Phoniatrica et Logopaedica, 63,* 57-64.

Kent-Walsh, J., Binger, C., & Hasham, Z. (2010). Effects of parent instruction on the symbolic communication of children using augmentative and alternative communication during storybook reading. *American Journal of Speech-Language Research, 19,* 97-107.

Kent-Walsh, J., Hasham, Z., & Stewart, J. (2004). Instructing parents to support children during story book reading. Paper presented at the annual convention of the American Speech-Language-Hearing Association, Philadelphia.

Kerlinger, F. N., & Lee, H. B. (2000). *Foundations of behavioral research* (4th ed.) New York: Harcourt Brace.

Kiran, S., & Roberts, P. M. (2010). Semantic feature analysis treatment in Spanish-English and French-English bilingual aphasia. *Aphasiology, 24,* 231-261.

Klompas, M., & Ross, E. (2004). Life experiences of people who stutter and the perceived impact of stuttering on quality of life: Personal accounts of South African individuals. *Journal of Fluency Disorders, 29,* 275-305.

Kohnert, K. (2010). Bilingual children with primary language impairment: Issues, evidence and implications for clinical actions. *Journal of Communication Disorders, 43(6),* 456-473.

Kohnert, K., & Derr, A. (2004). Language intervention with bilingual children. In B. Goldstein (Ed.), *Bilingual language development and disorders in Spanish-English speakers* (pp. 315-343). Baltimore: Brookes.

Kohnert, K., & Medina, A. (2009). Bilingual children and communication disorders: A 30-year research retrospective. *Seminars in Speech and Language, 30,* 219-233.

Kong, A. P. (2011). The main concept analysis in Cantonese aphasia oral discourse: External validation and monitoring chronic aphasia. *Journal of Speech, Language, and Hearing Research, 54,* 148-159.

Kummerer, E. (2010). Language intervention for Hispanic children with language learning disabilities: Evidence-based practice. *Current Topics in Review, 45,* 192-200.

Lim, V. P. C., Lincoln, M., Yiong Huak, C. & Onslow, M. (2008). Stuttering in English Mandarin bilingual speakers: The influence of language dominance on stuttering severity. *Journal of Speech, Language & Hearing Research, 51,* 1522-1537.

Lorenzen, B., & Murray, L. L. (2008). Bilingual aphasia: A theoretical and clinical review. *American Journal of Speech-Language Pathology, 17,* 299-317.

MacWhinney, B. (2000). *The CHILDES project: tools for analyzing talk* (3rd ed.). Hillsdale, NJ: Lawrence Erlbaum.

Mattes, L. J., & Omark, D. R. (1991). *Speech and language assessment for the bilingual handicapped.* San Diego: College-Hill Press.

Mayo, R., Holt, Y., & Zajac, D. J. (2007) Nasalance and velopharyngeal closure timing characteristics: A cross-cultural study. *ECHO: E-Journal for Black and Other Ethnic Group Research and Practices in Communication Sciences and Disorders, 3,* 9-24.

Mayo, R., Mayo, C. M., & Brock, K. D. (2006). Public knowledge of voice disorders: A survey of African Americans. *ECHO E-Journal for Black and Other Ethnic Group Research and Practices in Communication Sciences and Disorders, 2,* 9-26.

Molrine, C. J., & Pierce, R. S. (2002). Black and white adults' expressive language: Performance on three tests of aphasia. *American Journal of Speech-Language Pathology, 11,* 139-150.

Muma, J. (1992). The need for replication. *Journal of Speech & Hearing Research, 36,* 927-931.

Munoz, M. L., & Marquardt, T. P. (2008). The performance of neurological normal bilingual speakers of Spanish and English on the short version of the Bilingual Test of Aphasia. *Aphasiology, 22,* 3-19.

Munoz, M. L., Marquardt, T. P., & Copeland (1999). A comparison of the codeswitching patterns of aphasic and neurologically normal bilingual speakers of English and Spanish. *Brain and Language, 66,* 249-274.

Mupawose, A., & Broom, Y. (2010). Assessing cognitive-linguistic abilities in South African adults living with HIV: The Cognitive Linguistic Quick Test. *African Journal of AIDS Research, 9,* 147-152.

Oates, J., & Winkworth, A. (2008). Current knowledge, controversies and future directions on hyperfunctional voice disorders. *International Journal of Speech-Language Pathology, 10,* 267-277.

Olness, G. S., Matteson, S. E., & Stewart, C. T. (2010). "Let me tell you the point": How speakers with aphasia assign prominence to information in narratives. *Aphasiology, 24,* 697-708.

Olness, G. S., Ulatowska, H. K., Wertz, R. T., et al. (2002). Discourse elicitation with pictorial stimuli in African Americans and Caucasians with and without aphasia. *Aphasiology, 16,* 623-633.

Parette, P., Huer, M. B., & Wyatt, T. A. (2006). Young African American children with disabilities and augmentative and alternative communication issues. *Early Childhood Education Journal, 29,* 201-207.

Paradis, J. (2010). The interface between bilingual development and specific language impairment. *Applied Psycholinguistics, 31,* 227-252.

Paradis, M. (1987). *Assessment of bilingual aphasia.* Hillsdale, NJ: Lawrence Erlbaum.

Peña, E. D. (2000). Measurement of modifiability in children from culturally and linguistically diverse backgrounds. *Communication Disorders Quarterly, 21,* 87-97.

Peterson, C., & McCabe, A. (1983). *Developmental psycholinguistics: Three ways of looking at a child's narrative.* New York: Plenum.

Proctor, A., Yairi, E., Duff, M., & Jie, Z. Prevalence of stuttering in African American preschoolers. *Journal of Speech, Language & Hearing Research, 51,* 1465-1479.

Qualls, C. D. (2002). Recruitment of African American adults as research participants to a language in aging study: Example of a principled, creative, and culture-based approach. *Journal of Allied Health, 31,* 241-246.

Qualls, C. D. (2009, July). Recruiting participants to clinical practice research. Presentation at the 1st Annual Clinical Practice Research Institute, American Speech-Language-Hearing Association, Rockville MD.

Ross, K. B., & Wertz, R. T. (2003). Discriminative validity of selected measures for differentiating normal from aphasic performance. *American Journal of Speech-Language Pathology, 12(3):* 312-319.

Seymour, H., Roper, T. W., & de Villiers, J. (2003). *Diagnostic evaluation of language variation: Screening test.* San Antonio: Psychological Corporation.

Stockman, I. J. (2010). A review of developmental and applied language research on African American children: From a deficit to difference perspective on dialect differences. *Language, Speech, and Hearing Services in Schools, 41,* 23-38.

Stockman, I. J., Boult, J., & Robinson, G. C. (2008). Multicultural/multilingual instruction in educational programs: A survey of perceived faculty practices and outcomes. *American Journal of Speech-Language Pathology, 17,* 241-264.

Streit Olness, G., Ulatowska, H. K., Carpenter, C. M., et al. (2005). Holistic assessment of narrative quality: A social validation study. *Aphasiology, 19,* 251-262.

Summers, C., Bohman, T. M., Gillam, R. B., et al. (2010). Bilingual performance on nonword repetition in Spanish and English. *International Journal of Language & Communication Disorders, 45,* 480-493.

Terry, N. P, Connor, C. M., Thomas-Tate, S., & Love, M. (2010). Examining relationships among dialect variation, literacy skills, and school context in first grade. *Journal of Speech, Language, and Hearing Research, 53,* 126-145.

Tsai, W., & Chang, C. (2008). "But I first . . . and then he kept picking": Narrative skill in Mandarin-speaking children with language impairment. *Narrative Inquiry, 18,* 349-377.

Ulatowska, H. K., Olness, G. S. (2001). Dialectical variants of verbs in narratives of African Americans with aphasia: Some methodological considerations. *Journal of Neurolinguistics, 14,* 93-110.

Ulatowska, H. K., Olness, G. S., Wertz, R. T., et al. (2001). Comparison of language impairment, functional communication, and discourse measures in African-American aphasic and normal adults. *Aphasiology, 15,* 1007-1016.

Ulatowska, H. K., Reyes, B. A., Santos, T. O., & Worle, C. (2011). Stroke narratives in aphasia: The role of reported speech. *Aphasiology, 25,* 93-105.

Ulatowska, H. K., Streit Olness, G., Hill, C. L., et al. (2000). Repetition in narratives of African Americans: The effects of aphasia. *Discourse Processes, 30,* 265-283.

Ulatowska, H., Streit Olness, G., Wertz, R., et al. (2003). Relationship between discourse and Western Aphasia Battery performance in African Americans with aphasia. *Aphasiology, 17,* 511.

Ulatowska, H. K, Wertz, R. T., Chapman, S. B., et al. (2001). Interpretation of fables and proverbs by African Americans with and without aphasia. *American Journal of Speech-Language Pathology, 10,* 40-50.

Van Borsel, J., Maes, E., & Foulon, S. (2001). Stuttering and bilingualism: A review. *Journal of Fluency Disorders, 26,* 179-205.

Vieira, V. P., De Biase, N., Peccin, M. S., & Atallah, A. N. (2009). The research questions and methodological adequacy of clinical studies of the voice and larynx published in Brazilian and international journals. *Journal of Evaluation in Clinical Practice, 15,* 473-477.

Wertz, R, T., Auther, L. L, & Ross, K. B. (1997). Aphasia in African-American and Caucasians: Severity, improvement, and rate of improvement. *Aphasiology, 11,* 533-542.

Wertz, R. T., de Riesthal, M., Irwin, W. H., & Ross, K. B. (2009). Department of Veterans Affairs' contributions to treatment outcomes research in aphasia. *Aphasiology, 23(9),* 1158-1183.

Xue, S. A., Hao, G. J., P., & Mayo, R. (2006). Volumetric measurements of vocal tracts for male speakers from different races. *Clinical Linguistics & Phonetics, 9,* 691-702.

Yancey, A. K., Ortega, A. N., & Kumanyika, S. K. (2005). Effective recruitment and retention of minority research participants. *Annual Review of Public Health, 27,* 1-28.

U.S. Census Bureau. Available at: http://2010.census.gov/2010census/index.php.

ADDITIONAL RESOURCES

Evidence-based practice at the American Speech-Language-Hearing Association (ASHA). Available at: www.asha.org/members/ebp/. ASHA's National Center on Evidence-Based Practices (NCEP) provides information and education on EBP for communication sciences and disorders. Included on the site are an introduction to EBP, Web-based tutorials, a compendium of clinical practice guidelines and systematic reviews, evidence maps, ASHA/NCEP evidence-based systematic reviews, and a calendar of events.

Cochrane database of systematic reviews. Available at: www.cochrane.org/cochrane-reviews. This website houses a database of investigations on the effects of interventions for prevention, treatment, and rehabilitation. The reviews of the literature also assess the accuracy of a diagnostic test for a given condition in a specific patient group and setting. The abstracts and the plain language summaries of all Cochrane systematic reviews are free to the public.

International Brain Research Foundation. Available at: www.ibrfinc.org/. This nonprofit organization serves as a platform for the support of and collaboration with leading neuroscientists and research institutions around the world. The objectives are to create, operationalize, validate, and disseminate diagnostic and treatment protocols derived from innovative, novel research and translate those protocols into clinical practice for implementation with individuals afflicted with disorders, diseases, and injuries of the brain.

Multicultural Research and Resource Center at George Mason University. Available at: http://mrrc.gmu.edu/. The Multicultural Research and Resource Center (MRRC) consolidates and disseminates research on intercultural and cross-cultural inclusion and collaborates with academicians to develop curriculum that reflects the multicultural society within our local, regional, national, and international communities. The MRRC also offers students, faculty, and staff a cultural exchange opportunity abroad and always seeks to provide the Mason community with the ability to identify the many ways that oppression affects our communication with each other and the skills to shift prejudicial attitudes and behavior.

National Institutes of Health, National Institute for Deafness and Communication Disorders (NIDCD). Available at: www.nidcd.nih.gov/. The Institute conducts and supports research and research training related to disease prevention and health promotion; addresses special biomedical and behavioral problems associated with people who have communication impairments or disorders; and supports efforts to create devices that substitute for lost and impaired sensory and communication function.

Ethics in multicultural research. Trimble, J. E., & Fisher, C. B. (2006). *The handbook of ethical research with ethnocultural populations and communities.* Thousand Oaks, CA: Sage.

Index

Note: Page numbers followed by f indicate figure(s); t, table(s); b, box(es)